AUTISM
IMAGING
and
DEVICES

AUTISM IMAGING and DEVICES

Edited by
Manuel F. Casanova
Ayman El-Baz
Jasjit S. Suri

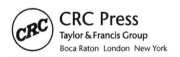

CRC Press
Taylor & Francis Group
Boca Raton London New York

CRC Press is an imprint of the
Taylor & Francis Group, an **informa** business

CRC Press
Taylor & Francis Group
6000 Broken Sound Parkway NW, Suite 300
Boca Raton, FL 33487-2742

First issued in paperback 2019

ISBN-13: 978-1-4987-0981-1 (hbk)
ISBN-13: 978-0-367-87210-6 (pbk)

Library of Congress Cataloging-in-Publication Data

Names: Casanova, Manuel F., editor. | El-Baz, Ayman S., editor. | Suri,
Jasjit S., editor.
Title: Autism imaging and devices / edited by Manuel F. Casanova, Ayman
El-Baz and Jasjit S. Suri.
Description: Boca Raton, FL : Taylor & Francis Group [2016]
Identifiers: LCCN 2016025919| ISBN 9781498709811 (hbk) | ISBN 9781498709828
(ebk)
Subjects: LCSH: Autism--Imaging. | Brain--Diseases--Diagnosis.
Classification: LCC RC386.6.D52 A98 2016 | DDC 616.85/882--dc23
LC record available at https://lccn.loc.gov/2016025919

Visit the Taylor & Francis Web site at
http://www.taylorandfrancis.com

and the CRC Press Web site at
http://www.crcpress.com

Contents

Preface ix

Contributors xi

1   **Present and future autism data science** 1
Nicholas Lange

2   **Twin research in autism spectrum disorder** . . . 15
Charlotte Willfors, Kristiina Tammimies, and
Sven Bölte

3   **Neurodevelopment of autism: The first three
years of life** 37
Meghan R. Swanson and Joseph Piven

4   **Anatomy of autism** 59
Verónica Martínez Cerdeño

5   **Neurobiology of imitation in autism** 75
Marco Iacoboni

6   **Neuroimaging biomarkers for autism
spectrum disorder** 95
Christine Ecker and Andre Marquand

7   **Structural magnetic resonance imaging of
autism spectrum disorder** 121
Rong Chen

8 **Atypical hemispheric asymmetries in autism spectrum disorders.** 135
Annukka Lindell

9 **Corpus callosum and autism** 157
Lawrence K. Fung and Antonio Hardan

10 **Macrocephaly and megalencephaly in autism spectrum disorder** 171
Lauren E. Libero, Christine W. Nordahl,
Deana D. Li, and David G. Amaral

11 **Imaging the striatum in autism spectrum disorder** 189
Adriana Di Martino, Eun Young Choi, Rebecca M.
Jones, F. Xavier Castellanos, and Ayman Mukerji

12 **GABA system dysfunction in autism and related disorders: From synapse to symptoms?** 219
Jamie Horder

13 **Imaging brain connectivity in autism spectrum disorder** 245
Robert Coben, Iman Mohammad-Rezazadeh,
Joel Frohlich, Joseph Jurgiel, and Giorgia Michelini

14 **Brain network organization in ASD: Evidence from functional and diffusion weighted MRI** 287
Ralph-Axel Müller and Ruth A. Carper

15 **Behavioral signal processing and autism: Learning from multimodal behavioral signals.** 319
Daniel Bone, Theodora Chaspari, and
Shrikanth Narayanan

16 **Behavior Imaging®: Innovative technology to
    enable remote autism diagnosis** 345
    N. Nazneen, Agata Rozga, Gregory D. Abowd,
    Christopher J. Smith, Ron Oberleitner,
    Rosa I. Arriaga, and Jasjit S. Suri

17 **Behavior Imaging®: Resolving assessment
    challenges for autism spectrum disorder
    in pharmaceutical trials.** 355
    Ron Oberleitner, Uwe Reischl, Kamilla G.
    Gazieva, N. Nazneen, Jasjit S. Suri, and
    Christopher J. Smith

18 **Virtual reality with psychophysiological
    monitoring as an approach to evaluate
    emotional reactivity, social skills, and joint
    attention in autism spectrum disorder.** 371
    Estate M. Sokhadze, Manuel F. Casanova,
    Desmond L. Kelly, Guela E. Sokhadze, Yi Li,
    Adel S. Elmaghraby, and Ayman S. El-Baz

19 **The impact of robots on children with autism
    spectrum disorder** 397
    Zhi Zheng, Esubalew Bekele, Amy Swanson,
    Amy Weitlauf, Zachary Warren, and Nilanjan Sarkar

20 **Using an ecological systems approach to
    target technology development for autism
    research and beyond** 419
    Rosa I. Arriaga

21 **Electrophysiology of error processing in
    individuals with autism spectrum disorder:
    A meta-analysis** 437
    Wen-Pin Chang

22 **Gamma abnormalities in autism spectrum
    disorders.** 457
    Gina Rippon

23   Repetitive transcranial magnetic stimulation
     (rTMS) effects on evoked and induced
     gamma frequency EEG oscillations in autism
     spectrum disorder 497
     Estate M. Sokhadze, Ayman S. El-Baz,
     Allan Tasman, Guela E. Sokhadze,
     Heba Elsayed M. Farag, and Manuel F. Casanova

     Index 537

Preface

In 2014, the Centers for Disease Control and Prevention (CDC) released data on an autism surveillance study. The new data estimated the prevalence of autism spectrum disorders (ASD) as 1 in 68 among 8-year-old children within multiple communities in the United States. The new figure was about 30% higher than the previous estimate they reported in 2012, and approximately 120% higher than the estimates for 2002. This provides for a rough 6%–15% increase each year during the last decade. Although the prevalence rates for ASD have significantly increased over the last few years, other figures have remained essentially unchanged. In this regard, ASD is five times as common in males as compared to females, and white children are more likely to have a diagnosis as compared to blacks and Hispanics.

The new prevalence rates offered by the CDC are not necessarily representative of what may be happening in the entire world or for that matter the United States. The survey only covered 11 communities within the United States. The fact that somewhat less than half of the children surveyed by the CDC were evaluated for developmental concerns by the time they were 3 years of age, and a diagnosis of ASD was not established until after age 4, underscores the need for early screening techniques. Indeed, there is a significant lag in time between when a parent raised concerns about their child's development and when they were diagnosed. This is of importance as the cost of lifelong care can be reduced with early diagnosis and intervention.

The new figures indicate that more than 3.5 million Americans live with an autism spectrum disorder. However, it is difficult to make sense of data when the same is determined solely by a review of records without having personally assessed a single child. Over the years, some have suggested that wider recognition, a shift in diagnosis from intellectual disability to ASD, and expanded diagnostic criteria may partially offset the reported rise in prevalence. Indeed, sometime in the early 1990s, when the rates for autism started to skyrocket, autism was associated with intellectual disability. Now, many of those surveyed have normal intelligence. Despite these criticisms, the weight of the evidence has led researchers to conclude that diagnosis at a younger age changes in diagnostic criteria, and inclusion of milder cases may account for some of the rise in prevalence but certainly not for all of it.

This rise in ASD prevalence is a worldwide phenomenon. Lower figures in some countries are usually due to the use of older screening instruments or a focus on the diagnosis of classical autism to the exclusion of the wider spectrum. When total population screening is performed, the prevalence may be even higher than that reported by the CDC. In South Korea, for example, an international team of investigators determined that the prevalence for ASD is 2.64% or 1 in 38 children aged 7–12 ($n \approx 55,000$).

Autism spectrum disorders transcend cultural and geographic boundaries and is a worldwide health problem. Some economists say that the cost associated with caring for people with autism in the United States could reach $260 billion this year, and that this figure could easily be eclipsed in the coming decade. The staggering number of patients and costs associated with caring for those with the condition clearly demand more research.

Research in autism will only be facilitated by conjoint international efforts, that is, bringing together multiple stakeholders. We need the coordinated efforts of many governments and agencies to promote research, follow the burden of the disease, provide resolution in terms of conflicting studies, disseminate truthful information, and collect data using agreed upon standardized measures. Probably the highest priority should be given to postmortem research, as it has the highest level of resolution and the one that most clearly will be able to elucidate any underlying pathophysiological mechanisms. Thus far, postmortem research indicates that autism is a neurodevelopmental condition affecting many different areas of the brain, primarily the cerebral cortex. The findings help explain the presence of seizures and sensory problems in ASD. More importantly, the research has helped establish a potential therapeutic intervention based on transcranial magnetic stimulation (TMS).

The authors of this book would like to join the efforts of Autism BrainNet in publicizing the enormous impact that postmortem research can have on the understanding and treatment of autism. We want to urge autistic individuals, families affected by autism, and unaffected people to register to donate brain tissue for research. Because brain tissue is so difficult to procure without advance planning, we are urging registration for Autism BrainNet by visiting http://takesbrains.org. Registration is not a binding decision to donate, but allows you access to updates on autism research, information about local activities of Autism BrainNet, and summaries of findings that are possible through brain tissue research.

Manuel F. Casanova, MD
Ayman S. El-Baz, PhD
Jasjit S. Suri, PhD, MBA

Contributors

Gregory D. Abowd
College of Computing
Georgia Institute of Technology
Atlanta, Georgia

David G. Amaral
M.I.N.D. Institute
University of California at Davis
Davis, California

Rosa I. Arriaga
School of Interactive
    Computing
Georgia Institute of Technology
Atlanta, Georgia

Esubalew Bekele
Robotics and Autonomous
    Systems Laboratory
Vanderbilt University
Nashville, Tennessee

Sven Bölte
Center of Neurodevelopmental
    Disorders
Karolinska Institutet
Solna, Sweden

Daniel Bone
Signal Analysis and Interpretation
    Laboratory
Department of Electrical
    Engineering
University of Southern California
Los Angeles, California

Ruth A. Carper
Brain Development Imaging
    Laboratory
San Diego State University
San Diego, California

Manuel F. Casanova
Departments of Pediatrics and
    Biomedical Sciences
University of South
    Carolina School of
    Medicine
Greenville, South Carolina

F. Xavier Castellanos
Child Study Center
NYU Langone Medical Center
New York, New York

and

Nathan S. Kline Institute for
    Psychiatric Research
Orangeburg, New York

Verónica Martínez Cerdeño
M.I.N.D. Institute
University of California
    at Davis
Davis, California

Wen-Pin Chang
Department of Occupational
    Therapy
Creighton University
Omaha, Nebraska

Theodora Chaspari
Signal Analysis and Interpretation
 Laboratory
Department of Electrical
 Engineering
University of Southern California
Los Angeles, California

Rong Chen
Department of Diagnostic
 Radiology and Nuclear
 Medicine
University of Maryland School of
 Medicine
Baltimore, Maryland

Eun Young Choi
Department of Pharmacology and
 Physiology
University of Rochester Medical
 Center
Rochester, New York

Robert Coben
NeuroRehabilitation and
 Neurpsychological
 Services, P.C.
Massapequa, New York

Adriana Di Martino
The Child Study Center
NYU Langone Medical Center
New York, New York

Christine Ecker
Department of Child & Adolescent
 Psychiatry, Psychosomatics and
 Psychotherapy
University Hospital Frankfurt am
 Main
Goethe-University
Frankfurt am Main, Germany

Ayman S. El-Baz
Department of Bioengineering
University of Louisville
Louisville, Kentucky

Adel S. Elmaghraby
Department of Computer
 Engineering and Computer
 Science
University of Louisville
Louisville, Kentucky

Heba Elsayed M. Farag
American Printing House for the
 Blind
Louisville, Kentucky

Joel Frohlich
Semel Institute for Neuroscience
 and Human Behavior
University of California at Los
 Angeles
Los Angeles, California

Lawrence K. Fung
Department of Psychiatry and
 Behavioral Sciences—Child
 and Adolescent Psychiatry
Stanford University School of
 Medicine
Stanford, California

Kamilla G. Gazieva
Master of Health Science Program
Department of Community and
 Environmental Health
Boise State University
Boise, Idaho

Antonio Hardan
Department of Psychiatry and
 Behavioral Sciences—Child and
 Adolescent Psychiatry
Stanford University
School of Medicine
Stanford, California

Jamie Horder
Department of Forensic and
 Neurodevelopmental
 Sciences
Institute of Psychiatry
King's College London
London, United Kingdom

Marco Iacoboni
Department of Psychiatry and
    Biobehavioral Sciences
Ahmanson-Lovelace Brain
    Mapping Center
David Geffen School of
    Medicine
University of California at Los
    Angeles
Los Angeles, California

Rebecca M. Jones
Center for Autism and the
    Developing Brain
Weill Cornell Medical College
New York, New York

Joseph Jurgiel
Department of Bioengineering
University of California at Los
    Angeles
Los Angeles, California

Desmond L. Kelly
Department of Pediatrics
University of South Carolina
    School of Medicine
Greenville, South Carolina

Nicholas Lange
Psychiatry and Biostatistics
Harvard Medical School
Boston, Massachusetts

Deana D. Li
M.I.N.D. Institute
University of California
    at Davis
Davis, California

Yi Li
Department of Computer
    Engineering and Computer
    Science
University of Louisville
Louisville, Kentucky

Lauren E. Libero
M.I.N.D. Institute
University of California
    at Davis
Davis, California

Annukka Lindell
Department of Psychology and
    Counselling
School of Psychology and Public
    Health
La Trobe University
Victoria, Australia

Andre Marquand
Donders Institute for
    Brain, Cognition and
    Behavior
Radboud University
Nijmegen, Netherlands

Giorgia Michelini
MRC Social, Genetic, and
    Developmental Psychiatry
Institute of Psychiatry
King's College London
London, United Kingdom

Iman Mohammad-Rezazadeh
Semel Institute for Neuroscience
    and Human Behavior
University of California at Los
    Angeles
Los Angeles, California

Ayman Mukerji
Child Study Center
NYU Langone Medical
    Center
New York, New York

Ralph-Axel Müller
Brain Development Imaging
    Laboratory
San Diego State University
San Diego, California

Shrikanth Narayanan
Signal Analysis and Interpretation
    Laboratory
Department of Electrical
    Engineering and Computer
    Science
University of Southern California
Los Angeles, California

N. Nazneen
School of Interactive Computing
Georgia Institute of Technology
Atlanta, Georgia

Christine W. Nordahl
M.I.N.D. Institute
University of California at Davis
Davis, California

Ron Oberleitner
Behavior Imaging Solutions Inc.
Boise, Idaho

Joseph Piven
Carolina Institute for
    Developmental Disabilities
University of North Carolina
Chapel Hill, North Carolina

Uwe Reischl
Master of Health Science
    Program
Department of Community and
    Environmental Health
Boise State University
Boise, Idaho

Gina Rippon
Department of Psychology
Aston University
Birmingham, United Kingdom

Agata Rozga
School of Interactive Computing
Georgia Institute of Technology
Atlanta, Georgia

Nilanjan Sarkar
Department of Mechanical
    Engineering
Vanderbilt University
Nashville, Tennessee

Christopher J. Smith
Director of Research
Southwest Autism Research &
    Resource Center
Phoenix, Arizona

Estate M. Sokhadze
Departments of Pediatrics and
    Biomedical Sciences
University of South Carolina
    School of Medicine
Greenville, South Carolina

Guela E. Sokhadze
Department of Anatomical
    Science and Neurobiology
University of Louisville
Louisville, Kentucky

Jasjit S. Suri
Neuroscience and Autism
    Division
Global Biomedical Technologies,
    Inc.
Roseville, California

Amy Swanson
Vanderbilt Kennedy Center
Vanderbilt University
Nashville, Tennessee

Meghan R. Swanson
Carolina Institute for
    Developmental Disabilities
University of North Carolina
Chapel Hill, North Carolina

Kristiina Tammimies
Center of Neurodevelopmental
    Disorders
Karolinska Institutet
Solna, Sweden

Allan Tasman
Department of Psychiatry and
   Behavioral Sciences
University of Louisville
Louisville, Kentucky

Zachary Warren
Division of Developmental
   Medicine
Vanderbilt University
Nashville, Tennessee

Amy Weitlauf
Division of Developmental
   Medicine
Vanderbilt University
Nashville, Tennessee

Charlotte Willfors
Center of Neurodevelopmental
   Disorders
Karolinska Institutet
Solna, Sweden

Zhi Zheng
Robotics and Autonomous
   Systems Laboratory
Vanderbilt University
Nashville, Tennessee

Chapter 1 Present and future autism data science

Nicholas Lange

Contents

Abstract 2
1.1   Introduction 2
    1.1.1   Seven important papers (out of so many more) 3
        1.1.1.1   Study design. 4
        1.1.1.2   Database design 5
        1.1.1.3   Sampling and screening. 5
        1.1.1.4   Randomization. 6
        1.1.1.5   Data entry and monitoring. 6
        1.1.1.6   Data analysis 6
        1.1.1.7   Publication 7
        1.1.1.8   Data sharing. 7
        1.1.1.9   Reproduction of central findings 7
        1.1.1.10 Planning the next study 7
1.2   Future of autism data science 7
    1.2.1   Data harmonization 7
        1.2.1.1   Some pros and cons of meta-analysis 8
        1.2.1.2   Planning multisite studies 9
    1.2.2   Data display and its diagnostic limitations. 9
        1.2.2.1   Is it possible to diagnose autism by brain
                  imaging?. 10
    1.2.3   Candidate phenotypes. 11
    1.2.4   Reporting results. 12
1.3   Concluding remarks 12
Acknowledgments 12
References 12

"Everything is related to everything else."

—Mahavira (599–527 BCE)
Anekāntavāda and Syādvāda

Abstract

This chapter begins with a critical look at the present state of autism data science in observational studies and clinical trials. It then proceeds to list the necessary steps in the proper application of autism data science for young researchers, and experienced researchers who may have seen this previously; it is worth taking another look. Multisite studies and cluster randomization methods are also discussed. It includes a section on the future state of autism imaging and its limits at present. The chapter concludes with some views and speculations on future improvement of autism data science.

1.1 Introduction

Autism data science is defined as the development and application of biostatistical methods for observations from scientific studies of the behavior and physical states of individuals with autism to serve the autism community in more effective ways in the present and future. Use of the terms "data analytics," "analytics," "bioinformatics," "biometrics," "knowledge engineering," "metric," and others is becoming more frequent than the terms "statistics" and "biostatistics," which may connote a static rather than dynamic measurement process to some; "data science" is the term adopted here.

When psychiatrist Leo Kanner first identified "early infantile autism" in 1943 through his astute observation of 11 children, he retracted his initial biological theory 6 years later. Since then, no valid alternative theory has yet emerged to take its place. The biological basis of autism has yet to be discovered. The last decade of autism research has shown that autism is not a static encephalopathy as thought previously by many, but a dynamic lifelong disorder with complex changes in behavior and the whole body and brain that themselves change over time from childhood into adulthood and old age (Frith 2013; Lange et al. 2015). Autism research began, as does much of science, as an attempt to explore a new and mysterious domain and describe what is observed. At first, it indeed seemed as though "everything is connected to everything else" due to major unknowns. Although Mahavira's ancient statement may be true in some abstract space, by careful observation, description, and analysis, science has evolved to a point; we have discovered that some "things" on the autism spectrum are more connected and less connected to other "things". Much of our progress over the last 70 years has been made possible by effective applications of the (Western) scientific method, in other words by applied statistics in autism research: autism data science.

The overarching aim of autism data science is to find the key that unlocks the data so it can impact individual lives. The essential benefits that autism data science provides are solid evidence to understand the brain and body mechanisms involved, the strength of longitudinal analysis to provide clinical and brain imaging phenotypes for genetic studies, and to contribute to the diagnosis, treatment, prognosis, and outcome of the disorder. This is the challenge; to determine the what are the developmental mechanisms that underlie the disorder throughout the life span. We refuse to wait 30 more years to find out.

This chapter aims to familiarize young researchers with effective applications of autism data science, to ask seasoned autism researchers to take another look, and to introduce and reintroduce autism data science to the autism community and the interested public. This chapter includes a short discussion of imaging neuroscience in autism research.

1.1.1 Seven important papers (out of so many more)

Leo Kanner's seminal paper and his follow-up report contain his careful and caring, sensitive and detailed observations of previously unnamed behavioral phenomena (Kanner 1943, 1971). No statistics were included in these reports; their inclusion would not have been possible, or irrelevant even if they were. Lotter (1966) provided the first epidemiological study of young children with autism. The landmark genetic twin study by Folstein and Rutter (1977) in England provided valuable epidemiological data on familial aggregation in the form of prose descriptions and summary tables. Their article also included a Fisher exact test of independence in a 2×2 contingency table of concordance and discordance in monozygotic and dizygotic twins; no additional hypotheses were tested. Further seminal epidemiologic information was provided by Fombonne (1999, 2003). By the time of the Bolton et al. (1994) case control family history study, autism data science had advanced to include extensive epidemiologic and summary tables, exact tests, logistic regression, estimation of standard errors robust to nonindependence, a partial Mann–Whitney U-test, and tests of multicollinearity. More recently, in schizophrenia research, Alexander-Bloch et al. (2014) estimated the growth curves of cortical thickness in 80,000 imaging locations across the cortex, in 212 individuals about half of whom had schizophrenia, in the age range 8–30 years, by use of semiparametric penalized spline generalized mixed-effect models to find that, in their words, "abnormal cortical development in schizophrenia may be modularized or constrained by the normal community structure of developmental modules of the human brain connectome." This finding has also been observed in autism. The complexity and heterogeneity of neuroimaging findings in individuals with autism spectrum disorder have suggested that many of the underlying alterations are subtle and involve many brain regions and networks. The ability to account for multivariate brain features and identify neuroimaging measures that characterize individual variation have thus become increasingly important for interpreting and understanding the effects of neurobiological mechanisms on behavioral anomalies central to the disorder. We have not yet learned as much about autism as we have about schizophrenia; research into other disorders is helping show

3

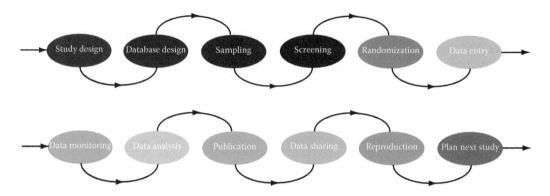

Figure 1.1 The sequential chain of necessary steps in the practice of autism data science.

us the way. The practice and quality of autism data science today falls far short of that in many other fields, such as Alzheimer's research, engineering, physics, chemistry, pharmaceutical research, and others. This is to be expected since we do not yet know what we are actually measuring. The present state of autism clinical trials is far behind the rigor of those in cancer research. Along with such articles as Alexander-Bloch et al. (2014) and many more not cited herein, there will continue to be exponential increases in the uses of novel methods for data collection (dynamic, static, wearable devices,…), tabulation (published, ongoing online, shared databases,…), display, and classical and novel biostatistical analysis; this is especially true in imaging neuroscience. As in all fields of science, we learn more about what we know, what we do not know, and what we have yet to learn. We have a long way to go, yet, still, in a sense, "everything is connected to everything else," almost.

Twelve necessary steps in the practice of autism data science are shown in Figure 1.1. The sequential ellipses may be new to some, and well known to others. Yet how many of these steps are practiced, and to what degree and quality? The steps shown in Figure 1.1 are relaxed for observational studies, and may vary across other types of studies; they are not intended to be universal. Our field is just beginning to travel along this scientifically acceptable road. The reader may find it useful to compare our current practice to that of cancer research trials as we traverse the ellipses.

1.1.1.1 Study design

- *Primary outcome measure.* The basic science researcher and trialist identify one, and only one, primary outcome measure. Only a few secondary outcome measures are stated. Each answers the question: Who, specifically, will benefit from the results, if any, of this study or trial? If the study is a clinical trial, then adherence to the 25-item CONSORT checklist and flow chart is mandatory (Schulz et al. 2010). Multiple "primary outcomes" and a plethora of secondary outcomes are discouraged. No aim is chosen based on data collected after the study begins. The narrative is succinct, crisp, and precise; it tells the story. Primary and secondary outcome measures are univariate (a single measurement per participant) or multivariate (many measurements per participant over time or other metameter, many at one time, or both). Univariate outcomes are chosen *a priori* when they are thought to be the most informative. For instance, although developmental domains coexist (general, behavioral, cognitive, sensual, etc.), the choice of one from which the primary outcome has been defined and its corresponding measurement may be best due to its specificity; others may best be designated secondary outcome measures. Overly complex multivariate measurements and biostatistical methods are discouraged when a simpler measurement or method will suffice.

- *Hypotheses.* All hypotheses are testable using the evidence generated by the study. The target population that may benefit from the trial is clearly defined. The primary testable hypothesis is linked to the primary outcome, and stated succinctly. Inclusion of a few testable subhypotheses are linked to the primary or secondary hypotheses as appropriate. Each testable hypothesis is stated in the science of the project for the nonexpert, and written in collaboration with the trialist(s) and biostatistician(s) involved. If for instance the goal is to study individual change over time in motor development, then a longitudinal sampling plan or mixed cross-sectional and longitudinal sampling plan is advisable. Ad hoc methods whose properties are not well understood are discouraged.

1.1.1.2 Database design   The database structure is described clearly, tightly aligned with the study design, and the database is built in collaboration with all investigators. It is relevant to ask why are we entering the data into the database. Even if one thinks that one knows all the answers that will be asked of the data, designing its base at the finest resolution to answer other questions that will very likely arise is important. Existing database designs and software are employed when possible. The biostatistician collaborates closely with the database manger as they tailor the database to provide the study's needs.

1.1.1.3 Sampling and screening   The target and sample populations are clearly defined. Participants are drawn at random from the target population whenever warranted. Inclusion and exclusion criteria and the enrollment procedure are stated clearly and applied strictly. For clinical trials, the necessary intent-to-treat (ITT) policy does not exclude participants who have had at least one measurement. To address generalizability, the researchers ask and answer the question: how can the results from this sample be applied to a different target population? Much more information can be provided here; additional considerations are described in many other reliable sources.

1.1.1.4 Randomization A randomization method for the study of two or more groups of participants is chosen in line with the testable hypotheses and sampling plan. The randomization method accounts for background measurements (such as demography, for example) that may influence the primary and secondary outcomes. Randomization schemes for multisite (cluster) studies are described in Section 1.1.2, "Planning Multisite Studies." Again, many such methods exist for many research scenarios common to autism research. The choice of an inadequate or inappropriate randomization method can sink the entire project before it even begins.

1.1.1.5 Data entry and monitoring This critical component follows directly from step 1.3 and is best pursued in a close alliance of the biostatistician and the database manager.

1.1.1.6 Data analysis The analytic methods are briefly described in plain English; it is not written for statisticians only. (Effective narration can be tricky here due to the high variability of readers, and reviewers writing a grant proposal.) A complete set of references to the relevant literature is provided; comprehensive literature search is essential. Univariate and multivariate models are employed as appropriate. The simplest, most powerful, and well-known methods, chosen by Occam's razor, are employed whenever possible. The use of more complex and less understood method is avoided when a simpler method is sufficient. Multivariate approaches are described clearly. Examples are provided when needed. No circular data analysis or "voodoo correlations" is performed (Kriegeskorte et al. 2009; Vul et al. 2009). Nonparametric methods are employed only when distributional assumptions of parametric approaches do not hold; parametric methods are more powerful when these assumptions hold (Altham 1984). Model selection is not based on any comparison of different p-values across options. Biostatistical models include all background measurements that are employed in randomization. To eschew serious bias, models that include an interaction, between treatment and group for instance, also include at least one of the main effects of the interaction; their absence must be justified *a priori* otherwise. Power considerations are based on parameter estimates derived from preliminary data, either from research team results or from relevant published literature when available. Acknowledge regression to the mean when present or possible.[*]

---

[*] Regression to the mean occurs when repeated measurements are made on the same participant or unit of observation, and was perhaps first acknowledged by Francis Galton, the inventor of regression. It is a type of selection bias and is the consequence of measurement error. There are customarily two sources of variation, random variation due to the act of taking repeated measurements of the participant (The Hawthorne effect, Heisenberg Uncertainty), and systematic variation due to the process being measured. Only random variation causes the regression to the mean effect. It can appear as an actual change, when, in fact, there is little or no change. Regression to the mean appears at the individual level and the group level. The effect is increased when random variation increases over time, and when subsets of participants or groups are selected based on baseline measurements. Its effects can be mitigated through better study design and use of appropriate mixed models and other statistical methods that address it directly.

1.1.1.7 Publication   The researchers tell us what they did and did *not* do. It is often best to wait until the submission of a manuscript to a peer-reviewed journal prior to presenting the results in public at scientific conferences.

1.1.1.8 Data sharing   The growing National Database for Autism Research (NDAR) is the required National Institute of Mental Health (NIMH) depository for National Institutes of Health (NIH)-funded autism research findings. The timing of study deposits allows for the original researchers to perform and publish the primary analysis. And the NIH is moving toward requiring that study results in an interpretable form are made publically available afterward.

1.1.1.9 Reproduction of central findings   Conducting reproducibility studies is not done as frequently as it needs to be, except perhaps in drug trials. Such efforts take precious time and funding away from being at the competitive edge. Yet autism data science needs to take this vital step in the scientific method to truly move the field forward. The NIMH guidelines on scientific rigor and reproducibility (NOT-OD-16-011) may increase this rate in the future, yet it must be raised much sooner, as close to the "here and now" as possible. If there is no change, our findings will continue to raise doubts in our own community and the scientific and lay communities at large. As the number of single and multisite autism observational studies and trials continues to soar, further disregard of this necessary step cannot be tolerated. The NIH spent $208,000,000 in FY2015 on autism research, and will spend an estimated $216,000,000 in FY2016. Are we employing and reporting statistical results derived rigorously and can they be replicated? Are the U.S. taxpayers receiving value for their money?

1.1.1.10 Planning the next study   The last step in the autism data science cycle research is to plan the next study based on the results of the completed study and relevant findings produced in the interim by other autism researchers.

1.2 Future of autism data science

The following is a brief discussion of a few possible future advances in autism data science. In essence, these topics point to the future improvement and effectiveness of autism data science.

1.2.1 Data harmonization

The human benefit in the here and now according to a well-defined and detailed target will be clearly stated as the primary intention of the study. There will be measureable study outcomes that are more specific than those for a general domain, population, or abstract ideal. Case-by-case evolution of the strategy will often take place; effective development is an iterative learning process. In each scenario, an unbiased panel of field experts, including a biostatistician, will decide which data to combine according to the prespecified clinical or research goal. Site-blinded quality assurance will be identified from within the panel of experts, and employed to develop and apply biostatistical methods to assess the magnitude of study inhomogeneity; this subcommittee will be allowed to propose modifications of the recommendations of other experts. The intended gains of a common data acquisition strategy for future studies will be weighed carefully against the present and future cost of freezing the technology and possible decreases in utility for pressing issues involving patients, participants, parents, and the general public. The biostatisticians will provide the most powerful analytic design(s) to test hypotheses. Preliminary data and estimates of the parameters to test the hypotheses will be provided and employed for empirically based power calculations. Some available designs, whose analytic power calculations are well known, are quite clever and surprisingly efficient (minimum sample size required) in some cases and will be applied effectively.

1.2.1.1 Some pros and cons of meta-analysis Meta-analysis is a systematic method for the analysis and rationalization of results from independent studies, taking into account all pertinent information (van Belle 2008). Meta-analyses attempt to mimic multisite studies, such as collaborative controlled clinical trials, to increase statistical power. The clinical benefits of combining studies to derive "one mega-database to rule them all," however, may not justify the effort and cost to build it. Aggregation of many small and heterogeneous data sets does not guarantee an increase in statistical power. Power could actually decrease. Data harmonization across sites will not settle on a strategy that yields the lowest performance for the sake of increasing overall sample size. Extraneous variability across multisite data sets can sink the combined data set when site differences are greater than the differences to be detected. This unfortunate scenario defeats the purpose and intention of retrospective and prospective multisite studies; the advisability of performing and reporting a meta-analysis will be scrutinized. According to some clinicians and researchers, hope is dwindling that the Autism Brain Imaging Data Exchange (ABIDE) data set for magnetic resonance (MR) brain images (Di Martino et al. 2014) results can provide clinically data truly more beneficial to patients because its phenotypic and imaging data are of such variable quality; others feel quite the opposite. Because the fleet moves only as fast as its slowest ship, autism data science will not settle for a combination of different imaging protocols and quality that yield poor clinical performance. If so, the fleet will never get anywhere.

The basic science and clinical validity and utility of any meta-analysis will depend strongly on the decisions of field experts on which data to combine and how to combine them (van Belle 2008). The success of such efforts will depend on two conditions applied impartially: the quality of each study must be ascertained prior to combination, and the studies to be combined must be homogeneous. The first condition will be met by expert review with specific reference to the overarching purpose and goal of the effort. This condition will be answered by the question: "Exactly what basic clinical scientific questions will the combined data be able to answer more effectively than if they are not combined?" The second condition will be met through the judicious application of empirical Bayes methods to assess the magnitude of inhomogeneity across the studies to be combined.[*]

1.2.1.2 Planning multisite studies   Multisite study protocols will be standardized by stipulating and enforcing the use of a fixed subset of parameter values across sites, as, for instance, is being done for the current Human Connectome Program and other similar present and future extensions. The resulting data will be easily understood and accessible to the general research scientist and interested citizen. Forward-thinking investments in computational resources, disk storage, and technical support will dramatically expand the number of investigators who will use the data sets. A central location for annotation of results (published and anecdotal) on a community forum will help to minimize duplication of effort and speed communication, analogous to *arxiv* in physics, particularly since not every observation may ultimately warrant formal publication in a peer-reviewed journal.

1.2.1.2.1 Multisite (cluster) sampling design   Large multisite cooperative studies will take precedence over many studies performed at a single site through dedication to cooperation over competition. Autism data science for multisite research requires different criteria than single-site designs. These studies typically have a three-level hierarchical data structure. In such studies, participants are nested in sites (level 1), and sites nested in treatments or exposures (level 2). Level 3 is the set of parameters drawn from a specified data-generating mechanism of a supra population. Randomization of participants to treatments within sites, rather than randomization of sites to treatments is becoming an useful alternate design. It will almost always be more informative for a total sample size of 600 to plan a sample of six sites with 100 participants each than to plan a sample of three sites with 200 participants each; Snijders (2005) provides some theory behind these ideas, and references to practical applications; more analytics need to be developed.

1.2.2 Data display and its diagnostic limitations

Graphics over numbers? For many, the processing and interpretation of numbers is difficult, and the use of graphics over tables has increased in recent decades. This practice promotes and increases innumeracy. The

---

[*] Draper et al. (1993), for instance, still very useful today, contains proper methods for meta-analysis, and important examples of the pros and cons when combining information; practical mathematical formulas are provided.

Oxford English Dictionary defines an image as "an artificial imitation or representation of the external form," a "copy," "likeness," "similitude," "semblance," "appearance," "shadow," namely not the real thing. In absence of the critical biology, brain and other imaging of the body seek to find evidence of autism etiology, and to further understand what goes askew during prenatal and very early childhood development that gives rise to the disorder. Some researchers today have exclaimed, however, that "science *is* imaging," a clear misconception regardless of how "real" the ever-improving spatiotemporal image resolution, brilliance of color, and attraction of animation appear to be. An image is a measurement, an organized set of numbers that represents observed objects. These numbers are nearly always transformed by complex image algebra, including smoothing, stretching, thresholding, mapping, layering, digital films and cartoons, and attractive coloring. These "enhanced" images generate strong visual and mental impressions. We forget about the numbers and the mathematical transformations employed and begin to see things that have not been observed in the real world. The neuropathology remains hidden outside the image. Regrettably, this illusion will continue to increase in future publications, grant proposals, and the media. This will be especially true in *imaging neuroscience.*

Part of the reason why autism remains so hard to pin down and treat is that we have yet to find any biological measurement, neither a gene nor gene set, to identify it with or without *a priori* knowledge of autism's presence or absence. Some genetic studies suggest that 400–600 genes or more may be involved as common variants (polymorphisms) and rare variants (mutations). The only candidate, yet nonspecific biomarker of autism to date is an elevated blood level of the neurotransmitter serotonin. Serotonin (5-hydroxytrypamine [5-HT]) is a brain chemical that plays an essential role in sleep, appetite, mood, anxiety, social affiliation, impulsivity, arousal, aggression, and reaction to stress. But low serotonin levels (hyperserotonemia) are hardly specific to autism. Tumors in the gastrointestinal tract and recreational drug use such as ecstasy and LSD also increase blood serotonin.

*1.2.2.1 Is it possible to diagnose autism by brain imaging?** A study published recently correctly identified 36 out of 39 children and adolescents with autism solely by the use of functional magnetic resonance imaging (fMRI). The researchers reported that as the subjects listened to their parents' voices, those with autism had lower brain activity in the superior temporal gyrus, a brain region involved in language reception, compared with controls. Although this finding makes sense, we should be cautious about its interpretation. This is not an autism-detecting brain scan. Language deficits are a core and defining feature of the disorder; one doesn't need a brain scan to show this. And there are many people

---

* Portions of this section have been modified from an article published previously in *Nature* (Lange 2012).

with language difficulties who do not have autism. Therefore, a technology that detects language problems doesn't move the ball toward a differential diagnosis. As result, in the view of this autism researcher, unless and until a stable biological basis for the cause(s) of autism is discovered, diagnosis of autism by brain imaging will not be possible. Autism clinicians need to know where and how to look prior to making a diagnosis.

Brain imaging does, of course, have a place in autism study. While it has little if any diagnostic utility at present, imaging technology has already helped us understand the disorder. Volumetric MRI has shown us that about one in five children (20%) with autism has an early abnormal enlargement of the brain that tends to stabilize during the first 18 months of life (Nordahl et al. 2011). Functional MRI has helped us learn where people with autism focus during social interaction, or when watching films with intense social content. Positron emission tomography (PET) has begun to show us differences between people with autism compared to typical controls in the distribution of serotonin and dopamine receptors—and of the evolving roles of serotonin throughout life.

Because autism is an individual heterogeneous disorder, its future data science will need to achieve the exceedingly difficult goals of a "stratified psychiatry." Stratified psychiatry refers to a newly proposed system for all psychiatric disorders in which homogeneous subgroups of individuals are defined by dimensional combinations of biological and behavioral features—such as an altered neurotransmitter pattern and a history of major depression—rather than by categorical criteria (Kapur et al. 2012). The NIH Research Domain Criteria (RDoC) are evolving continuously in this direction; the reader can follow at http://www.nimh.nih.gov/research-funding/rdoc/index.shtml to see just how.

1.2.3 Candidate phenotypes

What would it take to change autism clinical practice to include candidate imaging phenotypes? The answer is obvious: the discovery of a true biological marker (biomarker) of the disorder. Let it be clear, however, of Let the proper definition of a "biomarker" be clear. As formally defined, a biomarker is "a characteristic that is measured objectively and evaluated as an indicator of normal biological processes, pathogenic processes, or pharmacologic responses to a therapeutic intervention" (Biomarkers Definitions Working Group 2001). One may refer to a characteristic or phenotype as a biomarker "if it is minimally affected by the will, behavior, and attitudes of subjects or the evaluator or by transient environmental influences" (Kraemer 2002). Brain scans, whole-body scans, neuronal subtyping by brightfield and electron microscopy, for instance, and genetics, are signposts showing us where and how to look, see, ponder, hypothesize and test, and possibly treat. Such biological measurements and many others will (or may) one day be deemed autism phenotypes.

11

1.2.4 Reporting results

Abstract submissions, reports at conferences, submitted manuscripts, and the media will specify what type of trial or study was conducted. Is it Stage 0 (theoretical, speculative), Stage 1 (preclinical or preliminary findings), Stage 2 (validation study), or Stage 3 (clinical impact study)?

1.3 Concluding remarks

"Data?" "Statistics?" In the future, the "static" in "statistics" may become a contradiction in terms of sorts as autism data science becomes increasingly dynamic as scientists continue to employ more rapid and continuous devices having higher spatiotemporal resolution to analyze and synthesize what we can learn about an individual on the autism spectrum in order to enrich his or her life. I conclude with a puzzler, perhaps far-fetched at the moment. Autism devices may one day be able to place a newly improved, real-time, high-dimensional "living" brain simulation beside the living brain of a person with autism, and, as in the Ship of Theseus paradox and Turing's test, who will be able to discern which one is which?

Acknowledgments

The author thanks Brandon A. Zieliniski, MD, PhD, Jeffrey S. Andersen, MD, PhD, and Janet E. Lainhart, MD, for helpful suggestions that greatly improved this chapter, all of those who have taught me so much about autism, and Manny Casanova for his invitation to contribute to this book. He also thanks the many participants with autism and of typical development and their parents in the studies in which they have participated for their time, persistence, dedication, and resilience over many years.

References

Alexander-Bloch, A. F., P. T. Philip, J. Rapoport, H. McAdams, J. N. Giedd, E. T. Bullmore, and N. Gogtay. 2014. Abnormal cortical growth in schizophrenia targets normative modules of synchronized development. *Biol. Psychiatry* 76:438–46.

Altham, P. M. E. 1984. Improving the precision of estimation by fitting a model. *J. Royal Stat. Soc. Ser. B* 46:118–9.

Biomarkers Definitions Working Group. 2001. Biomarkers and surrogate endpoints: Preferred definitions and conceptual framework. *Clin. Pharmacol. Ther.* 69:89–95.

Bolton, P., H. Macdonald, A. Pickles, P. Rios, S. Goode, M. Crowson, A. Bailey, and M. Rutter. 1994. A case–control family history study of autism. *J. Child Psychol. Psychiatry* 35(5):877–900.

Di Martino, A., C.-G. Yan, Q. Li et al. 2014. The autism brain imaging data exchange: Towards a large-scale evaluation of the intrinsic brain architecture in autism. *Mol. Psychiatry* 19:659–67. doi: 10.1038/mp.2013.78.

Draper, D. et al. (eds) 1993. *On Combining Information: Statistical Issues and Opportunities for Research*. National Research Council report of the NRC/CATS, Committee, National Academy Press.

Folstein, S. and M. Rutter. 1977. Infantile autism: A genetic study of 21 twin pairs. *J. Child Psychol. Psychiatry Allied Discipl.* 18:297–321.

Fombonne, E. 1999. The epidemiology of autism: A review. *Psychological Medicine*. 29:769–86.

Fombonne, E. 2003. Epidemiological surveys of autism and other pervasive developmental disorders: An update. *J Autism Dev Disord*. 33:365. doi:10.1023/A:1025054610557.

Frith, U. 2013. A fundamental truth about developmental disorders. *Perspect. Psychol. Sci.* 8(6):670–2.

Kanner, L. 1943. Autistic disturbances of affective contact. *Nervous Child* 2:217–50.

Kanner, L. 1971. Follow-up study of eleven autistic children originally reported in 1943. *J. Autism Child. Schizophr.* 1(2):119–45.

Kapur, S., A. G. Phillips, and T. R. Insel. 2012. *Mol. Psychiatry*. doi: 10.1038/mp.2012.105.

Kraemer, H. C., S. K. Schultz, and S. Artndt. 2002. Biomarkers in psychiatry: Methodological issues. *Am. J. Geriatr. Psychiatry* 10(6):6532–659.

Kriegeskorte, N., W. K. Simmons, P. S. F. Bellgowan, and C. I. Baker. 2009. Circular analysis in systems neuroscience—The dangers of double dipping. *Nature Neuroscience*. 12(5):535–40.

Lange, N. 2012. Imaging autism. *Nature* 491:S17.

Lange, N., B. G. Travers, E. D. Bigler et al. 2015. Longitudinal volumetric brain changes in autism spectrum disorder ages 6–35 years. *Autism Research* 8(1):82–93.

Lotter, V. 1966. Epidemiology of autistic conditions in young children: I. Prevalence. *Soc. Psychiatry* 1:124–37.

Nordahl, C. W., N. Lange, D. D. Li, L. A. Barnett, A. Lee, M. H. Buonocore, T. J. Simon, S. Rogers, S. Ozonoff, and D. G. Amaral. 2011. Brain enlargement is associated with regression in preschool age boys with autism. *Proc. Natl. Acad. Sci.* 108(50):20195–200.

Schulz, K. F., D. G. Altman, and D. Moher. 2010. CONSORT 2010 statement: Updated guidelines for reporting parallel group randomised trials. *J. Pharmacol. Pharmacother*. 2010;1(2):100–7. doi: 10.4103/0976–500X.72352. PubMed PMID: 21350618; PMCID: PMC3043330.

Snijders, T. A. B. 2005. Power and sample size in multilevel linear models. In *Encyclopedia of Statistics in Behavioral Science*, vol. 3, eds. B. S. Everitt and D. C. Howell, 1570–3. Chichester: Wiley.

van Belle, G. 2008. *Statistical Rules of Thumb*, 2nd ed. New York: John Wiley & Sons.

Vul, E., C. Harris, P. Winkielman, and H. P. Puzzlingly. 2009. High correlations in fMRI studies of emotion, personality, and social cognition. *Perspectives on Psychological Science* 4(3):274–90. doi: 10.1111/j.1745-6924.2009.01125.x.

Chapter 2 Twin research in autism spectrum disorder

Charlotte Willfors, Kristiina Tammimies, and Sven Bölte

Contents

Abstract 15
2.1   Behavior genetics: Why conduct research on twins? 16
       2.1.1   Genetic influence 17
       2.1.2   Shared and nonshared variation 17
2.2   Twin studies 18
       2.2.1   Different twin designs 18
       2.2.2   Twin studies in ASD: What have we learned? 20
       2.2.3   Twin studies of ASD as a continuous trait 22
                2.2.3.1   The Missouri Twin Study 22
                2.2.3.2   The twin early development study 22
                2.2.3.3   The Child and Adolescent Twin Study
                           in Sweden. 25
       2.2.4   Twin studies of ASD symptoms in toddlers 26
       2.2.5   Discordant MZ twin pair design in ASD research. 26
       2.2.6   Twin studies in ASD and comorbidity 28
       2.2.7   Etiological overlap between different domains
                of symptoms 29
       2.2.8   Limitations of twin designs within ASD research 30
2.3   Summary and directions for future research 31
References 32

Abstract

Autism spectrum disorder (ASD) is a neurodevelopmental condition of multifactorial origin. Aside from clinically relevant ASD phenotypes qualifying for a categorical diagnosis, data increasingly support the notion of broader/extended phenotypes and traits of ASD that are continuously distributed in the general population, with variation in ASD traits determined by factors overlapping with the clinical phenotypes. Earlier twin studies confirmed repeatedly the genetic causes for ASD, with only modest environmental influences. Thus, ASD is considered one of the most heritable of psychiatric conditions with a heritability estimates between 80% and 90%. However, recent twin studies have suggested a stronger environmental influence on ASD etiologies. This chapter gives a short theoretical background on the basics of behavioral genetics and twin designs, summarizes the contribution of twin research to the knowledge of ASD etiologies, and discusses areas of interest for future twin research within the field of ASD.

2.1 Behavior genetics: Why conduct research on twins?

Behavior genetics assumes that individuals in a population differ for both genetic and nongenetic reasons. Different family-based studies are used to answer questions about the relative contributions of genes and environment. The underlying notion of these approaches is that if a trait or a disorder is heritable, individuals that are more genetically similar should also be more similar regarding that trait or disorder status. The two major designs in human behavioral genetics are adoption and twin studies. While studies applying the former design have decreased, the latter has increased during the last decades. The same is true for the number and quality of nationwide twin registries. There are two categories of environmental factors explored in behavioral genetics: environmental factors shared by family members (SE), making them similar, and environmental factors not shared (NSE), making family members different.

Plomin and Daniels (1987) were the first to claim that NSE are responsible for the majority of human behavior variation. They presumed that 40%–60% of the variation in personality, psychopathology, and cognitive abilities (after childhood) is owing to NSE. In order to understand how children in the same family can be different, they proposed a quantitative model to study the same trait in multiple children of the same family. This model comprises three components: (i) additive genetics, that is, the sum of all individual differences that are caused by independent effects of alleles or loci (heritability), (ii) common environment, that is, environmental factors that are shared between twins SE and (iii) environmental factors that are specific to each twin NSE (ACE model). This model has been demonstrated to be useful for explaining behavior variation in humans. In addition, two interesting findings have increased our understanding of how environmental factors affect human behavior and psychopathology. First, individuals growing up in the same family are not more similar than individuals growing up in different families on the majority of behavioral traits. This means that the environmental factors that make individuals different, NSE, are playing a larger role than the SE for most human behavior. Second, there is a genotype–environment correlation for most traits, meaning that the effect of an environmental exposure is dependent on a particular genotype.

2.1.1 Genetic influence

Not all genetic variation is additive. Nonadditive genetic variance is explained by factors that have nonlinear effect on the phenotype such as the interactions between alleles at the same locus, or on different loci (epistasis) and dominance. Additive genetic variation (narrow-sense heritability) can be considered as the proportion of the phenotype that can be predicted from the knowledge of the number of additive alleles (*A* versus *a* alleles) present in the genotype. Consider an *aa* individual to have zero *A* alleles, *Aa* has one *A* allele, and *AA* has two *A* alleles. Only, in the ideal case when alleles at a genetic locus are codominant, genes will act purely additive; if that is not the case, the dominant genetic effects will reduce the additive genetic variation. The nonadditive genetic influence of dominance can be estimated in twin models, called dominant genetic influence (D), and the model is then transformed into an ADE model.

The genetic causes of ASD are still only partly understood even though substantial progress has been made in recent years. A minority (~10%) of individuals with ASD have an identifiable single-gene disorder, such as fragile X, tuberous sclerosis, or neurofibromatosis, which may account for the phenotype. In addition, recent advances in genome-wide methods including detection of copy number variations (CNVs) and single nucleotide variants (SNVs) from sequencing studies have revealed multiple genes and variants with substantial risk for ASD (Geschwind and State 2015). The majority of findings have emerged from *de novo* CNVs and SNVs affecting genes involved in synaptic function, chromatin modification, and targets of the fragile X mental retardation protein. The recent estimates suggest the existence of hundreds of ASD risk genes (e.g., Pinto et al. 2014; Iossifov et al. 2014).

2.1.2 Shared and nonshared variation

Within twin designs, NSE is defined as all factors making siblings growing up in the same family different (e.g., epigenetic mechanisms, exposure of air pollution and heavy metals, somatic complications, traumatic life events, etc.). The definition of SE is nongenetic factors making twin siblings similar (e.g., parenting). Many environmental factors could potentially fall under both SE and NSE, depending on the trait studied. For example, a traumatic life event could be SE for one trait, making the siblings more similar for one phenotype, and NSE for another trait, making them more different for a second phenotype.

One of the most studied (social) environmental factors is parenting. Family studies of parenting show a correlation of $r = 0.25$ between siblings growing up in the same family (when reported by the children). Similar results have been shown for the effect of traumatic life events, that is, the events themselves are not causing the NSE effect but rather how they are experienced, which can highly differ between individuals (Plomin 2011).

Included in NSE are also nonheritable genetic mechanisms, that is, stochastic *de novo* mutations and environmentally influenced epigenetic mechanisms. In general, *de novo* mutations are not taken into account when estimating heritability in classic twin designs; however, these could be associated with environmental factors increasing the risk for ASD. For instance, the number of *de novo* mutations in the offspring's genome increases with advanced parental age and has been shown to be a risk factor for ASD (Parner et al. 2012; Kong et al. 2012; Ronemus et al. 2014). Epigenetic mechanisms, on the other hand, are defined as mechanisms other than those related to DNA that cause changes in an organism's gene expression and/or cellular phenotype. Even though there are no changes in the underlying DNA sequence of the organism, the epigenetic modifications may (or may not) remain through cell division and during the cell's life and last for multiple generations. In the literature of epigenetic effects on psychopathology, the focus has, to date, been mainly on processes causing alterations in gene expression on life course, not over multiple generations. Epigenetic changes occur via four principal mechanisms: covalent modifications of DNA (e.g., cytosine methylation), alteration of chromatin structure via histone modification, noncoding RNA products altering gene expression, and prion proteins. In ASD, evidence suggests a dysregulation of epigenetic markers or mechanisms, mainly DNA methylation (Smith et al. 2009; Wong et al. 2014; Loke et al. 2015). Whether these mechanisms are also inherited over multiple generations is still to be explored.

Environmental factors may be involved in the inception as well as the lifelong modulation of ASD (Herbert 2010). These include exposures to air pollution, maternal infection, low birth weight, organophosphates, and heavy metals associated with pathophysiology of ASD, including oxidative stress, neuroinflammation, and mitochondrial dysfunction (Chauhan and Chauhan 2006; Jung et al. 2013).

The other suggested environmental factors for ASD are underlying biochemical disturbances, such as abnormalities in glutathione, a critical antioxidant and detoxifier, which has been shown to be reversed by targeted nutritional interventions (Geraghty et al. 2010; Theije et al. 2011).

2.2 Twin studies

2.2.1 Different twin designs

Twin-based designs are powerful tools to investigate the relative contribution of genes and environment to behavioral variation. The classic twin design is based on comparisons between monozygotic (MZ) and dizygotic (DZ) twin pairs. MZ twins arise from the same zygote, while DZ twins arise from two separate zygotes and two different sperms. Hence, MZ twins have an identical nucleotide chromosomal DNA sequence, except for small errors of DNA replication, while the DZ twins share only 50% (on average) of the segregating DNA variation. Both MZ and DZ twin pairs growing up together, mainly share the same pre- and perinatal environment, as well as most family-related factors during childhood. Since MZ twins are genetically identical, except for rare post-twinning *de novo* mutations, all differences between the twins can be assumed to be due to NSE and/or measurement error (Plomin and Daniels 1987). As a result of this, if a phenotype is completely heritable, MZ pairs are estimated to be roughly twice as similar as DZ pairs. This gives a heritability coefficient of 1.0 for MZ pairs and 0.5 for DZ pairs. In a classic ACE model among twins, likelihood estimates based on the heredity coefficients are used to calculate how much of the phenotypic variance is due to genes, SE and NSE.

A powerful twin design to investigate environmental influences is to assess MZ twins reared apart. In the Minnesota Study of Twins Reared Apart, over 100 MZ and DZ twin pairs, separated from childhood and onward, were examined longitudinally (Bouchard et al. 1990). The results showed almost the same correlations between twin pairs reared apart as twin pairs growing up in the same family, on multiple measures (i.e., personality and temperament, occupational and leisure-time interests, social attitudes). Somewhat lower heritability (~70%) than expected from other studies was found for cognitive measures and intelligence. These results were replicated in a large Swedish sample of twins reared apart, the Swedish Adoption/Twin Study of Aging (SATSA). The results from the SATSA study showed SE to have an effect of less than 10% on personality traits (Pedersen et al. 1988).

Another design with the same aim is the assessment of MZ twins discordant for a phenotype, also called discordant MZ twin pair design, cotwin control design, or within-twin pair differences design (McGue et al. 2010). The measurement of how differences in exposure correlate with differences in outcome (differences in the phenotype) and cognitive and biological markers in the causal pathway can be identified, controlling for many environmental factors as well as for genetics. The design is very powerful for identifying biological and behavioral markers for a phenotype, although there are also some limitations to it (McGue et al. 2010). First, even though minor, there is a possibility for reverse causation. Second, the factors leading to differences in exposure may account for differences in outcome. Third, measurement error can result in differential decrease of effect estimates between MZ and DZ pairs in within-pair analyses. Finally, a main challenge is to identify twin pairs being discordant for a phenotype, which is assumed to be highly heritable, such as ASD.

2.2.2 Twin studies in ASD: What have we learned?

There are two behavior-genetic analytical approaches within ASD research, a categorical approach of strictly defined autism or ASD, and a continuous approach of autism traits in the total population. The first approach implies ASD to constitute a clinical entity with strict borders defined by severe symptoms related to social communication and interaction problems and repetitive and restricted behavioral patterns, qualitatively different from the normal population. Studies based on this approach have looked at either community-based clinical diagnoses, or golden standard assessments with the Autism Diagnostic Observation Schedule (ADOS; Lord et al. 1999) or the Autism Diagnostic Interview–Revised (ADI–R; Rutter et al. 2003), or screening instruments with validated cut-offs, such as the Autism-Tics, ADHD, and other Comorbidities inventory (A-TAC; Hansson et al. 2005). To estimate heritability a multifactorial threshold model is often used. This model assumes that multiple genetic and environmental factors of small effect sum up to an unobserved continuous trait called liability. Liability above a certain threshold value leads to disease in the model.

The second approach is to analyze continuous ASD trait data, with the so-called broader autism phenotype (BAP) as an intermediate presentation between the clinical and typical phenotypes (e.g., Ronald et al. 2005). Studies applying this approach have used quantitative trait measures such as the Social Responsiveness Scale (SRS; Constantino 2005), Autism Quotient (AQ; Baron-Cohen et al. 2001), or the Childhood Autism Spectrum Test (CAST; Williams et al. 2005). This approach demonstrates that autistic traits are approximating a continuous distribution in the general population, with categorical/clinical phenotypes forming the extreme end of the continuum. Studies supporting this approach have, for example, been comparing relatives to individuals with ASD with control families, and showed higher levels of autistic traits in ASD relatives, suggesting a shared etiology between extreme phenotypes and autistic traits (e.g., Constantino et al. 2006; Sandin et al. 2014).

The first twin study of ASD with reasonable power was published by Folstein and Rutter (1977). They aimed at recruiting all autistic twin pairs in the United Kingdom via child psychiatrists spread across the country, finally including 21 pairs (11 MZ and 10 DZ). Autism diagnosis was based on the criteria outlined by Kanner (1943), predominantly operationalizing core autism. The results were at the time groundbreaking, showing autism to be clearly influenced by genetic factors and that the same genetic factors seemed to be linked to a broader range of impairments. These results were replicated in two subsequent twin studies in the later 1980s (Ritvo et al. 1985; Steffenburg et al. 1989).

In the 1990s, the Folstein and Rutter sample was reassessed, including additionally identified pairs, ending up in a total sample of 44 pairs

(Bailey et al. 1995). The diagnosis in this study was based on ICD-10 criteria, and the results largely endorsed previous findings. Using liability threshold modeling, heritability was estimated to be 91%–93%. Slightly lower heritability estimates were reported in two later studies: one based on a Japanese sample and one on a Swedish sample. The Japanese study used a broader definition of ASD, including 45 twin pairs, with heritability estimates of 73% for males and 87% for females (Taniai et al. 2008). The Swedish sample was population-based including around 8000 pairs, and analyses using liability threshold modeling gave heritability estimates of 80%, a modest effect of NSE, and no effect of SE factors (Lichtenstein et al. 2010).

In contrast to these studies, all showing a strong genetic component, several more recent studies showed a substantially lower heritability for ASD. The first study assessed twins with ASD born in California between 1987 and 2004 (Hallmayer et al. 2011). This sample included 192 twin pairs and ASD diagnoses were confirmed by both ADOS and ADI–R assessments. Pairwise concordance between the affected twins and their co-twins, as well as classic ACE analysis and a liability-threshold model were calculated. The concordance results were similar to what had been showed in previous studies, with a concordance between 0.50 and 0.77 for MZ and between 0.21 and 0.36 for DZ (varying between males and females and strictly defined core autism and ASD). However, the heritability estimates based on the model fitting were lower. The strongest component was SE, estimated to be 55% for autism and 58% for ASD. Heritability estimates were 37% for autism and 38% for ASD. However, the confidence intervals were wide, showing a large uncertainty of the results.

The second study was based on a population cohort of >2 million children born in Sweden between 1982 and 2006, including 37,570 twins (Sandin et al. 2014). Also full siblings, half siblings, and cousins were included in the analysis. Within the sample were 312 DZ and 62 MZ twins with ASD diagnoses. The relative recurrence risk (RRR) was calculated measuring the relative risk of ASD in a participant with a sibling or a cousin with ASD in comparison with a participant with no diagnosed family member. Further, the heritability was estimated by model fitting statistics, again using a liability-threshold model. The RRR was 153.0 in MZ twins and 8.2 in DZ twins. The heritability analysis gave estimations of 50% for heritability and 50% for NSE, with no, or very small, influence of SE.

In a Danish population-based study, opposite results were found. A sample of same-sex twin pairs born in Denmark between 1988 and 1998 ($N = 5756$) were included in the study (Nordenbeak et al. 2014). The diagnoses were established by individual clinical assessments resulting in 36 pairs ASD pairs (13 MZ and 23 DZ). The results showed a concordance rate of 0.95 in MZ pairs and only 0.04 in DZ pairs, and no further analysis of heritability was done.

There have also been attempts to combine dimensionally measured traits and categorical diagnoses. In a sample recruited within the Interactive Autism Network (IAN), including 471 ASD pairs (Frazier et al. 2014), a categorical proband-wise concordance rate was calculated, using clinical diagnoses and scale cut-offs. Thereafter liability threshold parameters were calculated using maximum likelihood estimations. Regression analyses were used to assess the heritability and environmental influences at different levels of quantitatively assessed traits. The results yielded a higher heritability in more extreme phenotypes than in typical symptom levels. Heritability was estimated to be 21%–35%, with the rest of variance being attributable to NSE. However, the authors argue that the assumptions of the classic ACE model might not have been met, and that is why the results should be viewed cautiously.

2.2.3 Twin studies of ASD as a continuous trait

There are several twin registries established around the world, and in ASD research, these have been used mainly for quantitative trait analysis of ASD. Below is a nonexhaustive list of the most comprehensive twin collections that have been used to investigate ASD and autistic traits, and the results from these studies (Table 2.1).

2.2.3.1 The Missouri Twin Study   Three studies on ASD have been published from the Missouri Twin Study (Constantino and Todd 2000, 2003, 2005). Autistic traits were measured with the SRS, and structural equation modeling was used for analysis. The results varied slightly between the three studies. The first study showed autistic traits to be highly heritable in males, with an additive genetic influence of 76% and a moderate NSE influence of 24%. The second study showed a moderate heritability of 48% for both males and females, a moderate SE effect of 32%, and NSE effect of 20%. The last study, mainly including female pairs, gave a higher heritability estimation of 73%–87% across different sex and age groups. Interestingly, in this study, the inclusion of parental data in the structural equation model showed evidence for assortative mating. This was not investigated in the statistical models in the previous studies, and could explain the discrepancies between them. However, support for assortative mating has not been replicated in later twin studies including parental data (Hoekstra et al. 2007).

2.2.3.2 The twin early development study   The TEDS is a community-based twin sample from England and Wales, including all twins born between 1994 and 1996. The first study on ASD traits from TEDS examined a sample of >3000 twin pairs (Ronald et al. 2005). The results show a high heritability for both social and nonsocial behaviors (67%–76%), a modest influence of NSE (25%–38%), and a modest genetic overlap between social and nonsocial traits. Further studies based on the same sample, using the CAST (parent-report) for the assessment

Table 2.1 Twin Studies and ASD Heritability Estimates

Reference	Sample	Measures of ASD	Results	New Findings/ Conclusions
Folstein and Rutter (1977)	UK sample, 11 MZ and 10 DZ pairs	Diagnosis based on Kanner's description	Autism concordance: MZ 36%, DZ 0% BAP: MZ 82%, DZ: 10%	Strong genetic component for autism
Ritvo et al. (1985)	The UCLA Twin Registry 23 MZ, 17 DZ pairs	Diagnosis based on DSM-III for autism	Autism concordance: MZ 96%, DZ 24%	
Steffenburg et al. (1989)	Scandinavian sample, 11 MZ pairs, 10 DZ pairs, 1 set of triplets	Diagnosis based on DSM-III	Autism concordance: MZ 91%, DZ 0%	
Bailey et al. (1995)	Partly overlapping with Folstein and Rutter (see above) 25 MZ, 20 DZ, 2 sets of triplets	Diagnosis based on ICD-10	Autism concordance: MZ 60%, DZ 0%	
Constantino and Todd (2000)	Missouri Twin Study, 98 MZ, 134, DZ (males only)	SRS	Trait correlations: MZ 0.73, DZ 0.37 Heritability: 76%, NSE: 24%	ASD traits are highly heritable in males
Constantino and Todd (2003)	Missouri Twin Study, 268 MZ, 520 DZ	SRS	Trait correlations: MZ 0.73–0.79, DZ 0.37–0.63 Heritability: 48%, SE: 32%, NSE: 20%	Both shared and nonshared environmental components in ASD traits
Constantino and Todd (2005)	Missouri Twin Study, 89 MZ, 196 DZ	SRS	Heritability: 73%–87%, SE: 10–12%, NSE: 0% (males) and 17% (females)	ASD traits are highly heritable over the life span
Ronald et al. (2005)	TEDS, 3138 pairs	DSM-IV-based social and nonsocial questionnaires (parent- and teacher-report)	Heritability: 62%–67%, NSE: 25%–38% Overlap between social and nonsocial traits: 0.07–0.40 (genetic), 0.02–0.18 (NSE)	High heritability for both social and nonsocial traits, limited genetic overlap
Skuse et al. (2005)	Cardiff study of all Wales and North of England Twins, 278 MZ, 378 DZ	Social and communication disorder checklist (parent-report)	Trait correlations: MZ 0.73, DZ 0.38 Heritability: 74%, NSE 26%	High heritability for social cognitive skills
Ronald et al. (2006b)	TEDS, 3419 pairs	CAST (parent-report)	Heritability: 71%–77% for the three symptom domains	Limited genetic overlap between the different symptom domains
Hoekstra et al. (2007)	Sample based on the Dutch Twin Registry, 184 pairs 94 siblings, 128 parents of twins	AQ (self-report)	Heritability: 57%, NSE: 43%	No evidence for assortative mating

(Continued)

Table 2.1 (*Continued*) Twin Studies and ASD Heritability Estimates

Reference	Sample	Measures of ASD	Results	New Findings/ Conclusions
Ronald et al. (2008b)	TEDS 2586 pairs	CAST (parent-, teacher-, self-report	Heritability: 82%–87% (parent ratings), 69% (teacher ratings), 36%–47% (child self-ratings)	
Taniai et al. (2008)	Japanese sample 19 MZ, 26 DZ	Case vignettes CARS	ASD concordance: MZ 95%, DZ 31% Heritability: 73% (males), 87% (females) NSE: 13%–17%	No sex differences regarding heritability. Strong genetic component, modest effect of NSE
Rosenberg et al. (2009)	IAN, 67 MZ, 210 DZ	Caregiver-reported diagnosis	ASD concordance: MZ 88%, DZ 31%	Strong genetic component for ASD and modest effect of NSE
Edelson et al. (2009)	Boston University Twin Project, 145 MZ, 168 DZ	CBCL	Trait correlations: MZ 0.58, DZ 0.38 Heritability: 40%, SE: 20%, NSE: 40%	
Stilp et al. (2010)	The Wisconsin Twin Panel, 414 MZ, 797 DZ	Eight-item scale (parent-report)	Trait correlations: MZ 43%, DZ 20% Heritability: 44%, SE: 32%, NSE: 24%	
Ronald et al. (2010)	CATSS, 1788 MZ, 3752 DZ	A-TAC	Heritability: 49%–76%, NSE: 24%–51%	
Lichtenstein et al. (2010)	CATSS, MZ 2242, DZ 5740	A-TAC (parent-report)	ASD concordance: MZ 39%, DZ 15% Heritability: 80%, NSE: 20%	
Hallmayer et al. (2011)	Californian sample 54 MZ, 118 DZ	ADI–R, ADOS	Autism concordance: MZ 0.58–0.60, DZ 0.21–0.27 ASD: MZ 0.50–0.77, DZ 0.31–0.36 Heritability: 37% (autism), 38% (ASD), SE: 55% (autism), 58% (ASD)	First study showing a strong shared environmental component
Nordenbeak et al. (2014)	13 MZ, 23 DZ	Individual clinical assessments	ASD concordance: MZ 95%, DZ 4.3%	
Sandin et al. (2014)	MZ 14516, DZ 4169	National patient register data	Heritability: 50% NSE: 50%	Equally strong genetic and nonshared environmental effect, no shared environmental effect

(*Continued*)

Table 2.1 (*Continued*) Twin Studies and ASD Heritability Estimates

Reference	Sample	Measures of ASD	Results	New Findings/ Conclusions
Frazier et al. (2014)	IAN, 128 MZ, 440 DZ	SCQ, SRS, and caregiver-reported diagnosis	Heritability: 21%–35% NSE: 65%–79%	Higher heritability in the more extreme phenotypes than in typical symptom levels
Colvert et al. (2015)	TEDS, 6423 pairs	CAST, ADOS, ADI–R, best-estimate diagnosis	Heritability: 56%–95% NSE: <30%	

Notes: ASD = autism spectrum disorder; MZ = monozygotic; DZ = dizygotic; BAP = broader autism phenotype; UCLA = University of California, Los Angeles; DSM = Diagnostic and Statistical Manual; ICD = International Classification of Diseases; SRS = Social Responsiveness Scale; CBCL = Child Behaviour Check List; NSE = Nonshared environment; SE = Shared environment; TEDS = The Twins Early Development Study; CAST = The Childhood Autism Spectrum Test; AQ = Autism Quotient; CARS = Childhood Autism Rating Scale; IAN = The Interactive Autism Network; CATSS = The Child and Adolescent Twin Study in Sweden; A-TAC = Autism—Tics, ADHD and other Comorbidities Inventory; SCQ = Social Communication Questionnaire.

of ASD traits, included a similar number of twin pairs (Ronald et al. 2006a,b). The results confirmed a high heritability for overall autistic traits (81%–86%), as well as for extreme traits within the three symptom domains separately (social interaction, communication, and stereotyped and repetitive behavior). A later study of ~6000 twin pairs showed somewhat lower heritability levels (72% for males and 53% for females). No significant differences were found between heritability estimates in the general population compared to extreme phenotypes (Robinson et al. 2011), suggesting a shared etiology for extreme scores and normal variation. In a fourth study from the TEDS sample, the correlations between raters (parents, child, and teachers) were studied (Ronald et al. 2008b). The correlations were significant but moderate, showing a higher heritability in parent ratings (82%–87%) compared to teacher ratings (69%). A recent study from TEDS included a total sample of 6423 twin pairs. Subgroups from the sample were assessed with CAST, ADOS, ADI–R, the Development and Well-Being Assessment (DAWBA), as well as best estimate for clinical diagnosis. Heritability was calculated using liability threshold model fitting and a maximum likelihood method. Depending on which measures for ASD were used, the heritability estimates differed between 56% (ADI–R only) and 76%–95% (CAST, best-estimate diagnosis, ADOS, and DAWBA) (Colvert et al. 2015).

2.2.3.3 The Child and Adolescent Twin Study in Sweden   In Child and Adolescent Twin Study in Sweden (CATSS), twins are recruited from the Swedish Twin Registry and parents of all twins born in Sweden are contacted when the twins are aged 9 and 12 years. A standardized telephone interview, the A-TAC, is used, providing scores and cut-offs for several neurodevelopmental disorders including ASD (Anckarsäter et al. 2011). In a later study from the CATSS sample comprising >11,000 twin pairs, heritability was estimated to be 71% for autistic traits (Lundström et al. 2012). Both qualitative and quantitative cut-offs were used, pointing at similar heritability levels, again suggesting a shared etiology for autistic traits and clinical ASD phenotypes.

2.2.4 Twin studies of ASD symptoms in toddlers

Studies of autistic symptoms in toddlers indicate a lower heritability in young children compared to older children and adults (Edelson et al. 2009; Stilp et al. 2010). There are two North American studies of toddlers. The first is based on the Wisconsin Twin Panel including >1200 pairs assessed with eight items from the Modified Checklist for Autism in Toddlers (M-CHAT). The second is included in the Boston University Twin Project and assessed >300 pairs using the pervasive problem scale from Child Behavior Checklist (CBCL) as a measure of ASD. Both studies showed a moderate heritability (40%–44%) and significant SE and NSE influence on the measured ASD traits.

2.2.5 Discordant MZ twin pair design in ASD research

As mentioned earlier in this chapter, the discordant MZ twin pair design is powerful to identify the NSE factors. However, the design is challenging regarding the recruitment of large numbers of discordant MZ twin pairs in disorders with a strong genetic influence, such as ASD. A handful of studies have examined brain differences in ASD discordant pairs. Among those, Kates et al. (1998, 2004, 2009; Mitchell et al. 2009) published four studies on structural brain imaging in partly overlapping samples. The first study examined one MZ twin pair discordant for core autism. The co-twin was assessed as showing a BAP, and five typically developed singletons were included as controls. The results showed morphological differences between the affected twin and the co-twin, that is, smaller caudate, amygdala, and hippocampal volumes, as well as smaller cerebellar vermis lobules VI and VII. Both twins had reduced volumes of the superior temporal gyrus and the frontal lobe compared to the typically developing controls. The results suggest separate dysfunctional pathways; one subcortical network differentiating the twins from each other causing strictly defined autism, and one cortical network differentiating the twins from the controls causing BAP. In two later studies, these results were followed up in larger samples. The first of those included 16 MZ pairs (seven pairs clinically concordant for ASD, nine pairs discordant for core autism), and a control sample of 16 matched typically developed singletons. ASD was defined by ADI–R and ADOS assessments. The controls had no diagnoses, but the nonaffected co-twins within the discordant pairs, were classified as showing a BAP. The concordant as well as the discordant twin pairs showed concordance in cerebral gray and white matter volumes, but only the clinically concordant pairs exhibited concordance in cerebellar gray and white matter volumes. Within the discordant twin pairs, both the twins with autism and their co-twins exhibited frontal, temporal, and occipital white matter volumes that were lower than those of the controls. Also, the co-twins showed frontal, temporal, and occipital white matter volumes smaller than those of the controls (Kates et al. 2004). Focusing on cortical folding, 14 MZ pairs discordant for ASD were assessed, with the affected twins meeting the criteria for core autism. Fourteen typically developed singletons were included as additional controls. The results showed the patterns of cortical folding to be highly discordant within MZ pairs. In comparison to gender and aged matched controls, the twins with autism, as well as their co-twins, showed increased cortical folding in the right parietal lobe. Earlier findings of a robust association between intelligence and cortical folding in typically developed children were not found in the ASD discordant pairs. The authors suggested a disruption between cortical folding and intelligence in ASD (Kates et al. 2009). In an overlapping sample of the previously described studies, 14 MZ pairs and 14 age- and gender-matched singletons were assessed for volumetric differences in the brain. No areas in the brain differed in volumes between the twin pairs. In comparison to control singletons, dorsolateral prefrontal cortex volumes and anterior areas of the corpus callosum were significantly altered in autistic twins, and volumes of the posterior vermis were altered in both autistic twins and co-twins. The results indicate that the degree of within-pair neuroanatomic concordance varies by brain region. In the group of autism twins, dorsolateral prefrontal cortex, amygdala, and posterior vermis volumes were significantly associated with the severity of autism (Mitchell et al. 2009).

Differences in gene expression and methylation pattern have been examined in a sample of three male MZ twin pairs discordant for core autism (Hu et al. 2006; Nguyen et al. 2010). The co-twins did not meet the criteria for autism, but showed some autistic traits. For two of the three pairs, an unaffected sibling was included in the analysis. Moreover, two twin pairs being concordant for core autism but discordant for severity of language impairments were included, as well as one pair of typically developing twins having an autistic sibling. The aim of these two studies was to identify alterations in gene expression and methylation associated with ASD by analyzing lymphoblastoid cell lines derived from peripheral blood samples. The results showed the genes, being among the most differentially expressed and methylated, were important for development, function, and/or structure of the central nervous system. Many of the affected genes also map closely to chromosomal regions containing previously reported autism candidate genes. Two genes, B-cell CLL/lymphoma 2 (BCL2) and retinoic acid-related orphan receptor alpha (RORA), were further highlighted as higher methylation levels were confirmed in the affected twins compared with controls (Nguyen et al.

2010). The authors suggested that the findings might be used for developing a molecular screen for autism based on expressed biomarkers in an easily accessible tissue as peripheral blood lymphocytes.

Recently, a larger study analyzing 50 MZ twins from the TEDS cohort for the epigenome-wide methylation pattern was published (Wong et al. 2014). The authors provided multilevel analysis of methylation differences both within-pair and between groups associated with categorical ASD diagnosis as well as quantitatively rated autistic trait scores on the CAST. Within-twin pair analysis based on six discordant MZ pairs revealed the presence of multiple differentially methylated sites of which majority were family-specific. Based on the largest and most significant differences, the within-pair analysis resulted in a list of top 50 differentially methylated probes associated with ASD. Similarly, between-group analysis comparing autistic individuals with controls showed multiple sites with significant methylation differences, of which some were near genes earlier implicated in ASD etiology including *NRXN1* and *UBE3A*. Findings from this study underscore the heterogeneity of epigenetic factors that are potentially involved in the pathogenesis of ASD and show overlap with the earlier molecular genetic studies.

The Roots of Autism and ADHD Twin Study in Sweden (RATSS) is a MZ discordant twin pair design study with an ongoing data collection (Bölte et al. 2014; Mevel et al. 2015). In RATSS, multilevel data is collected on MZ twin pairs discordant for ASD, as well as different control pairs. The data collected includes an exhaustive behavioral phenotyping, dysmorphological assessments, multimodal neuroimaging, and biological sampling, that is, blood and saliva to assess genetic and epigenetic mechanisms, fibroblasts to derive induced pluripotent stem cells for the examinations of neural growth, teeth, hair, and urine to examine exposure to toxins, stool for microbiota analysis, and cerebrospinal fluid for assessments of inflammatory markers. In addition, medical records and a medical questionnaires are collected for identification of pre-, peri- and postnatal risk factors, as well as mapping the family history.

2.2.6 Twin studies in ASD and comorbidity

Comorbidity with other neurodevelopmental and psychiatric disorders is common in ASD. In a study using data from the Swedish CATSS cohort, 50% of the ASD cases had four or more coexisting conditions, and only 4% had no comorbid condition (Lundström et al. 2014), supporting the notion that different neurodevelopmental disorders have overlapping etiological pathways.

One of the most commonly diagnosed comorbid conditions in ASD is intellectual disability, with a genetic correlation around $r = 0.50$ (Matson and Shoemaker 2009). Molecular genetic studies have also pointed toward shared genetic etiology between the two disorders. In an exhaustive review of ASD genetics, Betancur (2011) found 103 disease genes and 44 genomic loci that have been associated with ASD or autistic behaviors and majority have been also implicated in intellectual disability. Recent large-scale sequencing studies have also shown that genes affected by rare penetrant *de novo* mutations in both disorders overlap significantly (Iossifov et al. 2014). Currently, three twin studies from different research groups have been exploring the etiological overlap between ASD and intellectual disability. Nishiyama et al. (2009) studied the overlap in a sample of 45 twin pairs in which at least one of the twins had an ASD diagnosis. They found a high overlap with a genetic correlation of $r = 0.95$ between the disorders. However, due to the small sample size, the confidence interval was large (CI 0.60–1.00). A considerable lower genetic correlation of 0.37 (CI 0.22–0.34) was found in a population-based twin study based on the TEDS sample (Hoekstra et al. 2009, 2010). Ronald and Hoekstra (2011) suggest that the difference between the studies could be explained by differences in the study design, investigating the diagnosis of ASD, or traits in the normal population. The differences might indicate that there are different genetic overlaps between ASD traits and IQ and to more extreme clinical ASD phenotypes and intellectual impairment.

Further, several studies have shown a considerable genetic overlap between ASD and ADHD. In a large population-based study of over 6000 twin pairs from the United Kingdom, a significant correlation was found between autistic and ADHD traits ($r = 0.51$–0.54), with similar results within the normative range and for more extreme phenotypes. These results suggest common genetic influences across autistic and ADHD traits, both for normal and the extreme behaviors (Ronald et al. 2008b). A slightly lower genetic overlap of 0.42 was found in a recent study in a Swedish sample (Lundström et al. 2014).

Anxiety disorders commonly co-occur with ASD. Findings from the TEDS sample show that autistic traits and anxiety-related behavior share some environmental pathways, but also that the genetic correlation differs with age. In middle childhood, a correlation of 0.12–0.18 has been found between ASD and anxiety disorders (Hallett et al. 2010), while other studies report a genetic correlation as high as $r = 0.50$–0.60 in both children and adults (Weisbrot et al. 2005; Lundström et al. 2011). Other conditions that have been proposed to have a genetic overlap with ASD are tics and developmental coordination disorder (Lichtenstein et al. 2010).

2.2.7 Etiological overlap between different domains of symptoms

ASD is characterized by a triad of symptoms in DSM-IV (social interaction, communication, stereotyped and repetitive behaviors), now condensed to a dyad of domains in DSM-V (social communication/interaction and stereotyped and repetitive behaviors). Several twin studies on large population-based samples have shown that the combined, as well as each separate domain of the triad of symptom domains to be highly heritable, with a modest-to-moderate NSE and almost no SE influence (Ronald et al. 2010). The majority of family studies of ASD support two or more domains constituting ASD, and indicate partly differing etiologies for them (Happé and Ronald 2008; Mandy and Skuse 2008). These results have been replicated in the normative range as well as in extreme phenotypes and for different age groups (Ronald et al. 2005, 2006a,b, Robinson et al. 2011).

2.2.8 Limitations of twin designs within ASD research

When applying twin design in psychiatric research, two assumptions are made. The first assumption is the equal environment assumption. It contains the notion of similarity of effects regarding environment for DZ and MZ pairs, meaning there is no systematic difference between how environmental factors affect both the twins in an MZ pair compared to a DZ pair. If this assumption is in any way violated, the heritability estimates would be affected, most likely leading to an overestimation of heritability. However, this assumption has been tested and proved to be reasonable for most traits (e.g., Derks et al. 2006). Possible exceptions are prenatal factors. MZ twins are often more affected by prenatal factors than DZ twins, particularly if the twins are sharing the same chorion. These pairs will, in most cases, experience a higher prenatal competition between them, which can result in greater differences, regarding, for example, birth weight.

The second assumption is assortative mating. In the classic twin design, a random partner selection is assumed, meaning that individuals would not choose partners that are phenotypically more similar to themselves. If this assumption is not met, the DZ pairs would share more than 50% of their genes, since the parents would be more genetically similar, while the genetic similarity would be unaltered for MZ twins. A few studies have investigated the degree of assortative mating in ASD, with mixed results (e.g., Constantino and Todd 2005). Ronald and Hoekstra (2011) argue that since the correlations are higher in studies using spouse reports (e.g., Virkud et al. 2009) than in studies using self-report (e.g., Hoekstra et al. 2010), the similarity between partners is more likely to be due to shared values and common beliefs than to shared genetic effects. More studies with a broader family design are needed to further investigate the occurrence of assortative mating and ASD traits.

An often-discussed limitation of twin design is how generalizable results from twin samples are to nontwin populations. It has been suggested that twinning could be a risk factor for ASD; however, when this hypothesis was tested in two UK population-based samples, no evidence was found to support such a twin bias. The CAST was used as a measure of autism traits and no significant differences between twins and singletons on neither CAST total scores nor standard errors. Equally, for ASD classification, it was found that the likelihood of scoring above ASD cut-off on CAST was significantly lower for twins compared to singletons (Curran et al. 2011). Other studies comparing twin populations with singletons have, for instance, shown that intelligence in twins does not differ from intelligence in the general population (Christiensen et al. 2006), overall supporting the generalizability of results from twin studies to the general population.

2.3 Summary and directions for future research

Twin designs are one of the most common designs in behavior genetics and have markedly contributed to the general understanding of the etiology of ASD as well as many other psychiatric disorders. The study by Folstein and Rutter (1977) presented for the first time solid evidence that ASD is a genetic disorder. These results were contrasting the dominating view at the time that autism was everything else but genetic (Hanson and Gottesman 1976). More recent studies have suggested an equally strong nongenetic component in the etiology of ASD (e.g., Hallmayer et al. 2011; Sandin et al. 2014). Even if there is evidence for SE to have a role in ASD, most twin studies indicate the effect of these factors to be limited, and NSE to be the most significant. There are two different approaches within behavioral genetic research in ASD, defining ASD as either a categorical clinical diagnosis or as continuously distributed traits in the general population. To date, the majority of twin studies show about the same heritability for ASD traits and for more extreme phenotypes (e.g., Ronald et al. 2006b). Several twin studies have investigated the overlap between behavioral domains of ASD. These studies show only a moderate genetic overlap between the domains of ASD symptoms, suggesting different etiology for the different areas of impairments (e.g., Ronald et al. 2005). Comorbidity is common in ASD, such as ADHD and intellectual disabilities, and twin researches suggest partly common etiological pathways for the disorders (Nishiyama et al. 2009; Lichtenstein et al. 2010; Ronald et al. 2014). More research is needed on overlaps between ASD and other neurodevelopmental disorders, for example, tics and other motor disorders, as well as the overlap with psychiatric disorders such as anxiety disorders.

Over a hundred different risk genes for ASD have been identified, especially those involved in synaptic functioning and chromatin modification (Betancur 2011; Geschwind and State 2015) with significant overlap with genes implicated in other neurodevelopmental disorders. Some genetic variants in ASD could be linked to an alteration of the vulnerability to environmental stressors and exposures, for example, random *de novo* mutations increasing with advanced parental age. Environmental factors may also act via epigenetic mechanisms and play an important role in

ASD. However, the exact mechanisms or processes leading to ASD are still largely unknown, and twin studies to date have mainly contributed to an estimation of the relative effect of genetics and environment, without any further specification of detailed pathologic pathways. A powerful but still rare design, which could contribute to the identification of the genetic as well as nonenvironmental factors, is the discordant MZ twin pair design. Thus, clinical studies assessing and combining discordancy data from multiple biological and behavioral levels in MZ and DZ twin pairs discordant for ASD are desirable. For instance, investigation of the full range genomic variation in the twins of interest, including putative post-twinning *de novo* mutations throughout the genome and possible rare high-risk mutations shared by the twins, is now fully possible with the advances in whole genome sequencing. Identification of these rare mutations coupled with of thorough analysis of epigenetic and gene expression differences can give insights into understanding the penetrance of certain mutations and relative contributions of gene × gene and gene × environmental interactions (Buil et al. 2015). To the authors' best knowledge, only one study has applied such a complex design (Bölte et al. 2014).

References

Anckarsäter, H., S. Lundström, L. Kollberg et al. 2011. The twin and adolescent twin study in Sweden (CATSS). *Twin Res. Hum. Genet.* 14:495–508.

Bailey, A., A. Le Couteur, I. Gottesman et al. 1995. Autism is a strongly genetic disorder: Evidence from a British twin study. *Psychol. Med.* 25:63–77.

Baron-Cohen, S., R. Wheelwright, J. Skinner, E. Martin, and E. Clubley. 2001. The autism-spectrum quotient (AQ): Evidence from Asperger syndrome/high-functioning autism, males and females, scientists and mathematicians. *J. Autism Dev. Disord.* 31:5–17.

Batancur, C. 2011. Etiological heterogeneity in autism spectrum disorders: More than 100 genetic and genomic disorders and still counting. *Brain Res.* 1380:42–77.

Bouchard, T. J., D. T. Lykken, M. McGue, N. L. Segal, and A. Tellegen. 1990. Sources of human psychological differences: The Minnesota Study of Twins Reared Apart. *Science* 250:223–50.

Bölte, S., C. Willfors, S. Berggren et al. 2014. The Roots of Autism and ADHD Twin Study in Sweden (RATSS). *Twin Res. Hum. Genet.* 3:164–76.

Buil, A., A. A. Brown, T. Lappalainen et al. 2015. Gene–gene and gene–environment interactions detected by transcriptome sequence analysis in twins. *Nat. Genet.* 47:88–91.

Chauhan, A. and V. Chauhan. 2006. Oxidative stress in autism. *Pathophysiology* 13:171–81.

Christiensen, K., I. Petersen, A. Skytthe, A. M. Herskind, M. McGue, and P. Bingley. 2006. Comparison of academic performance of twins and singletons in adolescence: Follow-up study. *Br. Med. J.* 333:1095–7.

Colvert, E., B. Tick, F. McEwen et al. 2015. Heritability of autism spectrum disorder in a UK population-based twin sample. *JAMA Psychiatry* 72:415–23.

Constantino, J. N. 2005. Social Responsiveness Scale (SRS). Los Angeles: Western Psychological Services.

Constantino, J. N., C. Lajonchere, M. Lutz et al. 2006. Autistic social impairment in the siblings of children with pervasive developmental disorders. *Am. J. Psychiatry* 163:294–6.

Constantino, J. N. and R. D. Todd. 2000. Genetic structure of reciprocal social behavior. *Am. J. Psychiatry* 157:2043–5.

Constantino, J. N. and R. D. Todd. 2003. Autistic traits in the general population— A twin study. *Arch. Gen. Psychiatry* 60:524–30.

Constantino, J. N. and R. D. Todd. 2005. Intergenerational transmission of sub-threshold autistic traits in the general population. *Biol. Psychiatry* 57:655–60.

Curran, S., K. Dworzynski, F. Happé et al. 2011. The major effect of twinning on autistic traits. *Autism Res.* 4:377–82.

Derks, E. M., C. V. Dolan, and D. Boomsma. 2006. A test of the equal environment assumption (EEA) in multivariate twin studies. *Twin Res. Hum. Genet.* 3:403–11.

Edelson, L. R. and K. J. Saudino. 2009. Genetic and environmental influences on autistic-like behaviors in 2-year-old twins. *Behav. Genet.* 39:255–64.

Folstein, S. and M. Rutter. 1977. Genetic influences and infantile autism. *Nature* 265:726–8.

Frazier, T., L. Thompson, E. A. Youngstrom et al. 2014. A twin study of heritable and shared environmental contributions to autism. *J. Autism Dev. Disord.* 44:2013–25.

Geraghty, M. E., J. Bates-Wall, K. Ratliff-Schaub, and A. E. Lane. 2010. Nutritional interventions and therapies in autism: A spectrum of what we know: Part 2. *Infant, Child, Adoles. Nutr.* 2:120–33.

Geschwind, D. H. and M. W. State. 2015. Gene hunting in autism spectrum disorder: On the path to precision medicine. *Lancet Neurol.* 14:1109–20.

Hallett, V., A. Ronald, F. Rijsdijk, and F. Happé. 2010. Association of autistic-like and internalizing traits during childhood: A longitudinal twin study. *Am. J. Psychiatry* 167:809–17.

Hallmayer, J., S. Cleveland, A. Torres et al. 2011. Genetic heritability and shared environmental factors among twin pairs with autism. *Arch Gen Psychiatry.* 68:1095–102.

Hanson, D. R. and I. Gottesman. 1976. The genetics, if any, of infantile autism and childhood schizophrenia. *J. Autism Childhood Schizophrenia* 3:209–34.

Hansson, S. L., A. A. Svanström Röjvall, M. Råstam, C. Gillberg, and H. Anckarsäter. 2005. Psychiatric telephone interview with parents for screening of autism—Tics, attention-deficit hyperactivity disorder and other comorbidities (A-TAC). *Br. J. Psychiatry* 187:262–7.

Happé, F. and A. Ronald. 2008. Fractionable autism triad: A review of evidence from behavioral, genetic, cognitive and neural research. *Neuropsychol. Rev.* 18:287–304.

Herbert, M. R. 2010. Contributions of the environment and environmentally vulnerable physiology to autism spectrum disorders. *Curr. Opin. Neurol.* 23:103–10.

Hoekstra, R. A., M. Bartels, C. J. H. Verweij, and D. I. Boomsma. 2007. Heritability of autistic traits in the general population. *Arch. Pediatr. Adoles. Med.* 161:372–7.

Hoekstra, R. A., F. Happé, S. Baron-Cohen, and A. Ronald. 2009. Association between extreme autistic traits and intellectual disability: Insights from a general population twin study. *Br. J. Psychiatry* 19:531–6.

Hoekstra, R. A., F. Happé, S. Baron-Cohen, and A. Ronald. 2010. Limited genetic covariance between autistic traits and intelligence: Findings from a longitudinal twin study. *Am. J. Med. Genet.* 153B:994–1007.

Hu, V.W., B. C. Frank, S. Heine, N. H. Lee, and J. Quackenbush. 2006. Gene expression profiling of lymphoblastoid cell lines from monozygotic twins discordant in severity of autism reveals differential regulation of neurologically relevant genes. *BMC Genom.* 7:118.

Iossifov, I., B. J. O'Roak, S. J. Sanders et al. 2014. The contribution of de novo coding mutations to autism spectrum disorder. *Nature* 515:216–21.

Jung, C. R., Y. T. Lin, and B. F. Hwang. 2013. Air pollution and newly diagnostic autism spectrum disorders: A population based cohort study in Taiwan. *PLoS One* 25:e75510.

Kanner, L. 1943. The autistic disturbances of affective contact. *Nervous Child* 2:217–50.

Kates, W. R., C. P. Burnette, S. Eliez et al. 2004. Neuroanatomic variation in immunozygotic twin pairs discordant for the narrow phenotype for autism. *Am. J. Psychiatry* 161:539–46.

Kates, W. R., I. Ikuta, and C. P. Burnette. 2009. Gyrification patterns in monozygotic twin pairs varying in discordance for autism. *Autism Res.* 2:267–78.

Kates, W. R., S. H. Mostofsky, A. W. Zimmerman, and M. M. Mazzocco. 1998. Neuroanatomical and neurocognitive differences in a pair of monozygous twins discordant for strictly defined autism. *Ann. Neurol.* 43:782–91.

Kong, A., M. L. Frigge, G. Masson et al. 2012. Rate of de novo mutations and the importance of father's age to disease risk. *Nature* 488:471–5.

Lichtenstein, P., E. Carlström, M. Råstam, C. Gillberg, and H. Anckarsäter. 2010. The genetics of autism spectrum disorder and related neuropsychiatric disorders in childhood. *Am. J. Psychiatry* 167:1357–63.

Loke, Y. J., A. J. Hannan, and J. M. Craig. 2015. The role of epigenetic change in autism spectrum disorders. *Front. Neurol.* 6:107.

Lord, C., M. Rutter, P. C. DiLavore, and S. Risi. 1999. *Autism Diagnostic Observation Schedule-WPS (ADOS-WPS)*. Los Angeles: Western Psychological Services.

Lundström, S., Z. Chang, N. Keres et al. 2011. Autistic-like traits and their associations with mental health problems in two nationwide twin cohorts of children and adults. *Psychol. Med.* 41:2423–33.

Lundström, S., Z. Chang, M. Råstam et al. 2012. Autism spectrum disorders and autistic like traits similar etiology in the extreme end and the normal variation. *Arch. Gen. Psychiatry* 69:46–52.

Lundström, S., A. Reichenberg, J. Melke et al. 2014. Autism spectrum disorders and coexisting disorders in a nationwide Swedish twin study. *J. Child Psychol. Psychiatry* 56:702–10.

Mandy, W. P. and D. H. Skuse. 2008. Research review: What is the association between the social-communication element of autism and repetitive interests, behaviors and activities? *J. Child Psychol. Psychiatry* 8:795–808.

Matson, J. and M. Shoemaker. 2009. Intellectual disability and its relationship to autism spectrum disorders. *Res. Dev. Disabilities* 30:1107–14.

McGue, M., M. Osler, and K. Christensen. 2010. Causal inference and observational research—The utility of twins. *Perspect. Psychol. Sci.* 5:546–56.

Mevel, K., P. Fransson, and S. Bölte. 2015. Multimodal brain imaging in autism spectrum disorders and promise of twin research. *Autism* 19:527–41.

Mitchell, S. R., A. L. Reiss, D. H. Tatusko et al. 2009. Neuroanatomic alterations and social and communication deficits in monozygotic twins discordant for autism disorder. *Am. J. Psychiatry* 166:917–25.

Nishiyama, T., H. Taniai, T. Miyachi, K. Ozaki, M. Tomita, and S. Sumi. 2009. Genetic correlation between autistic traits and IQ in a population-based sample of twin with autism spectrum disorders (ASDs). *J. Hum. Genet.* 54:56–61.

Nordenbaek. C., M. Jorgensen, K. Ohm Kyvik, and N. Bilenberg. 2014. A Danish population-based twin study on autism spectrum disorders. *Eur. Child Adoles. Psychiatry* 23:35–43.

Nguyen, A., T. A. Rauch, G. P. Pfeifer, and V. W. Hu. 2010. Global methylation profiling of lymphoblastoid cell lines reveals epigenetic contributions to autism spectrum disorders and a novel autism candidate gene, *RORA*, whose protein product is reduced in autistic brain. *FASEB J.* 24:3036–51.

Parner, E. T., S. Baron-Cohen, M. B. Lauritsen et al. 2012. Parental age and autism spectrum disorders. *Ann. Epidemiol.* 22:143–50.

Pedersen, N. L., R. Plomin, G. E. McClearn, and L. Friberg. 1988. Neuroticism, extroversion, and related traits in adult twins reared apart and reared together. *J. Personal. Social Psychol.* 6:950–7.

Pinto, D., E. Delaby, D. Merico et al. 2014. Convergence of genes and cellular pathways dysregulated in autism spectrum disorders. *Am. J. Hum. Genet.* 94:677–94.

Plomin, R. 2011. Commentary: Why are children in the same family so different? Non-shared environment three decades later. *Int. J. Epidemiol.* 40:582–92.

Plomin, R. and D. Daniels. 1987. Why are children in the same family so different from one another? *Behav. Brain Sci.* 10:1–16.

Ritvo, E. R., B. J. Freeman, A. Mason-Brothers, A. Mo, and A. M. Ritvo. 1985. Concordance for the syndrome of autism in 40 pairs of afflicted twins. *Am. J. Psychiatry* 142:74–7.

Robinson, E., K. C. Koenen, M. C. McCormick et al. 2011. Evidence that autistic traits show the same etiology in the general population and at the quantitative extremes (5%, 2.5% and 1%). *Arch. Gen. Psychiatry* 68:1113–21.

Ronald, A., F. Happé, P. Bolton et al. 2006a. Genetic heterogeneity between the three components of the autism spectrum: A twin study. *J. Am. Acad. Child Adoles. Psychiatry* 45:691–9.

Ronald, A., F. Happé, and R. Plomin. 2005. The genetic relationship between individual differences in social and nonsocial behaviors characteristics of autism. *Dev. Sci.* 5:444–58.

Ronald, A., F. Happé, T. S. Price, S. Baron-Cohen, and R. Plomin. 2006b. Phenotypic and genetic overlap between autistic traits at the extremes of the general population. *J. Am. Acad. Child Adoles. Psychiatry* 45:1206–14.

Ronald, A. and R. A. Hoekstra. 2011. Autism spectrum disorders and autistic traits: A decade of new twin studies. *Am. J. Med. Genet.* 156B:255–74.

Ronald, A., H. Larsson, H. Anckarsäter, and P. Lichtenstein. 2010. A Twin Study of Autism Symptoms in Sweden. *Mol. Psychiatry* 16:1039–47.

Ronald, A., H. Larsson, H. Anckarsäter, and P. Lichtenstein. 2014. Symptoms of autism and ADHD: A Swedish twin study examining their overlap. *J. Abnormal Psychol.* 2:440–51.

Ronald, A., F. Happé, and R. Plomin. 2008a. A twin study investigating the genetic and environmental aetiologies of parent, teacher and child ratings of autistic-like traits and their overlap. *Eur Child Adolsc Psychiatry.* 17:473–83.

Ronald, A., E. Simonoff, J. Kuntsi, P. Asherson, and R. Plomin. 2008b. Evidence for overlapping genetic influences on autistic and ADHD behaviors in a community twin sample. *J. Child Psychol. Psychiatry* 49:535–42.

Ronemus, M., I. Iossifov, D. Levy, and M. Wigler. 2014. The role of de novo mutations in the genetics of autism spectrum disorders. *Nat. Rev. Genet.* 15:133–41.

Rosenberg, R. E., J. K. Law, G. Yenokyan, J. McGready, W. E. Kaufmann, and P. A. Law. 2009. Characteristics and concordance of autism spectrum disorders among 277 twin pairs. *Arch. Pediat. Adoles. Med.* 163:907–14.

Rutter, M., A. Le Couteur, and C. Lord. 2003. *The Autism Diagnostic Interview, Revised (ADI-R).* Los Angeles: Western Psychological Services.

Sandin, S., P. Lichtenstein, R. Kuja-Halkola, H. Larsson, C. M. Hultman, and A. Reichenberg. 2014. The familial risk of autism. *J. Am. Med. Assoc.* 311:1770–7.

Smith, A. K., E. Mick, and S. V. Faraone. 2009. Advances in genetic studies of attention-deficit/hyperactivity disorder. *Curr. Psychiatry Rep.* 11:143–8.

Skuse, D. H., M. William, and J. Scourfield. 2005. Measuring autistic traits: Heritability and validity of the Social Communication Disorders Checklist. 187:586–72.

Steffenburg, S., C. Gillberg, L. Hellgren et al. 1989. A twin study of autism in Denmark, Finland, Iceland, Norway and Sweden. *J. Child Psychol. Psychiatry* 30:405–16.

Stilp, R. L. H., M. A. Gernsbacher, E. K. Schweigert, C. L. Arneson, and H. H. Goldsmith. 2010. Genetic variance for autism screening items in an unselected sample of toddler-age twins. *J. Am. Acad. Child Adoles. Psychiatry* 49:267–76.

Taniai, H., T. Nishiyama, T. Miyachi, M. Imaeda, and S. Sumi. 2008. Genetic influences on the broad spectrum of autism: Study of proband ascertained twins. *Am. J. Med. Genet.* 147B:844–9.

Theije, C., J. Wu, S. Lopes da Silva et al. 2011. Pathways underlying the gut-to-brain connection in autism spectrum disorder as future targets for disease management. *Eur. J. Pharmacol.* 668:570–80.

Virkud, Y. V., R. D. Todd, A. M. Abbachi, Y. Zhang, and J. N. Constantino. 2009. Familial aggregation of quantitative autistic traits in multiplex versus simplex autism. *Am. J. Med. Genet.* 150B:328–34.

Weisbrot, D. M., K. D. Gadow, C. J. DeVincent, and J. Pomeroy. 2005. The presentation of anxiety in children with pervasive developmental disorders. *J. Child Adoles. Psychopharmacol.* 15:477–96.

Williams, J., F. Scott, C. Stott et al. 2005. The CAST (Childhood Asperger Syndrome Test): Test accuracy. *Autism* 9:45–68.

Wong, C. C., E. L. Meaburn, A. Ronald et al. 2014. Methylomic analysis of monozygotic twins discordant for autism spectrum disorder and related behavioural traits. *Mol. Psychiatry* 19:495–503.

Chapter 3 Neurodevelopment of autism
The first three years of life

Meghan R. Swanson
and Joseph Piven

Contents

Abstract 37
3.1   Introduction 38
3.2   Structural magnetic resonance imaging 40
      3.2.1   Early brain overgrowth 40
      3.2.2   Surface area and cortical thickness 41
      3.2.3   Regional cortical differences in overgrowth 41
      3.2.4   Extra-axial fluid 43
      3.2.5   Cerebellum abnormalities 44
      3.2.6   Corpus callosum abnormalities 44
      3.2.7   Amygdala abnormalities 45
3.3   Diffusion tensor imaging 46
3.4   Conclusions and future directions 49
References 51

Abstract

The unfolding of behavioral features associated with autism spectrum disorder (ASD) occurs in the latter part of the first and in the second years of life. This dramatic shift in symptom presentation suggests underlying neuroanatomical and functional brain changes that either precede or co-occur with the emergence of aberrant behavioral features. In this chapter we will review recent literature on the neurodevelopment of ASD, particularly focusing on longitudinal studies since brain development is nonlinear during this time period. Key results to date include findings indicating that sometime before two years of age the brain undergoes a period of overgrowth. Infant-sibling research studies have identified abnormal development of white matter fiber tracts, corpus callosum size, and extra-axial fluid as early as six months of age. These findings indicate that it may be possible to use brain features in the first year of life to predict ASD, providing a means to identify infants for very early intervention studies with the hope of improving long-term outcomes.

3.1 Introduction

Autism spectrum disorder (ASD) is a neurodevelopmental disorder with a strong, but complex genetic basis; in families with one child with ASD, empirical evidence suggests that ASD recurrence risk for subsequently born children may be as high as 19% (Ozonoff et al. 2011), however epidemiological population-based estimates put recurrence risk closer to 10% (Sandin et al. 2014). Given this heightened recurrence rate, younger siblings of children with ASD are considered at high risk for developing ASD themselves during their first 3 years of life. Prospectively, following these infant siblings, employing the so-called "baby-sibling" paradigm provides an important approach to studying behavioral and brain development throughout the first 3 years of life in infants who go on to have ASD, in those who develop subthreshold but qualitatively similar behaviors, and in those at elevated familial risk who do not develop characteristics associated with ASD.

Behavioral results from infant-sibling studies have indicated that the defining behavioral characteristics of ASD unfold over the first few years of life. Social deficits associated with ASD are not commonly observed at 6 months of age. Typically, developing children are very social beings at 6 months of age, and generally indistinguishable from those who go on to have ASD. Repetitive behaviors associated with ASD have been reported to be present at 12 months of age in those who later meet criteria for ASD (Elison et al. 2014; Wolff et al. 2014; Filliter et al. 2015). Difficulties in other developmental areas, like motor skills, visual reception (Estes et al. 2015), and eye tracking of social scenes (Chawarska et al. 2013) and faces (Jones and Klin 2013), however, have been observed prior to the first birthday. ASD diagnoses at 24 months are highly stable; however, there are a number of children who do not meet diagnostic criteria until 36 months of age (Ozonoff et al. 2015). Further, there is evidence over the lifespan such that children diagnosed with ASD no longer meet the criteria for this condition as adults (Piven et al. 1996; Anderson et al. 2013; Fein et al. 2013).

The unfolding of ASD-associated behavioral features across the first 2 to 3 years of life marks the time when a child transitions from not having a clinically defined ASD to having ASD. This dramatic shift suggests underlying neuroanatomical and functional brain changes that either precede or co-occur with the emergence of aberrant behavioral features. Understanding the risk and protective factors for ASD that are present in early development will provide important insights into neural mechanisms and potentially provide insights relevant to early intervention. For example, the presence of some neural characteristics may be necessary but not sufficient for the development of ASD (e.g., those present in infants with high familial liability for ASD who both do and do not go on to develop ASD). See examples of this paradigm in Yuncel et al. (2014) and Kaiser et al. (2010), both studies show evidence for intermediate brain phenotypes in non-ASD relatives. Whereas other characteristics may be more specifically associated with the presence of the disorder but not seen in those who are unaffected but at high familial risk (Elison et al. 2013). To illustrate another possibility, we turn to schizophrenia research where cortical thickness was longitudinally measured to access occipito-temporal connectivity (Zalesky et al. 2015). Deficits in connectivity were found in children with childhood onset schizophrenia and their unaffected siblings; however, the deficits in the unaffected siblings normalized in mid-adolescence suggested resilience. This paradigm of searching for resiliency by studying unaffected high-risk siblings for risk signs that later resolve is largely nonexistent in ASD yet has the potential to make important contributions to our understanding of the neurobiology of this condition.

Characterizing early abnormal brain development is important as the first 3 years of life, and in particular the first year of life, is a time of great neural plasticity; hence intervention at this time theoretically would yield more optimal developmental outcomes for children with ASD than intervention at later ages. The potential power of intervention in the first year is highlighted by two recent studies. In one recent small pilot study, infants were identified as symptomatic for ASD at 7–15 months and provided with parent-mediated interventions. At 36 months, the treated infants were less symptomatic for ASD and developmental delay when compared to a control group of infant siblings who went on to have ASD but did not receive treatment (Rogers et al. 2014). Green et al. (2015) conducted a randomized control trial of high-risk siblings with treatment starting at age 7–10 months. When compared to infants in the control group, infants in the treatment groups showed fewer ASD risk behaviors and more attentiveness to their parents after the intervention.

In this chapter, particular focus will be given to early longitudinal studies. Brain development is both nonlinear and dynamic through the first 3 years of life and into early adulthood (Giedd et al. 1999; Deoni et al. 2014). Given the heterogeneity and nonlinear nature of brain development, cross-sectional studies spanning wide age ranges are vulnerable to having effects washed out simply due to study design. For example, adult studies have shown that cross-sectional analyses provide estimates of change that unreliably range from good to poor depending on the brain region, further indicating that cross-sectional studies are not a valid solution to studying early brain development (Raz et al. 2005; Pfefferbaum and Sullivan 2015).

Research on normative samples has highlighted the rapid brain growth occurring during the first 2 years of life. For example, from birth to 1 year, brain volume increases to 101% (Knickmeyer et al. 2008). Growth slows down after the first year with this volume increasing 15% in the second year (Knickmeyer et al. 2008). In terms of cortical structure, from birth to 2 years of age, the surface area increases 114% and cortical thickness increases 36%. At age two, cortical thickness is 97% of the adult values, whereas surface area is 69% (Lyall et al. 2014), indicating that after 2 years of age, expanding surface area is the primary contributor to increase cortical volume. Lyall et al. (2014) found clear regional differences in both cortical thickness and surface area expansion, but little overlap in regions across these two aspects of cortical structure, which may indicate differential affects from experience-dependent processes (Ebert and Greenberg 2013) mediated by both the environment as well as altered attention (Elison et al. 2013) and sensory processing (Estes et al. 2015) in the first year of life in those who go on to have developed ASD.

3.2 Structural magnetic resonance imaging

3.2.1 Early brain overgrowth

Large brain size in children with ASD is one of the most consistent neurodevelopmental phenomenon reported in psychiatric and psychological research. In the early 1990s, Piven and colleagues reported large brain size in adolescents and adults (Piven et al. 1995, 1996). This research spurred early studies measuring head circumference as a proxy of brain size; however, many of these studies utilized CDC norms as control samples and a recent systematic review revealed that these norms were falsely inflating group differences in head circumference (Raznahan et al. 2013).

In the early 2000s, researchers began collecting sMRI in children with ASD under 5 years of age to directly measure brain overgrowth patterns. Studies varied in their approach, with some applying a cross-sectional design (Courchesne et al. 2001; Sparks et al. 2002; Akshoomoff et al. 2004; Hazlett et al. 2005; Bloss and Courchesne 2007; Zeegers et al. 2009; Nordahl et al. 2012; Xiao et al. 2014), while others utilized longitudinal approaches to capture the developmental nature of brain development (Schumann et al. 2010; Hazlett et al. 2011; Nordahl et al. 2012; Shen et al. 2013). Generally speaking, the results indicated increased brain volume in children with ASD when compared to typically developing children (Courchesne et al. 2001; Sparks et al. 2002; Akshoomoff et al. 2004; Hazlett et al. 2005, 2011; Bloss and Courchesne 2007; Schumann et al. 2010; Nordahl et al. 2011, 2012; Shen et al. 2013) and children with developmental delay (Sparks et al. 2002; Xiao et al. 2014). Only one study did not find significant group differences in total brain volume; however, this cross-sectional study included a wide age range (2–7 years), which may have contributed to null results due to the non-linear nature of brain development during this age range (Zeegers et al. 2009).

Early cross-sectional studies by Courchesne et al. (2001) and Sparks et al. (2002) reported volume differences in 2 to 4 year olds with ASD when compared to controls. Since the early 2000s, a number of notable longitudinal studies have examined the developmental nature of early brain overgrowth in ASD. Three separate longitudinal studies following toddlers with ASD from 2 to 5 years found significantly larger brain volumes in ASD compared to typically developing controls, providing further support for the brain overgrowth taking place before 2 years of age (Schumann et al. 2010; Hazlett et al. 2011; Nordahl et al. 2012), see Figure 3.1 from Hazlett et al. (2011).

In the only report to date in infants, Shen et al. (2013) showed that the high-risk infants who went on to have ASD ($n = 10$) had a significantly faster growth trajectory for cerebral volume when compared to both high-risk infants who did not go on to have ASD and low-risk infants, and that by 12–15 months, high-risk infants who went on to have ASD had larger cerebral volumes when compared to the control groups. Two carefully controlled retrospective longitudinal studies of head circumference are in line with Shen and colleagues' findings; both studies found evidence of increased head circumference relative to local control samples occurring sometime after 12 months of age (Hazlett et al. 2005; Constantino et al. 2010). Together, these studies suggest that overgrowth occurs in the latter part of the first and the second years of life.

3.2.2 Surface area and cortical thickness

The overall volume of the cortex is determined by growth in the surface area and growth in cortical thickness, which are, in turn, determined by two genetically independent processes driven by different cellular mechanisms (Rakic 1995; Panizzon et al. 2009; Winkler et al. 2010). Studies investigating these two processes provide initial insights into the neurobiological mechanisms underlying the early overgrowth seen in children with ASD. Hazlett et al. (2011) found significantly increased surface area in frontal, temporal, and parietal lobes, but not cortical thickness, in 2 year olds with ASD when compared to control toddlers, a finding that is consistent with the minicolumn hypothesis of ASD (Casanova et al. 2006). A recent study by Ohta et al. (2015) confirmed these findings reporting increased surface area, but not cortical thickness in a large sample of 3-year-old boys with ASD. A third study did not find surface area differences; however, this study employed a cross-sectional design and included a wide age range (2–5 years) so it is plausible that study design and developmental effects could have washed out significant results (Raznahan et al. 2012).

3.2.3 Regional cortical differences in overgrowth

Several studies have attempted to further unpack the brain enlargement finding by investigating local areas of cortical enlargement. Carper and colleagues reported that 2- to 4-year-old boys with ASD displayed the greatest enlargement in white and gray matter in the frontal lobe when

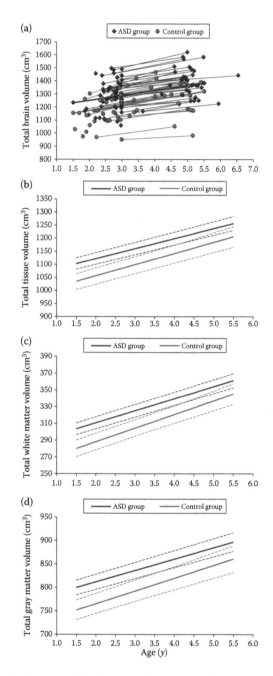

Figure 3.1 Trajectory of development: Total brain volume, total tissue volume, total white matter volume, and total gray matter volume. Panels show the subject trajectories (scatterplot) for total brain volume (a) and mean group trajectories with 95% confidence interval bands (dashed lines) for total tissue volume (b), total white matter volume (c), and total gray matter volume (d). ASD indicates autism spectrum disorder. (From Hazlett, H. C. et al. 2011. *Arch. Gen. Psychiatry* 68(5):467–76.)

compared to typically developing controls (Carper 2002; Carper and Courchesne 2005). Hazlett et al. (2005) found that when 18- to 35-month-old infants with ASD were compared to typically developing and developmentally delayed controls, they had larger gray and white matter volumes in frontal, temporal, parietal, and occipital lobes, with the largest increase in the temporal lobe. Later work by Xiao et al. (2014) and Hoeft et al. (2011) echoed these findings with reported higher gray and white matter volume localized in the superior temporal gyrus (STG) and superior temporal sulcus (STS), respectively. In adults with ASD, the STS has been shown to be thinner, suggesting that dynamic structural changes are occurring throughout the lifetime in this brain region (Hadjikhani et al. 2006).

The STG and STS are both biologically relevant areas for ASD. The STG contains the primary auditory cortex as well as Wernicke's areas (Brodmann 22p), making it an essential area for language comprehension. The STS separates the STG from the middle temporal gyrus, with putative involvement in the processing of biological motion and joint attention, the shared focus of two individuals (Adolphs 2003). It is common for children with ASD to have deficits or delays in both language and joint attention. So, neurobiological abnormality in the STS region could be a contributing factor to these early occurring ASD behavioral characteristics as there is a burst of language development in the first and second years, and joint attention first comes on line around 9 months of age and is fully in place by 15 months of age in typically developing children (Carpenter et al. 1998).

3.2.4 Extra-axial fluid

In Shen et al. (2013) infancy study, they also found increased extra-axial fluid from 6 to 24 months in infants who went on to have ASD, and increased extra-axial fluid was predictive of more severe autistic behaviors at the time of diagnosis. Extra-axial fluid is defined as increased cerebrospinal fluid (CSF) in the subarachnoid space. This study raised the question whether persistently elevated extra-axial CSF from 6 to 24 months is an early marker of altered neurodevelopment, and may be either a cause or consequence of the underlying pathology of ASD. Increased extra-axial fluid had been previously associated with impaired motor function and other learning disabilities (Nickel and Gallenstein 1987; Lorch et al. 2004; Hellbusch 2007). While normal CSF circulation is responsible for the removal of potentially neurotoxic waste products and inflammatory cytokines that accumulate in the brain (Johanson et al. 2008; Xie et al. 2013), altered CSF circulation and excessive CSF in the subarachnoid space may result in an accumulation of these metabolic by-products and cytokines (Johanson et al. 2008; Iliff et al. 2012). Indeed, altered composition of CSF has been shown to have a pathological effect on brain development (Mashayekhi et al. 2002; Lehtinen et al. 2011).

3.2.5 Cerebellum abnormalities

The cerebellum acts as a modulator for a diverse set of functional tasks, including motor control, posture, motor learning, as well as cognitive tasks, including language and attention. Most studies in older children and adults with ASD have reported larger cerebellum volume when compared to control participants (Fatemi et al. 2012); however, the literature in infants and toddlers has been less consistent with some groups reporting larger volumes (Sparks et al. 2002; Bloss and Courchesne 2007), while others do not find significant differences in cerebellum volumes (Hazlett et al. 2005; Webb et al. 2009; Zeegers et al. 2009). Inconsistent findings in substructures may in part be due to the methodological challenges associated with segmentation of these regions in young children (e.g., issues with delineating white and gray matter boundaries).

3.2.6 Corpus callosum abnormalities

The corpus callosum is a large commissural fiber tract connecting the right and left cerebral hemispheres, facilitating interhemispheric communication. Two recent studies have explored early structural abnormalities of the corpus callosum using longitudinal designs. The studies of Wolff et al. (2015) and Nordahl et al. (2015) highlight the importance of longitudinal data to understand the developmental processes. Taken together, these studies paint a picture of a dynamic corpus callosum that, relative to normative development, is larger in the first year of life, reaches normative sizes in the second year, and then becomes smaller sometime in the third year of life.

Wolff et al. (2015) prospectively studied infant-siblings of children with ASD from 6 to 24 months and found that starting at 6 months, infants who went on to have ASD had increased corpus callosum size when compared to infants who did not go on to have ASD, but by 24 months, significant group differences were no longer present (Figure 3.2). These early group differences were particularly robust in the anterior portion of the corpus callosum, which projects to the prefrontal cortex. Further, the volume of corpus callosum was found to be associated with repetitive behaviors. Nordahl et al. (2015) longitudinally followed preschool children aged from 3 to 5 years and found smaller corpus callosum volumes in regions projecting to the superior frontal cortex in children with ASD when compared to control children. The results also revealed region-specific sex differences with boys with ASD having smaller corpus callosum in areas projecting to orbitofrontal regions when compared to typically developing boys, whereas girls with ASD had smaller corpus callosum in areas projecting to anterior frontal and superior frontal regions when compared to typically developing females (see Figure 3.3; Nordahl et al. 2015). Like the Nordahl study, results from older children and adults with ASD consistently report smaller corpus callosum sizes

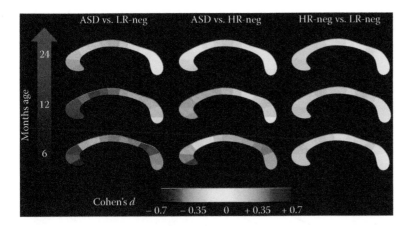

Figure 3.2 Six- and 12-month old infants who went on to have ASD had larger corpus callosum thickness in anterior regions when compared to infants in the control group. By 24 months, group differences were no longer present and the effect sizes across the corpus callosum were weak overall. (From Wolff, J. J. et al. 2015. *Brain*, May, awv118.)

when compared to control groups (Piven et al. 1997; Manes et al. 1999; Boger-Megiddo et al. 2006; Frazier et al. 2012).

3.2.7 Amygdala abnormalities

The amygdalae are a set of nuclei in the limbic system located deep medially within the temporal lobes that are functionally relevant for processing of emotions, motivation, and social cognition (Kandel et al. 2000; Kennedy et al. 2009). Several studies have reported large amygdala volumes relative to controls in infants and toddlers with ASD, even after controlling for total brain volume (Mosconi et al. 2009; Hoeft et al. 2011; Nordahl et al. 2012). To investigate the timing of amygdala enlargement, Nordahl et al. (2012) longitudinally investigated amygdala volume beginning at 37 months and then again 1 year later. Toddlers with ASD had larger amygdala volumes at both time points, but the relative difference in volume was greater at the second time point, indicating that between 3 and 4 years of life, the growth of amygdala seemed to speed up in children with ASD.

There is a dearth of knowledge surrounding the behavioral correlates and neurobiological underpinnings of this early amygdala overgrowth phenomenon. One study examining brain–behavior correlates showed that joint attention, a social attention skill that is a core deficit in ASD, is associated with amygdala volume overgrowth in 4 year olds with ASD (Mosconi et al. 2009). Amygdala volume was not associated with gestures, repetitive, or stereotyped behaviors. Joint attention requires attention to the eye region of the face, which might explain why amygdala volumes would be associated with joint attention, but not other clinical aspects of ASD (e.g., repetitive or stereotyped behaviors). In an attempt

45

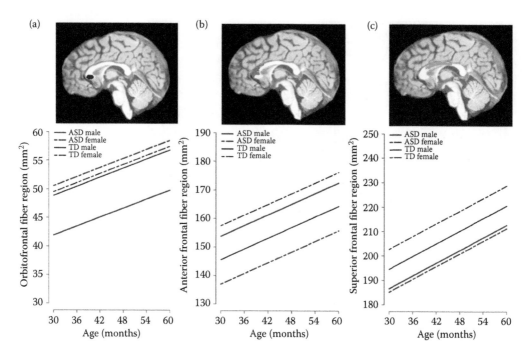

Figure 3.3 Region-specific sex differences in corpus callosum growth rates from 3–5 years indicated that the orbito-frontal region was smaller in males with ASD compared to control males (a), the anterior frontal region was smaller in females with ASD compared to control females (b), and the superior frontal region was smaller in males and females with ASD when compared to male and female control children (c). (From Nordahl, C. Wu. et al. 2015. *Mol. Autism* 6(1): 26.)

to examine the neurological underpinnings of early amygdala overgrowth, Breece et al. (2013) measured the frequency of myeloid dendritic cells as a metric of immune response in the gastrointestinal system in children who also participated in MRI scans. The results indicated that children with ASD had higher myeloid dendritic cells when compared to typically developing controls and that in children with ASD increased levels of myeloid dendritic cells were associated with enlarged amygdala volumes.

3.3 Diffusion tensor imaging

White matter fiber tracts allow the brain to communicate efficiently and process higher order cognitive functions. Given that individuals with ASD often have delays in language or other higher order cognitive processing, researchers have turned to DTI to investigate potential neural inefficiencies in individuals with ASD. In the following, we review literature from infants at high risk for ASD while then turning to the literature focusing on toddlers over 18 months of age. For a further review of DTI studies on individuals with ASD of all ages, see Travers et al. (2012), Hoppenbrouwers et al. (2014), and Conti et al. (2015).

Wolff et al. (2012) utilized an infant-sibling research design to longitudinally follow infants at high familial risk for ASD from 6 to 24 months of age with results showing widespread differences in major white matter fiber tract development across the brain in infants who went to have ASD when compared to infants who did not go on to have ASD. Infants who went on to have ASD showed higher FA at 6 months followed by blunted FA development such that by 24 months, they had lower FA values when compared to infants who did not go on to have ASD (see Figure 3.4 from Wolff et al. 2012). In another work by the same group, Elison and colleagues reported associations between visual orienting latencies and fiber properties of the splenium of the corpus callous in 7-month-old infants at low-familial risk for ASD; however this association was not found in infants who went on to have ASD (Elison et al. 2013). Infants who went on to have ASD also showed abnormal visual orienting, a foundational skill for early language development. These findings suggest that aberrant development in the splenium of the corpus callosum may result in atypical visual orienting, which, in turn, may impact language development.

In a previously described study (Section 3.2.6), Wolff et al. (2015) found that at 6-month-old infants who went on to have ASD had a larger anterior corpus callosum. DTI results from these infants indicated that radial diffusivity (RD), which is thought to approximate axon composition or density, accounted for a significant amount of variance in the size of callosal thickness. These results suggest that aberrant corpus callous area and thickness in the first year may be driven by density or packing of white matter fiber tracks or changes in fiber track axon diameter. DTI studies of older children have found higher fractional anisotropy in the corpus callosum when boys and girls with ASD were compared to children with developmental disabilities (Xiao et al. 2014) and when boys with ASD were compared to typically developing children (Nordahl et al. 2015). In a recent study by Solso and colleagues, young toddlers with ASD entered the study with higher FA in the anterior corpus callosum, but this effect dissipated after 3–4 years of age (Solso et al. 2015). Similar associations were found for the uncinate and arcuate fasciculi and the inferior frontal-superior tract. However, longitudinal data was only collected on 14 of 61 ASD toddlers and so conclusions about trajectories of FA development should be tempered.

DTI studies focused on children over 18 months have reported inefficiencies in white matter networks (Lewis et al. 2014) and abnormal diffusion metrics (Ben Bashat et al. 2007; Weinstein et al. 2011; Cascio et al. 2013; Xiao et al. 2014) when comparing children with ASD to matched controls. In terms of group differences in diffusion metrics, reported results have been inconsistent with some studies reporting lower global FA (Cascio et al. 2013) in children with ASD and others reporting higher

47

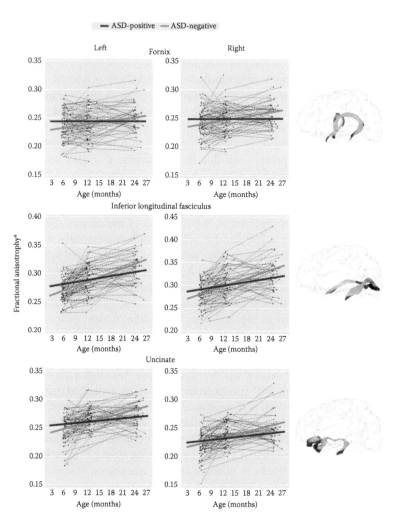

Figure 3.4 Trajectories of fractional anisotropy in limbic and association white matter fiber tracts in 92 high-risk infants (siblings of children already diagnosed with ASD. At age 12 months, N = 66. At age 24 months, N = 50). With and without evidence of ASD at 24 months of age (heavy lines represent mean values). [a] 0 = isotropic diffusion in fluid; 1 = strongly directional diffusivity in highly structured axonal bundles. (From Wolff, J. J. et al. 2012. *Am. J. Psychiatry* 169(6): 589–600.)

FA (Ben Bashat et al. 2007; Weinstein et al. 2011; Xiao et al. 2014). These inconclusive results may be due to the cross-sectional nature of these studies and the large range in chronological ages (1.5–6.5 years) in participant samples. A key point illustrated by Wolff et al.'s (2012) longitudinal study is that developmental brain trajectories of infants with and without ASD appear to be dynamic. A similarly dynamic development of white matter may be happening in years 2–5. The studies with younger samples (mean ages 2 and 3 years) reported higher FA values across the brain whereas the study by Cascio et al. (2013) reported on a much older sample (mean age 4.6 years) and results indicated lower FA across the brain. Lower FA has also been reported in a study on 5-year-old children with ASD (Billeci et al. 2012) and may reflect the functional underconnectivity often reported in older individuals with ASD (Just et al. 2004).

3.4 Conclusions and future directions

ASD is a lifelong disorder with a typical age of diagnosis around 4 years (Autism and Developmental Disabilities Monitoring Network 2014); however, behavioral features precede diagnosis by at least 2 years (Zwaigenbaum et al. 2005; Ozonoff et al. 2010). Backing up even further to birth to 2 years marks a time of tremendous change for children with ASD as they transition from not having behavioral features of ASD to having such features. The underlying neural development influencing these behavioral changes is not well understood. It is well established that sometime before 2 years of age, the brain undergoes a period of overgrowth, yet the ontogeny of this overgrowth and the long-term implications are currently unknown (Courchesne et al. 2001; Sparks et al. 2002; Akshoomoff et al. 2004; Hazlett et al. 2005; Bloss and Courchesne 2007; Schumann et al. 2010; Hazlett et al. 2011; Nordahl et al. 2011, 2012; Shen et al. 2013).

Although much remains unknown regarding the pathogenesis of ASD, the collection of studies reviewed in this chapter highlights the early onset and widespread nature of ASD-aberrant brain development. Postmortem studies of individuals with ASD have revealed abnormal neural structure however, to date samples have been relatively small (Buxhoeveden et al. 2006; Casanova et al. 2006; Tang et al. 2014). Casanova et al. (2006) reported smaller, but more numerous minicolumns in school-aged children with ASD when compared to typically developing controls. Cortical minicolumns are vertical columns that course through multiple layers of the cortex and grow from progenitor cells in the embryo. Interestingly, the results presented by Casanova et al. (2006) and Hazlett et al. (2011) are consistent as an increased number of minicolumns would, in turn, increase the brain's surface area and Hazlett and colleagues found an increase in brain surface area, but not cortical thickness in toddlers with ASD. Increased surface area is consistent with aberrant minicolumn morphology but it remains to be seen how those early observations will be understood given some recent conflicting data (McKavanagh et al. 2015). The studies by Hazlett et al. (2011) and Casanova et al. (2006) do present an interesting link between clinical imaging findings and postmortem studies. Early longitudinal data by Hazlett et al. (2011) as well as the recent single time point study by Ohta et al. (2015), which also reported increased surface area but not cortical thickness, provides important insights into the timing and sequence of these changes.

At the genetic level, gene mutations such as copy number variants (CNVs), deletion, and duplications have been shown to contribute to aberrant

49

brain development. The 16p11.2 CNV has been associated with ASD and individuals with this deletion present with increased head circumference (Shinawi et al. 2010; Zufferey et al. 2012; Qureshi et al. 2014), while some duplication carriers present with microcephaly (Shinawi et al. 2010; Jacquemont et al. 2011; Qureshi et al. 2014). Maillard et al. (2015) found gene dose-dependent associations between white and gray matter brain volumes in adults with 16p11.2 deletion, duplication, and control adults in an MRI study. Mouse models of 16p11.2 deletion have extended this work showing that a CNV at 16p11.2 results in altered cortical neurogenesis through enhanced neuronal differentiation and suppression of proliferation (Pucilowska et al. 2015). Patient populations with two other ASD-associated gene mutations, CHD8 and PTEN, have also displayed larger head circumferences when compared to controls (Bernier et al. 2014; Hobert et al. 2014; Mirzaa and Poduri 2014). While these findings are certainly promising, they are limited in scope to etiologically defined variants of ASD, and due to the complex nature of ASD may not be generalizable to the larger population of children and adults with "idiopathic" ASD.

Infant-sibling research designs have provided us with the earliest glimpse of the ASD brain in the first year of life and results from these studies have revealed that aberrant brain development is present in the first year of life in infants who go on to development ASD (Wolff et al. 2012, 2015; Shen et al. 2013). Early identification of aberrant brain development opens the door for very early intervention that could potentially improve long-term behavioral and cognitive outcomes for children with ASD. Hence infant-sibling studies have the potential to make important contributions to both the neurodevelopmental and clinical fields associated with ASD research. Given the promising research by Shen et al. (2013) and Wolff et al. (2012, 2015), we already have plausible targets to test prediction models including extra-axial fluid development, fiber tract development, and corpus callosum growth. A common theme across these targets is the equal importance placed on anatomical region and growth trajectory, further making the case for the necessity of longitudinal studies in early ASD research.

The literature on degenerative diseases illustrates an approach that can now be applied to ASD research. In Parkinson's disease, 50% of the dopamine receptors in the substantia nigra are diminished before the onset of motor symptoms associated with Parkinson's (Morrish et al. 1998). These findings have generated considerable research on utilizing medical imaging as a presymptomatic diagnostic tool for Parkinson's and other neurodegenerative disorders (Ba and Martin 2015). This model could be applied to ASD research with the potential of greater success than previously demonstrated with behavioral instruments (Turner-Brown et al. 2013).

From a neurodevelopmental perspective, intervening in the first year of life has potential for a large impact on later adaptive skills as this is the time of great neuroplasticity and a time when the brain overgrowth seen in ASD is only just beginning. The goal of early identification and intervention may perhaps be the most compelling reason to focus neurodevelopment research on infancy; however, without valid and effective intervention for infants, we may be getting the hypothetical cart before the horse. Although significant progress has been made in designing early interventions that are effective at reducing features associated with ASD (Magiati et al. 2012), there is only very preliminary evidence that intervention in the first year of life may ameliorate some features associated with ASD (Green et al. 2013; Rogers et al. 2014). Both very early intervention studies conducted to date utilized parent-mediated programs designed to optimize social interaction harnessing the activity-dependent neuronal development presumed to operate in ASD. Until Siller and Sigman (2002, 2008), the early social language environment was the third rail in ASD, perhaps such promising findings as those of Green et al. (2013) and Rogers et al. (2014) can serve as a bellwether of translational clinical research to focus on the social environment. Improving the long-term outcomes of children with ASD is a worthwhile goal that may be sped along with the help of diligent neuroimaging, with infant-sibling designs holding the key to intervention in the first year of life.

References

Adolphs, R. 2003. Cognitive neuroscience of human social behaviour. *Nat. Rev. Neurosci.* 4(3):165–78. doi: 10.1038/nrn1056.

Akshoomoff, N., C. Lord, A. J. Lincoln, R. Y. Courchesne, R. A. Carper, J. Townsend, and E. Courchesne. 2004. Outcome classification of preschool children with autism spectrum disorders using MRI brain measures. *J. Am. Acad. Child Adoles. Psychiatry* 43(3):349–57. doi: 10.1097/00004583-200403000-00018.

Anderson, D. K., J. W. Liang, and C. Lord. 2013. Predicting young adult outcome among more and less cognitively able individuals with autism spectrum disorders. *J. Child Psychol. Psychiatry Allied Disciplines* 55(5). doi: 10.1111/jcpp.12178.

Autism and Developmental Disabilities Monitoring Network. 2014. Prevalence of autism spectrum disorder among children aged 8 years—Autism and developmental disabilities monitoring network, 2010. *Morb. Mort. Wkly Rep.* 63 Suppl 2(2):1–21. doi: 24670961.

Ba, F. and W. R. Wayne Martin. 2015. Dopamine transporter imaging as a diagnostic tool for Parkinsonism and related disorders in clinical practice. *Parkinsonism Relat. Disord.* 21(2):87–94. doi: 10.1016/j.parkreldis.2014.11.007.

Ben Bashat, D., V. Kronfeld-Duenias, D. A. Zachor, P. M. Ekstein, T. Hendler, R. Tarrasch, A. Even, Y. Levy, and L. B. Sira. 2007. Accelerated maturation of white matter in young children with autism: A high B value DWI study. *NeuroImage* 37(1):40–47. doi: 10.1016/j.neuroimage.2007.04.060.

Bernier, R., C. Golzio, B. Xiong et al. 2014. Disruptive CHD8 mutations define a subtype of autism early in development. *Cell* 158(2):263–76. doi: 10.1016/j.cell.2014.06.017.

Billeci, L., S. Calderoni, M. Tosetti, M. Catani, and F. Muratori. 2012. White matter connectivity in children with autism spectrum disorders: A tract-based spatial statistics study. *BMC Neurol.* 12(Md):148.

Bloss, C. S. and E. Courchesne. 2007. MRI neuroanatomy in young girls with autism: A preliminary study. *J. Am. Acad. Child Adoles. Psychiatry* 46(4): 515–23. doi: 10.1097/chi.0b013e318030e28b.

Boger-Megiddo, I., D. W. W. Shaw, S. D. Friedman, B. F. Sparks, A. A. Artru, J. N. Giedd, G. Dawson, and S. R. Dager. 2006. Corpus callosum morphometrics in young children with autism spectrum disorder. *J. Autism Dev. Disord.* 36(6):733–39. doi: 10.1007/s10803-006-0121-2.

Breece, E., B. Paciotti, C. W. Nordahl, S. Ozonoff, J. A. Van de Water, S. J. Rogers, D. G. Amaral, and P. Ashwood. 2013. Myeloid dendritic cells frequencies are increased in children with autism spectrum disorder and associated with amygdala volume and repetitive behaviors. *Brain, Behav. Immunity* 31(July):69–75. doi: 10.1016/j.bbi.2012.10.006.

Buxhoeveden, D. P., K. Semendeferi, J. Buckwalter, N. Schenker, R. Switzer, and E. Courchesne. 2006. Reduced minicolumns in the frontal cortex of patients with autism. *Neuropathol. Appl. Neurobiol.* 32(5):483–91. doi: 10.1111/j.1365-2990.2006.00745.x.

Carpenter, M., K. Nagell, and M. Tomasello. 1998. Social cognition, joint attention, and communicative competence from 9 to 15 months of age. *Monogr. Soc. Res. Child Dev.* 63(4): i–vi, 1–143.

Carper, R. A. 2002. Cerebral lobes in autism: Early hyperplasia and abnormal age effects. *NeuroImage* 16(4):1038–51. doi: 10.1006/nimg.2002.1099.

Carper, R. A. and E. Courchesne. 2005. Localized enlargement of the frontal cortex in early autism. *Biol. Psychiatry* 57(2):126–33. doi: 10.1016/j.biopsych.2004.11.005.

Casanova, M. F., I. A. J. van Kooten, A. E. Switala, H. van Engeland, H. Heinsen, H. W. M. Steinbusch, P. R. Hof, J. Trippe, J. Stone, and C. Schmitz. 2006. Minicolumnar abnormalities in autism. *Acta Neuropathol.* 112(3): 287–303. doi: 10.1007/s00401-006-0085-5.

Cascio, C., M. Gribbin, S. Gouttard et al. 2013. Fractional anisotropy distributions in 2- to 6-year-old children with autism. *J. Intell. Disability Res.* 57(11):1037–49. http://doi.org/10.1111/j.1365-2788.2012.01599.x.

Chawarska, K., S. Macari, and F. Shic. 2013. Decreased spontaneous attention to social scenes in 6-month-old infants later diagnosed with autism spectrum disorders. *Biol. Psychiatry* 74(3):195–203. doi: 10.1016/j.biopsych.2012.11.022.

Constantino, J. N., P. Majmudar, A. Bottini, M. Arvin, Y. Virkud, P. Simons, and E. Spitznagel. 2010. Infant head growth in male siblings of children with and without autism spectrum disorders. *J. Neurodev. Disord.* 2(1):39–46. doi: 10.1007/s11689-009-9036-5.

Conti, E., S. Calderoni, V. Marchi, F. Muratori, G. Cioni, and A. Guzzetta. 2015. The first 1000 days of the autistic brain: A systematic review of diffusion imaging studies. *Front. Hum. Neurosci.* 9 (January). Frontiers: 159. doi: 10.3389/fnhum.2015.00159.

Courchesne, E., C. M. Karns, H. R. Davis et al. 2001. Unusual brain growth patterns in early life in patients with autistic disorder: An MRI study. *Neurology* 57(2):245–54. doi: 10.1212/WNL.57.2.245.

Deoni, S. C. L., J. O'Muircheartaigh, J. T. Elison, L. Walker, E. Doernberg, N. Waskiewicz, H. Dirks, I. Piryatinsky, D. C. Dean, and N. L. Jumbe. 2014. White matter maturation profiles through early childhood predict general cognitive ability. *Brain Struct. Function*, November. doi: 10.1007/s00429-014-0947-x.

Ebert, D. H. and M. E. Greenberg. 2013. Activity-dependent neuronal signalling and autism spectrum disorder. *Nature* 493(7432):327–37. doi: 10.1038/nature11860.

Elison, J. T., S. J. Paterson, J. J. Wolff et al. 2013. White matter microstructure and atypical visual orienting in 7-month-olds at risk for autism. *Am. J. Psychiatry* 170(8):899–908.

Elison, J. T., J. J. Wolff, J. S. Reznick et al. 2014. Repetitive behavior in 12-month-olds later classified with autism spectrum disorder. *J. Am. Acad. Child Adoles. Psychiatry* 53(11):1216–24. doi: 10.1016/j.jaac.2014.08.004.

Estes, A. M., L. Zwaigenbaum, H. Gu et al. 2015. Behavioral, cognitive, and adaptive development in infants with autism spectrum disorder in the first 2 years of life. *J. Neurodev. Disord.* 7(1):24. doi: 10.1186/s11689-015-9117-6.

Fatemi, S. H., K. A. Aldinger, P. Ashwood et al. 2012. Consensus paper: Pathological role of the cerebellum in autism. *Cerebellum* 11(3):777–807. doi: 10.1007/s12311-012-0355-9.

Fein, D., M. Barton, I.-M. Eigsti et al. 2013. Optimal outcome in individuals with a history of autism. *J. Child Psychol. Psychiatry* 54(2):195–205. doi: 10.1111/jcpp.12037.

Filliter, J. H., J. Longard, M. A. Lawrence, L. Zwaigenbaum, J. Brian, N. Garon, I. M. Smith, C. Roncadin, W. Roberts, and S. E. Bryson. 2015. Positive affect in infant siblings of children diagnosed with autism spectrum disorder. *J. Abnormal Child Psychol.* 43(3):567–75. doi: 10.1007/s10802-014-9921-6.

Frazier, T. W., M. S. Keshavan, N. J. Minshew, and A. Y. Hardan. 2012. A two-year longitudinal MRI study of the corpus callosum in autism. *J. Autism Dev. Disord.* 42(11): 2312–22. doi: 10.1007/s10803-012-1478-z.

Giedd, J. N., J. Blumenthal, N. O. Jeffries, F. X. Castellanos, H. Liu, A. Zijdenbos, T. Paus, A. C. Evans, and J. L. Rapoport. 1999. Brain development during childhood and adolescence: A longitudinal MRI study. *Nat. Neurosci.* 2(10):861–63. doi: 10.1038/13158.

Green, J., T. Charman, A. Pickles et al. 2015. Parent-mediated intervention versus no intervention for infants at high risk of autism: A parallel, single-blind, randomised trial. *The Lancet Psychiatry* 2(2):133–40. doi: 10.1016/S2215-0366(14)00091-1.

Green, J., M. W. Wan, J. Guiraud, S. Holsgrove, J. McNally, V. Slonims, M. Elsabbagh, T. Charman, A. Pickles, and M. H. Johnson. 2013. Intervention for infants at risk of developing autism: A case series. *J. Autism Dev. Disord.* 43(11):2502–14. doi: 10.1007/s10803-013-1797-8.

Hadjikhani, N., R. M. Joseph, J. Snyder, and H. Tager-Flusberg. 2006. Anatomical differences in the mirror neuron system and social cognition network in autism. *Cerebral Cortex* 16(9):1276–82. doi: 10.1093/cercor/bhj069.

Hazlett, H. C., M. Poe, G. Gerig, R. G. Smith, J. Provenzale, A. Ross, J. Gilmore, and J. Piven. 2005. Magnetic resonance imaging and head circumference study of brain size in autism: Birth through age 2 years. *Arch. Gen. Psychiatry* 62(12) 1366–76. doi: 10.1001/archpsyc.62.12.1366.

Hazlett, H. C., M. D. Poe, G. Gerig, M. Styner, C. Chappell, R. G. Smith, C. Vachet, and J. Piven. 2011. Early brain overgrowth in autism associated with an increase in cortical surface area before age 2 years. *Arch. Gen. Psychiatry* 68(5):467–76.

Hellbusch, L. C. 2007. Benign extracerebral fluid collections in infancy: Clinical presentation and long-term follow-up. *J. Neurosurg.* 107(2 Suppl):119–25. doi: 10.3171/PED-07/08/119.

Hobert, J. A., R. Embacher, J. L. Mester, T. W. Frazier, and E. Charis. 2014. Biochemical screening and PTEN mutation analysis in individuals with autism spectrum disorders and macrocephaly. *Eur. J. Hum. Genet.* 22(2):273–76. doi: 10.1038/ejhg.2013.114.

Hoeft, F., E. Walter, A. A. Lightbody, H. C. Hazlett, C. Chang, J. Piven, and A. L. Reiss. 2011. Neuroanatomical differences in toddler boys with fragile X syndrome and idiopathic autism. *Arch. Gen. Psychiatry* 68(3):295–305. doi: 10.1001/archgenpsychiatry.2010.153.

Hoppenbrouwers, M., M. Vandermosten, and B. Boets. 2014. Autism as a disconnection syndrome: A qualitative and quantitative review of diffusion tensor imaging studies" *Res. Autism Spectrum Disord.* 8(4):387–412. doi: 10.1016/j.rasd.2013.12.018.

Iliff, J. J., M. Wang, Y. Liao et al. 2012. A paravascular pathway facilitates CSF flow through the brain parenchyma and the clearance of interstitial solutes, including amyloid β. *Sci. Transl. Med.* 4(147):147ra111. doi: 10.1126/scitranslmed.3003748.

Jacquemont, S., A. Reymond, F. Zufferey et al. 2011. Mirror extreme BMI phenotypes associated with gene dosage at the chromosome 16p11.2 locus. *Nature* 478(7367):97–102. doi: 10.1038/nature10406.

Johanson, C. E., J. A. Duncan, P. M. Klinge, T. Brinker, E. G. Stopa, and G. D. Silverberg. 2008. Multiplicity of cerebrospinal fluid functions: New challenges in health and disease. *Cerebrospinal Fluid Res.* 5(January):10. doi: 10.1186/1743-8454-5-10.

Jones, W. and A. Klin. 2013. Attention to eyes is present but in decline in 2–6-month-old infants later diagnosed with autism. *Nature.* doi: 10.1038/nature12715.

Just, M. A., V. L. Cherkassky, T. A. Keller, and N. J. Minshew. 2004. Cortical activation and synchronization during sentence comprehension in high-functioning autism: Evidence of underconnectivity. *Brain: J. Neurol.* 127(Pt 8):1811–21. doi: 10.1093/brain/awh199.

Kaiser, M. D., C. M. Hudac, S. Shultz et al. 2010. Neural signatures of autism. *Proc. Natl. Acad. USA* 107(49):21223–28. doi: 10.1073/pnas.1010412107.

Kandel, E. R., J. H. Schwartz, and T. M. Jessell. 2000. *Principles of Neural Science*, 4th ed. New York: McGraw-Hill.

Kennedy, D. P., J. Gläscher, J. M. Tyszka, and R. Adolphs. 2009. Personal space regulation by the human amygdala. *Nat. Neurosci.* 12(10):1226–27. doi: 10.1038/nn.2381.

Knickmeyer, R. C., S. Gouttard, C. Kang, D. Evans, K. Wilber, J. K. Smith, R. M. Hamer, W. Lin, G. Gerig, and J. H. Gilmore. 2008. A structural MRI study of human brain development from birth to 2 years. *J. Neurosci.* 28(47):12176–82. doi: 10.1523/JNEUROSCI.3479-08.2008.

Lehtinen, M. K., M. W. Zappaterra, X. Chen et al. 2011. The cerebrospinal fluid provides a proliferative niche for neural progenitor cells. *Neuron* 69(5):893–905. doi: 10.1016/j.neuron.2011.01.023.

Lewis, J. D., A. C. Evans, J. R. Pruett et al. 2014. Network inefficiencies in autism spectrum disorder at 24 months. *Transl. Psychiatry* 4 (January): e388. doi: 10.1038/tp.2014.24.

Lorch, S. A., J. A. D'Agostino, R. Zimmerman, and J. Bernbaum. 2004. 'Benign' extra-axial fluid in survivors of neonatal intensive care. *Arch. Pediatr. Adolesc. Med.* 158(2):178–82. doi: 10.1001/archpedi.158.2.178.

Lyall, A. E., F. Shi, X. Geng, S. Woolson, G. Li, L. Wang, R. M. Hamer, D. Shen, and J. H. Gilmore. 2014. Dynamic development of regional cortical thickness and surface area in early childhood. *Cerebral Cortex* March, doi: 10.1093/cercor/bhu027.

Magiati, I., X. W. Tay, and P. Howlin. 2012. Early comprehensive behaviorally based interventions for children with autism spectrum disorders: A summary of findings from recent reviews and meta-analyses. *Neuropsychiatry*, 2(6):543–570. http://doi.org/10.2217/npy.12.59.

Maillard, A. M., A. Ruef, F. Pizzagalli et al. 2015. The 16p11.2 locus modulates brain structures common to autism, schizophrenia and obesity. *Mol. Psychiatry* 20(1):140–47. doi: 10.1038/mp.2014.145.

Manes, F., J. Piven, D. Vrancic, V. Nanclares, C. Plebst, and S. E. Starkstein. 1999. An MRI study of the corpus callosum and cerebellum in mentally retarded autistic individuals. *J. NeuroPsychiatry Clin. Neurosci.* 11(4):470–74.

Mashayekhi, F., C. E. Draper, C. M. Bannister, M. Pourghasem, P. J. Owen-Lynch, and J. A. Miyan. 2002. Deficient cortical development in the hydrocephalic texas (H-Tx) rat: A role for CSF. *Brain: J. Neurol.* 125(Pt 8):1859–74.

McKavanagh, R., E. Buckley, and S. A Chance. 2015. Wider minicolumns in autism: A neural basis for altered processing? *Brain: J. Neurol.* 138(Pt 7):2034–45. doi: 10.1093/brain/awv110.

Mirzaa, G. M. and A. Poduri. 2014. Megalencephaly and hemimegalencephaly: Breakthroughs in molecular etiology. *Am. J. Med. Genet.* 166C(2):156–72. doi: 10.1002/ajmg.c.31401.

Morrish, P. K., J. S. Rakshi, D. L. Bailey, G. V. Sawle, and D. J. Brooks. 1998. Measuring the rate of progression and estimating the preclinical period of Parkinson's disease with [18F]dopa PET. *J. Neurol., Neurosurg. Psychiatry* 64(3):314–19. doi: 10.1136/jnnp.64.3.314.

Mosconi, M. W., H. Cody-Hazlett, M. D. Poe, G. Gerig, R. Gimpel-Smith, and J. Piven. 2009. Longitudinal study of amygdala volume and joint attention in 2-to 4-year-old children with autism. *Arch. Gen. Psychiatry* 66(5):509–16. doi: 10.1001/archgenpsychiatry.2009.19.

Nickel, R. E. and J. S. Gallenstein. 1987. Developmental prognosis for infants with benign enlargement of the subarachnoid spaces. *Dev. Med. Child Neurol.* 29(2):181–86.

Nordahl, C. Wu, N. Lange, D. D. Li, L. A. Barnett, A. Lee, M. H. Buonocore, T. J. Simon, S. Rogers, S. Ozonoff, and D. G. Amaral. 2011. Brain enlargement is associated with regression in preschool-age boys with autism spectrum disorders. *Proc. Natl. Acad. Sci. USA* 108(50):20195–200. doi: 10.1073/pnas.1107560108.

Nordahl, C. Wu, A.-M. Iosif, G. S. Young et al. 2015. Sex differences in the corpus callosum in preschool-aged children with autism spectrum disorder. *Mol. Autism* 6(1): 26. doi: 10.1186/s13229-015-0005-4.

Nordahl, C. Wu, R. Scholz, X. Yang, M. H. Buonocore, T. Simon, S. Rogers, and D. G. Amaral. 2012. Increased rate of amygdala growth in children aged 2 to 4 years with autism spectrum disorders: A longitudinal study. *Arch. Gen. Psychiatry* 69(1):53–61. doi: 10.1001/archgenpsychiatry.2011.145.

Ohta, H., C. Wu Nordahl, A.-M. Iosif, A. Lee, S. Rogers, and D. G Amaral. 2015. Increased surface area, but not cortical thickness, in a subset of young boys with autism spectrum disorder. *Autism Res.: Off. J. Int. Soc. Autism Res.*, July. doi: 10.1002/aur.1520.

Ozonoff, S., A.-M. Iosif, F. Baguio et al. 2010. A prospective study of the emergence of early behavioral signs of autism. *J. Am. Acad. Child Adoles. Psychiatry* 49(3):256–66.e1–2. doi: 10.1016/j.jaac.2009.11.009.

Ozonoff, S., G. S. Young, A. S. Carter et al. 2011. Recurrence risk for autism spectrum disorders: A baby siblings research consortium study. *Pediatrics* 128(3):e488–95. doi: 10.1542/peds.2010-2825.

Ozonoff, S., G. S. Young, R. J. Landa et al. 2015. Diagnostic stability in young children at risk for autism spectrum disorder: A baby siblings research consortium study. *J. Child Psychol. Psychiatry, Allied Disciplines*, April. doi: 10.1111/jcpp.12421.

Panizzon, M. S., C. Fennema-Notestine, L. T. Eyler et al. 2009. Distinct genetic influences on cortical surface area and cortical thickness. *Cerebral Cortex* 19(11):2728–35. doi: 10.1093/cercor/bhp026.

Pfefferbaum, A. and E. V. Sullivan. 2015. Cross-sectional versus longitudinal estimates of age-related changes in the adult brain: Overlaps and discrepancies. *Neurobiol. Aging* 36(9):2563–67. doi: 10.1016/j.neurobiolaging.2015.05.005.

Piven, J., S. Arndt, J. Bailey, and N. Andreasen. 1996. Regional brain enlargement in autism: A magnetic resonance imaging study. *J. Am. Acad. Child Adoles. Psychiatry* 35(4):530–36. doi: 10.1097/00004583-199604000-00020.

Piven, J., S. Arndt, J. Bailey, S. Havercamp, N. C. Andreasen, and P. Palmer. 1995. An MRI study of brain size in autism. *Am. J. Psychiatry* 152(8):1145–49.

Piven, J., J. Bailey, B. J. Ranson, and S. Arndt. 1997. An MRI study of the corpus callosum in autism. *Am. J. Psychiatry* 154(8):1051–56.

Piven, J., J. Harper, P. Palmer, and S. Arndt. 1996. Course of behavioral change in autism: A retrospective study of high-IQ adolescents and adults. *J. Am. Acad. Child Adoles. Psychiatry* 35(4):523–29. doi: 10.1097/00004583-199604000-00019.

Pucilowska, J., J. Vithayathil, E. J. Tavares, C. Kelly, J. C. Karlo, and G. E. Landreth. 2015. The 16p11.2 deletion mouse model of autism exhibits altered cortical progenitor proliferation and brain cytoarchitecture linked to the ERK MAPK pathway. *J. Neurosci.: Off. J. Soc. Neurosci.* 35(7):3190–3200. doi: 10.1523/JNEUROSCI.4864-13.2015.

Qureshi, A. Y., S. Mueller, A. Z. Snyder et al. 2014. Opposing brain differences in 16p11.2 deletion and duplication carriers. *J. Neurosci.: Off. J. Soc. Neurosci.* 34(34):11199–211. doi: 10.1523/JNEUROSCI.1366-14.2014.

Rakic, P. 1995. A small step for the cell, a giant leap for mankind: A hypothesis of neocortical expansion during evolution. *Trends Neurosci.* 18(9):383–88.

Raz, N., U. Lindenberger, K. M. Rodrigue, K. M. Kennedy, D. Head, A. Williamson, C. Dahle, D. Gerstorf, and J. D. Acker. 2005. Regional brain changes in aging healthy adults: General trends, individual differences and modifiers. *Cerebral Cortex* 15(11):1676–89. doi: 10.1093/cercor/bhi044.

Raznahan, A., R. Lenroot, A. Thurm, M. Gozzi, A. Hanley, S. J. Spence, S. E. Swedo, and J. N. Giedd. 2012. Mapping cortical anatomy in preschool aged children with autism using surface-based morphometry. *NeuroImage* 2(January):111–19. doi: 10.1016/j.nicl.2012.10.005.

Raznahan, A., G. L. Wallace, L. Antezana et al. 2013. Compared to what? Early brain overgrowth in autism and the perils of population norms. *Biol. Psychiatry* 74(8):563–75. doi: 10.1016/j.biopsych.2013.03.022.

Rogers, S. J., L. Vismara, A. L. Wagner, C. McCormick, G. Young, and S. Ozonoff. 2014. Autism treatment in the first year of life: A pilot study of infant start, a parent-implemented intervention for symptomatic infants. *J. Autism Dev. Disord.*, September. doi: 10.1007/s10803-014-2202-y.

Sandin, S., P. Lichtenstein, R. Kuja-Halkola, H. Larsson, C. M. Hultman, and A. Reichenberg. 2014. The familial risk of autism. *JAMA* 311(17):1770–77. doi: 10.1001/jama.2014.4144.

Schumann, C. M., C. S. Bloss, C. C. Barnes et al. 2010. Longitudinal magnetic resonance imaging study of cortical development through early childhood in autism. *J. Neurosci.* 30(12):4419–27. doi: 10.1523/JNEUROSCI.5714-09.2010.

Shen, M. D., C. Wu Nordahl, G. S. Young, S. L. Wootton-Gorges, A. Lee, S. E. Liston, K. R. Harrington, S. Ozonoff, and D. G. Amaral. 2013. Early brain enlargement and elevated extra-axial fluid in infants who develop autism spectrum disorder. *Brain* 136(Pt 9):2825–35. doi: 10.1093/brain/awt166; 10.1093/brain/awt166.

Shinawi, M., P. Liu, S.-H. L. Kang et al. 2010. Recurrent reciprocal 16p11.2 rearrangements associated with global developmental delay, behavioural problems, dysmorphism, epilepsy, and abnormal head size. *J. Med. Genet.* 47(5):332–41. doi: 10.1136/jmg.2009.073015.

Siller, M. and M. Sigman. 2002. The behaviors of parents of children with autism predict the subsequent development of their children's communication. *J. Autism Dev. Disord.* 32(2):77–89.

Siller, M. and M. Sigman. 2008. Modeling longitudinal change in the language abilities of children with autism: Parent behaviors and child characteristics as predictors of change. *Developmental Psychology*, 44(6):1691–1704. doi: 10.1037/a0013771.

Solso, S., R. Xu, J. Proudfoot et al. 2015. DTI provides evidence of possible axonal over-connectivity in frontal lobes in ASD toddlers. *Biol. Psychiatry* July. doi: 10.1016/j.biopsych.2015.06.029.

Sparks, B. F., S. D. Friedman, D. W. Shaw et al. 2002. Brain structural abnormalities in young children with autism spectrum disorder. *Neurology* 59(2):184–92. doi: 10.1212/WNL.59.2.184.

Tang, G., K. Gudsnuk, S.-H. Kuo et al. 2014. Loss of mTOR-dependent macroautophagy causes autistic-like synaptic pruning deficits. *Neuron* 83(5):1131–43. doi: 10.1016/j.neuron.2014.07.040.

Travers, B. G., N. Adluru, C. Ennis, D. P. M. Tromp, D. Destiche, S. Doran, E. D. Bigler, N. Lange, J. E. Lainhart, and A. L. Alexander. 2012. Diffusion tensor imaging in autism spectrum disorder: A review. *Autism Res.* 5(5):289–313. doi: 10.1002/aur.1243.

Turner-Brown, L. M., G. T. Baranek, J. S. Reznick, L. R. Watson, and E. R. Crais. 2013. The first year inventory: A longitudinal follow-up of 12-month-old to 3-year-old children. *Autism: Int. J. Res. Pract.* 17(5):527–40. doi: 10.1177/1362361312439633.

Webb, S. J., B.-F. Sparks, S. D. Friedman, D. W. W. Shaw, J. Giedd, G. Dawson, and S. R. Dager. 2009. Cerebellar vermal volumes and behavioral correlates in children with autism spectrum disorder. *Psychiatry Res.* 172(1):61–67. doi: 10.1016/j.pscychresns.2008.06.001.

Weinstein, M., L. Ben-Sira, Y. Levy, D. A. Zachor, E. B. Itzhak, M. Artzi, R. Tarrasch, P. M. Eksteine, T. Hendler, and D. B. Bashat. 2011. Abnormal white matter integrity in young children with autism. *Hum. Brain Mapping* 32(4):534–43. doi: 10.1002/hbm.21042.

Winkler, A. M., P. Kochunov, J. Blangero, L. Almasy, K. Zilles, P. T. Fox, R. Duggirala, and D. C. Glahn. 2010. Cortical thickness or grey matter volume? The importance of selecting the phenotype for imaging genetics studies. *NeuroImage* 53(3):1135–46. doi: 10.1016/j.neuroimage.2009.12.028.

Wolff, J. J., K. N. Botteron, S. R. Dager et al. 2014. Longitudinal patterns of repetitive behavior in toddlers with autism. *J. Child Psychol. Psychiatry, Allied Disciplines* 55(8):945–53. doi: 10.1111/jcpp.12207.

Wolff, J. J., G. Gerig, J. D. Lewis et al. 2015. Altered corpus callosum morphology associated with autism over the first 2 years of life. *Brain*, May, awv118. doi: 10.1093/brain/awv118.

Wolff, J. J., H. Gu, G. Gerig et al. 2012. Differences in white matter fiber tract development present from 6 to 24 months in infants with autism. *Am. J. Psychiatry* 169(6): 589–600. doi: 10.1176/appi.ajp.2011.11091447.

Xiao, Z., T. Qiu, X. Ke et al. 2014. Autism spectrum disorder as early neurodevelopmental disorder: Evidence from the brain imaging abnormalities in 2–3 years old toddlers. *J. Autism Dev. Disord.* 44(7): 1633–40. doi: 10.1007/s10803-014-2033-x.

Xie, L., H. Kang, Q. Xu et al. 2013. Sleep drives metabolite clearance from the adult brain. *Science* 342(6156):373–77. doi: 10.1126/science.1241224.

Yucel, G. H., A. Belger, J. Bizzell, M. Parlier, R. Adolphs, and J. Piven. 2014. Abnormal neural activation to faces in the parents of children with autism. *Cerebral Cortex*, July. doi: 10.1093/cercor/bhu147.

Zalesky, A., C. Pantelis, V. Cropley, A. Fornito, L. Cocchi, H. McAdams, L. Clasen, D. Greenstein, J. L. Rapoport, and N. Gogtay. 2015. Delayed development of brain connectivity in adolescents with schizophrenia and their unaffected siblings. *JAMA Psychiatry*, July. doi: 10.1001/jamapsychiatry.2015.0226.

Zeegers, M., H. H. Pol, S. Durston, H. Nederveen, H. Schnack, E. van Daalen, C. Dietz, H. van Engeland, and J. K. Buitelaar. 2009. No differences in MR-based volumetry between 2- and 7-year-old children with autism spectrum disorder and developmental delay. *Brain Dev.* 31(10):725–30. doi: 10.1016/j.braindev.2008.11.002.

Zufferey, F., E. H. Sherr, N. D. Beckmann et al. 2012. A 600 Kb deletion syndrome at 16p11.2 leads to energy imbalance and neuropsychiatric disorders. *J. Med. Genet.* 49(10):660–68. doi: 10.1136/jmedgenet-2012-101203.

Zwaigenbaum, L., S. E. Bryson, T. Rogers, W. Roberts, J. Brian, and P. Szatmari. 2005. Behavioral manifestations of autism in the first year of life. *Int. J. Dev. Neurosci.* 23(2–3):143–52. doi: 10.1016/j.ijdevneu.2004.05.001.

Chapter 4 Anatomy of autism

Verónica Martínez Cerdeño

Contents

Abstract 59
4.1 Brain size 59
4.2 Cerebral cortex 60
4.3 Hippocampus 64
4.4 Subcortical regions 64
4.5 Cerebellum 65
4.6 Brain stem 66
4.7 Alteration in neuronal volumes 66
4.8 Alteration in brain connectivity 67
4.9 Conclusion 68
References 69

Abstract

The alteration in social interaction, communication, and repetitive and obsessive behaviors that are the hallmark of autism are a consequence of a series of anatomical and histological abnormalities in the cerebral cortex and other brain areas in patients with autism. However, due to the heterogeneous nature of this disorder, not all the subjects with autism suffer the same symptoms, indicating that their brain abnormalities vary in form and/or severity. The pathology reports of brains with autism by Bauman and Kemper gave us the first observations about the macro- and microscopical structure of the autistic brain. These observations were followed by anatomical studies that focused on individual brain areas and specific traits such as the size of brain nuclei or the number and size of neurons in a given structure. Most of the later studies were performed using unbiased stereological methods of cell number and volumes. Here, we will review the available data on the anatomy of autism from the macro- to microscopic characteristics present in this disorder.

4.1 Brain size

Initial observations of an increased head circumference and structural MRI studies suggested and increased volume of the brain in children with autism. Follow-up studies indicated that the abnormal regulation of brain growth in autism results in early overgrowth followed by abnormally slowed growth. This brain overgrowth in autistic children (2–3 years old) was explained by more cerebral (18%) and cerebellar (39%) white matter, and more cerebral cortical gray matter (12%) than in control children, whereas older autistic children and adolescents did not have such enlarged gray and white matter volumes (Courchesne et al. 2001). Further data revealed significantly increased total brain volume in autistic males but not females (Piven et al. 1996). An analysis of lobe sizes suggested that the increase in brain size in autism is the result of a pattern of enlargement of specific cortical lobes (Piven et al. 1996). Further studies corroborated Courchesne and Piven studies (Aylward et al. 2002; Herbert et al. 2003; Herbert et al. 2004; Hazlett et al. 2005; Palmen et al. 2005; Peterson et al. 2006; Ke et al. 2008; Freitag et al. 2009; Hardan et al. 2009; Ecker et al. 2012; Riedel et al. 2014). Children with FXS also have larger global brain volumes compared with controls and equal to that of children with idiopathic autism (Hazlett et al. 2012).

4.2 Cerebral cortex

Gyrification of the cerebral cortex has been shown to be abnormal in autism (Williams et al. 2015). High-resolution MRI studies demonstrated that children with more autistic traits present with widespread areas of decreased gyrification (Blanken et al. 2015). Cortical thickness abnormalities are also present in autism and are region-specific, vary with age, and may remain dynamic well into adulthood. MRI data from the Courchesne Lab indicated cortical volume loss in the parietal lobes of 43% (6–32 years old) of autistic patients (Courchesne et al. 1993). Matching these data, Hutsler and colleagues examined eight postmortem ASD individuals (15–45 years old) and age-matched controls using MRI and found that cortical thickness values significantly decreased with age in autistic cases when compared to control cases (Hutsler et al. 2007). However, available data varies from reductions (Scheel et al. 2011; Misaki et al. 2012; Ecker et al. 2013; Ecker et al. 2014) to increases on cortical thickness in autism, most prominently in the frontal and temporal lobes (Hardan et al. 2006; Hyde et al. 2010; Sato 2013; Foster et al. 2015). As an explanation to these contradictory data, it was suggested that abnormal cortical development in autism undergoes three distinct phases: accelerated expansion in early childhood, accelerated thinning in later childhood and adolescence, and decelerated thinning in early adulthood (Zielinski et al. 2014). Focal disruptions of cortical laminar architecture in the cortex of children with autism have been also reported. These include focal patches of abnormal laminar cytoarchitecture and cortical disorganization of neurons in prefrontal and temporal cortical tissue in children with autism (Stoner et al. 2014). In addition, pencil fibers were present within the prefrontal cortex (BA 47) of a 40-year-old woman diagnosed at an early age with autism and mental retardation (Hashemi et al. 2016a). Abnormalities in cortical minicolumns, the most basic functional unit in the cortex composed of neurons and circuits, have been well described. Casanova and colleagues measured minicolumns in the prefrontal and temporal lobes of nine brains of autistic patients and matched controls, and found significant differences in the number of minicolumns, in the horizontal spacing that separates cell columns, and in their internal structure. Specifically, cell columns in brains of autistic patients were more numerous, smaller, and less compact in their cellular configuration with reduced neuropil space in the periphery (Casanova et al. 2002, 2003). In a follow-up study including six age-matched pairs of autism patients and controls, they corroborated that minicolumnar width was decreased in autistic patients. An analysis of inter- and intra-cluster distances using Delaunay triangulation suggested that the overall increased cell density previously described in the autistic cortex is the result of a greater number of minicolumns; otherwise the number of cells per minicolumns appeared normal (Casanova et al. 2006). In addition, brains from seven autistic patients and an equal number of age-matched controls were analyzed showing that minicolumn dimensions varied according to neocortical area in autism. The greatest difference between autistic and control groups was observed in BA44 located in the prefrontal cortex. Casanova suggested that diminished minicolumnar width across deep and superficial neocortical layers most probably reflects the involvement of shared constituents among the different layers (Casanova et al. 2009). Overall, the cerebral cortex in autism presents with changes in cortical thickness, abnormal laminar cytoarchitecture, and smaller minicolumns. The cortical areas most affected by these changes seem to be located in the prefrontal and temporal lobes.

The understanding about the number of neurons present in the cerebral cortex in autism is limited. The available data is not consistent; however, this inconsistency could be explained by several variables such as the area of the cortex studied, the type of neuron quantified, the patients' age (children, adolescents, or adults), the number of subjects included in each study, and the method used for quantification, among others. One of the first postmortem reports in autism was by Aarkrog, which noticed "some cell increase" together with increases in the thickness of the cortical arteries and meninges (Aakrog 1968). Kemper and Bauman described an increase in cell density in the cortex in eight out of nine cases of autism (Kemper and Bauman 1998). Later stereological studies of prefrontal tissue from seven autistic and six control male children (2–16 years old) found that children with autism had 67% more neurons in the prefrontal cortex compared with control children. The authors suggested that previously demonstrated brain overgrowth in males with autism is the result of an abnormal excess number of neurons in the prefrontal cortex (Courchesne et al. 2011). However, Van Kooten and colleagues studied the fusiform gyrus in seven brains from male and female patients with autism (12.1 ± 2.8 years old) and 10 matched controls (30.1 ± 7.5 years old), and found that patients with autism showed significant reductions

61

in neuron densities in layer III, and total neuron numbers in layers III, V, and VI (van Kooten et al. 2008). None of these alterations were found in the primary visual cortex or in the whole cerebral cortex. Other studies did not find any difference in the number of neurons in the cortex between autism and control cases. Kim and colleagues analyzed nine subjects with autism and nine age-matched control subjects (13–56 years old) and did not find a significant difference in the number of supragranular or infragranular neurons in the superior temporal cortex in autism (Kim et al. 2015). Neuron quantification in the occipitotemporal gyrus in seven autism and seven control subjects (4–21 years old) found no significant differences in pyramidal neuron numbers in layers III, V, and VI in seven pairs of autism and control subjects (Uppal et al. 2014). However, this study found that the number of pyramidal neurons positively correlated with autism severity in the anterior mid-cingulate cortex (Uppal et al. 2014). While these studies show an increase, a decrease, or no change in the number of neurons, they differ in the age of the subjects, the cortical area studied, the quantification of total versus density of neurons, and the quantification of all neurons versus quantification of only pyramidal neurons. Studies of specific neuronal population have also been performed. Kennedy and Santos quantified von Economo neurons (VEN, also called spindle neurons). VENs are only present in hominids, elephants, and cetaceans, and only in the anterior cingulate cortex and the fronto-insular cortex. While Kennedy et al. did not find evidence of a change in VEN number in the frontoinsular cortex of four autistic and two control subjects (3–41 years old in autism; 4–75 years old in control) (Kennedy et al. 2007), Santos et al. found that patients with autism consistently had a significantly higher ratio of VENs to pyramidal neurons than control subjects—four cases with autism and three controls (4–14 years old) (Santos et al. 2011). In agreement Uppal, using stereological methods, determined that VEN numbers positively correlated with autism in the anterior mid-cingulate cortex (Uppal et al. 2014a,b). Simms and colleagues reported that, among nine autism cases, there were two subsets; three brains with significantly increased VEN density, and the remaining six cases with reduced VEN density compared to controls. Collectively, these findings may reflect the known heterogeneity in individuals with autism and variations in clinical symptomatology (Simms et al. 2009). One recent study analyzed interneuron subtypes in the postmortem cortex of 11 autistic cases and 10 control cases, and found that the number of parvalbumin-expressing interneurons in the three cortical areas analyzed (BA46, BA47, and BA9) were significantly reduced in autism compared with control cases. However, the number of calbindin-expressing and calretinin-expressing interneurons did not differ in the cortical areas examined. Parvalbumin-expressing interneurons in the cortex are basket and chandelier fast-spiking cells that synchronize the activity of pyramidal cells through perisomatic and axo-axonic inhibition. Therefore, the reduced number of parvalbumin+ interneurons could disrupt the balance of excitation/inhibition and alter gamma wave oscillations in the cerebral cortex of autistic subjects (Hashemi et al. 2016b). Cajal-Retzius cells, a specific type of interneurons in layer I of the cortex, were also evaluated in the superior temporal cortex of four autism and four control cases (13–57 years old), and the authors did not find any difference in the number of these cells between autistic and control cases (Camacho et al. 2014). In summary, studies have found an increase in the number or density of neurons in prefrontal cortex (Courchesne et al. 2011) and of pyramidal neurons in the mid-cingulate cortex (Uppal et al. 2014b), a decrease in neurons in the fusiform cortex (van Kooten et al. 2008), and no change in pyramidal neurons in the superior temporal cortex (Kim et al. 2015), the occipitotemporal cortex (Uppal et al. 2014a), or visual cortex (Uppal et al. 2014b). In addition, a decrease of PV-expressing interneurons has been described in the prefrontal cortex in autism. Some found an increase of VENs in frontoinsular cortex (Kennedy et al. 2007; Simms et al. 2009; Santos et al. 2011; Uppal et al. 2014a,b), while other found no change in these cells in the same region (Kennedy et al. 2007). No change was found in the number of Cajal-Retzius cells in the adult superior temporal cortex (Camacho et al. 2014). Many more similar studies need to be performed in order to understand neuronal number dynamics in the autistic cortex.

In addition to changes in number, pyramidal neurons have been shown to present with an altered morphology in autism. Hutsler and Zhang studied frontal, temporal, and parietal lobe regions using the Golgi method, and found that relative to controls, spine densities were greater in ASD subjects. In analyses restricted to the apical dendrites of pyramidal cells, greater spine densities were found predominantly within layer II of each cortical location and within layer V of the temporal lobe. High spine densities were associated with decreased brain weights and were most commonly found in ASD subjects with lower levels of cognitive functioning (Hutsler and Zhang 2010). Interestingly, these data contrast to that in most neurodevelopmental diseases that are associated to decreased numbers of pyramidal dendrites and spines.

Other cell types have been shown to be altered in the cerebral cortex in autism. Microglia, the immune cell of the nervous system, has been also implicated in the cortical pathology in autism. Microglia proliferate and increase their soma volume under injury and most pathological conditions. Activated microglia secrete inflammatory cytokines and actively phagocytize cells. Microglia appeared markedly activated in the dorsoprefrontal cortex of five of 13 autistic patients (3–41 years old), and marginally activated in an additional four. Many interactions were observed between near-distance microglia and neurons that appear to involve encirclement of the neurons by microglial processes. Analysis of a young subject subgroup suggested that this alteration might be present from an early age in autism. It was additionally observed that neuron–neuron clustering increased with advancing age in autism, suggesting a gradual loss of normal neuronal organization in this disorder (Morgan et al. 2010; Morgan et al. 2012). These data indicate that microglial activation might play a role in the pathogenesis of autism in a substantial proportion of patients. Alternatively, activation may represent a response of the innate neuroimmune system to synaptic, neuronal, or neuronal network disturbances, or reflect genetic and/or environmental abnormalities impacting multiple cellular populations. Alterations have been also described in the ependymal cells of the SVZ (Kotagiri et al. 2014).

Specific pathology related to comorbidities has also been described in autism. For example, an autistic woman in her twenties suffering from autism and presenting with self-injury behavior presented with numerous neurofibrillary tangles in the perirhinal and entorhinal cortex and a fewer number of tangles in the amygdala and in the prepiriform and orbito-frontal cortex. There were no neuritic plaques or amyloid deposits. These tangles probably resulted from self-injury behavior that included head banging (Hof et al. 1991).

4.3 Hippocampus

Little is known about the anatomy of the hippocampus in autism. MRI studies have found no alteration in the size of the hippocampus. Saitoh et al. described a lack of a significant difference in the cross-sectional size of the posterior hippocampal formation between autistic and normal cases (6–42 years old) (Saitoh et al. 1995; Saitoh and Courchesne 1998). These data were corroborated by other studies (Rojas et al. 2004). Bauman and Kemper found abnormal hippocampus, subiculum, and entorhinal cortex in the brain of a 29-year-old autistic man. Additional cases showed similar alterations. Bauman and Kemper first described increased cell density in the hippocampus in most of the cases of autism they analyzed (Bauman and Kemper 1985; Bauman 1994). Golgi analysis of CA1 and CA4 pyramidal neurons in two cases of infantile autism showed decreased complexity and extent of dendritic arbors (Raymond and Kemper 1996). Stereological techniques in five autistic (13–54 years old) and five control cases (14–63 years old) indicated a selective increase in the density of calbindin-immunoreactive interneurons in the dentate gyrus, an increase in calretinin-immunoreactive interneurons in area CA1, and an increase in parvalbumin-immunoreactive interneurons in areas CA1 and CA3 in the hippocampus of individuals with autism when compared with controls. These findings suggest that GABAergic interneurons may represent a vulnerable target in the brains of individuals with autism (Lawrence et al. 2010).

4.4 Subcortical regions

As in the case of the cerebral cortex, subcortical regions are also altered in autism, both in their anatomy and neuronal properties. The striatum has been shown enlarged in MRI studies in patients with autism (Sears et al. 1999; Hollander et al. 2005; Rojas et al. 2006; Langen et al. 2009). Accordingly, postmortem studies also showed an increase in the volumes of the caudate nucleus and nucleus accumbens by 22% and 34%, respectively, and a reduced numerical density of neurons in the nucleus accumbens and putamen by 15% and 13%, respectively (Wegiel et al. 2014). The first studies of the amygdala in autism noticed an increase in size and in cell density in the medially placed nuclei of the amygdala (Bauman 1994). However, later stereological quantifications showed that patients with autism have a similar size amygdala and amygdalar nuclei, and significantly fewer neurons overall and in its lateral nucleus in nine male autistic brains (3–47 years old) than in typically developing (10 males, 17–30 years old) patients (Schumann and Amaral 2006). Parallel studies showed a 12% reduction of neuronal density was limited to the lateral nucleus of the amygdala in 14 subjects with autism and 14 age-matched controls (4–60 years old) (Wegiel et al. 2014). Based on these studies, it is widely accepted that there is a reduction in cell number in the amygdala in autism. Follow-up stereological studies in subcortical regions demonstrated that in 14 of the 16 regions studied, the number of structures with a significant volume deficit was higher in 4- to 8-year-old subjects than in 30- to 60-year-old subjects (Wegiel et al. 2015). Other areas of the forebrain found to be abnormal in autism include septum and mammillary bodies described as apparently having increased cell density (Bauman 1994).

4.5 Cerebellum

MRI studies have described the presence of hypoplasia of posterior vermal lobules and cerebellar hemispheres in the majority of autistic patients examined, but also cerebellar hyperplasia of the posterior vermis in some cases (Courchesne et al. 1994; Saitoh et al. 1995; Scott et al. 2009). A study by Wegiel revealed focal disorganization of the flocculus cytoarchitecture, altered morphology, and spatial disorientation of Purkinje cells, deficit and abnormalities of granule, basket, stellate, and unipolar brush cells, and structural defects and abnormal orientation of Bergmann glia. These are indicators of profound disruption of the neural circuitry in autism (Wegiel et al. 2013). Ritvo showed that Purkinje cell counts were significantly lower in the cerebellar hemisphere and vermis in autistic subject in the comparison with control subjects (Ritvo et al. 2014). However, while the number of Purkinje cells has been unanimously shown to be decreased in autism (Ritvo et al. 1986; Whitney et al. 2008; Skefos et al. 2014), the number of other cerebellar cells such as basket cells and stellate cells has been found to be invariable in some cases of autism (Whitney et al. 2008). The loss of Purkinje cells is not accompanied by reactive gliosis, suggesting that the death of these cells is not related to age. Disturbances have also been observed in the cerebellar nuclei, including the fastigeal, globose, and emboliform nuclei. Neurons in these nuclei in adult brains have shown to be significantly decreased in number. In contrast, in children's brains these neurons have been found to be plentiful in number (Bauman 1994).

4.6 Brain stem

Initial descriptions reported that the number of neurons in the inferior olive is preserved in autism; however, there is a change in cell size (Bauman 1994). The inferior olive receives and sends fibers—climbing fibers—to the cerebellum, participating in motor, sensory, and cognitive tasks. The preservation of the olivary neurons in the face of a significant reduction in Purkinje cell number strongly supports a prenatal origin for the cerebellar abnormalities in autism (Bauman et al. 2005). Further studies described the presence of ectopic neurons lateral to the olives bilaterally in one case, and malformation of the olive in three cases, thus providing further pathological evidence for a prenatal onset of this disorder (Bailey et al. 1998). Other abnormalities described in the autistic brain stem include dysgenesis and reduction in neuronal number in the facial motor nucleus, and agenesis of the superior olivary nuclei in a case with autism and Moebius syndrome (Rodier et al. 1996).

4.7 Alteration in neuronal volumes

A good number of studies have shown a significantly smaller neuronal soma volume in the majority of the brain regions in autism, including various cortical and subcortical regions such as hippocampus, cerebellum, and brain stem (Bauman 1994; Raymond et al. 1996). In the cortex, a study that included seven patients with autism (12.1 ± 2.8 years old) and 10 matched controls (30.1 ± 7.5 years old) found significant reductions in mean perikaryal volumes of neurons in layers V and VI in the fusiform gyrus (Van Kooten et al. 2008). In addition, Casanova described smaller neuron and nucleolar cross-sections in the temporal and prefrontal cortices of autistic cases compared to controls (Casanova et al. 2003). VENs in the cingulate gyrus were also shown to be significantly decreased in cell size in layers I–III and layers V–VI of BA24b and in cell packing density in layers V–VI of BA24c (Simms et al. 2009). However, no significant differences were found in neuronal size in the prefrontal cortex in autism (Courchesne et al. 2011), in pyramidal neurons in layers III, V, and VI of the occipitotemporal gyrus (seven autism and seven control subjects, 4–21 years old) (Uppal et al. 2014a), nor in pyramidal volume in neurons of the supra and infragranular layers of the superior temporal cortex (nine autism [13–56 years old] vs. nine control [14–45 years old] cases) (Camacho et al. 2014). As in the case for studies on neuronal number in autism, these discrepancies in neuronal volume could be explained by several variables such as the specific area of the cortex examined and the age of the subjects included in each study. In the cerebellum, the average cross-sectional area of Purkinje cells of patients with autism was smaller by 24% when compared to the normal patients. Nevertheless, the authors pointed out that Purkinje cell atrophy in autism is heterogeneous among individuals diagnosed with this disorder (Fatemi et al. 2002). Multiple researchers corroborated these data (Whitney et al. 2008; Whitney et al. 2009; Skefos et al. 2014; Wegiel et al. 2014). Neurons in the cerebellar nuclei in adult brains have been shown to be small; however, the same neurons were found enlarged in children's brains (Bauman 1994). Small neuronal size was also observed in the medial septal nucleus and in the diagonal band of Broca, where reduced size soma was observed in patients older than 21 years of age (Kemper and Bauman 1998). Additional studies of neuronal size in 16 subcortical brain structures of 14 autistic and 14 control subjects (4–64 years old) indicated that the deficit of neuronal soma volume in children with autism was associated with deficits in the volume of the neuronal nucleus and cytoplasm (Wegiel et al. 2015). This study also revealed that the number of structures with a significant volume deficit decreased from fourteen in 4- to 8-year-old to four in the 36- to 60-year-old autistic subjects. These data reveal defects of neuronal growth in early childhood in autism and delayed upregulation of neuronal growth during adolescence and adulthood, reducing the neuron soma volume deficit in a majority of the examined regions (Wegiel et al. 2014). Overall, the soma and nuclear size of many neuronal populations in the autistic brain seem to be reduced, both in cortical and subcortical brain structures.

4.8 Alteration in brain connectivity

In addition to cell alterations, autism also presents with an alteration in the anatomy of brain connectivity, including a disconnection of long and short distance pathways and excessive connections between neighboring areas. All major tracts have been shown to be altered in autism, including the corpus callosum, internal capsule, and cerebellar peduncles. Multiple studies have demonstrated that the size of the corpus callosum (CC) is decreased in autism, suggesting an impaired interhemispheric communication (Piven et al. 1997; Manes et al. 1999; Hardan et al. 2000; Chung et al. 2004; Vidal et al. 2006; He et al. 2008; Casanova et al. 2011; El-Baz et al. 2011; Pryweller et al. 2014). One of the latest studies demonstrated that the reduction in size of the CC occurs over all of its subdivisions (genu, body, splenium) in patients with autism. Since the commissural fibers that traverse the different anatomical compartments of the CC originate in disparate brain regions, these data suggest the presence of widely distributed cortical abnormalities in people with autism (Casanova et al. 2011). However, adults with ASD show an inverse relation between CC size and callosal fiber length (Sundaram et al. 2008; Hong et al. 2011; Thomas et al. 2011; Billeci et al. 2012; Lewis et al. 2013). The internal capsule in all three segments, the cerebellar peduncles, and the right inferior longitudinal fasciculus are also altered in patients with autism (Brito et al. 2009; Sivaswamy et al. 2010; Shukla et al. 2010; Duerden et al. 2014; Koldewyn et al. 2014). Local connectivity is also disrupted in ASD across development, with the most pronounced differences occurring in childhood (Dajani 2015). Specifically, a reduced cortical functional connectivity in middle and superior temporal sulci and parietal lobule regions, lower local connectivity in sensory processing brain regions, and higher local connectivity in complex information processing regions is present in autism (Cheng et al. 2015).

Individual axons have been shown to have lower myelin thickness in autism, as is the case for the orbitofrontal cortex (Zikopoulos et al. 2010). Moreover, morphometric analysis of serotonin-stained axons in postmortem brain tissue from autism donors (2.8–29 years old) demonstrated that the number of serotonin axons was increased in two forebrain pathways (principal ascending fiber bundles of the medial and lateral forebrain bundles, and innervation of the amygdala and the piriform, superior temporal, and parahippocampal cortices), and terminal regions in cortex from autistic donors. In autistic donors, 8 years old and up, several types of dystrophic serotonin axons were seen in the termination fields. One class of these dystrophic axons, the thick heavily stained axons, was not seen in the brains of patients with neurodegenerative diseases (Azmitia et al. 2011a,b). Overall, the alteration of connectivity in the autistic brain is well accepted and documented, although many other studies are needed in order to complete our understanding of an alteration of specific short and long pathways present in autism.

4.9 Conclusion

Autism is characterized by anatomical disturbances in the cerebral cortex and subcortical brain areas, including cerebellum, limbic system structures, and many others. Cortical disturbances affect predominantly the prefrontal and temporal cortices. Altered regions in the limbic system include cingulated cortex, hippocampus, amygdala, and mammillary bodies, among others. Cortical disturbances include changes in cortical thickness, laminar disorganization, and changes in cell number and volume. Other brain regions also present with similar neuronal alterations. In addition, autism presents with a disconnection of long and short distance pathways. Due to the heterogeneity of the autism disorder, these disturbances vary from patient to patient. Many more studies are needed in order to clarify some aspects of the anatomy of autism and further our understanding of the underlying anatomy of this disorder. One of the current limiting factors in the pathway to unraveling the nature of autism is the lack of postmortem brain tissue available to perform these studies. More effort is needed to increase the number of brain donations of both autistic and control brains. Moreover, new protocols for sharing this tissue should be established within the scientific community to allow obtaining the maximum amount of knowledge from the reduced amount of tissue currently available for research.

References

Aakrog, T. 1968. Organic factors in infantile psychosis and borderline psychosis. Retrospective study of 45 cases subjected to pneumoencephalography. *Dan. Med. Bull.* 15:283–288.

Aylward, E. H., N. J. Minshew, K. Field, B. F. Sparks, and N. Singh. 2002. Effects of age on brain volume and head circumference in autism. *Neurology* 59(2):175–183.

Azmitia, E. C., J. S. Singh, X. P. Hou, and J. Wegiel. 2011a. Dystrophic serotonin axons in postmortem brains from young autism patients. *Anat. Rec. (Hoboken)* 294(10):1653–1662.

Azmitia, E. C., J. S. Singh, and P. M. 2011b. Whitaker-Azmitia. Increased serotonin axons (immunoreactive to 5-HT transporter) in postmortem brains from young autism donors. *Neuropharmacology* 60(7–8):1347–1354.

Bailey, A. L. P., A. Dean, B. Harding, I. Janota, M. Montgomery, M. Rutter, and P. Lantos. 1998. A clinicopathological study of autism. *Brain* 121(Pt 5):889–905.

Bauman, M. L. and T. L. Kemper. 1985. Histoanatomic observations of the brain in early infantile autism. *Neurology* 35(6):866–874.

Bauman, M. L. and T. L. Kemper 1994. Neuroanatomic observations of the brain in autism. In *The Neurobiology of Autism*, eds. M. L. Bauman and T. L. Kemper, 119–145. Baltimore, MD: Johns Hopkins University Press.

Bauman, M. L. and T. L. Kemper. 2005. Neuroanatomic observations of the brain in autism: A review and future directions. *Int. J. Dev. Neurosci.* 23(2–3):183–187.

Billeci, L., S. Calderoni, M. Tosetti, M. Catani, and F. Muratori. 2012. White matter connectivity in children with autism spectrum disorders: A tract-based spatial statistics study. *BMC Neurol.* 12:148.

Blanken, L. M., S. E. Mous, A. Ghassabian, et al. 2015. Cortical morphology in 6- to 10-year-old children with autistic traits: A population-based neuroimaging study. *Am. J. Psychiatry* 172(5):479–486.

Brito, A. R., M. M. Vasconcelos, R. C. Domingues, L. C. Jr. Hygino da Cruz, S. Rodrigues Lde, E. L. Gasparetto, and C. A. Calçada. 2009. Diffusion tensor imaging findings in school-aged autistic children. *J. Neuroimaging* 19(4):337–343.

Camacho, J., E. Ejaz, J. Ariza, S. C. Noctor, and V. Martinez-Cerdeno. 2014. RELN-expressing neuron density in layer I of the superior temporal lobe is similar in human brains with autism and in age-matched controls. *Neurosci. Lett.* 579:163–167.

Casanova, M. and J. Trippe. 2009. Radial cytoarchitecture and patterns of cortical connectivity in autism. *Philos. Trans. R. Soc. Lond. B Biol. Sci.* 364(1522):1433–1436.

Casanova, M. F., D. Buxhoeveden, A. E. Switala, and E. Roy. 2002. Longitudinal changes in cortical thickness in autism and typical development. *Neurology* 58(3):428–432.

Casanova, M. F., D. Buxhoeveden, and J. Gomez. 2003. Disruption in the inhibitory architecture of the cell minicolumn: Implications for autism. *Neuroscientist* 9(6):496–507.

Casanova, M. F., A. El-Baz, A. Elnakib et al. 2011. Quantitative analysis of the shape of the corpus callosum in patients with autism and comparison individuals. *Autism* 15(2):223–238.

Casanova, M. F., I. A. van Kooten, A. E. Switala et al. 2006. Minicolumnar abnormalities in autism. *Acta Neuropathol.* 112(3):287–303.

Cheng, W., E. T. Rolls, H. Gu, J. Zhang, and J. Feng. 2015. Autism: Reduced connectivity between cortical areas involved in face expression, theory of mind, and the sense of self. *Brain* 138(Pt 5):1382–1393.

Chung, M. K., K. M. Dalton, A. L. Alexander, and R. J. Davidson. 2004. Less white matter concentration in autism: 2D voxel-based morphometry. *Neuroimage* 23(1):242–251.

Courchesne, E., C. M. Karns, H. R. Davis et al. 2001. Unusual brain growth patterns in early life in patients with autistic disorder: An MRI study. *Neurology* 57(2):245–254.

Courchesne, E., P. R. Mouton, M. E. Calhoun et al. 2011. Neuron number and size in prefrontal cortex of children with autism. *JAMA* 306(18):2001–2010.

Courchesne, E., G. A. Press, and R. Yeung-Courchesne. 1993. Parietal lobe abnormalities detected with MR in patients with infantile autism. *Am. J. Roentgenol.* 160(2):387–393.

Courchesne, E., Saitoh, O., Yeung-Courchesne, R. et al. 1994. Abnormality of cerebellar vermian lobules VI and VII in patients with infantile autism: Identification of hypoplastic and hyperplastic subgroups with MR imaging. *Am. J. Roentgenol.* 162(1):123–130.

Dajani, D. R. U. L. 2015. Local brain connectivity across development in autism spectrum disorder: A cross-sectional investigation. *Autism Res.* 9(1):43–54.

Duerden, E. G., D. Card, S. W. Roberts et al. 2014. Self-injurious behaviours are associated with alterations in the somatosensory system in children with autism spectrum disorder. *Brain Struct. Funct.* 219(4):1251–1261.

Ecker, C., C. Ginestet, Y. Feng et al. 2013. Brain surface anatomy in adults with autism: The relationship between surface area, cortical thickness, and autistic symptoms. *JAMA Psychiat.* 70(1):59–70.

Ecker, C., A. Shahidiani, Y. Feng et al. 2014. The effect of age, diagnosis, and their interaction on vertex-based measures of cortical thickness and surface area in autism spectrum disorder. *J. Neural Transm.* 121(9):1157–1170.

Ecker, C., J. Suckling, S. C. Deoni et al. 2012. Brain anatomy and its relationship to behavior in adults with autism spectrum disorder: A multicenter magnetic resonance imaging study. *Arch. Gen. Psychiat.* 69(2):195–209.

El-Baz, A., A. Elnakib, M. F. Casanova et al. 2011. Accurate automated detection of autism related corpus callosum abnormalities. *J. Med. Syst.* 35(5):929–939.

Fatemi, S. H., A. R. Halt, G. Realmuto et al. 2002. Purkinje cell size is reduced in cerebellum of patients with autism. *Cell Mol. Neurobiol.* 22(2):171–175.

Foster, N. E., K. A. Doyle-Thomas, A. Tryfon et al. 2015. Structural gray matter differences during childhood development in autism spectrum disorder: A multimetric approach. *Pediatr. Neurol.* 53(4):350–9.

Freitag, C. M., E. Luders, H. E. Hulst et al. 2009. Total brain volume and corpus callosum size in medication-naive adolescents and young adults with autism spectrum disorder. *Biol Psychiat.* 66(4):316–319.

Hardan, A. Y., R. A. Libove, M. S. Keshavan, N. M. Melhem, and N. J. Minshew. 2009. A preliminary longitudinal magnetic resonance imaging study of brain volume and cortical thickness in autism. *Biol. Psychiat.* 66(4):320–326.

Hardan, A. Y., N. J. Minshew, and M. S. Keshavan. 2000. Corpus callosum size in autism. *Neurology* 55(7):1033–1036.

Hardan, A. Y., S. Muddasani, M. Vemulapalli, M. S. Keshavan, and N. J. Minshew. 2006. An MRI study of increased cortical thickness in autism. *Am. J. Psychiat.* 163(7):1290–1292.

Hashemi, E., J. Ariza, M. Lechpammer, S. C. Noctor, and V. Martínez-Cerdeño. 2016a. Abnormal white matter tracts resembling pencil fibers involving prefrontal cortex (Brodmann area 47) in autism: A case report. *J Med Case Rep.* 10(1):237.

Hashemi, E., J. Ariza, H. Rogers, S. C. Noctor, and V. Martínez-Cerdeño. 2016b. The number of parvalbumin-expressing interneurons is decreased in the prefrontal cortex in autism. *Cereb. Cortex.* 46(4):1307–1318.

Hazlett, H. C., M. Poe, G. Gerig et al. 2005. Magnetic resonance imaging and head circumference study of brain size in autism: Birth through age 2 years. *Arch. Gen. Psychiat.* 62(12):1366–1376.

Hazlett, H. C., M. D. Poe, A. A. Lightbody et al. 2012. Trajectories of early brain volume development in fragile X syndrome and autism. *J. Am. Acad. Child Adolesc. Psychiat.* 51(9):921–933.

He, Q., K. Karsch, and Y. Duan. 2008. Abnormalities in MRI traits of corpus callosum in autism subtype. *Conf. Proc. IEEE Eng. Med. Biol. Soc.* 3900–3903.

Herbert, M. R., D. A. Ziegler, N. Makris et al. 2004. Localization of white matter volume increase in autism and developmental language disorder. *Ann. Neurol.* 55(4):530–540.

Herbert, M. R., D. A. Ziegler, C. K. Deutsch et al. 2003. Dissociations of cerebral cortex, subcortical and cerebral white matter volumes in autistic boys. *Brain* (126(Pt 5)):1182–1192.

Hof, P. R., R. Knabe, P. Bovier, and C. Bouras. 1991. Neuropathological observations in a case of autism presenting with self-injury behavior. *Acta Neuropathol.* 82(4):321–326.

Hollander, E., E. Anagnostou, W. Chaplin et al. 2005. Striatal volume on magnetic resonance imaging and repetitive behaviors in autism. *Biol. Psychiat.* 58(3):226–232.

Hong, S., X. Ke, T. Tang et al. 2011. Detecting abnormalities of corpus callosum connectivity in autism using magnetic resonance imaging and diffusion tensor tractography. *Psychiat. Res.* 194(3):333–339.

Hutsler, J. J., T. Love, and H. Zhang. 2007. Histological and magnetic resonance imaging assessment of cortical layering and thickness in autism spectrum disorders. *Biol Psychiat.* 61(4):449–457.

Hutsler, J. J. and H. Zhang. 2010. Increased dendritic spine densities on cortical projection neurons in autism spectrum disorders. *Brain Res.* 1309:83–94.

Hyde, K. L., F. Samson, A. C. Evans, and L. Mottron. 2010. Neuroanatomical differences in brain areas implicated in perceptual and other core features of autism revealed by cortical thickness analysis and voxel-based morphometry. *Hum. Brain Mapp.* 31(4):556–566.

Ke, X., S. Hong, T. Tang et al. 2008. Voxel-based morphometry study on brain structure in children with high-functioning autism. *Neuroreport* 19(9):921–925.

Kemper, T. L. and M. Bauman. 1998. Neuropathology of infantile autism. *J. Neuropathol. Exp. Neurol.* 57(7):645–652.

Kennedy, D. P., K. Semendeferi, and E. Courchesne. 2007. No reduction of spindle neuron number in frontoinsular cortex in autism. *Brain Cogn.* 64(2):124–129.

Kim, E., J. Camacho, Z. Combs et al. 2015. Preliminary findings suggest the number and volume of supragranular and infragranular pyramidal neurons are similar in the anterior superior temporal area of control subjects and subjects with autism. *Neurosci. Lett.* 589:98–103.

Koldewyn, K. Y. A., S. Weigelt, H. Gweon, J. Julian, H. Richardson, C. Malloy, R. Saxe, B. Fischl, and N. Kanwisher. 2014. Differences in the right inferior longitudinal fasciculus but no general disruption of white matter tracts in children with autism spectrum disorder. *Proc. Natl. Acad. Sci. USA* 111(5):1981–1986.

Kotagiri, P. C. S., F. G. Szele, and M. M. Esiri. 2014. Subventricular zone cytoarchitecture changes in autism. *Dev. Neurobiol.* 74(1):25–41.

Langen, M., H. G. Schnack, H. Nederveen et al. 2009. Changes in the developmental trajectories of striatum in autism. *Biol. Psychiat.* 66(4):327–333.

Lawrence, Y. A., T. L. Kemper, M. L. Bauman, and G. J. Blatt. 2010. Parvalbumin-, calbindin-, and calretinin-immunoreactive hippocampal interneuron density in autism. *Acta Neurol. Scand.* 121(2):99–108.

Lewis, J. D., R. J. Theilmann, V. Fonov et al. 2013. Callosal fiber length and inter-hemispheric connectivity in adults with autism: Brain overgrowth and under-connectivity. *Hum. Brain Mapp.* 34(7):1685–1695.

Manes, F. P. J., D. Vrancic, V. Nanclares, C. Plebst, and S. E. Starkstein. 1999. An MRI study of the corpus callosum and cerebellum in mentally retarded autistic individuals. *J. Neuropsychiat. Clin. Neurosci.* 11(4):470–474.

Misaki, M., G. L. Wallace, N. Dankner, A. Martin, and P. A. Bandettini. 2012. Characteristic cortical thickness patterns in adolescents with autism spectrum disorders: Interactions with age and intellectual ability revealed by canonical correlation analysis. *Neuroimage* 60(3):1890–1901.

Morgan, J. T., G. Chana, I. Abramson, K. Semendeferi, E. Courchesne, and I. P. Everall. 2012. Abnormal microglial-neuronal spatial organization in the dorsolateral prefrontal cortex in autism. *Brain Res.* 1456:72–81.

Morgan, J. T., G. Chana, C. A. Pardo et al. 2010. Microglial activation and increased microglial density observed in the dorsolateral prefrontal cortex in autism. *Biol. Psychiat.* 68(4):368–376.

Palmen, S. J., H. E. Hulshoff Pol, C. Kemner et al. 2005. Increased gray-matter volume in medication-naive high-functioning children with autism spectrum disorder. *Psychol. Med.* 35(4):561–570.

Peterson, E., G. L. Schmidt, J. R. Tregellas et al. 2006. A voxel-based morphometry study of gray matter in parents of children with autism. *Neuroreport* 17(12):1289–1292.

Piven, J., S. Arndt, J. Bailey, and N. Andreasen. 1996. Regional brain enlargement in autism: A magnetic resonance imaging study. *J. Am. Acad. Child Adolesc. Psychiat.* 35(4):530–536.

Piven, J., J. Bailey, B. J. Ranson, and S. Arndt. 1997. An MRI study of the corpus callosum in autism. *Am. J. Psychiat.* 154(8):1051–1056.

Pryweller, J. R., K. B. Schauder, A. W. Anderson et al. 2014. White matter correlates of sensory processing in autism spectrum disorders. *Neuroimage Clin.* 6:379–387.

Raymond, G. V. B. M. and T. L. Kemper. 1996. Hippocampus in autism: A Golgi analysis. *Acta Neuropathol.* 91(1):117–119.

Riedel, A., S. Maier, M. Ulbrich et al. 2014. No significant brain volume decreases or increases in adults with high-functioning autism spectrum disorder and above average intelligence: A voxel-based morphometric study. *Psychiat. Res.* 223(2):67–74.

Ritvo, E. R., B. J. Freeman, A. Yuwiler et al. 1986. Fenfluramine treatment of autism: UCLA collaborative study of 81 patients at nine medical centers. *Psychopharmacol. Bull.* 22(1):133–140.

Rodier, P. M., J. L. Ingram, B. Tisdale, S. Nelson, and J. Romano. 1996. Embryological origin for autism: Developmental anomalies of the cranial nerve motor nuclei. *J. Comp. Neurol.* 370(2):247–261.

Rojas, D. C., E. Peterson, E. Winterrowd, M. L. Reite, S. J. Rogers, and J. R. Tregellas. 2006. Regional gray matter volumetric changes in autism associated with social and repetitive behavior symptoms. *BMC Psychiat.* 6:56.

Rojas, D. C., J. A. Smith, T. L. Benkers, S. L. Camou, M. L. Reite, and S. J. Rogers. 2004. Hippocampus and amygdala volumes in parents of children with autistic disorder. *Am. J. Psychiat.* 161(11):2038–2044.

Saitoh, O. C. E., B. Egaas, A. J. Lincoln, and L. Schreibman. 1995. Cross-sectional area of the posterior hippocampus in autistic patients with cerebellar and corpus callosum abnormalities. *Neurology* 45(2):317–324.

Saitoh, O. and E. Courchesne. 1998. Magnetic resonance imaging study of the brain in autism. *Psychiat. Clin. Neurosci.* 52 Suppl:S219–S222.

Santos, M., N. Uppal, C. Butti et al. 2011. Von Economo neurons in autism: A stereologic study of the frontoinsular cortex in children. *Brain Res.* 1380:206–217.

Sato, K. 2013. Placenta-derived hypo-serotonin situations in the developing forebrain cause autism. *Med. Hypoth.* 80(4):368–372.

Scheel, C., A. Rotarska-Jagiela, L. Schilbach et al. 2011. Imaging derived cortical thickness reduction in high-functioning autism: Key regions and temporal slope. *NeuroImage* 58(2):391–400.

Schumann, C. M. and D. G. Amaral. 2006. Stereological analysis of amygdala neuron number in autism. *J. Neurosci.* 26(29):7674–7679.

Scott, J. A., C. M. Schumann, B. L. Goodlin-Jones, and D. G. Amaral. 2009. A comprehensive volumetric analysis of the cerebellum in children and adolescents with autism spectrum disorder. *Autism Res.* 2(5):246–257.

Sears, L. L., C. Vest, S. Mohamed, J. Bailey, B. J. Ranson, and J. Piven. 1999. An MRI study of the basal ganglia in autism. *Prog. Neuropsychopharmacol. Biol. Psychiat.* 23(4):613–624.

Shukla, D. K., B. Keehn, A. J. Lincoln, and R. A. Muller. 2010. White matter compromise of callosal and subcortical fiber tracts in children with autism spectrum disorder: A diffusion tensor imaging study. *J. Am. Acad. Child Adolesc. Psychiat.* 49(12):1269–1278, 1278 e1261–e1262.

Simms, M. L., T. L. Kemper, C. M. Timbie, M. L. Bauman, and G. J. Blatt. 2009. The anterior cingulate cortex in autism: Heterogeneity of qualitative and quantitative cytoarchitectonic features suggests possible subgroups. *Acta Neuropathol.* 118(5):673–684.

Sivaswamy, L., A. Kumar, D. Rajan et al. 2010. A diffusion tensor imaging study of the cerebellar pathways in children with autism spectrum disorder. *J. Child Neurol.* 25(10):1223–1231.

Skefos, J., C. Cummings, K. Enzer et al. 2014. Regional alterations in Purkinje cell density in patients with autism. *PLoS One* 9(2):e81255.

Stoner, R., M. L. Chow, M. P. Boyle et al. 2014. Patches of disorganization in the neocortex of children with autism. *N. Engl. J. Med.* 370(13):1209–1219.

Sundaram, S. K., A. Kumar, M. I. Makki, M. E. Behen, H. T. Chugani, and D. C. Chugani. 2008. Diffusion tensor imaging of frontal lobe in autism spectrum disorder. *Cereb. Cortex* 18(11):2659–2665.

Thomas, C., K. Humphreys, K. J. Jung, N. Minshew, and M. Behrmann. 2011. The anatomy of the callosal and visual-association pathways in high-functioning autism: A DTI tractography study. *Cortex* 47(7):863–873.

Uppal, N., I. Gianatiempo, B. Wicinski et al. 2014a. Neuropathology of the postero-inferior occipitotemporal gyrus in children with autism. *Mol. Autism* 5(1):17.

Uppal, N., B. Wicinski, J. D. Buxbaum, H. Heinsen, C. Schmitz, and P. R. Hof. 2014b. Neuropathology of the anterior midcingulate cortex in young children with autism. *J. Neuropathol. Exp. Neurol.* 73(9):891–902.

van Kooten, I.A. P.S., P. von Cappeln, H. W. Steinbusch, H. Korr, H. Heinsen, P. R. Hof, H. van Engeland, and C. Schmitz. 2008. Neurons in the fusiform gyrus are fewer and smaller in autism. *Brain* 131(Pt 4):987–999.

Vidal, C.N., R. Nicolson, T. J. DeVito et al. 2006. Mapping corpus callosum deficits in autism: An index of aberrant cortical connectivity. *Biol Psychiat.* 60(3):218–225.

Wegiel, J., M. Flory, I. Kuchna et al. 2015. Neuronal nucleus and cytoplasm volume deficit in children with autism and volume increase in adolescents and adults. *Acta Neuropathol. Commun.* 3:2.

Wegiel, J., M. Flory, I. Kuchna et al. 2014. Stereological study of the neuronal number and volume of 38 brain subdivisions of subjects diagnosed with autism reveals significant alterations restricted to the striatum, amygdala and cerebellum. *Acta Neuropathol. Commun.* 2:141.

Wegiel, J., I. Kuchna, K. Nowicki et al. 2013. Contribution of olivofloccular circuitry developmental defects to atypical gaze in autism. *Brain Res.* 1512:106–122.

Whitney, E. R. K. T., M. L. Bauman, D. L. Rosene, and G. J. Blatt. 2008. Cerebellar Purkinje cells are reduced in a subpopulation of autistic brains: A stereological experiment using calbindin-D28k. *Cerebellum* 7(3):406–416.

Whitney, E. R., T. L. Kemper, D. L. Rosene, M. L. Bauman, and G. J. Blatt. 2009. Density of cerebellar basket and stellate cells in autism: Evidence for a late developmental loss of Purkinje cells. *J. Neurosci Res.* 87(10):2245–2254.

Williams, E. L. E.-B. A., M. Nitzken, A. E. Switala, and M. F. Casanova. 2012. Spherical harmonic analysis of cortical complexity in autism and dyslexia. *Trans. Neurosci.* 3(1):36–40.

Zielinski, B. A. P. M., J. A. Nielsen, A. L. Froehlich et al. 2014. Longitudinal changes in cortical thickness in autism and typical development. *Brain* 137(pt 6):1799–1812.

Zikopoulos, B. and H. Barbas. 2010. Changes in prefrontal axons may disrupt the network in autism. *J. Neurosci.* 30(44):14595–14609.

Chapter 5 Neurobiology of imitation in autism

Marco Iacoboni

Contents

Abstract 75
5.1 Introduction 75
5.2 Broken mirrors 76
    5.2.1 Imitation in ASD 76
    5.2.2 Mirror neurons 77
5.3 Imitation, MNS, and ASD 79
5.4 Unbroken? 81
    5.4.1 The imaging challenge 81
    5.4.2 The behavioral challenge 83
5.5 Taking control 84
    5.5.1 Pervasive mirroring 85
    5.5.2 Top-down and bottom-up 87
    5.5.3 The promise of noninvasive neuromodulation 89
5.6 Conclusion 91
References 91

Abstract

Recent work on the neurobiology of imitation in autism investigated early on deficits in the mirror neuron systems. This research also generated a number of criticisms. This chapter discussed this literature and concludes by reviewing more recent studies that focus on the complex interplay between imitation and its control. This more recent work promises to provide clues on potential interventions in autism that are tailored to the individual patients.

5.1 Introduction

Dysfunction in imitative behavior in autism has been reported a long time ago (Ritvo and Provence 1953). Yet the research on the neurobiology of imitation in autism did not pick up pace until approximately 10 or 15 years ago. The main reason for such a long incubation period is likely due to the inconvenient fact that the imitation impairment observed in autism had no easy way to fit the then dominant theoretical models of the condition. Some 25 years ago, however, converging research in the behavioral (Rogers and Pennington 1991) and brain sciences (di Pellegrino et al. 1992) ignited much interest in the role of impaired imitation in autism. After a brewing period of about 10 years, a hypothesis connecting the imitation deficit in autism to a specific neural system that had been recently discovered was proposed (Williams et al. 2001). Initial research on this hypothesis supported the main idea, and suggested a potential biomarker of the condition. This created excitement and generated further research, which is still very active today. Indeed, a PubMed search on imitation and autism returns 340 entries in early 2016, and more than a third of these entries were published in the previous 5 years.

This chapter is divided in three main parts. The first part is called "Broken Mirrors" and discusses briefly the early behavioral work on imitation in autism, the discovery of mirror neurons in monkeys and the subsequent research in humans, and the hypothesis of an impairment of mirror neurons in autism leading to imitative deficits in subjects with autism spectrum disorder (ASD). The second part is called "Unbroken?" and discusses some empirical challenges to the hypothesis of mirror neuron and even imitative deficits in autism. The last part is called "Taking Control" and discusses recent work on mirroring and its control that may inspire further research in the neurobiology of imitation in autism that could potentially lead to new forms of intervention.

5.2 Broken mirrors

5.2.1 Imitation in ASD

Observations and speculations regarding imitative impairment in autism date back more than 60 years (Ritvo and Provence 1953). The early behavioral studies faced two theoretical issues with no easy solution. First, imitation is an umbrella term covering many kinds of behaviors, which likely engage in various ways different sets of cognitive functions. Is imitative behavior in autism impaired across the board or is the impairment selective to certain kinds of imitation? The second one had to do with the type of processing that imitation deficits in autism reveal: Is it a general information processing disorder or is it a special one, associated with the social problems that subjects with autism typically experience? These are foundational questions with no easy answers and indeed they are still investigated today because they have not been conclusively solved.

The root of the problem is that imitation is a very complex behavior that cannot be easily reduced to a small set of operations. It is also a behavior that humans display in a number of domains, which are seemingly rather different. Imitating someone's voice and accent seems very different from imitating someone's posture and movement. Furthermore, imitation "in the wild" (i.e., during real-life events and situations) is inevitably very different from the kind of imitative tasks that can be performed in the lab. While the lab environment affords much better control over the behavior of the imitative subject, it is also a much more impoverished environment, compared to the richness and complexity of real-life contexts. Not surprisingly, results from empirical studies in the lab are not entirely concordant. The choice of the task matters, and the theory behind that choice matters too. These methodological issues have no easy solutions and they also affect the brain science literature on imitation in autism, as we will see later on in this chapter.

The early behavioral research on imitation impairments in autism also had another problem to face, which had to do with the rather limited knowledge on the neural correlates of imitative behavior in humans. Until some 25 years ago, the only relevant data were from neurological patients. While the neurological literature can obviously be quite illuminating on some functional aspects of behavior (we will see that it still is with regard to current brain research on imitation), it generally tends to provide fairly ambiguous information with regard to the neural systems and mechanisms associated with the behavior of interest. This is obviously due to the fact that naturally occurring lesions have a variety of locations and size, and that compensatory mechanisms that get into play after the lesion has occurred may complicate the behavioral correlates of the lesion. It is not surprising, then, that the early behavioral research on imitative impairments in autism had very little to say about the potential neural correlates of the impairment. This changed rather dramatically after the discovery of mirror neurons, which provided a compelling neural mechanism for imitative behavior.

5.2.2 Mirror neurons

In the early 1990s, a group of neurophysiologists that were investigating the single-cell properties of ventral premotor neurons in the macaque brain associated with grasping behavior reported a rather unexpected finding. Some of the grasping-related cells in the macaque premotor cortex were discharging not only when the subject was making a grasping action, but also when the monkey was observing another subject making the same action (di Pellegrino et al. 1992; Gallese et al. 1996). Sensory responses in premotor neurons had been previously described by the same group and other groups of neurophysiologists. However, previously reported sensory responses had been associated with much simpler stimuli. The perception of an action performed by someone else is a very complex type of perception, and yet the single-cell recordings from the ventral premotor cortex of the macaque brain were suggesting that the sensory "coding" of the premotor neurons was at the level of the whole action. These cells were eventually called mirror neurons because the sensory properties of the cells mirrored their motor properties. Or, to put it differently, the properties of these cells suggested that the monkey, when watching actions performed by others, was sort of seeing her own actions reflected by a mirror. The same group later reported that neurons in the inferior parietal cortex had also the same mirroring properties (Fogassi et al. 2005).

The discovery of mirror neurons was both serendipitous and exciting (serendipity and excitement often go together in scientific discoveries). Because of the excitement that propagated from the unexpected discovery of mirror neurons in monkeys, research in the human brain looking for similar mirroring phenomena started very early. Indeed, the very same group of neurophysiologists that discovered mirror neurons in monkeys reported the first findings in humans of a similar mirroring phenomenon (Fadiga et al. 1995). The scientists used transcranial magnetic stimulation (TMS), a tool that allows to stimulate the human brain noninvasively and painlessly. TMS was devised originally mostly to study human motor neurophysiology, and to replace the more painful (from the stimulated subject standpoint) transcranial electric stimulation. When TMS delivers a magnetic pulse over the motor cortex, it induces an electric current in the brain that stimulates the motor neurons and determines the contraction of muscles controlled by those neurons. The idea behind the first human study on neural mirroring was fairly simple. If humans have mirror neurons in their premotor cortex, the sight of someone else's action should activate these neurons. Since premotor neurons are only one synapse away from the motor cortex, the activation of a pool of premotor neurons should make the primary motor cortex more excitable. Hence, if a TMS pulse is delivered over the motor cortex while the stimulated subject is watching an action of someone else, there should be a bigger muscle contraction compared to watching a control visual stimulus that does not involve an action of someone else. Indeed, this was the case, and this finding and phenomenon (typically called "motor resonance" in this literature) has been replicated by many labs. Thus, TMS provided the first marker of mirror neuron activity in humans with the phenomenon of motor resonance.

Shortly thereafter, magnetoencephalography (MEG) and the much more scalable electroencephalography (EEG) provided the second marker of neural mirroring in humans. With both MEG and EEG, it is possible to record in central, sensory-motor brain regions, synchronized oscillating activity in the 10–20 Hz frequency range when subjects are at rest. When subjects make an action, this activity desynchronizes and subsequently synchronized activity reemerges when subjects stop moving. Obviously, the de-synchronization of these central rhythms is an indicator of motor activation. Then, if such de-synchronization also happens when subjects are not moving, but are watching actions of someone else (and does not happen during observation of control stimuli that do not involve actions of other people), it can be assumed that motor activation has been triggered by action observation. With both MEG and EEG, then, it is possible to measure a second marker of neural mirroring in humans. In the MEG literature, the parameter typically used to measure mirroring is called "beta rebound" (Hari et al. 1998), and quantifies the reappearance of oscillating activity around the 20 Hz frequency. In the EEG literature, the parameter typically used to measure mirroring is called "mu suppression" and quantifies the disappearance of oscillating activity around the 10 Hz frequency (Oberman et al. 2005).

Brain imaging provides the third marker of neural mirroring in humans. An early approach proposed to simply look at activation in premotor areas during both action execution and action observation (Rizzolatti et al. 1996). The brain imaging signal, however, comes from neurovascular coupling, that is, from the response in the vascular compartment to neural activation. As such, its spatial resolution is physiologically limited, and activation in the same voxels during action execution and action observation may be ambiguous. Most importantly, the physiological properties of mirror neurons seem to match very well the functional requirements of imitation, which is a pervasive and foundational human behavior that we use for learning, to connect with others, and for cultural transmission. For these reasons, we propose to use imitation tasks with functional magnetic resonance imaging (fMRI) to test whether human brain areas with mirror-like activity were involved in the imitative behavior (Iacoboni et al. 1999). The idea behind our first study was the following. If one looks at the discharge of mirror neurons in monkeys, one can see that mirror neurons discharge more strongly during action execution than during action observation (i.e., the firing rate change from baseline of the neuron is much higher for action execution than action observation) (Gallese et al. 1996). Hence, a mirror neuron area during action observation should have a signal increase in fMRI, which is lower than the signal increase during action execution. Most importantly, since imitation involves both observing and making an action, during imitation the same area should show an increased signal that resembles roughly the additive effect of the signal changes measured during action observation and action execution. Our first fMRI study on imitation in humans (the task was a simple finger movement task) reported two areas, in the frontal and parietal lobe, that had such a pattern of activity (Iacoboni et al. 1999). These areas were anatomically compatible with the two areas in the macaque brain in which mirror neurons had been previously recorded (Rizzolatti and Craighero 2004).

5.3 Imitation, MNS, and ASD

Shortly after we published out first fMRI study of imitation, a review article summarizing the previous behavioral studies on imitation in autism, the mirror neuron findings in macaques, and the brain imaging data in humans proposed the hypothesis of a mirror neuron dysfunction in autism (Williams et al. 2001). The main idea of this hypothesis was that a deficit in mirror neurons functions could potentially account for the imitation and social impairments in autism.

Links between imitation and social cognition had been proposed repeatedly. One of the most compelling empirical evidence in favor of this association had been provided by a study demonstrating that the more people imitate others during social interactions, the more they tend to be empathic (Chartrand and Bargh 1999). This suggested to us that mirror neuron areas and brain systems for emotions such as the limbic system had to be connected and communicate with each other. Anatomical data show that the insula is connected with both frontal and parietal mirror neuron areas and with the limbic system (Augustine 1985). This pattern of connectivity made the insula a good candidate for being part of a larger network including mirror neuron areas and limbic areas that supported empathy via imitation. To test this neural systems model, we used fMRI with an activation task that required healthy subjects to imitate facial emotional expressions. The results indeed supported the hypothesis that a circuitry including the inferior frontal mirror neuron area, the insula, and the amygdala was involved in our capacity to feel what others feel through imitation (Carr et al. 2003). Follow-up studies also demonstrated that the levels of activation in this circuitry during observation and imitation of facial emotional expressions correlated with self-reported empathy and social competence (Pfeifer et al. 2008).

On the basis of these results, we used the same activation task to test whether children with autism had reduced activity in the circuitry including the inferior frontal mirror neuron area, the insula, and the amygdala while observing and imitating facial emotional expressions. Indeed, compared to typically developing children, the children with autism demonstrated reduced activity in the inferior frontal mirror neuron area (Dapretto et al. 2006). Crucially, the reduced signal in the inferior frontal mirror neuron area in children with autism correlated with widely used clinical assessments of the severity of the condition. The more severe the autism, the more reduced the signal was in the inferior frontal mirror neuron area during observation and imitation of facial emotional expressions. These data suggested that markers of mirroring could potentially be markers of the severity of the autism condition in subjects with ASD (Iacoboni and Dapretto 2006).

Another group also reported that subjects with autism had reduced EEG mu suppression during observation of action compared to control subjects. This was an independent empirical finding—with a different marker—in support of the hypothesis of reduced mirroring in autism (Oberman et al. 2005). Obviously, after these two studies, the broken mirror hypothesis got traction and generated much interest and new research.

5.4 Unbroken?

For some time after the initial reports supporting the broken mirror hypothesis of autism, the hypothesis was some sort of media darling, being covered often by science reporters. Inevitably, when such high media attention to a scientific theory happens, some people feel that it is absolutely necessary to debunk the theory. This obviously happened also to the broken mirror hypothesis of autism. The challenges were mostly at two levels: whether the imaging data were convincing enough, and whether the behavioral data were really supporting an imitation deficit in autism. The two sections that form this middle part of the chapter address the merits of these challenges.

5.4.1 The imaging challenge

The first challenge that the broken mirror hypothesis of autism had to face on the imaging front was about the existence of mirror neurons in humans. If humans don't have mirror neurons, there can't be obviously an impairment of mirror neurons in autism. While this critique is actually rather tangential to the issue of imitation in autism, since it is such a foundational critique, it cannot be ignored. The critique on the imaging data was also curiously cavalier about the existence of the other two noninvasive markers of mirroring typically used in humans, the EEG mu suppression (and MEG beta rebound), and the "motor resonance" phenomenon observed with TMS. The main argument for focusing on brain imaging only seems to be based on the fact that brain imaging (fMRI) is more anatomically precise than EEG or TMS (Hamilton et al. 2007). We'll see at the beginning of the third part of this chapter that the anatomical precision is not much of a factor to be considered when studying neural mirroring with fMRI in humans, since reports of mirror neurons activity from single-cell recordings now include a number of neural systems encompassing three major lobes (the frontal lobe, the parietal lobe, and the temporal lobe). The pervasiveness of mirror neurons in a number of neural systems makes it difficult to "localize" mirror neuron responses with the use of anatomical information.

The main critique to the fMRI work on the mirror neurons system was that, in principle, there may be two completely different neuronal populations in the same area (say, premotor cortex): a population of motor neurons and a population of visual neurons. The motor neurons activate during action execution only and the visual neurons activate only during action observation. If these two functionally different neuronal populations coexist anatomically in the same area, with fMRI, one would see activation of the same voxels during both action execution and action observation, seemingly suggesting that a mirroring response is not there (Dinstein et al. 2008). When this critique was originally formulated, there was still no single-cell recording in humans, and the single-cell data were only recorded from the monkey brain. Monkey neurophysiologists, however, see very rarely responses in premotor areas that are exclusively visual. So, the critique seemed to be based on rather implausible physiological assumptions. However, a later depth electrode recording study in humans that indeed reported mirroring responses in the spiking activity of individual human cells (Mukamel et al. 2010), also reported an unexpectedly high number of purely visual neurons in frontal lobe areas of motor significance. Whether the difference between monkeys and humans in frequency of purely visual neurons in areas of motor significance is real or an artifact due to different recording practices (the study in humans has obviously many more limitations than the study in monkeys) is, at the moment, unclear. However, in light of the human data, the hypothesis of the two neuronal populations is not completely implausible.

The same group that raised this objection also proposed a solution to the problem. What was proposed was to use fMRI adaptation to truly image the activity of mirror neurons in humans exclusively (Dinstein et al. 2007). The use of fMRI adaptation had been proposed in the past to circumvent the limited spatial resolution of fMRI. The idea behind fMRI adaptation is that with clever experimental designs that repeat the presentation of stimuli in specific ways, it is possible to image only the population of neurons that are adapting to stimulus presentation. Unfortunately, this turned out not to be so simple and true even for populations of neurons that do adapt, like the MT motion direction selective cells (Bartels et al. 2008). But most importantly, in the case of mirror neurons, we now know that these cells do not adapt (Caggiano et al. 2013), at least for adaptation designs typically used in fMRI adaptation (Kilner et al. 2014). Hence, using fMRI adaptation paradigms to study mirroring responses makes very little sense, even though some studies seem to support this practice with results that seem in line with previous imaging findings using more traditional activation design (Kilner et al. 2009). It is at the moment unclear what is the neural origin of the adapting BOLD signal in these studies. It may reflect a decoupling between the spiking activity and the local field potential in the mirror neuron population.

A second, serious conceptual mistake that the fMRI adaptation literature on mirroring has made is related to the so-called cross-modal adaptation. The idea behind cross-modal adaptation is that mirror neurons are active during both action observation and action execution and seem to code specific actions. Thus, the observation of a grasping action preceded by the execution of the same action should show adaptation (Lingnau et al. 2009) (the cross-modal adaptation was proposed before single-cell recordings demonstrated lack of adaptation with two repetitions in mirror neurons). This was, however, conceptually wrong because it assumes that the functional locus of neuronal adaptation is at the level of its spiking output. Studies have, in contrast, shown that the locus of adaptation in truly adapting neurons is at a presynaptic level (Sawamura et al. 2006). Since the mirror neurons presumably receive presynaptic visual information from the temporal lobe during action observation but presynaptic prefrontal information about motor planning during action execution, there can't be presynaptic adaptation during "cross-modal" repetition, because the presynaptic inputs are different.

5.4.2 The behavioral challenge

The other challenge to the broken mirror hypothesis of autism comes from behavioral studies that fail to show imitation deficits in the ASD group compared to the control group (Sowden et al. 2015). There are many recently published studies on imitation in autism (sparked by the interest raised by the broken mirror hypothesis of autism) and this brief section does not intend to go over all this literature in detail. However, some important points need to be addressed here.

As we have discussed at the beginning of the chapter, imitation is an umbrella term for a number of behaviors, some very complex, some other simpler. Imitative behaviors and imitation tasks most likely engage diverse sets of cognitive and neural operations. It is unreasonable to expect similarity of performance across different kinds of imitation in autism. There will always be studies showing no imitation deficits in autism in some tasks, while other studies will show deficits. The unevenness of the reported results makes much more sense than seeing a consistent pattern across all studies, given the breadth and variety of tasks used and the broad phenotype of autism.

However, from this vast literature, some patterns do emerge. First, it is more likely to see imitation deficits in autism when tasks are more complex, more social, more linked to emotional behavior. It is less likely to see imitation deficits in autism for simpler tasks, tasks that have less social relevance, or tasks that do not tap onto emotional processing (Grecucci et al. 2013). It is also very likely that the lab environment is a much better context than real-life situation for the mind with autism. Thus, embedding imitation tasks into the lab makes it easier for subjects with autism to perform the task well. This does not guarantee, however, that when "in the wild," that is, in real-life situations, the same subjects can pick up and respond to social cues via imitative behavior as control subjects do. Imitation is a powerful way to connect with others, to learn from them, to conform to social expectations. It's rather effortless for most people, and indeed often people adopt imitative behaviors during social interactions in a prereflective, almost automatic way. Yet, a fluent and flexible imitative behavior does require complex streams of processing of sensory and motor information to be integrated with the emotional and reward value associated with it. The more complex is the scenario, the more likely it is that the imitative behavior may break down. But these complex scenarios are often left outside the lab. Failure to show an imitative deficit in a laboratory task often stripped down to very simple requirements can hardly deny the existence of imitative deficits in autism that had been noted many decades ago already. Furthermore, the beneficial effects of imitation-based interventions in autism are solid evidence that reinforcing imitative skills can only improve the clinical condition of the subject (Koehne et al. 2016).

There are two other important concepts to discuss in relation to imitative performance and its neural basis. Some of the behavioral studies on imitation in ASD make the unreasonable assumption that a lack of imitation deficit is evidence against the broken mirror hypothesis of autism (Sowden et al. 2015). This is a conceptual confusion of gigantic proportion. The assumption that lack of imitation deficits equals to normal functioning of mirror neurons relies on the notion that there is a one-to-one mapping between behavior and brain systems, such that one can look at behavior, and deduce the level of functioning of brain systems. It'd be nice if that were actually the case. We could throw away our magnets and scanners. But, unfortunately, it is not the case. There are compensatory mechanisms; there is neural plasticity. There is no way of looking at the imitative behavior of someone and inferring the level of functioning of her or his mirror neurons.

Indeed, in our first fMRI study on imitation of facial emotional expression in autism, we did see and report increased brain activity in the autism group compared to the typically developing group of subjects in some brain regions. We did interpret those findings as compensatory mechanisms (Dapretto et al. 2006). The reduced activity in the posterior part of the inferior frontal gyrus had to be compensated somehow, since our subjects with autism were able to perform the task. Obviously, we had to make sure that our subjects with autism were able to perform the task, as a difference in performance between the two groups of subjects would have made differences in brain activity uninterpretable. This does not mean, however, that the subjects with autism we studied in the scanner were skilled imitator that would have no problem imitating effortlessly and perhaps subconsciously other people during social interactions.

5.5 Taking control

From its outset, the research on the neurobiological mechanisms supporting imitation has been well aware that the spontaneous, prereflective imitation that humans display during social interactions requires mechanisms of control. While we unconsciously imitate others during social interactions, this imitative behavior is skillful enough not to get in the way of the social interaction. We do not mechanically and mindlessly parrot whatever the other person is doing and saying. We imitate others' postures and gestures and facial expressions and even language, but we do so subtly, in a nuanced, skillful way that gets often unnoticed at conscious level and facilitates human connection and bonding. How do we do that? The neurological literature has shown that there are neural mechanisms of imitation control. Patients with prefrontal lesions may exhibit "imitative behavior," the irresistible urge to imitate whatever the other person in front of them is doing. Patients already wearing glasses had the urge to put on themselves another pair of glasses only because they saw the doctor doing the same thing. These lesions tend to be large, which suggest that there are multiple control areas (Lhermitte et al. 1986; De Renzi et al. 1996). The research on imitation control has been inspired by these observations. However, this research has often been framed as if imitation control is something we consciously do. Yet, both our own phenomenology of social interactions and the imitation literature in neurological patients do suggest that the kind of control that keeps imitative behavior in check and makes it highly adaptive is very likely an "implicit" form of control, in which we don't have to make deliberations on how and when to control our tendency to imitate others.

How does this translate into neural mechanisms of imitation control, and control of mirror neuron activity? In recent years, some progress has been made on this front. And how does this research impact the research on autism and can potentially even suggest avenues for intervention and treatment? To start answering these questions, we first need to discuss the recent developments of the research on neural mirroring, which have important implications for the control of mirroring.

5.5.1 Pervasive mirroring

The single-unit recordings in macaques that led to the discovery of mirror neurons were performed in an area of the ventral premotor cortex (area F5 of the macaque brain) (di Pellegrino et al. 1992). After the initial recordings in F5, mirror neurons were also recorded in anterior areas of the inferior parietal lobule of the macaque (Fogassi et al. 2005). Single-cell recordings are time-consuming and complex, and can't obviously easily cover the whole brain, as brain imaging does. Also, neurophysiologists tend to record from very specific brain regions that they know well, rather than exploring a number of different brain areas they are not familiar with. The recordings in the anterior areas of the inferior parietal lobule of the macaque had been suggested by anatomical data that demonstrated that area F5 and the anterior inferior parietal cortex had many anatomical connections (Rizzolatti and Craighero 2004). They were also reinforced by physiological data on the properties of cells in the anterior inferior parietal cortex that demonstrated many grasping-related neurons in these areas, as in F5. On these anatomical and neurophysiological leads, it made sense to explore mirroring properties in the anterior inferior parietal lobule. Indeed,

85

such mirroring properties of neurons belonging to those areas were demonstrated in important studies.

Since area F5 and the connected anterior inferior parietal areas containing mirror neurons clearly belonged to a fronto-parietal circuitry for grasping-related behavior, for many years, the assumption of the neuroscience community had been that the mirror neuron system was a subsystem of these fronto-parietal circuits. All the imaging work in humans on mirroring had specifically looked for many years into the human homologues of those macaque areas to investigate mirror neuron responses in humans. Indeed, even now most of the imaging work on the mirror neuron system in autism is framed as if mirror neurons are only located in these fronto-parietal areas. This is, however, an oversight of recent developments in the single cell recordings work on neural mirroring that needs to be corrected. We have now compelling evidence of single-cell recordings demonstrating mirror neuron responses in a number of neural systems. In the macaque, the dorsal premotor cortex and the primary motor cortex have mirroring responses for reaching movements (Dushanova and Donoghue 2010). Also, the macaque lateral intraparietal area (LIP) that contains neurons controlling eye movements directed at attentionally salient stimuli has also mirroring responses for eye gaze of other individuals (Shepherd et al. 2009). Finally, the macaque ventral intraparietal area (VIP) that contains neurons with motor properties for arm, face, and neck movements that also have bimodal receptive fields for visual and tactile stimuli demonstrates also mirroring responses when the macaque is watching another individual being touched (Ishida et al. 2010). We now have also evidence from single-cell recordings in humans of mirror neurons in the medial frontal cortex and in the medial temporal cortex (Mukamel et al. 2010). Taken together, these findings show that mirror neurons are embedded in a large number of neural systems and mirror many different aspects of the actions of other people.

There are two main implications of these findings. First, the strategy of looking at specific anatomical regions to monitor mirror neuron activity with brain imaging (which can't record individual cells activity) is seriously problematic. It was problematic even before these new findings, but makes very little sense now. However, when it comes to imitative behavior, recent metadata do confirm the imitation circuitry that we had proposed early on in our imitation research (Caspers et al. 2010). It is likely that the activation pattern seen in imaging studies of imitation is dictated by the kinds of actions used in the experiment. Most imaging studies use either finger movements and hand actions or facial expressions. These are also the kinds of actions typically coded by the neurons in the fronto-parietal circuitry in which mirror neurons were originally found. It is not surprising to see corresponding human areas being active during the imitation of those kinds of actions. However, it is important to remember all the other neural systems with documented mirror neurons from single-cell recordings to avoid the mistake of considering only the grasping-related fronto-parietal circuitry the anatomical location of mirror neurons.

The second implication of the diffuse mirroring responses that recent studies suggest is relevant to the control of mirroring. Such diffuse mirroring constrains the type of control of mirroring that is required, since it determines how control areas can potentially transmit efficiently control signals to a number of diffuse brain areas. While there is still plenty of research that needs to be done on the control of mirroring and imitation, some data already available do support this flexible model of control of mirroring and imitation that requires both multiple control areas and parallel access to a number of cortical regions.

5.5.2 Top-down and bottom-up

Early imaging work on imitation control had suggested a role for the medial frontal cortex in controlling imitation (Brass et al. 2001). This finding was consistent with the neurological literature showing uncontrolled imitative behavior in patients with lesions in the frontal lobe. It is also consistent with more recent, more nuanced views on the neurobiology of imitation control. The study of imitation control is probably more important to research in autism than the study of imitation only. This is because while subjects with autism do show imitative deficits, they also show behaviors that demonstrate uncontrolled hyperimitation, such as echopraxia and echolalia. In light of these behaviors, it is possible to construe the imitative deficits in autism as part of a larger problem in imitation control.

While it is didactically useful to separate imitation and its control, however, very recent work suggests that perhaps one misses the point in focusing only on one of the two, either imitation or its control, because they are both heavily intertwined, as two continuous bottom-up and top-down processing streams. This concept does have implications also for interventions, as we will see in the last section of this part of the chapter.

Recent imaging evidence supports the idea that imitation control does require parallel access to a number of cortical areas in the human brain. In a recent study (Cross and Iacoboni 2013), the superior parietal cortex, the dorsal premotor cortex, the anterior insula, and the medial frontal cortex of both hemispheres demonstrated greater activity during imitation control compared to imitation (in the "imitation control" task subjects had to perform an action different from the one they were seeing). However, this same large network was also more active when subjects had to suppress the tendency to make an action spatially similar to a seen abstract spatial cue, thus suggesting that the increased activity in this large cortical network during imitation control was not specific to the suppression of imitation but rather to the suppression of any action that shared some similarity with visual stimuli of any kind. Nevertheless,

87

analysis of functional connectivity between this large cortical network and the rest of the brain demonstrated a selective increase in connectivity with thalamus and precuneus during imitation control. Thus, while levels of activation did not distinguish activity in this cortical network for prepotent action suppression, levels of functional connectivity with thalamus and precuneus indicated specificity for the control of imitation. The thalamic connectivity findings are especially of interest here, in light of the hypothesis that thalamo-cortical loops are especially important for flexible sensory-motor integration processes (Sherman and Guillery 2011). The findings of this study suggest that modulation of functional connectivity can be a powerful mechanism of control. In light of imaging data suggesting altered functional connectivity in autism, and the behavioral data suggesting altered control of imitation in ASD, this functional connectivity view of imitation control makes sense.

Recent studies in subjects with autism are consistent with this idea. Resting state fMRI has recently shown disrupted visuomotor functional connectivity in ASD, which is obviously important for imitation (Nebel et al. 2015). Another study has shown that subjects with autism, compared with control subjects, have reduced functional connectivity within the cortical circuitry for imitation that our early work had described, and increased connectivity between nodes of this circuitry and other cortical areas (Fishman et al. 2015). Furthermore, this study also demonstrated in ASD subjects altered structural connectivity within the imitation cortical circuitry that also correlated with clinical symptomatology.

One question that these studies left largely unexplored is whether and how much this matters to social competence and prosocial behavior, a dimension of high interest in autism. A recent study in healthy subjects suggests that the neural architecture of imitation and its control does matter for much more complex prosocial behavior (Christov-Moore and Iacoboni 2016). In this study, subjects first were studied with fMRI while they observed and imitated facial emotional expressions. After that, outside the scanner (indeed in a completely separate room) subjects played an economic game (the Dictator Game) that measures pure costly sharing, the sharing of money with strangers that has no strategic advantages. Correlation analyses between the brain activity during imitation of facial emotional expressions and sharing of money at the economic game demonstrated direct correlations between generosity and brain activity in brain areas that were engaged in mirroring the emotions, and inverse correlations in dorsolateral prefrontal cortex and medial prefrontal cortex, two areas classically associated with cognitive control, and specifically control of imitation in the case of medial prefrontal cortex. That is, the more subjects were mirroring in the scanner, the more they were generous later on at the economic game. Yet, the more they were controlling their mirroring in the scanner, the less they were generous at sharing money later on. These data do suggest relationships between imitation and its control and prosocial behavior.

Interestingly, connectivity data in autism do also suggest increased connectivity between prefrontal areas and the inferior frontal areas with mirroring properties we had identified in our imitation work (Shih et al. 2010). This increased connectivity may reflect increased control, which leads to reduced mirroring and imitation. Recent data from our lab suggest that it is possible to reduce such control, as we will see in the next section.

5.5.3 The promise of noninvasive neuromodulation

Two recent studies from our lab suggest that noninvasive neuromodulation can be used to modulate the control of imitation and prosociality. In the first study, we used fMRI while subjects were either imitating or "counterimitating" a finger movement (in this case, subjects were moving their finger in the opposite direction of the observed finger movement). Dynamic causal modeling analyses of the imaging data suggested that two areas in the medial prefrontal cortex were crucial in exerting imitative control over the posterior inferior frontal cortex area that our early work had associated with imitation (Cross et al. 2013) (a finding later confirmed by large meta-analyses of imaging studies of imitation and action observation) (Caspers et al. 2010).

A very recent study has used a type of very fast, patterned brain stimulation with TMS called theta burst stimulation (TBS) (Christov-Moore et al. 2016). The type of continuous TBS used in this study exerts inhibitory effects on the stimulated areas. Three groups of subjects were stimulated just before playing the Dictator Game. One group was stimulated over the MT/V5 complex, a major motion processing center in the human brain. This group was the control group. The other two groups were stimulated over the dorsolateral prefrontal cortex and the medial prefrontal cortex. The stimulation sites were determined by our previous study showing inverse correlations between these two areas and generosity at the Dictator Game (Christov-Moore and Iacoboni 2016). That is, we aimed at stimulating the peaks of such inverse correlation between brain activity during observation and imitation of facial emotional expressions and tendency to share money in costly altruism. The idea behind the study was that by inhibiting the activity in these areas, we would increase generosity. Indeed, this was the case, with interesting differences between the dorsolateral and medial prefrontal cortical areas stimulated. In this game, subjects share money with two types of players, players with high income and players with low income. Subjects generally tend to share more with players with low income, as players with high income are perceived not as in need of receiving money. Continuous TBS over the dorsolateral prefrontal cortex made subjects more generous with players of high income, whereas stimulation of the medial prefrontal cortex made subjects more generous with players of low income. These results suggest that while the dorsolateral prefrontal cortex exerts a type of "contextual" control (less perceived need does not require costly sharing, in this case), the medial prefrontal cortex seems to exert a form of tonic control on prosocial behavior, the type of control that determines our "baseline" generosity.

There is much interest now in the use of noninvasive neuromodulation in autism. This field is rapidly growing (Casanova et al. 2014; Oberman et al. 2015, 2016). The work on imitation and its control reviewed here suggests that by targeting with noninvasive neuromodulation cognitive control areas that seem to share control for imitation and prosocial behavior, it may be possible to improve social functioning in autism. This type of targeting, however, does require special care to maximize its potential effects, a type of care generally not used yet in noninvasive neuromodulation studies. For instance, our previous work had suggested that a crucial pathway for control of imitation and prosociality involves connections between the medial prefrontal cortex and the posterior inferior frontal cortex (Cross et al. 2013; Christov-Moore et al. 2016). In our TBS study over the two prefrontal areas, we had also obtained diffusion weighted imaging of most of our participating subjects. We

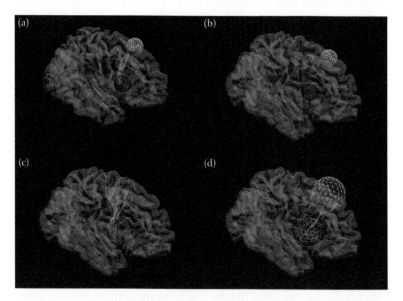

Figure 5.1 Variability in human white matter tracts and implications for TMS neuromodulation. When searching for white matter tracts connecting the dorsomedial prefrontal cortex (DMPFC) and the posterior inferior frontal gyrus (IFG) in a cohort of 60 healthy subjects, only in about half of these subjects, were the tracts visualized when using predefined coordinates (a). The remaining half did not show any tract (b). However, when keeping the same coordinates and enlarging the search, in these subjects, some tracts were visualizable (d). When exploring other cortical sites within the DMPFC, larger tracts were finally observed in these subjects (c). In these subjects, stimulating at predefined coordinates without knowing the underlying white matter anatomy may be less effective.

then decided to visualize the tracts connecting the targeted medial prefrontal area with the posterior inferior frontal cortex. However, only about half of the subjects had white matter tracts connecting the two areas with an origin at the site of stimulation. The remaining half had the white matter tracts connecting the medial prefrontal and the posterior inferior frontal cortex in neighboring cortical sites but not at the site of stimulation (see Figure 5.1). Also, the number of fibers differed widely between subjects. Since TMS effects spread through fiber tracts (the clearest example is the stimulation of the primary motor cortex and the subsequent motor evoked potential due to spreading of TMS effects through the corticospinal tract), all this information matters for effective neuromodulation. This means that an effective, personalized, precision noninvasive neuromodulation does ideally require multimodal imaging, including also diffusion MRI for better, more efficient targeting.

5.6 Conclusion

The study of the neurobiology of imitation in autism has generated much excitement in the last 15 years. A more mature research in this field should now take into account also the mechanisms of imitation control and their potential modulation. In order to do this more efficiently, it would be ideal to also use multimodal imaging for more rational targeting. Eventually, the study of the neurobiology of imitation and its control in autism, and also its response to neuromodulation, may become the type of research domain that NIMH has advocated recently for research in mental health. Subjects with autism may have reduced or dysfunctionally increased imitation that may originate from a number of potential interactions between areas with mirroring properties and areas of control. They may also respond in various ways to neuromodulation. Rather than asking the general, umbrella question of whether or not there is an imitation deficit in autism, future research should try to describe subtypes of autism on the basis of their imitative behavior and its control determined by the neural interactions between brain systems engaged in this behavior.

References

Augustine, J. R. 1985. The insular lobe in primates including humans. *Neurol. Res.* 7:2–10.

Bartels, A., N. K. Logothetis, and K. Moutoussis. 2008. fMRI and its interpretations: An illustration on directional selectivity in area V5/MT. *Trends Neurosci.* 31:444–53.

Brass, M., S. Zysset, and D. Y. von Cramon. 2001. The inhibition of imitative response tendencies. *Neuroimage* 14:1416–23.

Caggiano, V., J. K. Pomper, F. Fleischer, L. Fogassi, M. Giese, and P. Thier. 2013. Mirror neurons in monkey area F5 do not adapt to the observation of repeated actions. *Nat. Commun.* 4:1433.

Carr, L., M. Iacoboni, M. C. Dubeau, J. C. Mazziotta, and G. L. Lenzi. 2003. Neural mechanisms of empathy in humans: A relay from neural systems for imitation to limbic areas. *Proc. Natl. Acad. Sci. USA* 100:5497–502.

Casanova, M.F., M. K. Hensley, E. M. Sokhadze, A. S. El-Baz, Y. Wang et al. 2014. Effects of weekly low-frequency rTMS on autonomic measures in children with autism spectrum disorder. *Front. Hum. Neurosci.* 8:851.

Caspers, S., K. Zilles, A. R. Laird, and S. B. Eickhoff. 2010. ALE meta-analysis of action observation and imitation in the human brain. *NeuroImage* 50:1148–67.

Chartrand, T. L. and J. A. Bargh. 1999. The chameleon effect: The perception–behavior link and social interaction. *J. Personality Social Psychol.* 76: 893–910.

Christov-Moore, L. and M. Iacoboni. 2016. Self-other resonance, its control and prosocial inclinations: Brain–behavior relationships. *Hum. Brain Mapping* 37:1544–58.

Christov-Moore, L., T. Sugiyama, K. Grigaityte, and M. Iacoboni. 2016. Increasing generosity by disrupting prefrontal cortex. *Social Neurosci.*, 21:1–8. doi: 10.1080/17470919.2016.1154105.

Cross, K. A. and M. Iacoboni. 2013. Optimized neural coding? Control mechanisms in large cortical networks implemented by connectivity changes. *Hum. Brain Mapping* 34:213–25.

Cross, K. A., S. Torrisi, E. A. Losin, and M. Iacoboni. 2013. Controlling automatic imitative tendencies: Interactions between mirror neuron and cognitive control systems. *NeuroImage* 83:493–504.

Dapretto, M., M. S. Davies, J. H. Pfeifer, A. A. Scott, M. Sigman et al. 2006. Understanding emotions in others: Mirror neuron dysfunction in children with autism spectrum disorders. *Nat. Neurosci.* 9:28–30.

De Renzi, E, F. Cavalleri, and S. Facchini. 1996. Imitation and utilisation behaviour. *J. Neurol., Neurosurg. Psychiatry* 61:396–400.

Dinstein, I., U. Hasson, N. Rubin, and D. J. Heeger. 2007. Brain areas selective for both observed and executed movements. *J. Neurophysiol.* 98:1415–27.

Dinstein, I., C. Thomas, M. Behrmann, and D. J. Heeger. 2008. A mirror up to nature. *Curr. Biol.* 18:R13–8.

di Pellegrino, G., L. Fadiga, L. Fogassi, V. Gallese, and G. Rizzolatti. 1992. Understanding motor events: A neurophysiological study. *Exp. Brain Res.* 91:176–80.

Dushanova, J. and J. Donoghue. 2010. Neurons in primary motor cortex engaged during action observation. *Eur. J. Neurosci.* 31:386–98.

Fadiga, L., L. Fogassi, G. Pavesi, and G. Rizzolatti. 1995. Motor facilitation during action observation: A magnetic stimulation study. *J. Neurophysiol.* 73:2608–11.

Fishman, I., M. Datko, Y. Cabrera, R. A. Carper, and R. A. Müller. 2015. Reduced integration and differentiation of the imitation network in autism: A combined functional connectivity magnetic resonance imaging and diffusion-weighted imaging study. *Ann. Neurol.* 78:958–69.

Fogassi, L., P. F. Ferrari, B. Gesierich, S. Rozzi, F. Chersi, and G. Rizzolatti. 2005. Parietal lobe: From action organization to intention understanding. *Science* 308:662–7.

Gallese, V., L. Fadiga, L. Fogassi, and G. Rizzolatti. 1996. Action recognition in the premotor cortex. *Brain* 119:593–609.

Grecucci, A., P. Brambilla, R. Siugzdaite, D. Londero, F. Fabbro, and R. I. Rumiati. 2013. Emotional resonance deficits in autistic children. *J. Autism Dev. Disord.* 43:616–28.

Hamilton, A.F., R. M. Brindley, and U. Frith. 2007. Imitation and action understanding in autistic spectrum disorders: How valid is the hypothesis of a deficit in the mirror neuron system? *Neuropsychologia* 45:1859–68.

Hari, R., N. Forss, S. Avikainen, E. Kirveskari, S. Salenius, and G. Rizzolatti. 1998. Activation of human primary motor cortex during action observation: A neuromagnetic study. *Proc. Natl. Acad. Sci. USA* 95:15061–5.

Iacoboni, M. and M. Dapretto. 2006. The mirror neuron system and the consequences of its dysfunction. *Nat. Rev. Neurosci.* 7:942–51.

Iacoboni, M., R. P. Woods, M. Brass, H. Bekkering, J. C. Mazziotta, and G. Rizzolatti. 1999. Cortical mechanisms of human imitation. *Science* 286:2526–8.

Ishida, H., K. Nakajima, M. Inase, and A. Murata. 2010. Shared mapping of own and others' bodies in visuotactile bimodal area of monkey parietal cortex. *J. Cogn. Neurosci.* 22:83–96.

Kilner, J. M., A. Kraskov, and R. N. Lemon. 2014. Do monkey F5 mirror neurons show changes in firing rate during repeated observation of natural actions? *J. Neurophysiol.* 111:1214–26.

Kilner, J. M., A. Neal, N. Weiskopf, K. J. Friston, and C. D. Frith. 2009. Evidence of mirror neurons in human inferior frontal gyrus. *J. Neurosci.* 29:10153–9.

Koehne, S., A. Behrends, M. T. Fairhurst, and I. Dziobek. 2016. Fostering social cognition through an imitation- and synchronization-based dance/movement intervention in adults with autism spectrum disorder: A controlled proof-of-concept study. *Psychother. Psychosom.* 85:27–35.

Lhermitte, F., B. Pillon, and M. Serdaru. 1986. Human autonomy and the frontal lobes. Part I: Imitation and utilization behavior: A neuropsychological study of 75 patients. *Ann. Neurol.* 19:326–34.

Lingnau, A., B. Gesierich, and A. Caramazza. 2009. Asymmetric fMRI adaptation reveals no evidence for mirror neurons in humans. *Proc. Natl. Acad. Sci. USA* 106:9925–30.

Mukamel, R., A. D. Ekstrom, J. Kaplan, M. Iacoboni, and I. Fried. 2010. Single-neuron responses in humans during execution and observation of actions. *Curr. Biol.* 20:750–6.

Nebel, M. B., A. Eloyan, C. A. Nettles, K. L. Sweeney, K. Ament et al. 2015. Intrinsic visual-motor synchrony correlates with social deficits in autism. *Biol. Psychiatry* 79:633–41.

Oberman, L. M., P. G. Enticott, M. F. Casanova, A. Rotenberg, A. Pascual-Leone et al. 2016. Transcranial magnetic stimulation in autism spectrum disorder: Challenges, promise, and roadmap for future research. *Autism Res.* 9:184–203.

Oberman, L. M., E. M. Hubbard, J. P. McCleery, E. L. Altschuler, V. S. Ramachandran, and J. A. Pineda. 2005. EEG evidence for mirror neuron dysfunction in autism spectrum disorders. *Brain Res. Cogn. Brain Res.* 24:190–8.

Oberman, L. M., A. Rotenberg, and A. Pascual-Leone. 2015. Use of transcranial magnetic stimulation in autism spectrum disorders. *J. Autism Dev. Disord.* 45:524–36.

Pfeifer, J.H., M. Iacoboni, J. C. Mazziotta, and M. Dapretto. 2008. Mirroring others' emotions relates to empathy and interpersonal competence in children. *NeuroImage* 39:2076–85.

Ritvo, S. and S. Provence. 1953. From perception and imitation in some autistic children: Diagnostic findings and their contextual interpretation. *Psychoanal. Study Child* 8:155–61.

Rizzolatti, G. and L. Craighero. 2004. The mirror-neuron system. *Ann. Rev. Neurosci.* 27:169–92.

Rizzolatti, G., L. Fadiga, M. Matelli, V. Bettinardi, E. Paulesu et al. 1996. Localization of grasp representations in humans by PET: 1. Observation versus execution. *Exp. Brain Res.* 111:246–52.

Rogers, S. J. and B. F. Pennington. 1991. A theoretical approach to the deficits of infantile autism. *Dev. Psychopathol.* 3:137–62.

Sawamura, H., G. A. Orban, and R. Vogels. 2006. Selectivity of neuronal adaptation does not match response selectivity: A single-cell study of the FMRI adaptation paradigm. *Neuron* 49:307–18.

Shepherd, S. V., J. T. Klein, R. O. Deaner, and M. L. Platt. 2009. Mirroring of attention by neurons in macaque parietal cortex. *Proc. Natl. Acad. Sci. USA* 106:9489–94.

Sherman, S. M. and R. W. Guillery. 2011. Distinct functions for direct and transthalamic corticocortical connections. *J. Neurophysiol.* 106:1068–77.

Shih, P., M. Shen, B. Ottl, B. Keehn, M. S. Gaffrey, and R. A. Müller. 2010. Atypical network connectivity for imitation in autism spectrum disorder. *Neuropsychologia* 48:2931–9.

Sowden, S., S. Koehne, C. Catmur, I. Dziobek, and G. Bird. 2015. Intact automatic imitation and typical spatial compatibility in autism spectrum disorder: Challenging the broken mirror theory. *Autism Res.* 9:292–300.

Williams, J. H., A. Whiten, T. Suddendorf, and D. I. Perrett. 2001. Imitation, mirror neurons and autism. *Neurosci. Biobehav. Rev.* 25:287–95.

Chapter 6 Neuroimaging biomarkers for autism spectrum disorder

Christine Ecker and
Andre Marquand

Contents

Abstract 95
6.1 Introduction 96
6.2 Gold-standard diagnostic assessment tools for ASD and
    their limitations. 97
6.3 Neurobiological differences with ASD biomarker potential . . . 99
6.4 Advances in multivariate analytical techniques and
    predictive modeling as applied to neuroimaging data 100
6.5 Basic principles of multivariate pattern classification 102
    6.5.1 Acquisition of "training" data 103
    6.5.2 Feature extraction, feature selection, and
          dimensionality reduction 103
    6.5.3 Model training and optimization 104
    6.5.4 Validation using test data 104
6.6 The support vector machine. 106
6.7 Applications of multivariate pattern classification in ASD . . . 108
6.8 Current limitations to classification approaches. 111
6.9 Conclusions. 115
References 115

Abstract

Autism spectrum disorders (ASD) encompass a group of lifelong neuro-developmental conditions that are characterized by a triad of symptoms in impaired social communication, social reciprocity, and repetitive/stereotypic behavior. While the behavioral phenotype of ASD is well described, the search for autism biomarkers continues. Biomarker development has so far been hampered by the large degree of phenotypic complexity associated with ASD, and no "biological tests" yet exist that could facilitate case identification, or predict response to treatment.

However, recent studies utilizing novel analytical techniques with high exploratory and predictive power now hold promise for ASD biomarker development. In this chapter, we introduce the basic principles behind these so-called multivariate pattern classification (MVPC) approaches, and their application to neuroimaging data, and also review recent studies exploring their utility for biomarker development in the investigative (i.e., research) setting. Last, we will outline current limitations of MVPC and discuss several crucial research questions that need to be addressed first before these novel methods find their way into the real-world clinical practice.

6.1 Introduction

Autism spectrum disorder (ASD) comprises a group of heterogeneous neurodevelopmental conditions, which are typically characterized by a triad of symptoms consisting of (1) impaired communication, (2) social reciprocity, and (3) repetitive or stereotypic behavior (Wing 1997). There is increasing evidence to suggest that ASD is accompanied by neurodevelopmental differences in brain anatomy and connectivity, brain functioning, and neurochemistry (for review, see Amaral et al. 2008; Ecker et al. 2012a). Yet, the diagnosis of ASD remains to be based on clinical interviews and behavioral observations, and—unlike other areas of medicine—does not utilize biological markers. So far, the lack of such "biomarkers" for ASD has mainly been due to the genotypic and phenotypic complexity of the condition. Genetic studies suggest that ASD is not a single gene disorder but has a multifactorial genetic etiology (Abrahams and Geschwind 2008), which, in turn, leads to complex autistic phenotypes (see also Geschwind and Levitt 2007). For instance, it is known that autistic symptoms and traits are mediated by differences in multiple and spatially distributed neural systems, which result from an atypical developmental trajectory of brain maturation across the human life span (e.g., Courchesne 2002; Wallace et al. 2010; Zielinski et al. 2014). Due its phenotypic complexity, the neurobiology of ASD is thus inherently difficult to detect using conventional mass-univariate analytical approaches, which are predominantly based on mean differences between groups of individuals, and typically only consider a single neurobiological feature, rather than a set of multivariate biological measures. Moreover, conventional approaches to analyzing biological data are not well suited to making predictions at the level of individual patients, and are hence not informative for individuals of unknown diagnostic status. These conceptual issues have hampered the search for ASD biomarkers so far, and—until recently—little progress had been made toward identifying a set of biological measures that could be used for patient identification, stratification, and/or to predict the response to treatment.

Recent advances in analytical techniques, however, now make it possible to utilize complex biological data in order to make predictions. An important class of such techniques, known as multivariate pattern classification (MVPC) or "machine-learning" approaches, are currently being employed for biomarker development in various psychiatric disorders (reviewed in Klöppel et al. 2011; Orrù et al. 2012), predominantly using neuroimaging data coming from magnetic resonance imaging (MRI) or positron emission tomography (PET) studies, and are also becoming increasingly popular in the development for biomarkers for ASD (Ecker 2011; Ecker and Murphy 2014). While the implementation and application of these techniques in the everyday clinical practice remains a vision for the future, good progress has been made in exploring their clinical utility (e.g., for patient identification) in the research setting. The aims of this chapter are therefore (1) to highlight the clinical needs and limitations of gold-standard diagnostic assessments in ASD that could be overcome by the identification of biomarkers; (2) to introduce the basic concepts and methodological principles of MVPC as applied to neuroimaging data; (3) to review the progress that has been made so far in applying MVPC in the search of biomarkers for ASD; and (4) to outline some for the future challenges that have to be overcome first before biologically driven assessment tools for ASD find their way into clinical practice.

6.2 Gold-standard diagnostic assessment tools for ASD and their limitations

Due to the lifelong developmental nature of the condition, ASD is a disorder with particular clinical needs, not just in treating the often complex cluster of characteristic symptoms, but also in case identification. Despite the strong evidence for genetic and/or neurobiological underpinnings of ASD, the diagnosis and treatment of the condition is still solely based on symptomatology. Currently, ASD is being diagnosed with the help of two assessment tools, namely (1) the Autism Diagnostic Interview–Revised, ADI–R (Lord et al. 1994) and (2) the Autism Diagnostic Observation Schedule [ADOS; Lord et al. 1989]. The ADI–R is a semistandardized interview typically conducted with parents or carers of ASD individuals, and assesses the severity of autistic symptoms at the age of 4–5 years, which qualifies for a diagnosis of "childhood autism." The ADOS, on the other hand, is a semistructured assessment designed for use with the individual to be diagnosed, and assesses the severity of current autistic symptoms. Thus, the use of either ADI–R or ADOS can be problematic for diagnosing ASD in adult populations as (1) ADI–R assessments rely on the availability and reliability of an informant to give retrospective accounts of past autistic symptoms, which—in some cases—occurred many years ago; and (2) current symptoms assessed in adult samples are often masked by coping strategies developed across the human life span and potentially alleviated by treatments and interventions (e.g., social skills training or pharmacological interventions). It is therefore not uncommon for individuals to meet ADI–R but not ADOS diagnostic criteria during adulthood. Furthermore, certain cases present very specific difficulties for the behavioral diagnostic assessment of ASD, for example in case of severe co-occurring psychiatric disorders such as attention deficit hyperactivity disorder (ADHD), anxiety or mood disorders, and conduct disorders that—taken together—occur in up to 70% of people with ASD (Simonoff et al. 2008). A reliable diagnosis of ASD is also difficult to obtain in individuals with a learning disability, who make up approximately 40% of individuals on the low-functioning end of the ASD spectrum (Baird et al. 2006). Despite these limitations, however, diagnostic instruments such as the ADI–R and ADOS currently set the "gold standard" for diagnosing ASD in the general population, and for identifying "true positive" cases that will subsequently inform research into the etiology and neurobiology of ASD. While the behavioral diagnosis of ASD is highly advantageous in the clinical setting, as it can accommodate all variations of the autism spectrum regardless of their etiology and biological phenotype, for any biologist trying to determine the genetic and biological underpinning of ASD, starting with the behaviorally defined phenotype represents a heuristic challenge, which can also be compared with solving an inverse problem (i.e., similar behavioral or clinical symptoms may be explained by different genetic etiologies and different combinations of biological factors).

Indeed, there is strong evidence to suggest that ASD is a disorder with a large degree of genotypic and phenotypic heterogeneity. Genetic studies show that the genetic architecture of ASD is highly complex, and more than 100 disease genes and genomic loci have so far been implicated in the condition (Betancur 2011). It is estimated that about 10%–20% of the individuals with ASD have "syndromic" autism with an identified genetic etiology such as fragile X syndrome, tuberous sclerosis, or Rett syndrome (reviewed in Abrahams and Geschwind 2008). These autism-related monogenic syndromes share certain genetic variants with individuals with "idiopathic" or "nonsyndromic" autism for which there is no known etiology. Many of the genetic loci associated with ASD are, however, individually rare. For example, about 5%–10% of individuals with ASD have copy number variations (CNVs), which are genomic deletions and duplications, and that can either be inherited or occur *de novo* (Pinto et al. 2010). Based on these observations, ASD therefore does not follow a "common disease–common variant" model but rather a "common disease–multiple rare variants" model where a wide range of causative genetic variants can be found, each of which is individually rare and found in only a few people with the ASD (Betancur et al. 2009). Thus, while the gold standard behavioral diagnosis of ASD captures similar clinical phenotypes based on the classic triad of autistic symptoms, the genetic profile of individuals with ASD might actually be quite different. Moreover, the significant genotypic heterogeneity among individuals on the autism spectrum is also expected to elicit distinct neurobiological phenotypes, so that a diagnosis of ASD may potentially include different biological subgroups or "strata" of individuals with a shared neurobiological profile.

6.3 Neurobiological differences with ASD biomarker potential

Over the last decade, research into the neurobiology of ASD has high-lighted a range of neurobiological features in which individuals with ASD differ from neurotypical controls, and which may hence be utilized as potential biomarkers for the condition. Most of the neurobiological differences reported in ASD are localized in the brain itself and include measures of brain anatomy, connectivity, and brain functioning.

First, structural neuroimaging studies suggest that the brain in ASD undergoes an atypical developmental trajectory of brain maturation. Evidence for atypical neurodevelopment in ASD comes from several cross-sectional and longitudinal studies demonstrating that the brain in ASD is significantly enlarged during early childhood relative to typi-cally developing children (Piven et al. 1996; Courchesne et al. 2001). The early volumetric brain enlargement, which may have its origins even before the age of 2 years (Schumann et al. 2010), seems to persist until the age of 4–5 years, after which no significantly between-group differ-ences are typically observed (Hardan et al. 2009). These studies sug-gest that the brain in ASD might undergo a period of precocious brain overgrowth during early postnatal life—potentially driven by an accel-erated expansion of the cortical surface (Hazlett et al. 2011)—and that this period of accelerated growth is subsequently followed by a period of arrested growth or early decline during late childhood. Furthermore, during adolescence and adulthood, there are reports of accelerated corti-cal thinning in ASD individuals relative to controls (Wallace et al. 2010; Ecker et al. 2014), indicating that there are differences in brain devel-opment across the human life span in ASD. Such developmental dif-ferences are not restricted to individual brain regions but affect several large-scale neural systems, which are thought to mediate specific autistic symptoms and traits. For example, differences in regional brain anatomy in ASD have been reported in (1) fronto-temporal and fronto-parietal regions, (2) amygdala–hippocampal complex, (3) cerebellum, (4) basal ganglia, and (5) anterior and posterior cingulate regions (see Amaral et al. 2008 for a review). Such neuroanatomical differences in ASD may therefore also provide information that may be of diagnostic relevance.

Second, it has been suggested that the atypical development of the brain interferes with the development of brain connectivity in ASD (Geschwind and Levitt 2007), on the structural and functional level. For example, evidence for altered structural brain connectivity in ASD comes from neuroimaging studies investigating cortical white-matter show-ing, which show that individuals with ASD have spatially distributed reductions in white-matter volume during childhood, adolescence, and adulthood as measured using voxel-based morphometry (Waiter et al. 2005; McAlonan et al. 2009; Ecker et al. 2012b). Atypical structural connectivity in ASD has also been noted by numerous diffusion tensor imaging (DTI) studies, and particularly in fiber-tracts mediating autistic symptoms and traits (e.g., limbic pathways, frontostriatal circuitry, and corpus callosum) (e.g., Pugliese et al. 2009; Langen et al. 2011; Shukla et al. 2011). Taken together, these studies suggest that neuroanatomical differences in the brain in ASD are not restricted to gray matter only, but also include differences in the cortical white matter.

Last, it is also expected that the combined differences in gray and white matter affect brain functioning in ASD. Thus, a large number of functional MRI studies have examined the brain in ASD while participants perform a range of experimental tasks, most of which focus on socio-cognitive functions that relate to the cluster of behavioral symptoms typically observed in ASD (see above). For example, a large number of studies have reported reduced functional activation in ASD in brain regions comprising the "social brain network" during tasks related to (1) emotional processing or social cognition, including the amygdala, temporal–parietal junction, insula, and inferior frontal cortex (e.g., Castelli et al. 2002; Ashwin et al. 2007; Pelphrey et al. 2007; Koldewyn et al. 2011); (2) cognitive control and repetitive behaviors in the frontostriatal circuitry (e.g., Luna et al. 2002; Allen et al. 2004; Solomon et al. 2009); and (3) communication tasks in the language circuitry (e.g., Just et al. 2004; Eyler et al. 2012; Redcay et al. 2013). There is also strong support for differences in functional connectivity in the brain in ASD during the performance of many of the tasks listed above (e.g., Koshino et al. 2005; Just et al. 2007), and while the brain is "at rest" (e.g., Lai et al. 2010). Taken together, these previous neuroimaging studies suggest individuals with ASD differ significantly from typically developing controls in measures of brain anatomy, functioning, and brain connectivity. Using neuroimaging measures, it might therefore also be possible to distinguish individuals with ASD from typically developing controls, and to identify a set of biological markers that might provide meaningful prognostic/diagnostic information for ASD.

6.4 Advances in multivariate analytical techniques and predictive modeling as applied to neuroimaging data

The brain in ASD—and in other mental health conditions—has been investigated using a number of analytical techniques applied to magnetic resonance imaging (MRI) data in order to examine differences in brain anatomy, functioning, and connectivity. Most traditional techniques employed so-called mass-univariate approaches (e.g., statistical parametric mapping for functional MRI [Friston et al. 2004] data or voxel-based morphometry for structural MRI data [Ashburner and Friston 2000]), where each location in the brain is considered an independent spatial unit, and a separate statistical comparison is conducted at each voxel (or vertex) separately. While this approach significantly enhances the exploratory power over a region of interest analysis, corrections for multiple comparisons are required to limit the occurrence of false-positives (Genovese et al. 2002). Thus, mass-univariate approaches may be too conservative to detect the subtle morphological differences that are expected on the systems level, as is the case in ASD. Moreover, conventional approaches are ill-suited to describe individual cases, as statistical comparisons are conducted on the group level (e.g., using a general linear model [GLM]), and where statistical inferences are on the basis of population means, to which all individuals contribute equally, regardless of their interindividual differences in symptom severity, symptom profile, or demographic variables. Thus, conventional approaches to analyzing MRI data do not lend themselves naturally to making inferences about individual cases.

Some multivariate approaches, on the other hand, are optimized for making prediction at the level of individuals based on the intercorrelational structure in a large and potentially complex (e.g., multimodal) set of variables, which is often an intrinsic characteristic of biological data. In the context of functional brain imaging, these techniques have also been described as "brain-reading" or "brain-decoding" methods (Cox and Savoy 2003), and are a particular application of a wider group of techniques known collectively as supervised machine learning or multivariate pattern classification (MVPC). In brief, the basic idea of supervised machine learning is to train a computer algorithm to learn a decision function that predicts a categorical or continuous variable based on a set of labeled examples ("training phase"). Once such a decision function has been learned, it can then be applied on new individuals with potentially unknown labels to make a prediction ("testing phase") (Figure 6.1). Training ideally occurs in a well-characterized sample. In a classification context, where subjects are divided into two or more classes (e.g., patients and controls), this is achieved by finding a decision boundary or "hyperplane" that discriminates between different classes in a way that is in some sense optimal. Multivariate regression is a slightly more general problem and involves predicting a continuous outcome (e.g., symptom severity) in place of a class label. A key feature of pattern classification algorithms is their potential to detect distributed, complex and potentially multimodal patterns of potentially subtle abnormalities that cannot be easily identified with univariate methods. This makes supervised machine-learning approaches particularly well suited to the search for autism biomarkers, which could subsequently used for case identification, patient stratification, or for the prediction of clinical outcomes.

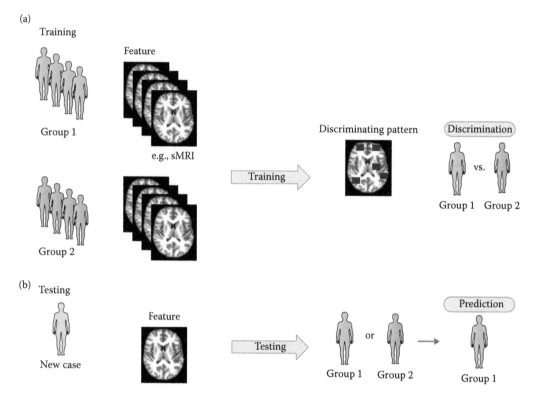

Figure 6.1 Basic principle of multivariate pattern classification as applied to neuroimaging data. (a) The classifier is initially on a well-characterized sample of biological data to derive a discriminative pattern of features that maximally separate the groups (i.e., "training" phase). (b) The pattern can then be used to predict group membership of a new set of data (i.e., "training" phase).

6.5 Basic principles of multivariate pattern classification

There are many different algorithms that have been used to perform multivariate pattern classification (MVPC) on neuroimaging data, which include the support vector machine (SVM) (e.g., Mourão-Miranda et al. 2009), Gaussian processes (GP) (e.g., Marquand et al. 2010; Doyle et al. 2013), random forests (e.g., Langs et al. 2011), and neural networks (e.g., Polyn et al. 2005) in addition to extensions of classical statistical techniques including linear discriminant analysis (e.g., Cox and Savoy 2003) and penalized logistic regression (e.g., Ryali et al. 2010). These approaches are commonly applied at either the whole-brain level, at the region/network of interest level, or by sweeping a local classifier across all brain voxels ("searchlight" approaches; Kriegeskorte et al. 2006). For clinical problems, including ASD, whole-brain classifiers are common and in this domain different classification algorithms often yield similar accuracy. The choice of which classification algorithm to employ therefore usually rests on the additional benefits provided by the different algorithms. For clinical problems, probabilistic predictions are often beneficial (see below), as are methods that provide a representation of the discriminating pattern that is sparse in the voxel or vertex space, which can help interpretation. Despite differences in the algorithms employed, most classification models follow a similar analytical pipeline that includes the following four steps.

6.5.1 Acquisition of "training" data

MVPC is a data-driven approach for the automated prediction of one of more classes (or groups) in which the decision boundary between classes is established based on a set of examples or training data. Any classifier can therefore only be as accurate as the labels assigned to the initial training set used for establishing the decision boundary and can also be influenced by the signal-to-noise ratio of the MRI image. It is thus essential that the training data includes well-characterized patients (i.e., true positive cases), which were initially identified using gold-standard assessment tools, in addition to neurotypical controls that do not have a clinical diagnosis (i.e., true negative cases). When establishing a classifier for ASD, it is thus essential to ensure that all cases meet ADOS and/or ADI–R cut-offs, which qualifies for a gold-standard diagnosis of ASD, while neurotypicals should have a few autistic symptoms and traits. This way, the resulting classifier will reflect properties in the training data that are related—if not specific—to ASD. In addition, careful acquisition, preprocessing, and quality control of MRI images are important for maximizing the accuracy of the trained classifier.

6.5.2 Feature extraction, feature selection, and dimensionality reduction

An important property of modern machine-learning methods is their ability to make accurate predictions in high-dimensional settings. This means that a large number of (biological) features can potentially be employed for the separation of individual classes. However, as biological data tends to be very high-dimensional in nature (e.g., large number of voxels in MRI image or large number of single nucleotide polymorphisms (SNP) in an SNP array) of which only a subset are assumed to be informative, it is common to include steps for feature extraction and/or feature selection. Feature extraction refers to the creation of new features from the raw data, aiming to summarize the data in a more informative way. Common approaches for feature extraction in neuroimaging data include parcellating the raw data into regions or networks based on a functional or anatomical atlas or performing a data decomposition such as principal or independent component analysis prior to classification (e.g., Mourão-Miranda et al. 2005; Anderson et al. 2010). In contrast to feature extraction, feature selection aims to remove as many noninformative features as possible while retaining features that carry discriminative information, thereby increasing the signal-to-noise ratio. In some, but not all cases, this is beneficial, depending on the particular feature selection approach employed and whether the underlying signal is distributed or focal. Again, many approaches have been demonstrated including hypothesis-driven, *a priori* selection of features expected to be of relevance to a particular disorder and data-driven approaches for selecting the optimal numbers of features prior to or as a part of the classification procedure (see Mwangi et al. 2014 for a review). Feature extraction and feature selection techniques are also often combined in the same analysis. In any case, the aim of this step is to generate a compact set of discriminative features that can be employed for training the classification model instead of the raw input data (see also Klöppel et al. 2011).

6.5.3 Model training and optimization

In this step, the decision boundary that best discriminates between the classes is identified in the training data, using the selected set of features. Depending on the specific classification approach, the decision boundary is found based on different criteria (e.g., maximum margin classification for the support vector machine, or probability theory for Gaussian process classification). These are described in further detail below. The set of parameters defining the decision boundary are optimized, ultimately aiming to find the model that generalizes accurately to new samples. This involves optimizing the parameters of the classification model itself, as well as additional parameters (often called hyperparameters), which might govern, for example, the degree of regularization applied to the classifier or the number of features selected. These additional parameters are often optimized by maximizing a measure of accuracy derived from the training set. In neuroimaging, most studies using MVPC tune and also validate classifier performance using the leave-one-out cross-validation approach, which provides a relatively unbiased estimate of the true generalization performance. Here, the classifier is trained repeatedly in an iterative fashion. In each iteration, one data set—or a data pair (e.g., patient and control)—are left out of the training set and the classifier is retrained using the remaining $n - 1$ pairs, where n denotes the total number of case control pairs. The model (or the set of parameters) that gives the best accuracy is then chosen as the final model.

6.5.4 Validation using test data

Once the optimal set of parameters defining the decision boundary has been identified, the model is validated or "tested" on a subset of the training data (see cross-validation above), or on a new and independent test data set (i.e., testing phase). If validation was performed using the leave-one-out approach, the model will be used to predict class membership of the sample pair that was left out in each iteration, and the accuracy of the classifier can then be determined based on the proportion of observations that were correctly classifier into their respective classes (e.g., patient or control group). In addition, the sensitivity and specificity and positive/negative predictive value (PPV/NPV) of the classifier are generally defined as

$$\text{Sensitivity} = \text{TP}/(\text{TP} + \text{FN})$$
$$\text{Specificity} = \text{TN}/(\text{TN} + \text{FP})$$
$$\text{PPV} = \text{TP}/(\text{TP} + \text{FP})$$
$$\text{NPV} = \text{TN}/(\text{TN} + \text{FN})$$

where TP is the number of true positives (i.e., the number of patients correctly classified as patients); TN is the number of true negatives (i.e., the number of controls correctly classified as controls); FP is the number of false-positives (i.e., the number of controls classified as patients); and FN is the number of false-negatives (i.e., the number of patients classified as controls). Additional measures such as receiver operating characteristic curves may also be useful to assess the classification performance across a range of decision thresholds.

An important issue for clinical studies is that class proportions may be unbalanced in that the training set may contain different numbers of each class. To avoid overly optimistic estimates of classifier performance in such cases, it is important to evaluate the classifier using statistics that accommodate class imbalance, for example the balanced accuracy (the mean of sensitivity and specificity [see Brodersen et al. 2010]). An illustration of the basic analysis pipeline for MVPC is provided in Figure 6.2.

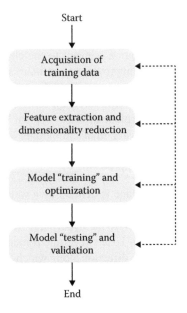

Figure 6.2 Processing steps involved in multivariate pattern classification.

6.6 The support vector machine

As an illustrative example, we consider one of the most widely used machine-learning techniques in neuroimaging, the support vector machine (SVM). The SVM is an algorithm that shows good categorical classification performance and has so far predominantly been used to distinguish patients from controls (i.e., binary outcomes or two-group classification). In the context of SVM, each MRI image is treated as a point in a high dimensional space, where the number of dimensions could, for example, equal the number of voxels in the image. The task of classifying the images into two classes can thus be viewed as a task of finding a separating hyperplane or a decision boundary, which is comparable to a diagnostic cut-off that separates patients from controls. In the training phase (see above), the algorithm finds a hyperplane that separates the examples in the input space according to their class labels. The classifier is trained by providing examples of the form <x,c>, where x represents a spatial pattern (e.g., gray matter image) and c is the class label (e.g., patient or control). Depending on the machine-learning method applied, there are many possible decision boundaries or hyperplanes. The SVM algorithm, however, is a "maximum margin classifier" (Vapnik 2000), where the margin is the distance from the separating hyperplane to the closest training examples. Thus, the SVM finds an optimal hyperplane in the sense that it is the one with the maximal margin (i.e., greater separation between the classes). By maximizing the margin between classes in the training set, it is hoped that the classifier will also show good generalization to unseen or future samples. The training examples that lie on the margin are the support vectors, which define the decision boundary or the hyperplane. Conceptually, the support vectors are also the data points, which are the most difficult to classify and also the points that carry all information relevant to the classification problem. The test margin of a data point provides a summary score for a particular individual and indicates how "prototypical" the individual is with regard to its respective class or diagnostic category. Thus, individuals located in close proximity of the hyperplane are less "typical" for their individual class and are harder to classify than individuals located further away from the decision boundary. Figure 6.3 illustrates an SVM classification for a two-group classification problem.

Mathematically, the hyperplane is defined by a weight vector **w** and an offset b. The weight vector is a linear combination of the support vectors and is normal (i.e., orthogonal) to the hyperplane. If the input space is an MRI image with a total of n voxels (i.e., one dimension per voxel), the weight vector **w** indicates the direction along which the classes are maximally separated. In case of a linear SVM, any hyperplane can also be written as a set of points **x** (e.g., voxel 1 to n) with $\mathbf{w} \cdot \mathbf{x} - b = 0$. Thus, the weight vector will also have n elements—one weight per voxel and can be used to generate a map of the most discriminating regions, which is also referred to as a discrimination map. However, because the classifier

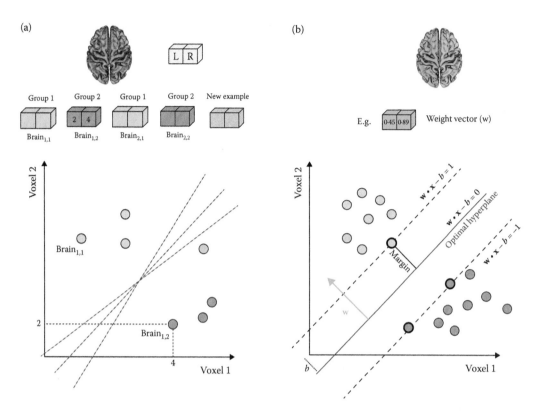

Figure 6.3 Two-group classification and support vector machine. (a) Illustration of a classification problem between two groups (e.g., patients vs. controls) for the simplified case of only two voxels (e.g., one data point per hemisphere). Each axis represents one voxel or hemisphere. Each symbol represents a brain image (e.g., gray matter map). The blue circles represent the images of controls (group 1), and the pink images represent images of patients (group 2). The dashed lines represent hyperplanes that correctly classify the groups. (b) Illustration of a hyperplane determined by the support vector machine (SVM) algorithm. The optimal hyperplane (red line) is the one with a margin of separation between the two classes. The symbols at the margin (thick outline) are the "support vectors." The separating hyperplanes are described by a learning weight vector **w**, which indicates the contribution of each voxel to the overall discrimination, and an offset *b*.

is multivariate by nature and also considers inter-regional correlations, the distribution of weights over all voxels should be interpreted as a distributed spatial pattern by which the groups differ. It does not provide inference about focal effects in the way that a GLM does. Hence, an individual voxel or brain regions may have high discriminative power due to two reasons: (1) there is a difference in mean volume or intensity measure useful to discriminate the groups, or (2) the region provides discriminative information mediated by its correlations with other features. Thus, discriminative networks resulting from MVPC should only be interpreted as spatially distributed "patterns" with discriminative information rather than making assumptions on their constituent parts (e.g., individual brain region). However, despite these limitations to the interpretability of multivariate prediction models, discrimination maps make it possible to differentiate between voxels or brain regions with high or low contributions to the overall classification accuracy, and hence highlight the relative importance of individual regions to distinguishing patients from controls in light of multivariate and complex biological data. While the biological plausibility and clinical relevance of multivariate patterns need to be confirmed by alternative analytical approaches (e.g., GLM), MVPC nevertheless offers significant exploratory power, in particular for conditions that involve multiple and correlated neural systems such as ASD.

6.7 Applications of multivariate pattern classification in ASD

There are an increasing number of publications applying multivariate pattern classification techniques in the investigative setting in order to assist the clinical diagnosis and prognosis of various psychiatric conditions, most of which employ the SVM. For example, neuroimaging-based pattern classification has been demonstrated to be sufficiently sensitive to separate patients with Alzheimer's disease (AD) from cognitively unaffected controls (Davatzikos et al. 2008), and to predict the conversion of mild cognitive impairment (MC) to AD (Davatzikos et al. 2011). In the ASD research, machine learning has also been applied to separate individuals with ASD from TD controls (i.e., for case identification). For example, Ecker et al. (2010b) explored the diagnostic value of whole-brain structural MRI scans representing regional gray and white matter volume for the identification of male adults with ASD using SVM. In a sample of 22 individuals with ASD and 22 matched controls, SVM correctly classified individuals with ASD and controls into their respective diagnostic categories in 87% of the cases, at a sensitivity of 0.88 and a specificity of 0.86 (Ecker et al. 2010b). In addition, Ecker et al. demonstrated that the test margins of each individual data set (i.e., the level of confidence with which an individual can be classified) were positively correlated with the severity of current autistic symptoms, thus suggesting that SVM may be able to capture ASD along a continuum, which is also reflected in its neuroanatomical imprint. The implementation of such a quantitative "dimensional" approach (rather than a simple binary or categorical classification) is very important as it enables machine-learning methods to provide an actual "biomarker," which acts as a quantitative indicator of a biologic or pathogenic process rather than simply testing for the existence/absence of a pathological phenotype.

In a second, independent sample of male adults with ASD, Ecker et al. (2010a) also employed a multiparameter classification approach to separate individuals with ASD from TD controls. Here, a set of five morphological features including volumetric and geometric features characterizing brain anatomy was employed to find a spatially distributed pattern of brain regions with maximal discriminative power. It was demonstrated that the ability of individual cortical features to discriminate between groups was highly variable across features and brain regions. For example, while SVM was able to identify individuals with ASD at a sensitivity and specificity of up to 0.90 and 0.80 overall in the left hemisphere (overall accuracy ~85%), accuracies based on features in the right hemisphere were not much more accurate than chance (i.e., overall accuracy was 65%). The best classification performance was obtained using cortical thickness measures in the left hemisphere, resulting in accuracies of up to 90%. Most importantly, however, this study also provided first steps toward addressing important question of the "clinical specificity" of automated neuroimaging-based classification approaches (i.e., although SVM may be able to distinguish individuals with ASD from controls, the classifier might not necessarily utilize neuroanatomical information that is specific to ASD rather than representing neurodevelopmental conditions in general).

Thus, to examine the clinical specificity of the automated approach, the authors utilized the established ASD classifier to predict group membership of individuals with attention deficit hyperactivity disorder (ADHD), which is highly comorbid with ASD (Simonoff et al. 2008), and may therefore serve as a neurodevelopmental control group. On the basis of the neuroanatomical information available for the left hemisphere, 78.9% of individuals with ADHD were allocated to the control category, and not to the ASD category, while the right hemisphere allocated cases with ADHD with approximately equal frequencies to both groups (Ecker et al. 2010a). Thus, it seems that a biological classifier that is highly accurate for ASD (i.e., 85% for left hemisphere vs. 65% for right hemisphere) is also more specific to the disorder than a classifier that displays low accuracies for the condition in the first place. Future research is, however, needed to determine how well MRI-based classifiers are able to separate individuals with ASD from the wide range of comorbid conditions—in addition to ADHD—typically observed in the clinical setting (e.g., social anxiety or obsessive-compulsive disorders, conduct disorders, etc. [Simonoff et al. 2008]), in order to establish the general clinical specificity of MRI-based classification approaches for ASD. For this, approaches that aim to directly discriminate between multiple conditions will be preferred to binary classification (e.g., Lim et al. 2013).

These original reports in male adults with ASD and TD controls, which provided "proof-of-concept," are also now supported by several other neuroimaging studies reporting similar classification accuracies have in younger age-groups (Jiao et al. 2010; Uddin et al. 2011; Wee et al. 2014), females with ASD (Calderoni et al. 2012), individuals with autism-related conditions such as fragile X syndrome (Hoeft et al. 2011), and using neuroimaging data coming from different image modalities and/

or multiple image parameters. For example, Anderson et al. (2011) utilized resting-state functional connectivity fMRI data to classify male adolescents with ASD, which is a finding that has recently been confirmed using a probabilistic neural network (Iidaka 2015). There are also reports that individuals with ASD may be identified based on their respective pattern of differences in structural white-matter connectivity as measured by diffusion tensor imaging (DTI) (Lange et al. 2010; Ingalhalikar et al. 2011), or in perfusion measures as measured by positron emission tomography (PET) (Duchesnay et al. 2011). Taken together, these studies add to the suggestion that there may be meaningful diagnostic information for ASD in measures of brain anatomy, functioning, and brain connectivity, and that high classification accuracies can be found in males with ASD and other autistic subgroups (e.g., females with ASD, children, or adolescents). However, it is important to note that a particular classifier is specific to the training sample (e.g., male adults with ASD and controls) and may not be generalizable to other groups of individuals (e.g., females with the condition). It is hence important to acquire a variety of different training samples that are expected to best reflect the neurobiological characteristics of different groups of individuals.

There are also a number of recent studies demonstrating that MVPC might be used to predict continuous outcome measures in addition to the traditional binary classification. For instance, Sato et al. (2013) used support vector regression to predict the severity of current autistic symptoms as measured by the Autism Diagnostic Observation Schedule utilizing inter-regional correlations of cortical thickness measures in a sample of individuals with ASD. Similarly, Coutanche et al. (2011) demonstrated that the severity of clinical symptoms might be predicted using multivoxel pattern analysis (MVPA) as applied to functional MRI data examining the neural basis for face processing. As mentioned above, the prediction of quantitative outcomes measures or multiple classes (e.g., multiple groups of patients) is of importance as it allows automated approaches to capture ASD along a continuum, rather than within an individual diagnostic category, which adds to the conceptual relevance and clinical importance of MVPC to ASD.

Last, due to the phenotypic complexity of the condition, it is unlikely that ASD can be linked to a single biomarker. Instead, ASD biomarkers are most likely to be multivariate and complex, encompassing data from different aspects of neurobiology as well as genetics. Several recent approaches have thus aimed at integrating information across multiple biological measures in order to improve diagnostic accuracy. For example, Wee et al. (2014) demonstrated that the integration of regional and interregional features via multikernel learning can significantly improve the classification performance for ASD as compared with using either regional or interregional features alone. A multimodal "fusion" approach combining magnetoencephalography (MEG) and DTI data was also employed by Ingalhalikar et al. (2014) in order to discriminate between individuals with and without language impairment. Here, the outputs from the MEG- and DTI-based classifiers were fused using a weighted aggregation giving an aggregate probabilistic score for each subject, which provided a higher classification accuracy in comparison with single modality classifiers. There is also some evidence to suggest that genetic models may add significant predictive value to neuroimaging-driven classifiers and may even outperform neuroanatomical classifiers for ASD in some circumstances (Jiao et al. 2011). Thus, the development of novel approaches to MVPC will be crucial in the future to enhance the flexibility and generalizability of findings across various groups of individuals, and to overcome some of the current limitation of conventional machine-learning approaches. Moreover, it is also possible that different sets of biomarkers may be suited to different clinical decisions and to different types of patients. For example, predicting quantitative measures of symptom severity may be achieved more effectively using different types of features than would be optimal for predicting a binary class decision.

6.8 Current limitations to classification approaches

While pattern classification approaches hold promise for assisting the behavioral diagnosis of ASD or for predicting clinical outcomes (e.g., response to treatment), several crucial issues will need to be addressed first before these methods find their way into everyday clinical practice. Notably, it will be crucial to address the clinical specificity of automated, biologically driven approaches by validating them in the real-world clinical setting. For example, although MVPC might be successful at distinguishing individuals with ASD from TD controls in the research setting, it is currently unknown how well MRI-based classification models will function in heterogeneous, real-world populations of individuals on the autism spectrum, and in distinguishing individuals with ASD from related comorbid conditions that typically present in the everyday mental health setting (see above). The acquisition of testing samples acquired in the real-world clinical setting and comprising samples that are independent of the actual testing data thus constitutes a crucial next step toward developing ASD biomarkers for clinical applications. Similarly, it will be important to acquire carefully controlled training samples that allow, for example, comorbidities and clinical variability to be modeled explicitly. A limitation with most current studies is that they have employed binary classification to separate, for example, ASD patients and controls. As noted, the real-world decision problem is much more complex, that is, it is not sufficient only to discriminate ASD patients from controls. Instead, what is required is a differential diagnosis enabling ASD patients to be separated from controls, from other patient groups and from patients with

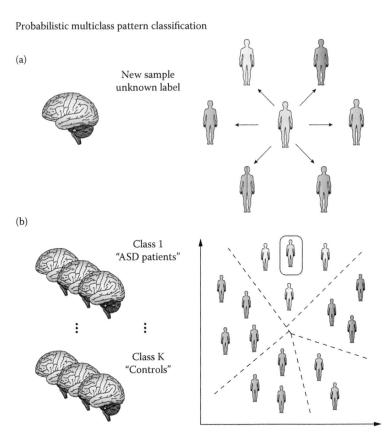

Probabilistic multiclass pattern classification

(a)

New sample
unknown label

(b)

Class 1
"ASD patients"

⋮   ⋮

Class K
"Controls"

Figure 6.4 Multiclass classification for a differential diagnosis of ASD.
(a) Each color represents a different group of individuals with different
diagnostic labels (e.g., ADHD, OCD, etc.). The two-colored example
represents a class of individuals with two comorbid conditions (e.g., ASD
and ADHD). (b) During testing, a new data set is compared to diagnostic
class and allocated to the best-fitting category.

comorbidities. While the methodological machinery for such multiclass
classification (Figure 6.4) has been demonstrated for other disorders (e.g.,
Lim et al. 2013; Marquand et al. 2013), a lack of suitably large and carefully controlled data sets has precluded more widespread application of
these techniques to ASD and related neurodevelopmental disorders. The
issue of comorbidities, in particular, has received little attention to date.
To address these problems, it is necessary to acquire carefully controlled
prospective samples containing a sufficient proportion of members of
each class to enable machine-learning techniques to be applied.

Another crucial issue that is not well addressed by most current techniques is to provide mechanisms to accommodate variability in prior class
frequencies (Bishop 2006). For example, in most clinical studies, classifiers are trained on samples with approximately balanced classes. That is,

the frequency of patients is approximately the same as the frequency of controls. This is very different from both the prevalence of ASD in the general population and the proportion of ASD cases that can be expected in specialist mental health settings. The prevalence of ASD in the general population is estimated to be approximately 1% (Baird et al. 2006), which means that there are 99 times more individuals that do not have a diagnosis of ASD than individuals with a diagnosis of ASD. On the one hand, training a classifier using the true class frequencies is highly suboptimal because many fewer cases than controls can be included in the training set, leading to poor coverage of the ASD phenotype. Even more problematical, is that in practice, it is difficult to prevent the classifier from reaching the trivial solution of always predicting the larger class (which would yield 99% accuracy in this case). On the other hand, training a classifier using a balanced sample and then applying it to a setting with class frequencies that do reflect disease prevalence leads to a classifier that provides an unacceptably high false-positive rate (or equivalently, a very low PPV), rendering it almost useless in practice. Fortunately, probabilistic classifiers provide a simple way to overcome these limitations. In comparison to conventional SVM-type classification, it is possible to recalibrate probabilistic predictions (e.g., from GPCs) to compensate for variable class priors. This ensures that inference remains coherent even if the frequency of each class in the test data is substantially different from the class frequencies in the training data (Svensén and Bishop 2007). A proof of concept of this idea was demonstrated for neuroimaging by Hahn et al. (2013). However, it is clear that work remains to be done to validate and translate this approach to ASD. Moreover, existing methods are also ill-suited to deal with the large degree of interindividual variability in biological measures that are typically observed in ASD. Probabilistic pattern classification, on the other hand, makes it possible to quantify predictive confidence, which can indicate whether a prediction is confident enough to be considered definitive, or whether further investigation is warranted (Figure 6.5). For example, a high predictive confidence (e.g., 90%) for a single class (e.g., ASD) in comparison to alternative classes (e.g., ADHD, OCD, etc.) may indicate a typical or "pure" diagnosis of ASD without comorbidities, whereas a medium predictive confidence for 60% for ASD and 40% for ADHD may indicate an ASD case with comorbid ADHD. It will thus be important in the future to explore the clinical utility of probabilistic pattern classification methods in addition to conventional SVM-type approaches in order to fully establish the translational research potential of MVPC in the clinical setting.

It is also important to note that MRI-based classifiers are theoretically not expected to perform better than "gold-standard" tools. For example, studies suggest that MRI-based classifiers provide accuracies for ASD that compare well with the behaviorally guided diagnostic tools, which provide accuracies of ~80% on average (see above for references). However, it is important to note that the accuracy of any biologically driven classifier can never exceed the sensitivity and specificity of the

113

Predictive confidence in the prediction of multiple classes

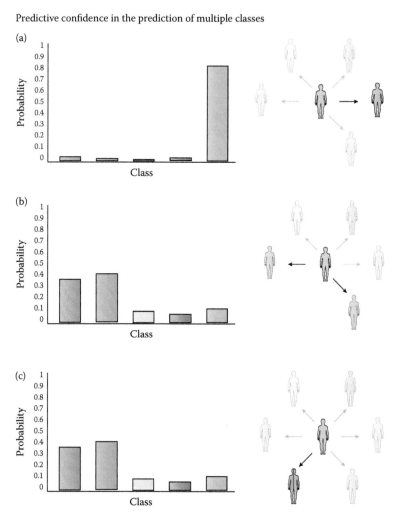

Figure 6.5 Predictive confidence for class membership as quantified using probabilistic pattern classification to indicate whether a prediction is confident enough to be considered definite. (a) High predictive confidence for a single class and hence confident assignment to one class, or equal confidence for multiple classes (b) indicating a potential comorbid diagnosis (c).

diagnostic gold standard that was used to define the sample of true positives and true negatives in the training set. Thus, if a classifier is trained on the basis of cases identified by ADOS or ADI–R gold standards, the maximal power a classification approach could reach is equal to the accuracy of ADOS and/or ADI–R. Therefore, an interesting area of future research could be to employ classification models that are tolerant to labeling errors in the training set (e.g., Kim and Ghahramani 2008; Frénay and Verleysen 2014). In such contexts, disagreement between the clinical diagnostic labels and the predictions from neurobiologically derived biomarkers could provide important insights into the underlying disease pathology. From a practical standpoint, this also implies that biologically driven approaches should not be used instead of the conventional gold-standard assessment tools for ASD but rather in addition to the behavioral gold standard assessment, especially in cases where insufficient clinical data is available to warrant a diagnosis of ASD.

6.9 Conclusions

Over the last two decades, neuroimaging approaches have had a crucial role in identifying the large-scale neural substrates that underlie autistic symptoms and traits. However, the role of neuroimaging in mental health research is currently transitioning from a basic scientific research tools to a clinical application that might inform the assessment and treatment of ASD in the future. While the behavioral diagnosis of ASD is invaluable in the clinical setting, it is also often problematic, particularly in adults where individuals have developed coping strategies across the life span that mask current symptoms, or where informants are no longer available to give reliable clinical accounts. The clinical usefulness of neuroimaging-based multivariate pattern classification approaches is therefore currently being explored for patient identification in the research setting. However, the clinical implementation of these approaches remains dependent on their clinical validation, which will be a crucial next step in the search for ASD biomarkers.

References

Abrahams, B. S. and D. H. Geschwind. 2008. Advances in autism genetics: On the threshold of a new neurobiology. *Nat. Rev. Genet.* 9:341–55. doi: 10.1038/nrg2346.

Allen, G., R.-A. Müller, and E. Courchesne. 2004. Cerebellar function in autism: Functional magnetic resonance image activation during a simple motor task. *Biol. Psychiatry* 56:269–78. doi: 10.1016/j.biopsych.2004.06.005.

Amaral, D. G., C. M. Schumann, and C. W. Nordahl. 2008. Neuroanatomy of autism. *Trends Neurosci.* 31:137–45. doi: 10.1016/j.tins.2007.12.005.

Anderson, A., I. D. Dinov, J. E. Sherin, J. Quintana, A. L. Yuille, and M. S. Cohen. 2010. Classification of spatially unaligned fMRI scans. *NeuroImage* 49:2509–19. doi: 10.1016/j.neuroimage.2009.08.036.

Anderson, J. S., J. A. Nielsen, A. L. Froehlich et al. 2011. Functional connectivity magnetic resonance imaging classification of autism. *Brain* 13:3739–51. doi: 10.1093/brain/awr263.

Ashburner, J. and K. J. Friston. 2000. Voxel-based morphometry—The methods. *NeuroImage* 11:805–21. doi: 10.1006/nimg.2000.0582.

Ashwin, C., S. Baron-Cohen, S. Wheelwright, M. O'Riordan, and E. T. Bullmore. 2007. Differential activation of the amygdala and the "social brain" during fearful face-processing in Asperger syndrome. *Neuropsychologia* 45:2–14. doi: 10.1016/j.neuropsychologia.2006.04.014.

Baird, G., E. Simonoff, A. Pickles, S. Chandler, T. Loucas, D. Meldrum, and T. Charman. 2006. Prevalence of disorders of the autism spectrum in a population cohort of children in South Thames: The Special Needs and Autism Project (SNAP). *Lancet* 368:210–15. doi: 10.1016/S0140-6736(06)69041-7.

Betancur, C. 2011. Etiological heterogeneity in autism spectrum disorders: More than 100 genetic and genomic disorders and still counting. *Brain Res.* 1380:42–77. doi: 10.1016/j.brainres.2010.11.078.

Betancur, C., T. Sakurai, and J. D. Buxbaum. 2009. The emerging role of synaptic cell-adhesion pathways in the pathogenesis of autism spectrum disorders. *Trends Neurosci.* 32(7): 402–12. doi: 10.1016/j.tins.2009.04.003.

Bishop, C. M. 2006. *Pattern Recognition and Machine Learning.* New York: Springer.

Brodersen, K. H., C. S. Ong, and K. E. Stephan. 2010. The balanced accuracy and its posterior distribution. *Int. Conf. Pattern Recog.* 20:3121–4.

Calderoni, S., A. Retico, L. Biagi, R. Tancredi, F. Muratori, and M. Tosetti. 2012. Female children with autism spectrum disorder: An insight from mass-univariate and pattern classification analyses. *NeuroImage* 59:1013–22. doi: 10.1016/j.neuroimage.2011.08.070.

Castelli, F., C. Frith, F. Happé, and U. Frith. 2002. Autism, Asperger syndrome and brain mechanisms for the attribution of mental states to animated shapes. *Brain* 125:1839–49.

Courchesne, E. 2002. Abnormal early brain development in autism. *Mol. Psychiatry* 7(Suppl 2):S21–3. doi: 10.1038/sj.mp.4001169.

Courchesne, E., C. M. Karns, H. R. Davis et al. 2001. Unusual brain growth patterns in early life in patients with autistic disorder: An MRI study. *Neurology* 57:245–54.

Coutanche, M. N., S. L. Thompson-Schill, and R. T. Schultz. 2011. Multi-voxel pattern analysis of fMRI data predicts clinical symptom severity. *NeuroImage* 57:113–23. doi: 10.1016/j.neuroimage.2011.04.016.

Cox, D. D. and R. L. Savoy. 2003. Functional magnetic resonance imaging (fMRI) "brain reading": Detecting and classifying distributed patterns of fMRI activity in human visual cortex. *NeuroImage* 19:261–70.

Davatzikos, C., P. Bhatt, L. M. Shaw, K. N. Batmanghelich, and J. Q. Trojanowski. 2011. Prediction of MCI to AD conversion, via MRI, CSF biomarkers, and pattern classification. *Neurobiol. Aging* 32:2322.e19–27. doi: 10.1016/j.neurobiolaging.2010.05.023.

Davatzikos, C., S. M. Resnick, X. Wu, P. Parmpi, and C. M. Clark. 2008. Individual patient diagnosis of AD and FTD via high-dimensional pattern classification of MRI. *NeuroImage* 41:1220–27. doi: 10.1016/j.neuroimage.2008.03.050.

Doyle, O. M., J. Ashburner, F. O. Zelaya, S. C. R. Williams, M. A. Mehta, and A. F. Marquand. 2013. Multivariate decoding of brain images using ordinal regression. *NeuroImage* 81:347–57. doi: 10.1016/j.neuroimage.2013.05.036.

Duchesnay, E., A. Cachia, N. Boddaert, N. Chabane, J.-F. Mangin, J.-L. Martinot, F. Brunelle, and M. Zilbovicius. 2011. Feature selection and classification of imbalanced datasets: Application to PET images of children with autistic spectrum disorders. *NeuroImage* 57:1003–14. doi: 10.1016/j.neuroimage.2011.05.011.

Ecker, C. 2011. Autism biomarkers for more efficacious diagnosis. *Biomarkers Med.* 5:193–95. doi: 10.2217/bmm.11.13.

Ecker, C., A. Marquand, J. Mourão-Miranda et al. 2010a. Describing the brain in autism in five dimensions—Magnetic resonance imaging-assisted diagnosis of autism spectrum disorder using a multiparameter classification approach. *J. Neurosci.* 30:10612–23. doi: 10.1523/JNEUROSCI.5413-09.2010.

Ecker, C. and D. Murphy. 2014. Neuroimaging in autism—From basic science to translational research. *Nat. Rev. Neurol.* 10:82–91. doi: 10.1038/nrneurol.2013.276.

Ecker, C., V. Rocha-Rego, P. Johnston, J. Mourão-Miranda, A. Marquand, E. M. Daly, M. J. Brammer, C. Murphy, D. G. Murphy, and the MRC AIMS Consortium. 2010b. Investigating the predictive value of whole-brain structural MR scans in autism: A pattern classification approach. *NeuroImage* 49:44–56. doi: 10.1016/j.neuroimage.2009.08.024.

Ecker, C., W. Spooren, and D. G. M. Murphy. 2012a. Translational approaches to the biology of autism: False dawn or a new era? *Mol. Psychiatry* 18:435–42. doi: 10.1038/mp.2012.102.

Ecker, C., A. Shahidiani, Y. Feng et al. 2014. The effect of age, diagnosis, and their interaction on vertex-based measures of cortical thickness and surface area in autism spectrum disorder. *J. Neural Transmission* 121:1157–70. doi: 10.1007/s00702-014-1207-1.

Ecker, C., J. Suckling, S. C. Deoni et al. 2012b. Brain anatomy and its relationship to behavior in adults with autism spectrum disorder: A multicenter magnetic resonance imaging study. *Arch. Gen. Psychiatry* 69:195–209. doi: 10.1001/archgenpsychiatry.2011.1251.

Eyler, L. T., K. Pierce, and E. Courchesne. 2012. A failure of left temporal cortex to specialize for language is an early emerging and fundamental property of autism. *Brain* 135:949–60. doi: 10.1093/brain/awr364.

Frénay, B. and M. Verleysen. 2014. Classification in the presence of label noise: A survey. *IEEE Trans. Neural Networks Learning Systems* 25:845–69. doi: 10.1109/TNNLS.2013.2292894.

Friston, K. J., A. P. Holmes, K. J. Worsley, J. P. Poline, C. D. Frith, and R. S. J. Frackowiak. 2004. Statistical parametric maps in functional imaging: A general linear approach. *Hum. Brain Mapping* 2:189–210. doi: 10.1002/hbm.460020402.

Genovese, C. R., N. A. Lazar, and T. Nichols. 2002. Thresholding of statistical maps in functional neuroimaging using the false discovery rate. *NeuroImage* 15:870–78. doi: 10.1006/nimg.2001.1037.

Geschwind, D. H. and P. Levitt. 2007. Autism spectrum disorders: Developmental disconnection syndromes. *Curr. Opin. Neurobiol.* 17:103–11. doi: 10.1016/j.conb.2007.01.009.

Hahn, T., A. F. Marquand, M. M. Plichta et al. 2013. A novel approach to probabilistic biomarker-based classification using functional near-infrared spectroscopy. *Hum. Brain Mapping* 34:1102–14. doi: 10.1002/hbm.21497.

Hardan, A. Y., R. A. Libove, M. S. Keshavan, N. M. Melhem, and N. J. Minshew. 2009. A preliminary longitudinal magnetic resonance imaging study of brain volume and cortical thickness in autism. *Biol. Psychiatry* 66:320–26. doi: 10.1016/j.biopsych.2009.04.024.

Hazlett, H. C., M. D. Poe, G. Gerig, M. Styner, C. Chappell, R. G. Smith, C. Vachet, and J. Piven. 2011. Early brain overgrowth in autism associated with an increase in cortical surface area before age 2 years. *Arch. Gen. Psychiatry* 68:467–76. doi: 10.1001/archgenpsychiatry.2011.39.

Hoeft, F., E. Walter, A. A. Lightbody, H. C. Hazlett, C. Chang, J. Piven, and A. L. Reiss. 2011. Neuroanatomical differences in toddler boys with fragile X syndrome and idiopathic autism. *Arch. Gen. Psychiatry* 68:295–305. doi: 10.1001/archgenpsychiatry.2010.153.

Iidaka, T. 2015. Resting state functional magnetic resonance imaging and neural network classified autism and control. *Cortex* 63:55–67. doi: 10.1016/j.cortex.2014.08.011.

Ingalhalikar, M., D. Parker, L. Bloy, T. P. L. Roberts, and R. Verma. 2011. Diffusion based abnormality markers of pathology: Toward learned diagnostic prediction of ASD. *NeuroImage* 57:918–27. doi: 10.1016/j.neuroimage.2011.05.023.

Ingalhalikar, M., W. A. Parker, L. Bloy, T. P. L. Roberts, and R. Verma. 2014. Creating multimodal predictors using missing data: Classifying and subtyping autism spectrum disorder. *J. Neurosci. Methods* 235:1–9. doi: 10.1016/j.jneumeth.2014.06.030.

Jiao, Y., R. Chen, X. Ke, L. Cheng, K. Chu, Z. Lu, and E. H. Herskovits. 2011. Predictive models for subtypes of autism spectrum disorder based on single-nucleotide polymorphisms and magnetic resonance imaging. *Adv. Med. Sci.* 56:334–42. doi: 10.2478/v10039-011-0042-y.

Jiao, Y., R. Chen, X. Ke, K. Chu, Z. Lu, and E. H. Herskovits. 2010. Predictive models of autism spectrum disorder based on brain regional cortical thickness. *NeuroImage* 50:589–99. doi: 10.1016/j.neuroimage.2009.12.047.

Just, M. A., V. L. Cherkassky, T. A. Keller, R. K. Kana, and N. J. Minshew. 2007. Functional and anatomical cortical underconnectivity in autism: Evidence from an fMRI study of an executive function task and corpus callosum morphometry. *Cerebral Cortex* 17:951–61. doi: 10.1093/cercor/bhl006.

Just, M. A., V. L. Cherkassky, T. A. Keller, and N. J. Minshew. 2004. Cortical activation and synchronization during sentence comprehension in high-functioning autism: Evidence of underconnectivity. *Brain* 127:1811–21. doi: 10.1093/brain/awh199.

Kim, H. C. and Z. Ghahramani. 2008. Outlier robust Gaussian process classification. *Lecture Notes Comput. Sci.* 5342:896–905. doi: 10.1007/978-3-540-89689-0_93.

Klöppel, S., A. Abdulkadir, C. R. Jack, N. Koutsouleris, J. Mourão-Miranda, and P. Vemuri. 2011. Diagnostic neuroimaging across diseases. *NeuroImage* 61:457–63. doi: 10.1016/j.neuroimage.2011.11.002.

Koldewyn, K., D. Whitney, and S. M. Rivera. 2011. Neural correlates of coherent and biological motion perception in autism. *Dev. Sci.* 14:1075–88. doi: 10.1111/j.1467-7687.2011.01058.x.

Koshino, H., P. A. Carpenter, N. J. Minshew, V. L. Cherkassky, T. A. Keller, and M. A. Just. 2005. Functional connectivity in an fMRI working memory task in high-functioning autism. *NeuroImage* 24:810–21. doi: 10.1016/j.neuroimage.2004.09.028.

Kriegeskorte, N., R. Goebel, and P. Bandettini. 2006. Information-based functional brain mapping. *Proc. Natl. Acad. Sci. USA* 103:3863–68. doi: 10.1073/pnas.0600244103.

Lai, M.-C., M. V. Lombardo, B. Chakrabarti, S. A. Sadek, G. Pasco, S. J. Wheelwright, E. T. Bullmore, S. Baron-Cohen, MRC AIMS Consortium, and J. Suckling. 2010. A shift to randomness of brain oscillations in people with autism. *Biol. Psychiatry* 68:1092–99. doi: 10.1016/j.biopsych.2010.06.027.

Lange, N., M. B. Dubray, J. E. Lee et al. 2010. Atypical diffusion tensor hemispheric asymmetry in autism. *Autism Res.* 3:350–58. doi: 10.1002/aur.162.

Langen, M., A. Leemans, P. Johnston, C. Ecker, E. Daly, C. M. Murphy, F. Dell'acqua, S. Durston, the AIMS Consortium, and Declan G. M. Murphy. 2011. Fronto-striatal circuitry and inhibitory control in autism: Findings from diffusion tensor imaging tractography. *Cortex* 48:183–93. doi: 10.1016/j.cortex.2011.05.018.

Langs, G., B. H. Menze, D. Lashkari, and P. Golland. 2011. Detecting stable distributed patterns of brain activation using Gini contrast. *NeuroImage* 56:497–507. doi: 10.1016/j.neuroimage.2010.07.074.

Lim, L., A. Marquand, A. A. Cubillo, A. B. Smith, K. Chantiluke, A. Simmons, M. Mehta, and K. Rubia. 2013. Disorder-specific predictive classification of adolescents with attention deficit hyperactivity disorder (ADHD) relative to autism using structural magnetic resonance imaging. *PLoS One* 8:e63660. doi: 10.1371/journal.pone.0063660.

Lord, C., M. Rutter, and A. Le Couteur. 1994. Autism diagnostic interview-revised: A revised version of a diagnostic interview for caregivers of individuals with possible pervasive developmental disorders. *J. Autism Dev. Disord.* 24:659–85.

Lord, C., M. Rutter, S. Goode, J. Heemsbergen, H. Jordan, L. Mawhood, and E. Schopler. 1989. Autism Diagnostic Observation Schedule: A standardized observation of communicative and social behavior. *J. Autism Dev. Disord.* 19:185–212.

Luna, B., N. J. Minshew, K. E. Garver, N. A. Lazar, K. R. Thulborn, W. F. Eddy, and J. A. Sweeney. 2002. Neocortical system abnormalities in autism: An fMRI study of spatial working memory. *Neurology* 59:834–40.

Marquand, A. F., M. Filippone, J. Ashburner, and M. Girolami. 2013. Automated, high accuracy classification of Parkinsonian disorders: A pattern recognition approach. *PLoS One* 8:e69237.

Marquand, A., M. Howard, M. Brammer, C. Chu, S. Coen, and J. Mourão-Miranda. 2010. Quantitative prediction of subjective pain intensity from whole-brain fMRI data using Gaussian processes. *NeuroImage* 49:2178–89. doi: 10.1016/j.neuroimage.2009.10.072.

McAlonan, G. M., C. Cheung, V. Cheung, N. Wong, J. Suckling, and S. E. Chua. 2009. Differential effects on white-matter systems in high-functioning autism and Asperger's syndrome. *Psychol. Med.* 39:1885–93. doi: 10.1017/S0033291709005728.

Mourão-Miranda, J., A. L. W. Bokde, C. Born, H. Hampel, and M. Stetter. 2005. Classifying brain states and determining the discriminating activation patterns: Support vector machine on functional MRI data. *NeuroImage* 28:980–95. doi: 10.1016/j.neuroimage.2005.06.070.

Mourão-Miranda, J., C. Ecker, J. R. Sato, and M. Brammer. 2009. Dynamic changes in the mental rotation network revealed by pattern recognition analysis of fMRI data. *J. Cogn. Neurosci.* 21:890–904. doi: 10.1162/jocn.2009.21078.

Mwangi, B., T. S. Tian, and J. C. Soares. 2014. A review of feature reduction techniques in neuroimaging. *Neuroinformatics* 12:229–44. doi: 10.1007/s12021-013-9204-3.

Orrù, G., W. Pettersson-Yeo, A. F. Marquand, G. Sartori, and A. Mechelli. 2012. Using support vector machine to identify imaging biomarkers of neurological and psychiatric disease: A critical review. *Neurosci. Biobehav. Rev.* 36:1140–52. doi: 10.1016/j.neubiorev.2012.01.004.

Pelphrey, K. A., J. P. Morris, G. McCarthy, and K. S. Labar. 2007. Perception of dynamic changes in facial affect and identity in autism. *Social Cogn. Affective Neurosci.* 2:140–49. doi: 10.1093/scan/nsm010.

Pinto, D., A. T. Pagnamenta, L. Klei et al. 2010. Functional impact of global rare copy number variation in autism spectrum disorders. *Nature* 466:368–72. doi: 10.1038/nature09146.

Piven, J., S. Arndt, J. Bailey, and N. Andreasen. 1996. Regional brain enlargement in autism: A magnetic resonance imaging study. *J. Am. Acad. Child Adoles. Psychiatry* 35:530–36. doi: 10.1097/00004583-199604000-00020.

Polyn, S. M., V. S. Natu, J. D. Cohen, and K. A. Norman. 2005. Category-specific cortical activity precedes retrieval during memory search. *Science* 310:1963–66. doi: 10.1126/science.1117645.

Pugliese, L., M. Catani, S. Ameis, F. Dell'acqua, M. T. de Schotten, C. Murphy, D. Robertson, Q. Deeley, E. Daly, and D. G. M. Murphy. 2009. The anatomy of extended limbic pathways in Asperger syndrome: A preliminary diffusion tensor imaging tractography study. *NeuroImage* 47:427–34. doi: 10.1016/j.neuroimage.2009.05.014.

Redcay, E., D. Dodell-Feder, P. L. Mavros, M. Kleiner, M. J. Pearrow, C. Triantafyllou, J. D. Gabrieli, and R. Saxe. 2013. Atypical brain activation patterns during a face-to-face joint attention game in adults with autism spectrum disorder. *Hum. Brain Mapping* 34:2511–23. doi: 10.1002/hbm.22086.

Ryali, S., K. Supekar, D. A. Abrams, and V. Menon. 2010. Sparse logistic regression for whole-brain classification of fMRI data. *NeuroImage* 51:752–64. doi: 10.1016/j.neuroimage.2010.02.040.

Sato, J. R., M. Queiroz Hoexter, P. P. de Magalhães Oliveira, M. J. Brammer, MRC AIMS Consortium, D. Murphy, and C. Ecker. 2013. Inter-regional cortical thickness correlations are associated with autistic symptoms: A machine-learning approach. *J. Psychiatry Res.* 47:453–59. doi: 10.1016/j.jpsychires.2012.11.017.

Schumann, C. M., C. S. Bloss, C. C. Barnes et al. 2010. Longitudinal magnetic resonance imaging study of cortical development through early childhood in autism. *J. Neurosci.* 30:4419–27. doi: 10.1523/JNEUROSCI.5714-09.2010.

Shukla, D. K., B. Keehn, and R.-A. Müller. 2011. Tract-specific analyses of diffusion tensor imaging show widespread white matter compromise in autism spectrum disorder. *J. Child Psychol. Psychiatry* 52:286–95. doi: 10.1111/j.1469-7610.2010.02342.x.

Simonoff, E., A. Pickles, T. Charman, S. Chandler, T. Loucas, and G. Baird. 2008. Psychiatric disorders in children with autism spectrum disorders: Prevalence, comorbidity, and associated factors in a population-derived sample. *J. Am. Acad. Child Adolescent Psychiatry* 47:921–29. doi: 10.1097/CHI.0b013e318179964f.

Solomon, M., S. J. Ozonoff, S. Ursu, S. Ravizza, N. Cummings, S. Ly, and C. S. Carter. 2009. The neural substrates of cognitive control deficits in autism spectrum disorders. *Neuropsychologia* 47:2515–26. doi: 10.1016/j.neuropsychologia.2009.04.019.

Svensén, M. and C. M. Bishop. 2007. *Pattern Recognition and Machine Learning: Solutions to Exercises.* New York: Springer.

Uddin, L. Q., V. Menon, C. B. Young, S. Ryali, T. Chen, A. Khouzam, N. J. Minshew, and A. Y. Hardan. 2011. Multivariate searchlight classification of structural magnetic resonance imaging in children and adolescents with autism. *Biol. Psychiatry* 70:833–41. doi: 10.1016/j.biopsych.2011.07.014.

Vapnik, V. 2000. *The Nature of Statistical Learning Theory.* New York: Springer Science & Business Media.

Waiter, G. D., J. H. G. Williams, A. D. Murray, A. Gilchrist, D. I. Perrett, and A. Whiten. 2005. Structural white matter deficits in high-functioning individuals with autistic spectrum disorder: A voxel-based investigation. *NeuroImage* 24:455–61. doi: 10.1016/j.neuroimage.2004.08.049.

Wallace, G. L., N. Dankner, L. Kenworthy, J. N. Giedd, and A. Martin. 2010. Age-related temporal and parietal cortical thinning in autism spectrum disorders. *Brain* 133:3745–54. doi: 10.1093/brain/awq279.

Wee, C.-Y., L. Wang, F. Shi, P.-T. Yap, and D. Shen. 2014. Diagnosis of autism spectrum disorders using regional and interregional morphological features. *Hum. Brain Mapping* 35:3414–30.

Wing, L. 1997. The autistic spectrum. *Lancet* 350:1761–66. doi: 10.1016/S0140-6736(97)09218-0.

Zielinski, B. A., M. B. D. Prigge, J. A. Nielsen et al. 2014. Longitudinal changes in cortical thickness in autism and typical development. *Brain* 137:1799–1812. doi: 10.1093/brain/awu083.

Chapter 7 Structural magnetic resonance imaging of autism spectrum disorder

Rong Chen

Contents

Abstract 121
7.1   Introduction 122
7.2   ROI-based morphometry 122
7.3   Voxel-based morphometry 124
7.4   Surface-based morphometry 126
7.5   Tensor-based morphometry 126
7.6   Structural brain network........................... 127
7.7   Structural MR-based predictive models................. 128
7.8   Conclusion, new developments and future directions 129
References 130

Abstract

Recent advances in the understanding of structural MRI correlates of ASD reveal some patterns. Cross-sectional region-of-interest-based studies reported changes in total brain volume and the corpus callosum volume. Longitudinal region-of-interest-based studies reported subjects with ASD had atypical cortical thickness trajectories. Voxel-based morphometry-based studies reported increased gray matter volume and reduced gray matter density in the frontal and temporal lobes. Surface-based morphometry-based studies reported that regions in the temporal lobe showed thinner cortex in the ASD group. For brain network analysis, structural covariance analysis-based studies found atypical anatomical connectivity patterns in ASD. For predictive modeling, structural MR-based predictive models can accurately differentiate individuals with ASD from normal controls.

7.1 Introduction

Autism spectrum disorder (ASD) (Rapin 1997; Geschwind and Levitt 2007; Chen et al. 2011) refers to a diverse group of developmental conditions, characterized by these core features: (1) impairment in reciprocal social interactions, (2) verbal and nonverbal communication deficits, (3) repetitive behavior, and (4) narrow and intense interest. ASD occurs in about 1% of the general population (Nygren et al. 2012). About 40% of ASD individuals have significant cognitive deficits (Bauman 2010). ASD is characterized by heterogeneity and affects individuals differently. It may be caused by many different underlying biological processes and developmental pathways (Walsh et al. 2011).

Magnetic resonance (MR) imaging can noninvasively examine brain structure and function *in vivo*, and may provide information to facilitate diagnosis and treatment of ASD. T1-weighted structural MR imaging is widely used to investigate brain morphology because of its high-contrast sensitivity and spatial resolution. It entails no radiation exposure, which is an important consideration for children and adolescents (Eliez and Reiss 2000).

T1-weighted structural MRI is used in ASD studies to understand brain morphological changes and atypical anatomical connectivity patterns and to provide imaging biomarkers for diagnosis or patient stratification. Figure 7.1 summarizes existing structural MR research in ASD. Brain morphological changes in ASD can be examined by region-of-interest (ROI)-based methods, which are often hypothesis-driven, or by more automated whole brain voxel-wise analysis methods including voxel-based morphometry (VBM), surface-based morphometry, and tensor-based morphometry. These analytic methods are sensitive to detecting morphological changes in ASD, and consistently found such changes in individuals with ASD. Using machine-learning methods, predictive models can be constructed to distinguish ASD and controls at the individual level. Structural MR-based network analysis method is based on structural covariance and provides information on interregional anatomical associations for ASD. Collectively, these structural MR-based studies can reveal the neuroanatomical substrates of ASD.

7.2 ROI-based morphometry

ROI-based morphometry studies define ROIs based on expert knowledge or a brain atlas, calculate features such as volume, thickness, or curvature for each ROI, and then perform statistical analysis. Relative to voxel-wise analysis, ROI-based morphometry studies have the potential to increase statistical power in detecting morphological changes in ASD by aggregating voxels into ROIs. However, depending on the degree of automation, the ROI delineation process may be labor-intensive and

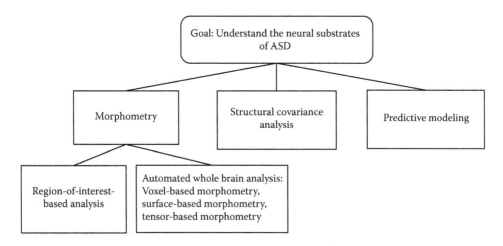

Figure 7.1 Structural MR research in ASD.

time-consuming. An inherent bias in ROI-based analysis is that such studies depend on the ROIs chosen by investigators.

ROI-based studies consistently report changes in both total brain and corpus callosum volumes. Young children with ASD (ages 18 months to 4 years) have 5%–10% abnormal enlargement in brain volumes, compared to those of typical development (Courchesne et al. 2001; Amaral et al. 2008). The enlargement in brain volume involves gray matter (GM) and white matter (WM) (Amaral et al. 2008). Whether this enlargement persists into later childhood and adolescence is not clear (Courchesne et al. 2001; Aylward et al. 2002). A meta-analysis of cross-sectional brain size showed that the period of greatest brain enlargement in ASD is during the toddler years (Redcay and Courchesne 2005). One hypothesis of the neuropathology of ASD is that the brain undergoes a period of precocious growth during early postnatal life, then a reduced age-related growth (Courchesne et al. 2003). MRI studies of total brain volume in early childhood support this theory.

The corpus callosum is the largest WM structure in the human brain. Its primary function is to facilitate the communication between two hemispheres in order to produce seamless motor, sensory, and cognitive functions. Structural MR studies demonstrate reduced corpus callosum volumes in individuals with ASD (Egaas et al. 1995; Piven et al. 1997; Hardan et al. 2000; Casanova et al. 2009; Keary et al. 2009; Frazier et al. 2012). In a study comprised of 32 individuals with ASD (mean age = 20 years, standard deviation (SD) = 10) and 34 age-, gender-, and intelligence quotient (IQ)-matched controls, Keary et al. (2009) reported that the ASD group displayed reductions in total corpus callosum volumes and in several of its subdivisions; and the corpus callosum volumetric alterations were associated with performance on several cognitive tests including the Tower of Hanoi tests.

The above mentioned ROI-based studies are cross-sectional, and cannot provide direct evidence of aberrant growth trajectories in ASD. Longitudinal studies can directly assess the age-related morphological changes. In a longitudinal study of brain growth in toddlers with ASD (Schumann et al. 2010), structural MR data of 41 toddlers with ASD (mean age = 48 months) and 41 age- and sex-matched controls were obtained. Fifteen toddlers with ASD and 12 controls had one MR scan. For other subjects, multiple MR scans were obtained. Cerebral GM, cerebral WM, frontal GM, temporal GM, cingulate GM, and parietal GM volumes showed abnormal growth rates in toddlers with ASD. A recent longitudinal study examined age-related cortical thickness changes in subjects with ASD (Zielinski et al. 2014). Three hundred forty-five MR scans were obtained from 97 males with ASD (mean age = 16.8 years; range 3–36 years) and 60 males with typical development (mean age = 18 years; range 4–39 years), with an average interscan interval of 2.6 years. The brain was parcellated into 34 ROIs using FreeSurfer and mean cortical thickness was calculated for each ROI. It was found that group differences in cortical thickness varied by developmental stages: accelerated expansion in early childhood, accelerated thinning in later childhood, and reduced thinning in early adulthood. The changes in age-related trajectory were also region-specific.

To investigate the growth of corpus callosum volumes in youths with autism, Frazier et al. (2012) examined MR data of 23 male children with ASD and 23 age- and gender-matched controls, at baseline and 2-year follow-up. The baseline mean age for ASD was 10 years. They found persistent reductions in total corpus callosum volumes in ASD children relative to controls.

7.3 Voxel-based morphometry

VBM generates voxel-wise morphometric feature maps such as GM volume maps using tissue segmentation and image registration and then quantifies changes in GM volume or density between groups in a voxel-wise manner. Relative to ROI-based methods, VBM is fully automated and capable of providing objective whole-brain analysis. However, in contrast to ROI-based methods, VBM may deliver lower statistical power because of the stringent multiple comparisons to control false-positives. Additionally, VBM is sensitive to noise and registration uncertainty.

We reviewed 15 VBM studies for ASD (age range 8.8–32 years) (Abell et al. 1999; McAlonan et al. 2002, 2005, 2008; Boddaert et al. 2004; Kwon et al. 2004; Waiter et al. 2004, 2005; Rojas et al. 2006; Bonilha et al. 2008; Ke et al. 2008; Hyde et al. 2010; Toal et al. 2010; Uddin et al. 2011; Ecker et al. 2012). The findings are summarized at the lobar level, instead of the voxel or brain regional level, in order to increase statistical power. In our analysis, we distinguished VBM studies focusing on GM

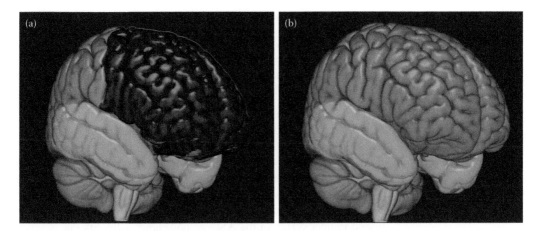

Figure 7.2 Findings of the voxel-based (a) and surface-based (b) morphometry studies of ASD. (a): VBM studies report increased GM volume and reduced GM density in the frontal and temporal lobes. (b): Surface-based morphometry studies report that regions in the temporal lobe showed thinner cortexes in the ASD group.

volumes and those on GM densities (or concentrations, probabilities) because GM volumes and densities are two kinds of morphological features. There are seven GM density-based and eight volume-based studies. We observed several consistent patterns. For the frontal lobe, five out of eight GM volume-based studies reported increased GM volume in the ASD group; while four out of seven GM density-based studies reported reduced GM density. For the temporal lobe, four out of eight GM volume-based studies reported the ASD group demonstrated GM volume enlargement; while four out of seven density-based studies found that ASD subjects had reduced GM density. For the parietal lobe, four out of eight GM volume-based studies found that GM volumes were increased in the ASD group. The findings of the occipital and limbic lobes were heterogeneous. In summary, existing studies report increased GM volumes and reduced GM densities in the frontal and temporal lobes in patients with ASD (Figure 7.2a). Based on experimental animal studies, lesion studies in human patients, and functional imaging studies, many brain regions in the frontal and temporal lobes have been implicated in social impairment, communication deficit, and repetitive behavior (Amaral et al. 2008).

A typical VBM study of ASD was the one undertaken by Bonilha et al. (2008). In this study, Bonilha et al. assessed GM and WM volume differences in 12 male ASD subjects (mean age = 12.4 years) and 16 age-matched male controls. Using VBM implemented in SPM5, they found that the ASD group exhibited increased GM volumes in the medial and dorsolateral frontal areas, in the lateral and medial parts of the temporal lobes, in the parietal lobes, cerebellum, and claustrum. ASD subjects also showed decreased WM volumes in the frontal, parietal, temporal, and occipital lobes.

7.4 Surface-based morphometry

The intrinsic topology of the cerebral cortex is that of a 2D sheet with a highly folded and curved geometry. Surface-based morphometry focuses on cortical topographic measurements such as cortical thickness and curvature and provides information complementary to that provided by VBM.

We reviewed seven studies centered on cortical thickness (Hadjikhani et al. 2006; Hardan et al. 2006; Hyde et al. 2010; Jiao et al. 2010; Wallace et al. 2010; Scheel et al. 2011; Mak-Fan et al. 2012). These studies used surface-based morphometry tools such as FreeSurfer to calculate cortical thickness and then performed whole-brain vertex-wise or regional analysis. Although the findings in these studies are somewhat inconsistent, some trends are clear. Four out of seven studies reported that regions in the temporal lobe showed thinner cortex in the ASD group (Figure 7.2b). Six out of seven studies found no change in the cortical thickness in the occipital lobe.

Scheel et al. (2011) assessed the difference in cortical thickness between 28 subjects with high-functioning ASD (18 males, mean age 33 [SD 10]) and 28 age-, sex-, handedness-, and IQ-matched controls. Using FreeSurfer, they found that the ASD group exhibited reduced cortical thickness in the posterior superior temporal sulcus of the left hemisphere.

Many surface-based morphometry studies center on the age effect in ASD. One hypothesis is that cortical thickness in the ASD group may follow a pattern in which early overgrowth is followed by prematurely arrested growth. Wallace et al. (2010) assessed differences in cortical thickness between high-functioning males with ASD ($n = 41$, mean age = 16.8 years) and age-, handedness, and IQ-matched typically developing males ($n = 40$, mean age = 17.0 years). A significant age × diagnosis interaction was found in the left fusiform/inferior temporal cortex. The ASD group had a thinner cortex in this region with increasing age to a greater degree than did controls.

A novel method to explore intrinsic brain connectivity based on attributes extracted from surface-based morphological features is reported in Ecker et al. (2013). Ecker et al. assessed 34 male, right-handed adults with ASD (mean age = 26 years) and 34 age- and full scale IQ-matched controls. The mean separation distance is the average geodesic distance from a vertex to the rest of the surface, and estimates the global intrinsic wiring cost. Local intrinsic wiring costs were estimated by radius function and perimeter function. Significantly reduced global and local intrinsic wiring costs were found in the ASD group. Differences in global and local wiring costs were primarily in the fronto-temporal regions.

7.5 Tensor-based morphometry

Both tensor-based morphometry and VBM measure the volume changes. In tensor-based morphometry, the signals analyzed are generated based on the registration of the images, rather than on aligned segmented GM. Tensor-based morphometry does not require that GM be perfectly registered. Therefore, the advantage of tensor-based morphometry over VBM is that false-positive findings due to systematic group differences in registration errors are less likely. Brun et al. (2009) used tensor-based morphometry to analyze T1-weighted MR images of 24 male children with ASD (mean age 9.5 years [SD 3.2]) and 26 age-matched controls. They detected significant GM volume deficits in the bilateral parietal, left temporal, and left occipital lobes. They also detected trend-level cerebral WM volume excesses and volume deficits in the cerebellar vermis. This pattern may indicate impaired neuronal connectivity, resulting from aberrant myelination and/or an inflammatory process.

7.6 Structural brain network

Several functional MR and diffusion tensor imaging-based neuroimaging studies reveal brain structural and functional connectivity changes in ASD. Recently, structural MR has been used to investigate network architecture in ASD. The most widely used structural MR-based network analysis method is structural covariance analysis, which provides information on interregional anatomical associations. A metric of structural covariance measures the correlation between regional morphological features. For example, to study the default-mode network, one may first choose a seed vertex in the default-mode network based on existing publications and then calculate a correlation coefficient between the cortical thickness of the seed vertex and that of another vertex, across subjects. Condition-by-covariance analyses to detect connectivity changes between ASD and controls may also be performed.

Several studies used structural covariance analysis to explore the anatomical connectivity patterns in ASD (Zielinski et al. 2012; Bernhardt et al. 2013; Sharda et al. 2016). Zielinski et al. (2012) used structural covariance analysis to examine the default-mode network and salient network in 49 male ASD subjects (mean age = 13.3 years [SD 5.1]) and 49 age- and IQ-matched male controls. They used seed ROI-based methods. Seed ROIs were selected within right fronto-insular cortex (for the salient network), and right posterior cingulate cortex (for the default-mode network). Condition-by-covariance analyses were performed in which the mean seed GM intensity was the variable of interest, and the grouping variable was disease/controls. They found that the salient network demonstrated restricted extent and distribution in ASD, and the default-mode network showed overgrowth in discrete posterior regions in ASD. Bernhardt et al. (2013) used structural covariance analysis to examine sociocognitive networks in 16 ASD subjects (mean age = 34.8 years [SD 13.3]) and 16 age-, sex- and IQ-matched controls. Seed ROIs were in the dorsomedial prefrontal cortex, and temporo-parietal junction, which are associated with theory of mind, and the fronto-insular cortex, which is associated with interception of emotion and empathy. They found that ASD showed reduced covariance in networks centered on the dorsomedial prefrontal cortex and temporo-parietal junction, but not within fronto-insular networks.

7.7 Structural MR-based predictive models

MR-based predictive models can be used for diagnosis and patient stratification. Compared to traditional statistical analysis methods such as the t-test, which provides group-level analysis, predictive modeling can provide a score at the individual level representing the probability that a subject belongs to the patient group, or the degree of symptom severity. Structural MR-based predictive modeling usually involves three steps. First, features are extracted from structural MR images; then a predictive model (a classifier) is constructed using machine-learning algorithms; finally, the resulting predictive model is evaluated and validated. Several studies centered on structural MR-based predictive models of ASD to distinguish ASD and normal controls (Akshoomoff et al. 2004; Ecker et al. 2010a,b; Jiao et al. 2010; Uddin et al. 2011). For these studies, the mean age for the ASD group ranged from 6 to 33 years. The sensitivity, specificity, and accuracy of these predictive models are in the range of [0.77, 0.95], [0.75, 0.92], and [0.81, 0.87], respectively. Overall, structural MR-based predictive models can accurately differentiate individuals with ASD from normal controls.

The performance of a predictive model is critically affected by morphological feature types. Jiao et al. compared thickness-based diagnostic models to those based on structure volumes (Jiao et al. 2010). Four machine-learning techniques were used to generate predictive models. They found thickness-based classification was superior to volume-based classification, for each combination of classifier and performance metric. For thickness-based classification, logistic model trees achieved the highest accuracy (0.87). For volume-based classification, logistic model trees achieved the highest accuracy (0.74).

Because different kinds of imaging features have different neuropathological and genetic underpinnings, combining them may generate a superior predictive model than using them individually. Ecker et al. (2010a) used five morphological parameters—cortical thickness, radial curvature, average convexity, metric distortion, and pial area—to distinguish 20 male ASD (mean age = 33 years (SD 11); full-scale IQ > 75) and 20 age-, sex-, handedness-, and full-scale IQ-matched controls. They found that for the left hemisphere, the performance of a classifier using all five parameters was accuracy = 0.85, sensitivity = 0.90, and specificity = 0.80; for the right hemisphere, the performance of a classifier using all parameters was accuracy = 0.65, sensitivity = 0.60, and specificity = 0.70. For both left and right hemispheres, the classifier using all parameters usually has a higher accuracy than that using a single parameter. The only exception is for the left hemisphere, cortical thickness-based classification achieved an accuracy of 0.90, which is higher than using all parameters. This study suggests that combining different morphological features may improve classification accuracy.

7.8 Conclusion, new developments, and future directions

Recent advances in the understanding of structural MRI correlates of ASD reveal several patterns:

1. Cross-sectional ROI-based studies reported changes in total brain volume and the corpus callosum volume.
2. Longitudinal ROI-based studies reported ASD subjects had atypical cortical thickness trajectories. The cortical thickness trajectory differences between ASD and typical development varied by developmental stages.
3. VBM studies reported increased GM volume and reduced GM density in the frontal and temporal lobes.
4. Surface-based morphometry studies reported that regions in the temporal lobe showed thinner cortex in the ASD group.
5. Structural covariance analysis-based studies found atypical anatomical connectivity patterns in ASD.
6. Structural MR-based predictive models can accurately differentiate individuals with ASD from normal controls.

Different MR imaging technologies can provide complementary information about a brain disorder or cognitive process. Multimodal brain imaging plays an important role in revealing structure–structure (e.g., GM and WM) or structural–functional (e.g., GM and resting-state functional MR) associations. In a multimodal imaging study, Itahashi et al. (2014) examined structural MRI and diffusion tensor imaging data acquired from 46 adult males with ASD (mean age = 30.5 years) and 46 age- and full-scale IQ-matched controls. Using linked independent component analysis, they found two composite components that showed significant between-group differences. One composite component was significantly correlated with age. In the other component, subjects with ASD showed decreased GM volumes in multiple regions, including the bilateral fusiform gyri, bilateral orbitofrontal cortices, and bilateral pre- and postcentral gyri. These GM changes were associated with a pattern of decreased fractional anisotropy in several WM tracts. This multimodal imaging study showed that different brain morphology alternations may co-occur in specific brain regions.

Genetic factors play an important role in ASD (Geschwind 2011). Imaging-genetics studies can reveal intermediate phenotypes of ASD. The concept of intermediate phenotype assumes that genes do not code for psychopathology but mediate risk for symptom expression through their effect on neural systems (Meyer-Lindenberg and Weinberger 2006; Ameis and Szatmari 2012). Structural variation in the neurexin-1 gene increases the risk for ASD. Vineskos et al. examined morphological features in 53 healthy individuals (18–59 years of age). These subjects were genotyped at 11 single nucleotide polymorphisms of the neurexin-1 gene. Compared to nonrisk homozygotes, subjects who were homozygous for the rs1045881C risk allele had reduced frontal lobe WM volume and thalamic volume.

To date, most morphometry studies including VBM, surface-based morphometry, and tensor-based morphometry are mass-univariate. These studies cannot reveal interactions among the brain regions. Multivariate analysis can be used to detect interactions among the brain regions. Multivoxel pattern analysis (MVPA) is a multivariate approach to detect differences between conditions by focusing on the analysis and comparison of distributed patterns. It has been used to distinguish ASD and controls (Uddin et al. 2011). Another method for multivariate morphometric analysis is graphical model-based multivariate analysis (GAMMA) (Chen and Herskovits 2005, 2012). GAMMA is based on Bayesian network modeling. MVPA is based on a support vector machine, which is a black-box approach. Relative to MVPA, the model generated by GAMMA is more declarative. That is, the model is easy to understand and visualize. Multivariate analysis such as MVPA and GAMMA may shed light on the heterogeneity problem involved in studying ASD.

There are many conflicting findings regarding structural MR changes in individuals with ASD. Numerous factors such as inclusion and exclusion criteria, population age, MR acquisition parameters, image processing methods, feature extraction procedures, analytic methods used to detect group differences, and sample sizes may have contributed to disparities. Standardized image acquisition and image processing procedures could help investigators to reduce variability in structural MR studies of ASD and lead to more comparable results across studies. Autism Brain Imaging Data Exchange (ABIDE) is a consortium of investigators to which members contribute structural and resting-state MR data from ASD subjects and controls using similar clinical and imaging protocols. Analyzing data from this consortium using standardized image processing and statistical analysis methods (univariate or multivariate) may help clarify conflicting findings from the previous studies.

References

Abell, F., M. Krams, J. Ashburner, R. Passingham, K. Friston, R. Frackowiak, F. Happe, C. Frith, and U. Frith. 1999. The neuroanatomy of autism: A voxel-based whole brain analysis of structural scans. *NeuroReport.* 10:1647–51.

Akshoomoff, N., C. Lord, A. J. Lincoln, R. Y. Courchesne, R. A. Carper, J. Townsend, and E. Courchesne. 2004. Outcome classification of preschool children with autism spectrum disorders using MRI brain measures. *J. Am. Acad. Child. Adolesc. Psychiatry* 43:349–57.

Amaral, D. G., C. M. Schumann, and C. W. Nordahl. 2008. Neuroanatomy of autism. *Trends Neurosci.* 31:137–45.

Ameis, S. H. and P. Szatmari. 2012. Imaging-genetics in autism spectrum disorder: Advances, translational impact, and future directions. *Front. Psychiatry* 3:46.

Aylward, E. H., N. J. Minshew, K. Field, B. F. Sparks, and N. Singh. 2002. Effects of age on brain volume and head circumference in autism. *Neurology* 59:175–83.

Bauman, M. L. 2010. Medical comorbidities in autism: Challenges to diagnosis and treatment. *Neurotherapeutics* 7:320–7.

Bernhardt, B. C., S. L. Valk, G. Silani, G. Bird, U. Frith, and T. Singer. 2013. Selective disruption of sociocognitive structural brain networks in autism and alexithymia. *Cereb. Cortex* 24:3258–67.

Boddaert, N., N. Chabane, H. Gervais et al. 2004. Superior temporal sulcus anatomical abnormalities in childhood autism: A voxel-based morphometry MRI study. *NeuroImage* 23:364–9.

Bonilha, L., F. Cendes, C. Rorden, M. Eckert, P. Dalgalarrondo, L. M. Li, and C. E. Steiner. 2008. Gray and white matter imbalance—Typical structural abnormality underlying classic autism? *Brain Dev.* 30:396–401.

Brun, C. C., R. Nicolson, N. Lepore et al. 2009. Mapping brain abnormalities in boys with autism. *Hum. Brain Mapp.* 30:3887–900.

Casanova, M. F., A. El-Baz, M. Mott, G. Mannheim, H. Hassan, R. Fahmi, J. Giedd, J. M. Rumsey, A. E. Switala, and A. Farag. 2009. Reduced gyral window and corpus callosum size in autism: Possible macroscopic correlates of a minicolumnopathy. *J. Autism Dev. Disord.* 39:751–64.

Chen, R. and E. H. Herskovits. 2005. Graphical-model based morphometric analysis. *IEEE Trans. Med. Imaging* 24:1237–48.

Chen, R. and E. H. Herskovits. 2012. Graphical model based multivariate analysis (GAMMA): An open-source, cross-platform neuroimaging data analysis software package. *Neuroinformatics* 10:119–27.

Chen, R., Y. Jiao, and E. H. Herskovits. 2011. Structural MRI in autism spectrum disorder. *Pediatr. Res.* 69:63R–8R.

Courchesne, E., R. Carper, and N. Akshoomoff. 2003. Evidence of brain overgrowth in the first year of life in autism. *JAMA* 290:337–44.

Courchesne, E., C. M. Karns, H. R. Davis et al. 2001. Unusual brain growth patterns in early life in patients with autistic disorder: An MRI study. *Neurology* 57:245–54.

Ecker, C., A. Marquand, J. Mourao-Miranda et al. 2010a. Describing the brain in autism in five dimensions—Magnetic resonance imaging-assisted diagnosis of autism spectrum disorder using a multiparameter classification approach. *J. Neurosci.* 30:10612–23.

Ecker, C., V. Rocha-Rego, P. Johnston, J. Mourao-Miranda, A. Marquand, E. M. Daly, M. J. Brammer, C. Murphy, and D. G. Murphy. 2010b. Investigating the predictive value of whole-brain structural MR scans in autism: A pattern classification approach. *Neuroimage* 49:44–56.

Ecker, C., L. Ronan, Y. Feng et al. 2013. Intrinsic gray-matter connectivity of the brain in adults with autism spectrum disorder. *Proc. Natl. Acad. Sci. USA* 110:13222–7.

Ecker, C., J. Suckling, S. C. Deoni et al. 2012. Brain anatomy and its relationship to behavior in adults with autism spectrum disorder: A multicenter magnetic resonance imaging study. *Arch. Gen. Psychiat.* 69:195–209.

Egaas, B., E. Courchesne, and O. Saitoh. 1995. Reduced size of corpus callosum in autism. *Arch. Neurol.* 52:794–801.

Eliez, S. and A. L. Reiss. 2000. MRI neuroimaging of childhood psychiatric disorders: A selective review. *J. Child. Psychol. Psychiat.* 41:679–94.

Frazier, T. W., M. S. Keshavan, N. J. Minshew, and A. Y. Hardan. 2012. A two-year longitudinal MRI study of the corpus callosum in autism. *J. Autism. Dev. Disord.* 42:2312–22.

Geschwind, D. H. 2011. Genetics of autism spectrum disorders. *Trends. Cogn. Sci.* 15:409–16.

Geschwind, D. H. and P. Levitt. 2007. Autism spectrum disorders: Developmental disconnection syndromes. *Curr. Opin. Neurobiol.* 17:103–11.

Hadjikhani, N., R. M. Joseph, J. Snyder, and H. Tager-Flusberg. 2006. Anatomical differences in the mirror neuron system and social cognition network in autism. *Cereb. Cortex* 16:1276–82.

Hardan, A. Y., N. J. Minshew, and M. S. Keshavan. 2000. Corpus callosum size in autism. *Neurology* 55:1033–6.

Hardan, A. Y., S. Muddasani, M. Vemulapalli, M. S. Keshavan, and N. J. Minshew. 2006. An MRI study of increased cortical thickness in autism. *Am. J. Psychiat.* 163:1290–2.

Hyde, K. L., F. Samson, A. C. Evans, and L. Mottron. 2010. Neuroanatomical differences in brain areas implicated in perceptual and other core features of autism revealed by cortical thickness analysis and voxel-based morphometry. *Hum. Brain Mapp.* 31:556–66.

Itahashi, T., T. Yamada, M. Nakamura et al. 2014. Linked alterations in gray and white matter morphology in adults with high-functioning autism spectrum disorder: A multimodal brain imaging study. *Neuroimage Clin.* 7:155–69.

Jiao, Y., R. Chen, X. Ke, K. Chu, Z. Lu, and E. H. Herskovits. 2010. Predictive models of autism spectrum disorder based on brain regional cortical thickness. *NeuroImage* 50:589–99.

Ke, X., S. Hong, T. Tang, B. Zou, H. Li, Y. Hang, Z. Zhou, Z. Ruan, Z. Lu, G. Tao, and Y. Liu. 2008. Voxel-based morphometry study on brain structure in children with high-functioning autism. *NeuroReport* 19:921–5.

Keary, C. J., N. J. Minshew, R. Bansal, D. Goradia, S. Fedorov, M. S. Keshavan, and A. Y. Hardan. 2009. Corpus callosum volume and neurocognition in autism. *J. Autism Dev. Disord.* 39:834–41.

Kwon, H., A. W. Ow, K. E. Pedatella, L. J. Lotspeich, and A. L. Reiss. 2004. Voxel-based morphometry elucidates structural neuroanatomy of high-functioning autism and Asperger syndrome. *Dev. Med. Child Neurol.* 46:760–4.

Mak-Fan, K. M., M. J. Taylor, W. Roberts, and J. P. Lerch. 2012. Measures of cortical grey matter structure and development in children with autism spectrum disorder. *J. Autism Dev. Disord.* 42:419–27.

McAlonan, G. M., V. Cheung, C. Cheung, J. Suckling, G. Y. Lam, K. S. Tai, L. Yip, D. G. M. Murphy, and S. E. Chua. 2005. Mapping the brain in autism. A voxel-based MRI study of volumetric differences and intercorrelations in autism. *Brain* 128:268–76.

McAlonan, G. M., E. Daly, V. Kumari et al. 2002. Brain anatomy and sensorimotor gating in Asperger's syndrome. *Brain* 125:1594–606.

McAlonan, G. M., J. Suckling, N. Wong, V. Cheung, N. Lienenkaemper, C. Cheung, and S. E. Chua. 2008. Distinct patterns of grey matter abnormality in high-functioning autism and Asperger's syndrome. *J. Child Psychol. Psychiatry* 49:1287–95.

Meyer-Lindenberg, A. and D. R. Weinberger. 2006. Intermediate phenotypes and genetic mechanisms of psychiatric disorders. *Nat. Rev. Neurosci.* 7:818–27.

Nygren, G., M. Cederlund, E. Sandberg, F. Gillstedt, T. Arvidsson, I. Carina Gillberg, G. Westman Andersson, and C. Gillberg. 2012. The prevalence of autism spectrum disorders in toddlers: A population study of 2-year-old Swedish children. *J. Autism Dev. Disord.* 42:1491–7.

Piven, J., J. Bailey, B. J. Ranson, and S. Arndt. 1997. An MRI study of the corpus callosum in autism. *Am. J. Psychiat.* 154:1051–6.

Rapin, I. 1997. Autism. *N. Engl. J. Med.* 337:97–104.

Redcay, E. and E. Courchesne. 2005. When is the brain enlarged in autism? A meta-analysis of all brain size reports. *Biol. Psychiat.* 58:1–9.

Rojas, D. C., E. Peterson, E. Winterrowd, M. L. Reite, S. J. Rogers, and J. R. Tregellas. 2006. Regional gray matter volumetric changes in autism associated with social and repetitive behavior symptoms. *BMC Psychiatry* 6:56.

Scheel, C., A. Rotarska-Jagiela, L. Schilbach, F. G. Lehnhardt, B. Krug, K. Vogeley, and R. Tepest. 2011. Imaging derived cortical thickness reduction in high-functioning autism: Key regions and temporal slope. *Neuroimage* 58:391–400.

Schumann, C. M., C. S. Bloss, C. C. Barnes et al. 2010. Longitudinal magnetic resonance imaging study of cortical development through early childhood in autism. *J. Neurosci.* 30:4419–27.

Sharda, M., B. S. Khundrakpam, A. C. Evans, and N. C. Singh. 2016. Disruption of structural covariance networks for language in autism is modulated by verbal ability. *Brain Struct. Funct.* 221(2):1017–32.

Toal, F., E. M. Daly, L. Page et al. 2010. Clinical and anatomical heterogeneity in autistic spectrum disorder: A structural MRI study. *Psychol. Med.* 40:1171–81.

Uddin, L. Q., V. Menon, C. B. Young, S. Ryali, T. Chen, A. Khouzam, N. J. Minshew, and A. Y. Hardan. 2011. Multivariate searchlight classification of structural magnetic resonance imaging in children and adolescents with autism. *Biol. Psychiatry* 70:833–41.

Waiter, G. D., J. H. G. Williams, A. D. Murray, A. Gilchrist, D. I. Perrett, and A. Whiten. 2004. A voxel-based investigation of brain structure in male adolescents with autistic spectrum disorder. *Neuroimage* 22:619–25.

Waiter, G. D., J. H. G. Williams, A. D. Murray, A. Gilchrist, D. I. Perrett, and A. Whiten. 2005. Structural white matter deficits in high-functioning individuals with autistic spectrum disorder: A voxel-based investigation. *Neuroimage* 24:455–61.

Wallace, G. L., N. Dankner, L. Kenworthy, J. N. Giedd, and A. Martin. 2010. Age-related temporal and parietal cortical thinning in autism spectrum disorders. *Brain* 133:3745–54.

Walsh, P., M. Elsabbagh, P. Bolton, and I. Singh. 2011. In search of biomarkers for autism: Scientific, social and ethical challenges. *Nat. Rev. Neurosci.* 12:603–12.

Zielinski, B. A., J. S. Anderson, A. L. Froehlich et al. 2012. scMRI reveals large-scale brain network abnormalities in autism. *PLoS One* 7:e49172.

Zielinski, B. A., M. B. Prigge, J. A. Nielsen et al. 2014. Longitudinal changes in cortical thickness in autism and typical development. *Brain* 137:1799–812.

Chapter 8 Atypical hemispheric asymmetries in autism spectrum disorders

Annukka Lindell

Contents

Abstract 135
8.1 Language 137
    8.1.1 Structural lateralization for language 137
    8.1.2 Functional lateralization for language 140
8.2 Emotion 144
    8.2.1 Functional lateralization for emotion 145
8.3 Faces 147
    8.3.1 Structural lateralization for faces 148
    8.3.2 Functional lateralization for faces 149
8.4 Conclusion 151
References 151

Abstract

One of the most striking characteristics of the human brain is its lateral division into two halves. Though the two sides of the brain appear superficially symmetrical, the brain is both structurally and functionally asymmetric. Hemispheric lateralization is a fundamental principle of nervous system organization and is evident throughout the animal kingdom (Ocklenburg and Güntürkün 2012). In the typical human brain, the left and right hemispheres are specialized for different cognitive functions, enhancing information processing efficiency.

With the invention and availability of new imaging technologies, our appreciation for the complex networks that control cognitive functions continues to grow. Such technologies have made it apparent that neural networks distributed across both hemispheres of the brain are active during cognitive processing. For example, though it was once popularly believed that the left hemisphere was "verbal" and the right hemisphere was "nonverbal" (a concept known as "hemisphericity"), the notion that any one function is governed solely by a single hemisphere was debunked in the scientific literature in the 1980s and has been consigned to history. However, while both hemispheres are involved in cognitive processing, the relative distribution of activation of networks distributed across the left and right hemispheres is asymmetric: the brain is functionally lateralized. Thus, during language processing, we typically see relatively greater activation in the left than right fronto-temporo-parietal network, whereas looking at faces prompts more activation in the right than left fusiform gyrus. These patterns of activation are taken to index the relative contributions of the two sides of the brain to a given process, allowing us to conclude that in the typical brain, language is functionally lateralized to the left, and face processing to the right, hemisphere.

However, the brains of people with neurodevelopmental disorders, such as autism spectrum disorder (ASD), show markedly different patterns of hemispheric lateralization. Aberrant patterns of hemispheric asymmetry are considered a risk factor in ASD, dyslexia, schizophrenia, Down's syndrome, specific language impairment, and attention deficit hyperactivity disorder (ADHD) (Smalley et al. 2004; Moncrieff 2010; see Klimkeit and Bradshaw 2006, for a review). These disorders share more than just atypicalities in lateralization: there is a high degree of comorbidity, both in behavioral characteristics and diagnoses, suggesting a degree of shared etiology (Knaus et al. 2010). Thus, given that atypically reduced or reversed lateralization is known to impair information processing and is evident in ASD, examination the of the hemispheric lateralization in people with ASD can help shed light on the relationship between anomalous cortical lateralization and symptomatology.

This chapter will focus on hemispheric asymmetries for three cardinal cognitive functions: language, emotion, and face processing. These functions were selected because they are characteristically impaired in people with ASD, and are typically lateralized to the left (language) and right (emotion, face processing) hemispheres. Consequently, they have been the subject of much investigation, seeking to establish the relationship between hemispheric asymmetry and behavioral outcomes in people with ASD. The research reviewed in this chapter confirms that atypically reduced or reversed structural and functional lateralization is typical in people with ASD.

It is important to note that in this chapter, the term "lateralized" is used to describe relative rather than absolute lateralization (e.g., describing language function as being lateralized to the left hemisphere should not be taken to imply that language is solely a function of the left hemisphere). Instead, lateralization indicates that one side of the brain plays a greater role in a given cognitive process than the other, that is, their involvement is asymmetric.

8.1 Language

Language is the paradigmatic lateralized function. Though the idea that different regions of the brain are specialized for different types of function is now taken for granted, this knowledge is comparatively new. French neurosurgeon Paul Broca (1865) first suggested that the brain is lateralized for articulate language, based on his observation of patients with speech impairments. At autopsy, he noticed a pattern: patients who presented with speech problems had damage to the left hemisphere. In the 150 years since Broca's discovery, confirmatory research has grown, indicating that though both sides of the brain contribute to language processing (see Lindell 2006), the left hemisphere is undoubtedly the superior language processor in the typical brain.

As left hemisphere lateralization is typically associated with normal language function, it follows that atypical language lateralization may compromise language ability. And indeed, people with developmental disorders that impair language function, including dyslexia (Xu et al. 2015), ADHD (Hale et al. 2005), and specific language impairment (Hodge et al. 2010), show evidence of reduced and/or reversed left hemisphere lateralization for language.

Language and communication impairments form a core diagnostic criterion in ASD, and additionally play a key prognostic role (Herbert et al. 2002). For example, in children with ASD, the early presence of speech (before age 5, Mody and Belliveau 2012; before age 2, Mayo et al. 2013) is considered the strongest predictor of favorable outcomes. Given that atypical language lateralization has been linked to language impairment, research has sought to investigate the relationships between language lateralization and behavioral outcomes, seeking to establish the link between atypical hemispheric asymmetry and language deficits in ASD.

8.1.1 Structural lateralization for language

In the typically developing brain, a network of fronto-temporo-parietal regions appears vital for normal language processing (Figure 8.1). This network includes Broca's area (inferior frontal gyrus; controls speech planning and production) and Wernicke's area (posterior superior temporal gyrus, supramarginal and middle temporal gyri; stores the sound patterns of words), and is left lateralized in the majority of the population. However, lateralization varies with handedness: 96% of strong right handers, 85% of mixed handers, and 73% of strong left handers are left lateralized for speech (Knecht et al. 2000).

Research using structural magnetic resonance imaging (MRI) to examine the architecture of the brain confirms that both the left hemisphere frontal and temporo-parietal regions are structurally atypical in people with ASD (e.g., Knaus et al. 2010). Whereas typically developing boys

137

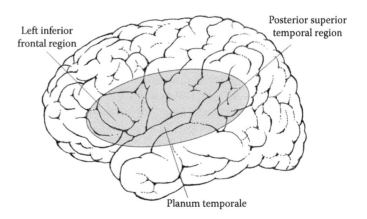

Figure 8.1 Fronto-temporo-parietal network involved in typical language processing. (Brain illustration courtesy of Michael Lindell.)

(aged 7–11) have 17% greater volume in the left inferior lateral frontal (Broca's area) and posterior superior temporal (Wernicke's area) regions, boys with ASD have 27% greater matter in the right hemisphere analogues of these areas (Herbert et al. 2005). Gage et al. (2009) similarly reported that children with ASD show a rightward asymmetry in the posterior superior temporal gyrus and planum temporale, indicating a reversal of typical left lateralization. Other studies have indicated a reduced, rather than reversed, leftward asymmetry in the planum temporale in children (aged 5–16) and adults with ASD (Rojas et al. 2002, 2005). Given that stronger language ability is associated with a relatively greater volume in the left than right hemisphere frontal and temporal regions (Morgan and Hynd 1998), the fact that children with ASD show reduced or reversed hemispheric asymmetries in these regions is likely to play a causal role in the language problems that characterize the disorder.

McAlonan et al.'s (2008) structural imaging research speaks directly to the relationship between atypical hemisphere asymmetries in ASD and language impairment. They assessed gray matter volumes in the left frontal region in children (aged 7–16) with high functioning autism, Asperger's syndrome, and typically developing controls. The scans confirmed a negative correlation between gray matter volume in the left inferior frontal gyrus and delayed age of acquisition (phrase speech) only in children with high functioning autism and language impairment. Given that this relationship was not evident in children with Asperger's syndrome, these data suggest that atypical lateralization in the left frontal region is associated with language impairment broadly, rather than ASD specifically.

Further evidence confirming that reduced left frontal matter is linked to poorer language outcomes is presented by De Fossé et al. (2004). They examined structural asymmetries in boys with ASD (aged 6–13);

crucially, they compared boys with ASD with and without language impairment, providing a strong test of the hypothesized causal role of atypical hemispheric asymmetry in language-processing deficits in ASD. The data of De Fossé et al. confirmed that language-impaired boys with ASD had greater volume in the right than left frontal region (i.e., reversed asymmetry). Critically, the frontal asymmetries of boys with ASD who did not exhibit language impairments were indistinguishable from the typically developing controls: both groups had greater matter in the left frontal region (Figure 8.2). As such, these data appear consistent with the findings of McAlonan et al. (2008), indicating that reduced left frontal volume is a correlate of language impairment, rather than ASD specifically.

This conclusion appears consistent with the findings of Brieber et al. (2007). They examined structural frontal asymmetries in adolescents (aged 10–16) with ASD and typically developing controls. The results indicated no frontal volume differences between the two groups, a finding that may be explained by examining the composition of the ASD sample. Though Brieber et al. did not directly assess language impairment,

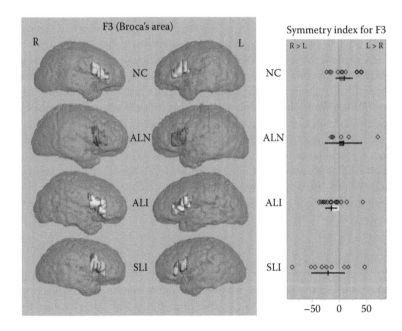

Figure 8.2 Reduced asymmetry in Broca's area in people with ASD with language impairment (ALI) and people with ASD without language impairment (ALN) in comparison with normal controls. (NC; De Fossé, L. et al., Language-association cortex asymmetry in autism and specific language impairment. *Ann. Neurol.* 2004. 56. 757–766. doi: 10.1002/ana.20275. Copyright Wiley-VCH Verlag GmbH & Co. KGaA. Reproduced with permission of John Wiley & Sons in the format reuse in a book/e-book via Copyright Clearance Center.)

their ASD sample comprised predominantly (87%) adolescents with Asperger's syndrome. By definition, language delay is not a characteristic of Asperger's syndrome, and indeed, McAlonan et al. (2008) reported that the left frontal matter reduction noted in children with high-functioning autism was not present in children with Asperger's syndrome. The absence of reduced/reversed frontal asymmetry in the sample of Brieber et al. thus offers further evidence supporting the notion that atypical left frontal asymmetries are characteristic of language impairment, rather than ASD.

These regional atypicalities should be viewed within the context of overall cortical enlargement and macrocephaly (e.g., Courchesne et al. 2003). A number of studies indicate that people with ASD show increased brain volumes in comparison with controls, evident in the first few years of life (Courchesne et al. 2001) and extending into adulthood (Hardan et al. 2001; though see Aylward et al. 2002). It is worth noting that the direction of the asymmetry in overall lobe volume is not necessarily consistent with that seen regionally (Hazlett et al. 2006). De Fossé et al. (2004), Herbert et al. (2002), and McAlonan et al. (2008) all reported regionally reduced left frontal volume in people with ASD and language impairment. In contrast, Hazlett et al.'s investigation of gray matter lobe volumes in men with ASD (aged 13–29) and typical controls indicated an exaggerated left hemisphere bias in the frontal and temporal lobes in the ASD sample (participants' specific diagnosis and language abilities were not reported). As this study assessed lobular but not regional lateralization, we cannot determine whether this overall leftward lobe asymmetry masks a reduced/reversed asymmetry in the left inferior frontal region; theoretically, both atypical asymmetries may present simultaneously. However, these data demonstrate that atypical structural asymmetries are present in the brains of people with ASD, both regionally and at the lobe level. Whether the structural atypicalities in language-related regions influence functional lateralization for language processing in ASD will be explored in the next section.

8.1.2 Functional lateralization for language

Although the atypicalities in structural lateralization for language in people with ASD do not necessitate that functional lateralization for language will be similarly atypical, abnormalities in structural lateralization make the recruitment of alternate networks to support language function more likely. And indeed, functional imaging research confirms that across a broad range of both receptive and expressive language tasks, the brains of people with ASD show anomalous functional asymmetries. As such, the functional imaging data appear consistent with the structural imaging data, indicating that language lateralization patterns are reduced or reversed in ASD.

Early PET research by Müller et al. (1999) used sentence processing tasks to assess patterns of activation in high-functioning adults with ASD and typical controls. As predicted, people with ASD showed reduced activation in the left frontal region in comparison with controls (see also Just et al. 2004). Imaging during other discourse tasks, such as phrase recognition, indicates that while people with ASD and typical controls show comparable activation in the left frontal region, the tasks prompt reduced activation in the left insula and increased activation in the right hemisphere analogue of Wernicke's area in the ASD group (Anderson et al. 2010). Although these studies fail to show a consistent pattern of reduced/reversed activation across tasks, the findings are consistent insuggesting that the brains of people with ASD show atypical patterns of lateralized activation during language processing.

Clever research by Harris et al. (2006) indicates that people with ASD show similar patterns of activation in Broca's area during semantic and perceptual judgments, indicating a lack of specificity. In the typical brain, semantic processing prompts activation in Broca's area but perceptual processing does not; Harris et al. found reduced activation in Broca's area in the ASD group during semantic processing and importantly, that the reduced level of activation in the region was akin to that prompted by a perceptual task (Figure 8.3). This lack of difference in activation during perceptual and semantic processing suggests a lack of functional specificity. As behavioral performance for the ASD and typical groups did not differ, the findings of Harris et al. suggest that high-functioning people with ASD recruit alternate neural networks to perform semantic judgment tasks, despite the fact that the left frontal regions that typically mediate semantic processing are not similarly sensitive in people with ASD, and the activation of an alternate network allows comparable performance in this instance.

EEG studies suggest that children with ASD have right, rather than left, hemisphere dominance for language tasks (e.g., Dawson et al. 1982). This aberrant pattern of activation appears to be evident very early in a child's development, suggesting potential diagnostic utility. For example, Seery et al. (2013) reported that infants (aged 6–12 months) at high risk of developing ASD failed to show a lateralized response to speech sounds, in marked contrast with the left lateralized activation patterns observed in low-risk infants. As children with ASD grow, the reduced asymmetry may develop into a reversed, right hemisphere asymmetry for language processing (Dawson et al. 1982), unlike typically developing children. The data of Flagg et al. (2005) support this notion. Their cross-sectional MEG investigation assessed cortical activation in children with ASD (aged 8–17) and typically developing controls, as they were presented with vowel stimuli in a passive auditory presentation paradigm. While young children in both groups showed bilateral patterns of activation, the older typical developing children showed a left lateralized pattern of activation whereas the older children with ASD instead showed right

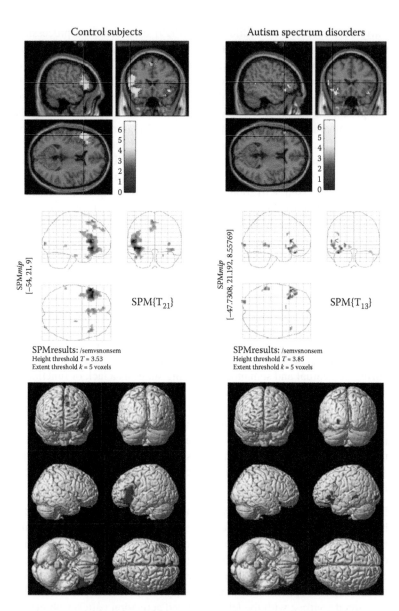

Figure 8.3 Activation for Semantic > Perceptual word processing tasks shows reduced activation in Broca's area in people with ASD in comparison with typical controls. (Reprinted from *Brain Cogn.* 61, Harris, G.J. et al., Brain activation during semantic processing in autism spectrum disorders via functional magnetic resonance imaging, 54–68, doi: 10.1016/j.bandc.2005.12.015, Copyright 2006, with permission from Elsevier. Reproduced with permission of Elsevier in the format reuse in a book/e-book via Copyright Clearance Center.)

lateralized activation. Findings of Eyler et al.'s (2012) findings suggest that the deficiencies in activation are particularly pronounced in the left anterior temporal region in children with ASD, with overactivation in the analogous right hemisphere region. Overall, these data suggest that functional lateralization for language in children with ASD becomes increasingly aberrant during the course of development, though longitudinal investigation is needed to confirm this speculation.

Research adopting behavioral techniques to probe language lateralization in ASD is consistent with the functional imaging data, indicating atypical lateralization. Hemispheric asymmetries for receptive language can be assessed using dichotic listening—a simple behavioral paradigm in which two different stimuli are presented simultaneously to the left and right ears; participants are instructed to report what was heard. As the auditory pathways are under predominant contralateral control, a right ear bias indicates a left hemisphere advantage for the task. Whereas typically developing children exhibit a right ear dichotic listening advantage, consistent with left hemisphere lateralization, children with ASD favor the left ear for verbal stimuli, indicating an atypical right hemisphere advantage for language processing (Blackstock 1978; Prior and Bradshaw 1979). Recent dichotic listening data again indicate atypical lateralization in ASD, reporting that boys (aged 6) with ASDs (high-functioning autism, Asperger's syndrome, and pervasive developmental disorder, not otherwise specified) show no ear preference for verbal stimuli, in contrast with the right ear advantage shown by typical controls (Martínez-Sanchis et al. 2014). Given that all the ASD samples tested by Martínez-Sanchis et al. were dominantly right-handed, and hence highly likely to show left hemisphere lateralization, these behavioral data indicate abnormal functional lateralization for language in children with ASD.

The structural imaging research suggested a causal relationship between atypical lateralization for language and poorer language outcomes. Not surprisingly, the functional imaging data confirm this relationship (e.g., Dawson et al. 1986, 1989). For example, at age 1–3 years, ERP research shows that the brains of typically developing children show different responses to known and unknown words in a focused, left parietal electrode site (Coffey-Corina et al. 2008). At the same age, not only do lower functioning children with ASD show a more right lateralized pattern of activation than either higher functioning children with ASD or typical controls, but the difference in response to known and unknown words was distributed across multiple right hemisphere electrode sites. These findings indicate that poorer language outcomes are linked to atypical lateralization of activation, with more diffuse rather than focused activation in the right, rather than left, hemisphere in lower functioning infants with ASDs.

The neuroimaging data are thus consistent with the structural imaging data: people with ASD show atypical functional asymmetries for language processing, with reduced left hemisphere and/or reversed patterns of activation. Again, the data suggest that poorer language outcomes are linked to more deviant patterns of functional lateralization. Whether the increased recruitment of the right hemisphere during language processing is the cause or the effect of atypical structural lateralization remains to be determined (Lindell et al. 2009; Lindell and Hudry 2013). Theoretically, an atypical hemispheric asymmetry present at birth could serve to catalyze greater right hemisphere involvement in language processing, with atypical structure promoting atypical functional activation. Atypical structural asymmetries could also develop as a result of experience: right hemisphere language homologues may increase in volume to compensate for deficient responses in the left-hemisphere language regions. Lindell and Hudry's (2013) model of language lateralization in ASD proposes a bidirectional relationship between abnormal structural and functional lateralization: in ASD, an initial genetic or environmental atypicality leads to abnormal structural lateralization, which, in turn, catalyzes atypical functional activation in response to language; the attenuated left hemisphere response to language in ASD further consolidates anomalous structural lateralization. Again, longitudinal research is needed to clarify both the cause and development of atypical functional asymmetries for language processing in people with ASD.

8.2 Emotion

While language has received the greatest amount of research attention, it is not the only lateralized function in the human brain. Following observation of patients following unilateral brain damage, English neurologist John Hughlings-Jackson (1874/1915) noted that patients with damage to the left hemisphere retained their ability to produce emotional speech. This faculty was lost in patients who suffered right hemisphere damage, suggesting that emotion was a function of the right hemisphere. Although a number of different models of emotion lateralization have since been proposed (see Demaree et al. 2005; Harmon-Jones et al. 2010; Rutherford and Lindell 2011), the right hemisphere is still widely regarded to play the dominant role in emotion processing (Lindell 2013). Consequently, patients with right hemisphere damage have greater difficulty than patients with left hemisphere damage in identifying, matching, and discriminating facial emotions (see Abbott et al. 2014).

There's no question that emotion plays a fundamental role in everyday communication and social interaction. Understanding others' emotions and determining their mental states rests on the ability to accurately perceive, recognize, and interpret facial expressions and prosodic cues in speech. Understanding emotion is therefore a key component in the theory of mind. Deficits in the expression, perception, and recognition of emotion, and challenges in understanding others' mental states, are all notable diagnostic criteria in ASDs. Although the body of research-assessing emotion lateralization in ASD is smaller than that devoted to the investigation of language lateralization (indeed, structural imaging data assessing emotion-processing regions are notably absent), the available data offer further evidence of atypical hemispheric asymmetries in people with ASDs.

8.2.1 Functional lateralization for emotion

The brain regions surrounding the superior temporal sulcus, including the superior, middle, and inferior temporal gyri, are thought to be responsible for processing emotional facial expressions (e.g., Haxby et al. 2000). And indeed, functional imaging investigations of emotion processing suggest atypical lateralization of activation in these areas in people with ASD. Using an implicit presentation of emotional faces (happy and angry), Leung et al.'s (2015) magnetoencephalography (MEG) data indicated that high-functioning adolescents with ASD show atypically reduced right hemisphere activation accompanied by increased left hemisphere activation in homologous regions (Figure 8.4). Whereas happy faces prompt right inferior and middle temporal activation in the typically developing controls, happy faces prompt greater left activation (superior, middle, and inferior temporal regions) in homologous temporal regions. Viewing angry faces similarly prompted overactivation in the left middle and inferior temporal areas, and hypoactivation in homologous right temporal regions. Leung et al. (2015) suggest that the difficulties that people with ASD have in processing affect may be attributed to "increased left hemispheric lateralization at the expense of typical right hemispheric or bilateral processing" (p. 209).

Functional imaging during emotional prosody tasks indicates that people with ASD show broader patterns of activation than typically developing controls, echoing the language findings. For example, Eigsti et al. (2012) used fMRI to examine activation during a task that implicitly assessed emotional prosody. High-functioning adolescents with ASD and typically developing controls were asked to listen to sentences and make semantic judgments; the sentences varied in emotional prosody (angry vs. neutral). There were no group differences in the behavioral findings, yet activation in response to prosody (incidental to the explicit task) revealed that the equivalent behavioral performance resulted from reliance on different cortical networks. Whereas both groups of participants demonstrated right-lateralized activation in the superior temporal gyrus in response to emotional prosody, participants with ASD additionally demonstrated activation across a range of other regions bilaterally, including bilateral parahippocampal gyri, the left globus pallidis, and the right middle frontal gyrus. As such, these data indicate that the brains of people with ASD show a more diffuse pattern of activation in response to emotional prosody than seen in typical development.

145

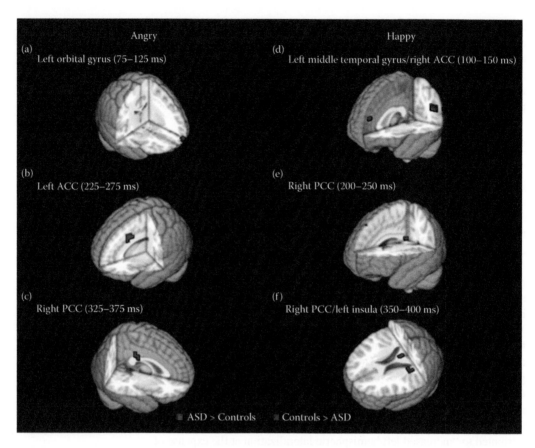

Figure 8.4 Reduced right hemisphere activation during emotion processing in people with ASD in comparisons with typical controls. (From Leung, R.C. et al. *NeuroImage: Clin.* 7, 203–212, 2015. doi: 10.1016/j.nicl.2014.11.009. Unmodified image reproduced with permission CC-BY http:// creativecommons.org/licenses/by-nc-nd/3.0/legalcode.)

Whereas a right ear advantage indicates left hemisphere superiority for language function in dichotic listening studies, this paradigm can also be used to assess emotion lateralization by varying the stimuli used. For example, lateralization of emotion can be investigated by using nonsense stimuli that vary in emotional prosody. Baker et al. (2010) compared dichotic listening performance in children and adolescents with high-functioning ASD and typically developing controls. Nonsense passages spoken in different emotional tones (happy, sad, angry, neutral) were simultaneously delivered to the left and right ears and participants were asked to identify the emotions presented. Both ASD and typical developing groups demonstrated a left ear advantage, consistent with right-hemisphere advantage for interpreting emotion. Importantly, there was no indication of an interaction, thus the magnitude of the advantage was not reduced for the ASD group, offering no evidence of aberrant hemispheric asymmetry for emotional prosody. As similar investigation has yet to be conducted examining people with lower-functioning ASDs, the possibility that atypical asymmetries for emotion (and emotional prosody in particular) evince only in those with more profound ASDs cannot be ruled out.

Visual half-field investigations also offer evidence of atypical lateralization for emotion processing in ASD. The paradigm relies on the projection of the visual fields: stimuli presented in the left visual field are initially projected to the right hemisphere, thus a left visual field advantage for a task implies right hemisphere superiority. Whereas typical controls show a left visual field (right hemisphere) advantage for emotion in the universal chimeric face task, children with ASDs show a less lateralized pattern of performance, akin to that expected for much younger children (Taylor et al. 2012). Consistently, other studies indicate that people with Asperger's syndrome fail to show a left visual field (i.e., right hemisphere) advantage for emotion recognition, unlike typically developing controls (Shamay-Tsoory et al. 2010), again indicating atypically reduced hemispheric asymmetries.

Given the emotion-processing impairments that characterize the ASD, atypical patterns of emotion lateralization are expected. If the brains of people with ASD show reduced lateralization for emotion processing, and activate less specific neural networks when processing emotion, it is not surprising that performance is compromised. In keeping with the language-processing investigations, the emotion-processing research suggests a failure of cortical specialization and atypical recruitment alternate brain regions in ASDs, suggesting widespread aberration in lateralization. That said, the number of available studies is small; a surprising number of imaging investigations of emotion processing in ASDs fail to assess left and right hemisphere differences in activation. Given that structural and functional atypicalities in lateralization in ASD show promise as potential biomarkers of ASD (Lindell and Hudry 2013), it is important that hemispheric comparisons are more regularly drawn in imaging investigations.

8.3 Faces

In addition to impairments in language and emotion processing, difficulties in processing faces form one of the core symptoms of ASDs. And indeed, deficits in face processing are likely to further compromise language and emotion processing, given the vital role played by the face in communicating both verbal and nonverbal information during social interactions. Whereas language processing is predominantly controlled by the left hemisphere, face processing is strongly right lateralized in the majority of the typical population (see Haxby et al. 2000, for review). The right fusiform gyrus is larger than the corresponding left hemisphere region in the typical population (Pierce et al. 2001), and viewing

147

faces consistently prompts heightened activation in this region (e.g., Kanwisher et al. 1999). Congruently, damage to the right fusiform gyrus is associated with problems in recognizing faces (e.g., De Renzi et al. 1994). As such deficits are rarely evident when the analogous left hemisphere region alone is damaged, face processing is considered strongly right lateralized. However, following the patterns noted for language and emotion processing, people with ASD show patterns of atypical cortical lateralization for face processing.

8.3.1 Structural lateralization for faces

Given that face-processing deficits are such a striking component of the symptomatology of ASD, surprisingly few studies have directly assessed structural asymmetries in the fusiform gyrus: researchers have instead focused on functional activation. The available structural research is mixed, with some studies reporting increased, and others reporting decreased (to the extent of complete reversal), rightward fusiform gyrus asymmetries.

Herbert et al. (2002) found evidence of reversed asymmetry in the fusiform gyrus of people with ASD, with greater matter on the left rather than right side. This pattern was not restricted to the fusiform region: Herbert et al. found that the brains of people with ASD had a greater number of regions with a rightward volumetric bias, in direct contrast with the brains of controls, which had a greater number of regions with a leftward volumetric bias.

However, other structural imaging studies report very different patterns. Pierce et al. (2001) found that people with ASD showed a similar rightward bias in fusiform gyrus volume to that seen in typical controls. Although overall fusiform gyrus volume was reduced in the ASD group (8% smaller than controls), volume in the region was not significantly different from the control group. In a marked contrast, whereas Pierce et al. reported a nonsignificant decrease in fusiform gyrus volume in people with ASD, Waiter et al. (2004) reported a significant increase in right fusiform gyrus volume in people with ASD. Thus with available investigations indicating a normal rightward fusiform asymmetry (Pierce et al. 2001), an increased rightward fusiform asymmetry (Waiter et al. 2004), and a reversed leftward fusiform asymmetry (Herbert et al. 2002), it's something of an understatement to say that the available data are "inconclusive."

Beyond gross regional anatomy, fine-grained postmortem structural examination of the fusiform gyrus in people with autism does suggest neuropathological abnormality. Specifically, van Kooten et al. (2008) found that the fusiform gyrus in people with ASD contains a smaller number and volume of neurons, and reduced neuron density, in comparison with typical controls. Despite this, the overall volume of the fusiform gyrus did not differ between people with ASD and typical controls.

This suggests that overall similarities in gross brain volume may mask dissimilarities in the underlying neuronal composition, highlighting the need for more fine-grained analysis of cortical composition. However, it should be noted that van Kooten et al. (2008) had access to only one hemisphere from each of their participants (four left and three right hemispheres for the ASD group; four left and six right hemispheres for the control group), and the researchers did not draw any comparisons between left and right hemisphere volumes or neuronal composition. As such, further investigation is clearly needed as relative differences in left/right hemisphere fusiform gyrus volume and composition cannot be assessed from single hemisphere investigations.

The limited research examining structural lateralization for face processing in people with ASD fails to paint a clear picture, and it would be premature to draw firm conclusions based on the data. Though it appears probable that the fusiform gyrus in people with ASD is atypically lateralized, whether that atypicality manifests in increased rightward, or reversed and increased leftward, asymmetry remains to be determined. Fortunately, a far greater body of research has assessed functional lateralization for face processing in people with ASD, allowing clearer conclusions to be drawn.

8.3.2 Functional lateralization for faces

One of the most consistent findings in the neuroimaging literature is that the fusiform gyrus responds preferentially to faces (e.g., Kanwisher et al. 1999). However, in keeping with the evidence of structural abnormality in people with ASD, fusiform gyrus hypoactivation has been repeatedly reported when people with ASD view faces (e.g., Critchley et al. 2000; Pierce et al. 2001; Deeley et al. 2007). As the right fusiform response in people with ASD is relatively stronger for familiar than stranger faces (Hadjikhani et al. 2004; Pierce et al. 2004), right fusiform hypoactivation may well reflect strong influences of attention and motivation to neuronal responses to faces in ASD (i.e., disinterest in/attention to faces attenuates the response, hence hypoactivation).

Faces not only prompt atypically reduced right fusiform gyrus activation in ASD: faces activate alternate right hemisphere brain regions. Using fMRI to assess patterns of activation in response to faces and objects, Schultz et al. (2000) found that people with ASD showed less activation in response to faces in the right fusiform gyrus. This reduced fusiform activation was accompanied by an increased activation in the right inferior temporal gyrus, a region that responds preferentially to objects in the typical population. Their data indicate remarkable similarity in the regions that show heightened activation in response to faces in ASD and objects in the typical population. As Schultz et al. suggest, these findings imply that perceptual processing of faces in people with ASD is more like the perceptual processing of objects seen in the typical population,

149

hence the reduction/absence of right fusiform activation in response to faces (see also Hubl et al. 2003). Koshino et al. (2008) offer further support for this notion, finding that the location of right fusiform activation differed between ASD and control groups, being displaced toward the inferior temporal gyrus (Figure 8.5). Overall then, these data imply that people with ASD are using atypical strategies, and consequently activating aberrant brain regions, when processing faces.

Bailey et al. (2005) offer further evidence indicating abnormal cortical organization in people with ASD. They used MEG to assess both the spatial location and time course of activation as adults with ASD and typical controls categorized and identified stimuli (faces vs. mugs). The neural response to faces in the ASD group did not differ from the control group in terms of timing of activation; however, the location and strength of activation were anomalous. The neuronal response to faces was weaker in the ASD group, and though right lateralized, showed greater overlap with the pattern of activation in response to mugs, activating extrastriate regions. As such, Bailey et al.'s data again indicate that people with ASD are engaging similar brain regions to process both faces and objects, consistent with previous reports. These findings may help explain why training interventions designed to improve recognition of facial affect fail to increase activation in the fusiform gyrus in people with ASD (Bölte et al. 2006). If people with ASD adopt different strategies, and engage alternate brain regions, when processing faces, training/interventions are likely to consolidate the existing atypical face-processing networks, rather than catalyze recruitment of the

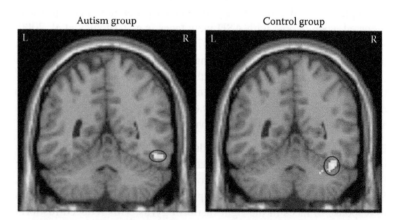

Figure 8.5 Right hemisphere activation in response to faces in ASD and control groups. Note that activation in ASD is reduced and displaced in comparison with activation in the control group. (From Koshino, H. et al. *Cerebral Cortex*, 2008, doi: 10.1093/cercor/bhm054, Oxford University Press, by permission of Oxford University Press. Reproduced with permission of Oxford University Press in the format reuse in a book/ e-book via Copyright Clearance Center.)

face-processing regions engaged in the typically developing population, hence the absence of change in fusiform activation in response to faces following intervention (Bölte et al. 2006).

Overall, the functional imaging data examining face processing indicate reduced lateralization and reliance on alternate neural networks in people with ASD. In ASD, faces activate regions recruited for object recognition in the typically developing population, including the inferior temporal gyrus (Figure 8.5), consistent with the idea that people with ASD process faces using a featural, rather than configural, recognition strategy (e.g., Deruelle et al. 2008).

8.4 Conclusion

The research reviewed in this chapter suggests that the neural networks controlling language, face, and emotion processing are atypically lateralized in people with ASD. As a rule of thumb, the ASD brain is hypolateralized: it shows reduced activation in the brain regions typically responsible for language, emotion, and face processing, and instead activates additional/alternate brain regions, not activated in the neurotypical population. The fact that asymmetries are atypical across such a broad range of cognitive functions implies pervasive, rather than regionally or functionally specific, neural system disorganization. Although atypical lateralization is likely just one index of more widespread neural system abnormality, it shows suggestive promise as a potential biomarker of ASD (see Lindell and Hudry, 2013). However, further systematic investigation is needed, given the heterogeneity in findings (presumably a reflection of the heterogeneity that characterizes ASD). As Pierce and Courchesne (2000) note, "different individuals with autism have different patterns of functional deviation [...]. Some may show activation reduction in normal locations, while other may show abnormal hemispheric asymmetry of activation, and still others may show robust activation but in aberrant or scattered cortical locations" (p. 345). Though such individual differences may hold the key for explaining differences in ASD presentation, intervention efficacy, and outcomes, this area of research has yet to be systematically explored. Such systematic investigation into hemispheric asymmetries may help facilitate earlier identification and diagnosis, enhancing outcomes for people with ASD.

References

Abbott, J. D., T. Wijeratne, A. Hughes, D. Perre, and A. K. Lindell. 2014. The perception of positive and negative facial expressions by unilateral stroke patients. *Brain and Cognition* 86:42–54.

Anderson, J. S., N. Lange, A. Froehlich et al. 2010. Decreased left posterior insular activity during auditory language in autism. *Am. J. Neuroradiol.* 31:131–9. doi: 10.3174/ajnr.A1789.

Aylward, E. H., N. J. Minshew, K. Field, B. F. Sparks, and N. Singh. 2002. Effects of age on brain volume and head circumference in autism. *Neurology* 59(Suppl 2):175–83. doi: 10.1212/WNL.59.2.175.

Bailey, A. J., S. Braeutigam, V. Jousmäki, and S. J. Swithenby. 2005. Abnormal activation of face processing systems at early and intermediate latency in individuals with autism spectrum disorder: A magnetoencephalographic study. *Eur. J. Neurosci.* 21:2575–85. doi: 10.1111/j.1460-9568.2005.04061.x.

Baker, K. F., A. A. Montgomery, and R. Abramson. 2010. Perception and lateralization of spoken emotion by youths with high-functioning forms of autism. *J. Autism Dev. Disord.* 40:123–9. doi: 10.1007/s10803-009-0841-1.

Blackstock, E. G. 1978. Cerebral asymmetry and the development of early infantile autism. *J. Autism Childhood Schizophr.* 8:339–53.

Bölte, S., D. Hubl, S. Feineis-Matthews, D. Prulovic, T. Dierks, and F. Poustka. 2006. Facial affect recognition training in autism: Can we animate the fusiform gyrus? *Behav. Neurosci.* 120:211–6. doi: 10.1037/0735-7044.120.1.211.

Brieber, S., S. Neufang, N. Bruning et al. 2007. Structural brain abnormalities in adolescents with autism spectrum disorder and patients with attention deficit/hyperactivity disorder. *J. Child Psychol. Psychiatry* 48:1251–8. doi: 10.1111/j.1469-7610.2007.01799.x.

Broca, P. 1865. Sur la siege de la faculté du langage articulé. *Bull. Soc. Anthropologie Paris.* 6:377–93.

Coffey-Corina, S., D. Padden, and P. K. Kuhl. 2008. ERPs to words correlate with behavioral measures in children with autism spectrum disorder. *J. Acoust. Soc. Am.* 123:3742. doi: 10.1121/1.2935280.

Courchesne, E., R. Carper, and N. Akshoomoff. 2003. Evidence of brain overgrowth in the first year of life in autism. *J. Am. Med. Assoc.* 290:337–44. doi: 10.1001/jama.290.3.337.

Courchesne, E., C. Karns, H. Davis et al. 2001. Unusual brain growth patterns in early life in patients with autistic disorder: An MRI study. *Neurology* 57:245–54. doi: 10.1212/WNL.57.2.245.

Critchley, H. D., E. M. Daly, E. T. Bullmore et al. 2000. The functional neuroanatomy of social behaviour changes in cerebral blood flow when people with autistic disorder process facial expressions. *Brain* 123:2203–12. doi: 10.1093/brain/123.11.2203.

Dawson, G., C. Finley, S. Philips, and L. Galpert. 1986. Hemispheric specialization and the language abilities of autistic children. *Child Dev.* 57:1440–53. doi: 10.2307/1130422.

Dawson, G., C. Finley, S. Philips, and A. Lewy. 1989. A comparison of hemispheric asymmetries in speech-related brain potentials of autistic and dysphasic children. *Brain Lang.* 37:26–41. doi: 10.1016/0093-934X(89)90099-0.

Dawson, G., S. Warrenburg, and P. Fuller. 1982. Cerebral lateralization in individuals diagnosed as autistic in early childhood. *Brain Lang.* 15:353–68. doi: 10.1016/0093-934X(82)90065-7.

De Fossé, L., S. M. Hodge, N. Makris et al. 2004. Language-association cortex asymmetry in autism and specific language impairment. *Ann. Neurol.* 56:757–66. doi: 10.1002/ana.20275.

De Renzi, E., D. Perani, G. A. Carlesimo, M. C. Silveri, and F. Fazio. 1994. Prosopagnosia can be associated with damage confined to the right hemisphere—An MRI and PET study and a review of the literature. *Neuropsychologia* 32:893–902. doi: 10.1016/0028-3932(94)90041-8.

Deeley, Q., E. M. Daly, S. Surguladze et al. 2007. An event related functional magnetic resonance imaging study of facial emotion processing in Asperger syndrome. *Biol. Psychiatry* 62:207–17. doi: 10.1016/j.biopsych.2006.09.037.

Demaree, H. A., E. Everhart, E. A. Youngstrom, and Harrison, D. W. 2005. Brain lateralization of emotional processing: Historical roots and a future incorporating "dominance." *Behavioural and Cognitive Neuroscience Review* 4:3–20.

Deruelle, C., C. Rondan, X. Salle-Collemiche, D. Bastard-Rosset, and D. Da Fonséca. 2008. Attention to low- and high-spatial frequencies in categorizing facial identities, emotions and gender in children with autism. *Brain Cogn.* 66:115–23. doi: 10.1016/j.bandc.2007.06.001.

Eigsti, I. M., J. Schuh, R. T. Schultz, and R. Paul. 2012. The neural underpinnings of prosody in autism. *Child Neuropsychol.* 18:600–17. doi: 10.1080/09297049.2011.639757.

Eyler, L.T., K. Pierce, and E. Courchesne. 2012. A failure of left temporal cortex to specialize for language is an early emerging and fundamental property of autism. *Brain* 135:949–60. doi: 10.1093/brain/awr364.

Flagg, E. J., J. E. Oram Cardy, W. Roberts, and T. P. L. Roberts. 2005. Language lateralization development in children with autism: Insights form the late field magnetoencephalogram. *Neurosci. Lett.* 386:82–7. doi: 10.1016/j. neulet.2005.05.037.

Gage, N. M., J. Juranek, P. A. Filipek, K. Osann, P. Flodman, A. L. Isenberg, and M. A. Spence. 2009. Rightward hemispheric asymmetries in auditory language cortex in children with autistic disorder: An MRI investigation. *Journal of Neurodevelop. Disord.* 1:205–14. doi: 10.1007/s11689-009-9010-2.

Hadjikhani, N., R. M. Joseph, J. Snyder et al. 2004. Activation of the fusiform gyrus when individuals with autism spectrum disorder view faces. *NeuroImage* 22:1141–50. doi: 10.1016/j.neuroimage.2004.03.025.

Hale, T. S., J. T. McCracken, J. J. McGough et al. 2005. Impaired linguistic processing and atypical brain laterality in adults with ADHD. *Clin. Neurosci. Res.* 5:255–63. doi: 10.1016/j.cnr.2005.09.006.

Hardan, A. Y., N. J. Minshew, M. Mallikarjuhn, and M. S. Keshavan. 2001. Brain volume in autism. *J. Child Neurol.* 16:421–4. doi: 10.1177/088307380101600607.

Harmon-Jones, E., P. A. Gable, and C. K. Peterson. 2010. The role of asymmetric frontal cortical activity in emotion-related phenomena: A review and update. *Biological Psychology* 84:451–62.

Harris, G. J., C. F. Chabris, J. Clark, T. Urban, I. Aharon, S. Steele, L. McGrath, K. Condouris, and H. Tager-Flusberg. 2006. Brain activation during semantic processing in autism spectrum disorders via functional magnetic resonance imaging. *Brain Cogn.* 61:54–68. doi: 10.1016/j.bandc.2005.12.015.

Haxby, J. V., E. A. Hoffman, and M. I. Gobbini. 2000. The distributed human neural system for face perception. *Trends Cogn. Sci.* 4:223–33. doi: 10.1016/ S1364-6613(00)01482-0.

Hazlett, H. C., M. D. Poe, G. Gerig, R. G. Smith, and J. Piven. 2006. Cortical gray and white brain tissue volume in adolescents and adults with autism. *Biol. Psychiatry* 59:1–6. doi: 10.1016/j.biopsych.2005.06.015.

Herbert, M. R., G. J. Harris, K. T. Adrien et al. 2002. Abnormal asymmetries in language association cortex in autism. *Ann. Neurol.* 52:588–96. doi: 10.1002/ ana.10349.

Herbert, M. R., D. A. Ziegler, C. K. Deutsch et al. 2005. Brain asymmetries in autism and developmental language disorder: A nested whole-brain analysis. *Brain* 128:213–26. doi: 10.1093/brain/awh330.

Hodge, S. M., N. Makris, D. N. Kennedy, V. S. Caviness Jr., J. Howard, L. McGrath, S. Steele, J. A. Frazier, H. Tager-Flusberg, and G. J. Harris. 2010. Cerebellum, language, and cognition in autism and specific language impairment. *J. Autism Dev. Disord.* 40:300–16. doi: 10.1007/s10803-009-0872-7.

Hubl, D., S. Bölte, S. Feinis-Matthews et al. 2003. Functional imbalance of visual pathways indicates alternative face processing strategies in autism. *Neurology* 61:1232–7. doi: 10.1212/01.WNL.0000091862.22033.1A.

Just, M. A., V. L. Cherkassky, T. A. Keller, and N. J. Minshew. 2004. Cortical activation and synchronization during sentence comprehension in high-functioning autism: Evidence of underconnectivity. *Brain* 127:1811–21. doi: 10.1093/ brain/awh199.

Kanwisher, N. D. Stanley, and A. Harris. 1999. The fusiform face area is selective for faces not animals. *NeuroReport* 10(1):183–7.

Klimkeit, E. I. and J. L. Bradshaw. 2006. Anomalous lateralisation in neurodevelopmental disorders. *Cortex* 42:113–6. doi: 10.1016/S0010-9452(08)70334-4.

Knaus, T. A., A. M. Silver, M. Kennedy, K. A. Lindgren, K. C. Dominick, J. Siegel, and H. Tager-Flusberg. 2010. Language laterality in autism spectrum disorder and typical controls: A functional, volumetric, and diffusion tensor MRI study. *Brain Lang.* 112:113–20. doi: 10.1016/j.bandl.2009.11.005.

Knecht, S., B. Dräger, M. Deppe, L. Bobe, H. Lohmann, A. Flöel, E. B. Ringelstein, and H. Henningsen. 2000. Handedness and hemispheric language dominance in healthy humans. *Brain* 123:2512–8. doi: 10.1093/brain/123.12.2512.

Koshino, H., R. K. Kana, T. A. Keller, V. L. Cherkassky, N. J. Minshew, and M. A. Just. 2008. fMRI investigation of working memory for faces in autism: Visual coding and underconnectivity with frontal areas. *Cereb. Cortex* 18:289–300. doi: 10.1093/cercor/bhm054.

Leung, R. C., E. W. Pang, D. Cassel, J. A. Brian, M. L. Smith, and M. J. Taylor. 2015. Early neural activation during facial affect processing in adolescents with autism spectrum disorder. *NeuroImage: Clin.* 7:203–12. doi: 10.1016/j.nicl.2014.11.009.

Lindell, A. K. 2006. In your right mind: Right hemisphere contributions to human language processing and production. *Neuropsychol. Rev.* 16:131–48. doi: 10.1007/s11065-006-9011-9.

Lindell, A. K. and K. Hudry. 2013. Atypicalities in cortical structure, handedness, and functional lateralization for language in autism spectrum disorders. *Neuropsychol. Rev.* 23:257–70. doi: 10.1007/s11065-013-9234-5.

Lindell, A. K., K. Notice, and K. Withers. 2009. Reduced language processing asymmetry in non-autistic individuals with high levels of autism traits. *Laterality* 14:457–72. doi: 10.1080/13576500802507752.

Martínez-Sanchis, S., M. C. Bernal, A. Costa, and M. Gadea. 2014. Abnormal linguistic lateralization and sensory processing in high functioning children with autism spectrum conditions. *J. Behav. Brain Sci.* 4:432–42. doi: 10.4236/jbbs.2014.49042.

Mayo, J., C. Chlebowski, D. A. Fein, and I. M. Eigsti. 2013. Age of first words predicts cognitive ability and adaptive skills in children with ASDs. *J. Autism Dev. Disord.* 43:253–64. doi: 10.1007/s10803-012-1558-0.

McAlonan, G. M., J. Suckling, N. Wong, V. Cheung, N. Lienenkaemper, C. Cheung, and S. E. Chua. 2008. Distinct patterns of grey matter abnormality in high-functioning autism and Asperger syndrome. *J. Child Psychol. Psychiatry* 49:1287–95. doi: 10.1111/j.1469-7610.2008.01933.x.

Mody, M. and J. W. Belliveau. 2012. Speech and language impairments in autism: Insight from behavior and neuroimaging. *North Am. J. Med. Sci.* 5:157–61. doi: 10.7156/v5i3p157.

Moncrieff, D. W. 2010. Hemispheric asymmetry in pediatric developmental disorders: Autism, attention-deficit/hyperactivity disorder, and dyslexia. In *The Two Halves of the Brain*, eds. K. Hugdahl and R. Westerhausen, 561–601. Cambridge, MA: MIT Press.

Morgan, A. E. and G. W. Hynd. 1998. Dyslexia, neurolinguistic ability, and the anatomical variation of the planum temporale. *Neuropsychol. Rev.* 8:79–93. doi: 10.1023/A:1025609216841.

Müller, R. A, M. E. Behen, R. D. Rothermel, D. C. Chugani, O. Muzik, T. J. Mangner, and H. T. Chugani. 1999. Brain mapping of language and auditory perception in high-functioning autistic adults: A PET study. *J. Autism Dev. Disord.* 29:19–31. doi: 10.1023/A:1025914515203.

Ocklenburg, S. and O. Güntürkün. 2012. Hemispheric asymmetries: The comparative view. *Front. Psychol.* 3:5. doi: 10.3389/fpsyg.2012.00005.

Pierce, K. and E. Courchesne. 2000. Exploring neurofuncitonal organization of face processing in autism. *Arch. Gen. Psychiatry* 57:344–6. doi: 10.1001/archpsyc.57.4.344.

Pierce, K., F. Haist, F. Sedaghar, and E. Courchesne. 2004. The brain response to personally familiar faces in autism: Findings of fusiform activity and beyond. *Brain* 127:2703–16. doi: 10.1093/brain/awh289.

Pierce, K., R. A. Müller, J. Ambrose, G. Allen, and E. Courchesne. 2001. Face processing occurs outside the fusiform "face area" in autism: Evidence from functional MRI. *Brain* 124:2059–73.

Prior, M. and J. Bradshaw. 1979. Hemispheric functioning in autistic children. *Cortex* 15:73–81. doi: 10.1016/S0010-9452(79)80008-8.

Rojas, D. C., S. D. Bawn, T. L. Benkers, M. L. Reite, and S. J. Rogers. 2002. Smaller left hemisphere planum temporale in adults with autistic disorder. *Neurosci. Lett.* 323:237–40. doi: 10.1016/S0304-3940(02)00521-9.

Rojas, D. C., S. L. Camou, M. L. Reite, and S. J. Rogers. 2005. Planum temporale volume in children and adolescents with autism. *J. Autism Dev. Disord.* 35:479–86. doi: 10.1007/s10803-005-5038-7.

Rutherford, H. J. and A. K. Lindell. 2011. Thriving and Surviving: Approach and avoidance motivation and lateralisation. *Emotion Review* 3(3):333–43.

Schultz, R. T., I. Gauthier, A. Klin et al. 2000. Abnormal ventral temporal cortical activity during face discrimination among individuals with autism and Asperger syndrome. *Arch. Gen. Psychiatry* 57:331–40. doi: 10.1001/archpsyc.57.4.331.

Seery, A. M., V. Vogel-Farley, H. Tager-Flusberg, and C. A. Nelson. 2013. Atypical lateralization of ERP response to native and non-native speech in infants at risk for autism spectrum disorder. *Dev. Cogn. Neurosci.* 5:10–24. doi: 10.1016/j.dcn.2012.11.007.

Shamay-Tsoory, S. G., E. Gev, J. Aharon-Peretz, and N. Adler. 2010. Brain asymmetry in emotional processing in Asperger syndrome. *Cogn. Behav. Neurol.* 23:74–84. doi: 10.1097/WNN.0b013e3181d748ec.

Smalley, S. L., S. K. Loo, M. H. Yang, and R. M. Cantor. 2004. Towards localizing genes underlying cerebral asymmetry and mental health. *Am. J. Med. Genet.* 135B:79–84. doi: 10.1002/ajmg.b.30141.

Taylor, S., L. Workman, and H. Yeomans. 2012. Abnormal patterns of cerebral lateralisation as revealed by the universal chimeric faces task in individuals with autistic disorder. *Laterality* 17:428–37. doi: 10.1080/1359650X.2010.521751.

van Kooten, I. A. J., S. J. M. C. Palmen, P. von Cappeln et al. 2008. Neurons in the fusiform gyrus are fewer and smaller in autism. *Brain* 131:987–99. doi: 10.1093/brain/awn033.

Waiter, G. D., J. H. G. Williams, A. D. Murray et al. 2004. A voxel-based investigation of brain structure in male adolescents with autism spectrum disorder. *NeuroImage* 22:619–25.

Xu, M., J. Yang, W. T. Siok, and L. H. Tan. 2015. Atypical lateralization of phonological working memory in developmental dyslexia. *J. Neurolinguist.* 33:67–77. doi: 10.1016/j.jneuroling.2014.07.004.

Chapter 9 Corpus callosum and autism

Lawrence K. Fung and
Antonio Hardan

Contents

Abstract 157
9.1   Introduction 158
9.2   Anatomy of the corpus callosum 158
9.3   Corpus callosum in idiopathic autism 159
     9.3.1   Cross-sectional area and volume of the corpus
          callosum 159
     9.3.2   Shape and symmetry of the corpus callosum 161
     9.3.3   Integrity and anatomical connectivity of the corpus
          callosum 162
     9.3.4   Functional connectivity of the corpus callosum 163
9.4   Corpus callosum in neurogenetic syndromes exhibiting
     social deficits 163
     9.4.1   Agenesis of the corpus callosum 163
     9.4.2   Neurofibromatosis type 1 164
     9.4.3   Velocardiofacial syndrome (VCFS) 164
     9.4.4   Williams syndrome. 165
9.5   Animal models with abnormalities of the corpus callosum 165
9.6   Summary and future directions 166
References 166

Abstract

The corpus callosum (CC) is the largest white matter structure connecting the left and right hemispheres of the human brain. Many studies have revealed that the topology, integrity, and connectivity of the CC of individuals with autism spectrum disorder (ASD) are different from neurotypical controls. In addition to ASD, various neurogenetic syndromes exhibiting social interaction deficits (e.g., neurofibromatosis type 1) also manifest abnormalities of the CC. Although much evidence supports the association of CC abnormalities with the ASD phenotype, abnormal CC is still not a pathognomonic sign of ASD. Much research is needed to further our understanding of the role of CC in the pathophysiology of ASD.

9.1 Introduction

The corpus callosum (CC) is the largest interhemispheric bundle between the left and right hemispheres of the human brain. CC has been suggested to facilitate long-distance integration of information flow from various sensory cortices within large brains (Mihrshahi 2006). Consistent with this hypothesis, increases in CC area and number of callosal fibers are correlated with increases in cortical volume across species (Rilling and Insel 1999), showing that increase in the size of CC is crucial in larger brains such as those in humans. When long-distance tracts such as CC are disrupted, significant negative consequences in neurobiological functions are predicted, as in the case of autism spectrum disorder (ASD). In this chapter, we will start with a general introduction on the neuroanatomy of CC. We will elaborate on various lines of evidence showing that CC of individuals with ASD differs from neurotypical controls in terms of its size, shape, symmetry, integrity, and connectivity. We will then explore specific conditions that affect CC, including agenesis of corpus callosum, neurofibromatosis, 22q11.2 deletion syndrome, and Williams syndrome. We will describe animal models of abnormalities of CC. Finally, we will describe the limitations of current approaches and potential future avenues to study CC.

9.2 Anatomy of the corpus callosum

The CC is a topographically organized anatomical structure in the brain. Fibers connecting a given cortical area are adjacent to the corresponding part of CC. The major parts of CC include the rostrum (Region 1), genu (Region 2), body (Regions 3–5), isthmus (Region 6), and splenium (Region 7) (see Figure 9.1). The rostrum connects the caudal-orbital prefrontal cortex and inferior premotor cortex (Hardan et al. 2000). The genu, which is the anterior one-sixth of the CC, primarily connects prefrontal association areas (Hofer and Frahm 2006), as well as the anterior inferior parietal regions (de Lacoste et al. 1985). The anterior part of the body of CC (Region 3) connects premotor and supplementary motor cortices. The midbody of CC (Regions 4 and 5) connects primary motor areas (Hofer and Frahm 2006). Toward the posterior of the callosum, the isthmus (Region 6) connects primary motor and primary sensory areas (Wahl et al. 2007). The anterior splenium (Region 7a) connects the association areas of the parietal and temporal lobes (Huang et al. 2005; Hofer and Frahm 2006). Finally, the posterior splenium (Region 7b) connects the occipital lobes (Huang et al. 2005; Hofer and Frahm 2006). The fibers of the genu and rostrum are generally thin, poorly myelinated, and slow-conducting, while the fibers of the posterior midbody and posterior splenium are thick, highly myelinated, and fast-conducting (Aboitiz et al. 1992). The rapid conduction via large fibers in the posterior parts of the CC aids in fusing lateralized sensory input (Aboitiz et al. 1992).

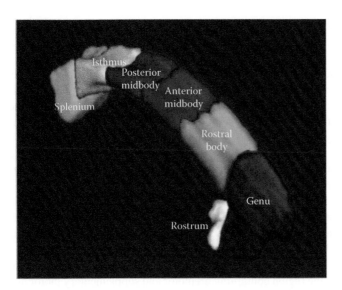

Figure 9.1 Subregions of the corpus callosum (CC) based on the organization according to Witelson. Regions denote anatomic label (cortical regions). Region 1 = rostrum (caudal-orbital prefrontal, inferior premotor); region 2 = genu (prefrontal, anterior inferior parietal); region 3 = rostral body (premotor, supplementary motor); regions 4 and 5 = midbody (primary motor); region 6 = isthmus (primary motor, primary sensory); region 7a = anterior splenium (association areas of temporal and parietal); region 7b = posterior splenium (occipital).

9.3 Corpus callosum in idiopathic autism

To study the pathology of CC in individuals with ASD, investigators have characterized this anatomical structure with various methodologies. The earliest attempts focused on measuring the size of the mid-sagittal area of CC and its subregions by structural magnetic resonance imaging (MRI). Later on, the shape and symmetry of the CC were studied. More recently, the integrity and anatomic connectivity of the white matter structure of CC was elucidated by diffusion tensor imaging (DTI) and related techniques, while functional connectivity of the CC was investigated by functional MR methodologies. We will summarize some of the key findings in ASD in this section.

9.3.1 Cross-sectional area and volume of the corpus callosum

Corpus callosum was first studied about 20 years ago when overall reduction in the mid-sagittal CC cross-sectional area was found in individuals with ASD (age range 3–45 years) as compared to age-matched neurotypical controls (Egaas et al. 1995). This reduction was found to be more pronounced in the posterior regions of the CC. Similar findings

159

were replicated by Piven et al. in a group of adolescents and young adults (Piven et al. 1997). In contrast to findings from Piven and Egaas, Hardan et al. found that the anterior (instead of the posterior) half of CC was smaller in adolescents and young adults with ASD, compared to age- and IQ-matched controls (Hardan et al. 2000). The greatest reduction in CC area in participants with ASD was found in the genu (region 2) of the CC. Significant reduction of total CC area was also found in young children (3–4 years old) with ASD, as compared to typically developing children, when adjusted for increased cerebral volume (Boger-Megiddo et al. 2006). Meta-analysis of the cross-sectional area of CC from 10 studies totaling 253 individuals (children, adolescents, and adults) with ASD and 250 age-matched healthy control subjects revealed a reduction of the total CC area in the ASD group with medium effect size (Frazier and Hardan 2009). Frazier and Hardan showed regional reductions in size with the magnitude of the effect decreasing posteriorly. The rostral body of CC (Region 3) showed the largest effect, indicating greatest reduction in the region containing premotor and supplementary motor neurons (Frazier and Hardan 2009).

Despite overwhelming agreement in reduction of CC cross-sectional area in individuals with ASD, a recent study did not support this finding in high-functioning adults with ASD (mean full-scale IQ = 125), as compared to age-matched controls (mean full-scale IQ = 135) (Tepest et al. 2010). Previous studies reporting a decrease in the size of the CC tended to include more children, and more importantly, recruited participants with full-scale IQ that tended to be lower 91 (Piven et al. 1997); 100 (Hardan et al. 2000). This inconsistency highlights, once again, the heterogeneity of ASD and the need to include large sample size with a wide age range and variable level of cognitive functioning.

In the past 10 years, the size of CC was also determined by novel volumetric methods. Compared to age- and IQ-matched controls, individuals with autism (age 8–45 years) were found to have reductions in total volume of the CC and several of its subdivisions (especially isthmus) (Keary et al. 2009). Decrease in total CC volume was also replicated in children (age 8–13 years; Hardan et al. 2009), as well as medication-naïve adolescents and adults (Freitag et al. 2009) with ASD. Using statistical maps of the CC, Vidal et al. revealed significant reductions in the volumes of both the splenium and genu of the CC in boys (mean age 10 years) with ASD (Vidal et al. 2006).

As ASD is a neurodevelopmental disorder, attempts have been made to chart the size of the CC over time. Volumetric measurements were also made in a recent longitudinal study of CC size in ASD (Frazier et al. 2012). In this 2-year longitudinal MRI study, persistent reductions in CC volumes were found in male children (age ~10 years at the start of the study) with ASD compared to age-matched controls. The rostral body was the only region showing normalization of size over time. Using a cross-sectional design, Prigge et al. examined the developmental trajectories of mid-sagittal CC area in children and adults with ASD (Prigge et al. 2013), and supported the potential for maturational abnormalities in CC in individuals with ASD.

Correlations between several neuropsychological test performance and CC measurements were found (Keary et al. 2009). CC volume reductions were correlated with poor performance on several neurocognitive tests including social deficits, repetitive behaviors, and sensory abnormalities (Hardan et al. 2009). While total CC volume was found to correlate positively with IQ in neurotypical controls, this relationship did not appear to be significant in individuals with ASD (Freitag et al. 2009).

9.3.2 Shape and symmetry of the corpus callosum

In addition to area and volume of CC, novel methodologies have been used to characterize the abnormalities in CC of individuals with ASD. The length, but not the width, of the CC was found to be shorter in children with ASD (He et al. 2008). The distance between the interior genu and the posterior-most section of the CC was also found to be shorter in children with ASD (He et al. 2010). An early study reported that there were no differences in shape between the CC of control individuals with benign macrocephaly and individuals with macrocephaly and ASD (Rice et al. 2005). However, He et al. reported significant global shape differences in the anterior lower body and posterior bottom, and there was a local shape difference in the anterior bottom (He et al. 2010). Sophisticated shape modeling of the CC has also been used to fit the contours of the structure and successfully capture the geometric features of the CC in individuals with ASD. Farag et al. employed the Bezier curve to connect the vertices of the contours of the CC, and coefficients of Bernstein polynomials to describe the geometric features of the CC. Together with descriptors derived from the Fourier transform, the coefficients of Bernstein polynomials were able to differentiate between the shape of the CC in individuals with ASD and that in neurotypical controls (Farag et al. 2010).

Using a novel quantitative paradigm to describe the shape of the CC in patients with ASD and typical control individuals, Cananova et al. found that the CC was significantly reduced in size throughout the entire structure, with the biggest differences at the splenium (Casanova et al. 2011). These investigators also found that there was a gradient of severity spanning the rostral-caudal axis of the left side of the CC. This finding appears to be consistent with the left hemisphere dysfunction theory of autism, which states that individuals with ASD have more deficits in functions ascribed to the left hemisphere (e.g., language, nonverbal communication). This theory was also supported by the asymmetry of the CC in adolescents with ASD (Floris et al. 2013).

161

9.3.3 Integrity and anatomical connectivity of the corpus callosum

Although the first study examining the integrity of CC by MRI did not show significant abnormalities in NMR signal intensity in the structure of individuals with ASD (Belmonte et al. 1995), many more studies using more modern techniques (e.g., diffusion tensor imaging [DTI]) have shown significant differences in this white matter structure. Alexander et al. found that adolescents with ASD exhibited smaller CC volumes, higher mean diffusivity, lower fractional anisotropy (FA), and increased radial diffusivity (Alexander et al. 2007). These findings were especially significant for a subgroup of participants with ASD and lower performance IQ. Shukla et al. replicated the finding of reduced FA, increased radial diffusion in all segments of the CC, and reduced axial diffusion in children with ASD, compared with those in TD children (mean age: 13 years; [Shukla et al. 2010]). Using DTI tractography and tract-based spatial statistics (TBSS), Kumar et al. replicated the finding of lower FA in children (mean age: 5 years) with ASD (Kumar et al. 2010). Furthermore, compared to neurotypical children, the ASD group was shown to have increased length and density of fibers in the CC. Increase in the density of callosal fibers was also shown in high-functioning children (Hong et al. 2011) and adults (Thomas et al. 2011) with ASD. Using DTI tractography, the lengths of callosal fibers originating from all areas of cortex in adults with ASD were determined (Lewis et al. 2013). Callosal fiber length (controlled for intracranial volume) was found to correlate directly with radial diffusivity, but inversely with CC size. Using magnetization transfer imaging, a novel MR technology allowing indirect measurement of myelin, Gozzi et al. demonstrated increases in myelin density around the CC in the brains of children with ASD (Gozzi et al. 2012).

Employing a cohort sequential design, Travers et al. conducted the only longitudinal DTI study of CC (Travers et al. 2015). This study revealed a different developmental trajectory of white matter microstructure in the anterior CC (genu and body) of individuals with ASD in comparison to typically developing controls, suggesting abnormal brain maturation in these regions. The developmental trajectories were most atypical in the youngest participants (<10 years of age). While decreased FA was found across all three subregions of the CC in the ASD group, increased mean diffusivity, radial diffusivity, and axial diffusivity were demonstrated in the posterior CC.

In addition to demonstrating abnormalities in anatomical connectivity in the CC (smaller CC and shorter fiber lengths), various studies have reported correlations between microstructural properties of CC and specific behavioral measures. For example, in a group of 7-month-old infants, Elison et al. recently found that visual orienting latencies were uniquely associated with the microstructural organization (especially radial diffusivity) of the splenium of the CC in low-risk infants, but this association was not apparent in infants later classified as having an ASD (Elison et al. 2013). However, in older children with ASD (mean age 9.5 years), Hanaie et al. found that the FA of the splenium of the CC was inversely correlated with sociocommunicative deficits (as measured by Autism Diagnostic Observation Schedule–Generic), but not to motor deficits in ASD (Hanaie et al. 2014).

9.3.4 Functional connectivity of the corpus callosum

Major cognitive hypotheses in ASD such as the complex information processing theory (Minshew et al. 2002) suggest the possibility of underdevelopment of connections in the brains of individuals with ASD. In a functional MRI study of an executive function task, Just et al. demonstrated cortical underconnectivity in the frontal-parietal network of individuals with ASD, and the correlation between functional connectivity in the frontal-parietal network and the area of the genu of the CC (Just et al. 2007). In another study, Anderson et al. constructed spatial maps of correlation between homologous voxels in each hemisphere, and revealed significant reduction in interhemispheric correlation in the sensorimotor cortex, anterior insula, fusiform gyrus, superior temporal gyrus, and superior parietal lobule (Anderson et al. 2011). As the affected regions have specific functional relevance to ASD, these findings suggest that transcallosal connectivity is reduced most in regions with functions associated with behavioral abnormalities in ASD.

9.4 Corpus callosum in neurogenetic syndromes exhibiting social deficits

Abnormal CC has been reported in various neurogenetic syndromes, including agenesis of the corpus callosum (AgCC), neurofibromatosis type 1 (NF1), velocardiofacial syndrome (VCFS), Williams syndrome (WS), Turner syndrome, 16p11.2 deletion syndrome, and haploinsufficiency of *ARID1B*. Here we will describe the abnormalities found in individuals with AgCC, NF1, VCFS, and WS.

9.4.1 Agenesis of the corpus callosum

Although the abnormalities of the CC appear to be a feature of some individuals with ASD, people with complete or partial absence of the CC did not appear to have more symptoms than those with ASD. When children with AgCC were compared to children with ASD, the former was found to have less impairment in attention, anxiety/depression, social function, and unusual thoughts as measured by the Child Behavior Checklist (Badaruddin et al. 2007). However, like individuals with ASD, some young people with AgCC showed theory of mind- and

163

emotion-processing deficits (Booth et al. 2011). In a recent study using the Autism Spectrum Quotient (AQ), Lau et al. screened a large cohort with AgCC ($n = 106$), and revealed that 45% of children, 35% of adolescents, and 18% of adults had scores that exceeded the predetermined ASD-screening cut-off (Lau et al. 2013). Furthermore, individuals with AgCC appeared to have reduced sensory registration and increased auditory-processing difficulties as compared to neurotypical controls (Demopoulos et al. 2015). In contrast with the above findings, Paul et al. found that the presence of residual CC did not associate with more current ASD symptoms. When comparing adults with AgCC and age-matched adults with ASD, no relationship between IQ and ASD symptomatology was found in the group with AgCC (Paul et al. 2014).

9.4.2 Neurofibromatosis type 1

Neurofibromatosis type 1 is a neurogenetic disorder that exhibits findings on skin (cafe-au-lait macules, neurofibromas, and axillary or inguinal freckling), eye (Lisch nodules), and brain (optic glioma). NF1 is an autosomal dominant disorder caused by mutations of the *NF1* gene. Several investigations have reported abnormalities in CC in individuals with NF1. Kayl et al. (2000) reported enlarged total CC area, rostral body area, anterior and posterior midbody area, but no change in posterior CC (isthmus and splenium). Wignall et al. (2010) found that the length and total cross-sectional area of the CC were larger in adults with NF-1 compared with typical controls. DTI studies revealed decreased FA of the CC in adults (Zamboni et al. 2007) and children (Filippi et al. 2013) with NF1.

9.4.3 Velocardiofacial syndrome (VCFS)

Velocardiofacial syndrome (aka 22q11.2 deletion syndrome, DiGeorge syndrome, Shprintzen syndrome) is a chromosomal disorder characterized by cardiac anomaly, dysmorphic facial features, thymic aplasia, cleft palate, hypocalcemia, and hypoparathyroidism. Antshel et al. reported that the CC of children with VCFA was more arched (Antshel et al. 2005). Compared to neurotypical control participants, children with VCFS were shown to have a larger CC area (Antshel et al. 2005) and increased fractional anisotropy in the CC (Simon et al. 2005). The increased sizes in CC in the VCFS group were found to associate with polymorphisms within the candidate genes: *COMT* (rs4680), *ZDHHC8* (rs175174), and *UFD1L* (rs5992403) (Shashi et al. 2012).

Interestingly, children with VCFS and comorbid attention deficit hyperactivity disorder (ADHD) had smaller total CC (especially for the splenium and genu) than children with VCFS alone (Simon et al. 2005). This finding is consistent with the smaller size of CC found in a meta-analysis of the size of CC in 284 individuals with ADHD (Hutchinson et al. 2008). In addition to the total CC area, specific regional areas of

CC were found to correlate with cognitive function in enumeration tasks for children with the VCFS (e.g., response time was inversely correlated with the size of the genu) (Machado et al. 2007).

9.4.4 Williams syndrome

Williams syndrome is a rare neurogenetic disorder, caused by deletion of a region on chromosome 7 consisting of approximately 26–28 genes. WS's cognitive-behavioral profile includes intellectual disability, attention deficits, and aberrant social behavior (e.g., hypersociability). Sampaio et al. found decreased CC cross-sectional area and volume in individuals with WS (Sampaio et al. 2013). The CC in WS is shorter but thicker throughout all subregions. Furthermore, the CC of in WS was characterized by a larger bending angle and more curved in the posterior part of the structure. Martens et al. found that callosal thickness was significantly reduced in the splenium of individuals with Williams syndrome individuals compared to controls (Martens et al. 2013). Furthermore, these investigators also found that the callosal area was smaller in left-handed patients with Williams syndrome than their right-handed counterparts, with opposite findings observed in the control group.

9.5 Animal models with abnormalities of the corpus callosum

Animal models with CC abnormalities are emerging tools for dissecting the pathogenesis of ASD in the context of the disruption of the development of CC. An example is the completely acallosal BTBR T⁺tpr3tf/J (BTBR) mice, which is an animal model of ASD with strong face validity (Meyza et al. 2013). By using resting-state functional MRI (rsfMRI), Sforazzini et al. showed that BTBR mice exhibited impaired intrahemispheric connectivity in fronto-cortical, but not in posterior sensory cortical areas (Sforazzini et al. 2016). Using the same animal model, 29 candidate genes were found to associate with synaptic activity, axon guidance, and neural development (Jones-Davis et al. 2013), consistent with a role for these processes in modulating CC development and aspects of ASD-relevant behaviors in the BTBR mouse.

While BTBR mice offers unique opportunities to test hypotheses that require a complete absence of the CC, mouse models that mimic the reduction in size of the CC in humans with ASD may also be useful. Reduced size of the CC was found to be associated with low sociability in the BALB/cJ inbred mouse strain (Fairless et al. 2008). This animal model was recently used in a longitudinal *in vivo* diffusion tensor imaging study, which revealed significant differences in FA and mean diffusivity values between BALB/cJ and control mice in most white and gray matter areas between postnatal days 30 and 90 (Kumar et al. 2012).

9.6 Summary and future directions

This chapter summarizes the phenomenology of the structural and functional anatomy of CC in ASD and other neurogenetic syndromes with ASD features. Overall, various converging lines of empirical evidence have supported the importance of CC in the pathophysiology of ASD. In order to determine if the phenomenological findings are causal to or associated with the behavioral symptoms in ASD, various investigators have examined the relationships between behavioral symptoms manifested in neurogenetic syndromes and alterations in the CC. While abnormalities of the CC were present in many of these syndromes, abnormal CC is also not a pathognomonic sign of ASD or deficits in social interactions.

Where do we go from here? What do we learn from the abnormalities of CC in individuals with ASD? Is the development of CC a mediator of the pathophysiology of ASD? Can the abnormalities of CC be used as part of biosignatures for subtypes of ASD? Can we develop treatments based on the understanding of the pathobiology of CC in ASD? Is it possible that abnormalities in the CC are indeed clues to molecular mechanisms underlying the ASD phenotype? In a recent study, RNA sequencing of the CC from postmortem samples of patients with ASD demonstrated extensive gene misexpression in a specific module of proteins (Li et al. 2014). Specifically, the expression of this module (containing 119 member genes, including *SHANK2*, *SHANK3*, *NLGN1*, *NLGN3*, *SEMA4C*), but not synaptic genes in general or known ASD candidate genes, was significantly altered in the CC of the ASD patients relative to the matched controls. This study delineates a specific molecular network involved in ASD, uncovers candidate genes for this disorder, and suggests the importance of the CC in the pathophysiology of ASD.

In order to understand the pathogenesis of ASD, investigators in the field have started charting the developmental trajectories of the brain in many different ways. We predict that future studies in charting the developmental trajectories of CC anatomically and functionally with novel noninvasive magnetic resonance imaging as well as molecular neuroimaging will advance our understanding of the role of the CC in pathobiology of ASD. We also anticipate that animal models such as the BTBR and BALB/cJ mice may be viable options for evaluating preclinical efficacy of novel pharmacologic interventions. Finally, while we are accumulating evidence in the importance of the CC in the pathobiology of ASD, we also appreciate that ASD is a complex neurodevelopmental disorder with multiple etiologies. Therefore, abnormalities in the CC may be key for some but not all subtypes of ASD. Future research will help determine more precisely the role of CC in the pathogenesis and pathophysiology of ASD.

References

Aboitiz, F., A. B. Scheibel, R. S. Fisher, and E. Zaidel. 1992. Fiber composition of the human corpus callosum. *Brain Res.* 598:143–53.

Alexander, A. L., J. E. Lee, M. Lazar et al. 2007. Diffusion tensor imaging of the corpus callosum in autism. *NeuroImage* 34:61–73.

Anderson, J. S., T. J. Druzgal, A. Froehlich et al. 2011. Decreased interhemispheric functional connectivity in autism. *Cerebral Cortex* 21:1134–46.

Antshel, K. M., J. Conchelos, G. Lanzetta, W. Fremont, and W. R. Kates. 2005. Behavior and corpus callosum morphology relationships in velocardiofacial syndrome (22q11.2 deletion syndrome). *Psychiatry Res.* 138:235–45.

Badaruddin, D. H., G. L. Andrews, S. Bolte, K. J. Schilmoeller, G. Schilmoeller, L. K. Paul, and W. S. Brown. 2007. Social and behavioral problems of children with agenesis of the corpus callosum. *Child Psychiatry Hum. Dev.* 38:287–302.

Belmonte, M., B. Egaas, J. Townsend, and E. Courchesne. 1995. NMR intensity of corpus callosum differs with age but not with diagnosis of autism. *NeuroReport* 6:1253–6.

Boger-Megiddo, I., D. W. Shaw, S. D. Friedman, B. F. Sparks, A. A. Artru, J. N. Giedd, G. Dawson, and S. R. Dager. 2006. Corpus callosum morphometrics in young children with autism spectrum disorder. *J. Autism Dev. Disord.* 36:733–9.

Booth, R., G. L. Wallace, and F. Happe. 2011. Connectivity and the corpus callosum in autism spectrum conditions: Insights from comparison of autism and callosal agenesis. *Prog. Brain Res.* 189:303–17.

Casanova, M. F., A. El-Baz, A. Elnakib, A. E. Switala, E. L. Williams, D. L. Williams, N. J. Minshew, and T. E. Conturo. 2011. Quantitative analysis of the shape of the corpus callosum in patients with autism and comparison individuals. *Autism* 15:223–38.

de Lacoste, M. C., J. B. Kirkpatrick, and E. D. Ross. 1985. Topography of the human corpus callosum. *J. Neuropathol. Exp. Neurol.* 44:578–91.

Demopoulos, C., M. S. Arroyo, W. Dunn, Z. Strominger, E. H. Sherr, and E. Marco. 2015. Individuals with agenesis of the corpus callosum show sensory processing differences as measured by the sensory profile. *Neuropsychology.* 29(5):751–8.

Egaas, B., E. Courchesne, and O. Saitoh. 1995. Reduced size of corpus callosum in autism. *Arch. Neurol.* 52:794–801.

Elison, J. T., S. J. Paterson, J. J. Wolff et al. 2013. White matter microstructure and atypical visual orienting in 7-month-olds at risk for autism. *Am. J. Psychiatry* 170:899–908.

Fairless, A. H., H. C. Dow, M. M. Toledo, K. A. Malkus, M. Edelmann, H. Li, K. Talbot, S. E. Arnold, T. Abel, and E. S. Brodkin. 2008. Low sociability is associated with reduced size of the corpus callosum in the BALB/cJ inbred mouse strain. *Brain Res.* 1230:211–7.

Farag, A., S. Elhabian, M. Abdelrahman, J. Graham, A. Farag, D. Chen, and M. F. Casanova. 2010. Shape modeling of the corpus callosum. *Conf. Proc. IEEE Eng. Med. Biol. Soc.* 2010:4288–91.

Filippi, C. G., R. Watts, L. A. Duy, and K. A. Cauley. 2013. Diffusion-tensor imaging derived metrics of the corpus callosum in children with neurofibromatosis type I. *Am. J. Roentgenol.* 200:44–9.

Floris, D. L., L. R. Chura, R. J. Holt, J. Suckling, E. T. Bullmore, S. Baron-Cohen, and M. D. Spencer. 2013. Psychological correlates of handedness and corpus callosum asymmetry in autism: The left hemisphere dysfunction theory revisited. *J. Autism Dev. Disord.* 43:1758–72.

Frazier, T. W. and A. Y. Hardan. 2009. A meta-analysis of the corpus callosum in autism. *Biol. Psychiatry* 66:935–41.

Frazier, T. W., M. S. Keshavan, N. J. Minshew, and A. Y. Hardan. 2012. A two-year longitudinal MRI study of the corpus callosum in autism. *J. Autism Dev. Disord.* 42:2312–22.

Freitag, C. M., E. Luders, H. E. Hulst, K. L. Narr, P. M. Thompson, A. W. Toga, C. Krick, and C. Konrad. 2009. Total brain volume and corpus callosum size in medication-naive adolescents and young adults with autism spectrum disorder. *Biol. Psychiatry* 66:316–9.

Gozzi, M., D. M. Nielson, R. K. Lenroot, J. L. Ostuni, D. A. Luckenbaugh, A. E. Thurm, J. N. Giedd, and S. E. Swedo. 2012. A magnetization transfer imaging study of corpus callosum myelination in young children with autism. *Biol. Psychiatry* 72:215–20.

Hanaie, R., I. Mohri, K. Kagitani-Shimono, M. Tachibana, J. Matsuzaki, Y. Watanabe, N. Fujita, and M. Taniike. 2014. Abnormal corpus callosum connectivity, socio-communicative deficits, and motor deficits in children with autism spectrum disorder: A diffusion tensor imaging study. *J. Autism Dev. Disord.* 44:2209–20.

Hardan, A. Y., N. J. Minshew, and M. S. Keshavan. 2000. Corpus callosum size in autism. *Neurology* 55:1033–6.

Hardan, A. Y., M. Pabalan, N. Gupta, R. Bansal, N. M. Melhem, S. Fedorov, M. S. Keshavan, and N. J. Minshew. 2009. Corpus callosum volume in children with autism. *Psychiatry Res.* 174:57–61.

He, Q., Y. Duan, K. Karsch, and J. Miles. 2010. Detecting corpus callosum abnormalities in autism based on anatomical landmarks. *Psychiatry Res.* 183:126–32.

He, Q., K. Karsch, and Y. Duan. 2008. Abnormalities in MRI traits of corpus callosum in autism subtype. *Conf. Proc. IEEE. Eng. Med. Biol. Soc.* 2008:3900–3.

Hofer, S. and J. Frahm. 2006. Topography of the human corpus callosum revisited—Comprehensive fiber tractography using diffusion tensor magnetic resonance imaging. *NeuroImage* 32:989–94.

Hong, S., X. Ke, T. Tang, Y. Hang, K. Chu, H. Huang, Z. Ruan, Z. Lu, G. Tao, and Y. Liu. 2011. Detecting abnormalities of corpus callosum connectivity in autism using magnetic resonance imaging and diffusion tensor tractography. *Psychiatry Res.* 194:333–9.

Huang, H., J. Zhang, H. Jiang, S. Wakana, L. Poetscher, M. I. Miller, P. C. van Zijl, A. E. Hillis, R. Wytik, and S. Mori. 2005. DTI tractography based parcellation of white matter: Application to the mid-sagittal morphology of corpus callosum. *NeuroImage* 26:195–205.

Hutchinson, A. D., J. L. Mathias, and M. T. Banich. 2008. Corpus callosum morphology in children and adolescents with attention deficit hyperactivity disorder: A meta-analytic review. *Neuropsychology* 22:341–9.

Jones-Davis, D. M., M. Yang, E. Rider et al. 2013. Quantitative trait loci for interhemispheric commissure development and social behaviors in the BTBR T(+) tf/J mouse model of autism. *PLoS One* 8:e61829.

Just, M. A., V. L. Cherkassky, T. A. Keller, R. K. Kana, and N. J. Minshew. 2007. Functional and anatomical cortical underconnectivity in autism: Evidence from an FMRI study of an executive function task and corpus callosum morphometry. *Cereb. Cortex* 17:951–61.

Kayl, A. E., B. D. Moore, 3rd, J. M. Slopis, E. F. Jackson, and N. E. Leeds. 2000. Quantitative morphology of the corpus callosum in children with neurofibromatosis and attention-deficit hyperactivity disorder. *J. Child. Neurol.* 15:90–6.

Keary, C. J., N. J. Minshew, R. Bansal, D. Goradia, S. Fedorov, M. S. Keshavan, and A. Y. Hardan. 2009. Corpus callosum volume and neurocognition in autism. *J. Autism Dev. Disord.* 39:834–41.

Kumar, A., S. K. Sundaram, L. Sivaswamy, M. E. Behen, M. I. Makki, J. Ager, J. Janisse, H. T. Chugani, and D. C. Chugani. 2010. Alterations in frontal lobe tracts and corpus callosum in young children with autism spectrum disorder. *Cereb. Cortex* 20:2103–13.

Kumar, M., S. Kim, S. Pickup, R. Chen, A. H. Fairless, R. Ittyerah, T. Abel, E. S. Brodkin, and H. Poptani. 2012. Longitudinal in-vivo diffusion tensor imaging for assessing brain developmental changes in BALB/cJ mice, a model of reduced sociability relevant to autism. *Brain. Res.* 1455:56–67.

Lau, Y. C., L. B. Hinkley, P. Bukshpun et al. 2013. Autism traits in individuals with agenesis of the corpus callosum. *J. Autism Dev. Disord.* 43:1106–18.

Lewis, J. D., R. J. Theilmann, V. Fonov, P. Bellec, A. Lincoln, A. C. Evans, and J. Townsend. 2013. Callosal fiber length and interhemispheric connectivity in adults with autism: Brain overgrowth and underconnectivity. *Hum. Brain Mapp.* 34:1685–95.

Li, J., M. Shi, Z. Ma, S. Zhao, G. Euskirchen, J. Ziskin, A. Urban, J. Hallmayer, and M. Snyder. 2014. Integrated systems analysis reveals a molecular network underlying autism spectrum disorders. *Mol. Syst. Biol.* 10:774.

Machado, A. M., T. J. Simon, V. Nguyen, D. M. McDonald-McGinn, E. H. Zackai, and J. C. Gee. 2007. Corpus callosum morphology and ventricular size in chromosome 22q11.2 deletion syndrome. *Brain Res.* 1131:197–210.

Martens, M. A., S. J. Wilson, J. Chen, A. G. Wood, and D. C. Reutens. 2013. Handedness and corpus callosal morphology in Williams syndrome. *Dev. Psychopathol.* 25:253–60.

Meyza, K. Z., E. B. Defensor, A. L. Jensen, M. J. Corley, B. L. Pearson, R. L. Pobbe, V. J. Bolivar, D. C. Blanchard, and R. J. Blanchard. 2013. The BTBR T+ tf/J mouse model for autism spectrum disorders—in search of biomarkers. *Behav. Brain Res.* 251:25–34.

Mihrshahi, R. 2006. The corpus callosum as an evolutionary innovation. *J. Exp. Zool. B. Mol. Dev. Evol.* 306:8–17.

Minshew, N. J., J. Sweeney, and B. Luna. 2002. Autism as a selective disorder of complex information processing and underdevelopment of neocortical systems. *Mol. Psychiatry* 7(Suppl 2):S14–5.

Paul, L. K., C. Corsello, D. P. Kennedy, and R. Adolphs. 2014. Agenesis of the corpus callosum and autism: A comprehensive comparison. *Brain* 137:1813–29.

Piven, J., J. Bailey, B. J. Ranson, and S. Arndt. 1997. An MRI study of the corpus callosum in autism. *Am. J. Psychiatry* 154:1051–6.

Prigge, M. B., N. Lange, E. D. Bigler et al. 2013. Corpus callosum area in children and adults with autism. *Res. Autism. Spectr. Disord.* 7:221–34.

Rice, S. A., E. D. Bigler, H. B. Cleavinger, D. F. Tate, J. Sayer, W. McMahon, S. Ozonoff, J. Lu, and J. E. Lainhart. 2005. Macrocephaly, corpus callosum morphology, and autism. *J. Child. Neurol.* 20:34–41.

Rilling, J. K. and T. R. Insel. 1999. Differential expansion of neural projection systems in primate brain evolution. *NeuroReport* 10:1453–9.

Sampaio, A., S. Bouix, N. Sousa, C. Vasconcelos, M. Fernandez, M. E. Shenton, and O. F. Goncalves. 2013. Morphometry of corpus callosum in Williams syndrome: Shape as an index of neural development. *Brain Struct. Funct.* 218:711–20.

Sforazzini, F., A. Bertero, L. Dodero, G. David, A. Galbusera, M. L. Scattoni, M. Pasqualetti, and A. Gozzi. 2016. Altered functional connectivity networks in acallosal and socially impaired BTBR mice. *Brain Struct. Funct.* 221(2):941–954.

Shashi, V., A. Francis, S. R. Hooper, P. G. Kranz, M. Zapadka, K. Schoch, E. Ip, N. Tandon, T. D. Howard, and M. S. Keshavan. 2012. Increased corpus callosum volume in children with chromosome 22q11.2 deletion syndrome is associated with neurocognitive deficits and genetic polymorphisms. *Eur. J. Hum. Genet.* 20:1051–7.

Shukla, D. K., B. Keehn, A. J. Lincoln, and R. A. Muller. 2010. White matter compromise of callosal and subcortical fiber tracts in children with autism spectrum disorder: A diffusion tensor imaging study. *J. Am. Acad. Child. Adolesc. Psychiatry* 49:1269–78, 78 e1–2.

Simon, T. J., L. Ding, J. P. Bish, D. M. McDonald-McGinn, E. H. Zackai, and J. Gee. 2005. Volumetric, connective, and morphologic changes in the brains of children with chromosome 22q11.2 deletion syndrome: An integrative study. *Neuroimage* 25:169–80.

Tepest, R., E. Jacobi, A. Gawronski, B. Krug, W. Moller-Hartmann, F. G. Lehnhardt, and K. Vogeley. 2010. Corpus callosum size in adults with high-functioning autism and the relevance of gender. *Psychiatry Res.* 183:38–43.

Thomas, C., K. Humphreys, K. J. Jung, N. Minshew, and M. Behrmann. 2011. The anatomy of the callosal and visual-association pathways in high-functioning autism: A DTI tractography study. *Cortex* 47:863–73.

Travers, B. G., P. M. Tromp do, N. Adluru et al. 2015. Atypical development of white matter microstructure of the corpus callosum in males with autism: A longitudinal investigation. *Mol. Autism* 6:15.

Vidal, C. N., R. Nicolson, T. J. DeVito et al. 2006. Mapping corpus callosum deficits in autism: An index of aberrant cortical connectivity. *Biol. Psychiatry* 60:218–25.

Wahl, M., B. Lauterbach-Soon, E. Hattingen, P. Jung, O. Singer, S. Volz, J. C. Klein, H. Steinmetz, and U. Ziemann. 2007. Human motor corpus callosum: Topography, somatotopy, and link between microstructure and function. *J. Neurosci.* 27:12132–8.

Wignall, E. L., P. D. Griffiths, N. G. Papadakis, I. D. Wilkinson, L. I. Wallis, O. Bandmann, P. E. Cowell, and N. Hoggard. 2010. Corpus callosum morphology and microstructure assessed using structural MR imaging and diffusion tensor imaging: Initial findings in adults with neurofibromatosis type 1. *AJNR. Am. J. Neuroradiol.* 31:856–61.

Zamboni, S. L., T. Loenneker, E. Boltshauser, E. Martin, and K. A. Il'yasov. 2007. Contribution of diffusion tensor MR imaging in detecting cerebral microstructural changes in adults with neurofibromatosis type 1. *AJNR. Am. J. Neuroradiol.* 28:773–6.

Chapter 10 Macrocephaly and megalencephaly in autism spectrum disorder

Lauren E. Libero, Christine W. Nordahl, Deana D. Li, and David G. Amaral

Contents

Abstract 171
10.1   Introduction. 172
10.2   Studies of macrocephaly. 172
10.3   Studies of megalencephaly 173
10.4   Brain enlargement in a subsample of individuals with ASD. . 175
10.5   Sex differences 176
10.6   Body size. 177
10.7   Normalization of brain size 178
10.8   Neurobiology of brain enlargement 178
10.9   Microcephaly 181
10.10 Conclusion. 181
References 182

Abstract

The very earliest description by Kanner indicated that large head size was associated with autism spectrum disorder. Yet, since then, opinion has ranged from those who argue that head and brain size is a general feature of autism spectrum disorder (ASD) to those who posit that this association is an artifact. We selectively review the literature on macrocephaly and megalencephaly in ASD and come to the conclusion that head and brain enlargement is characteristic of only a subset of approximately 15% of males with ASD. It appears that this is much less common in females. Moreover, the widespread notion that early macrocephaly and megalencephaly is followed by normalization of head/brain size is not supported by essential longitudinal studies. Given that an enlarged brain is a feature of one form of ASD, the critical remaining issues are what causes the abnormal brain enlargement and whether this has consequences on the clinical and cognitive outcomes of the affected individuals.

10.1 Introduction

In the seminal description of autism (Kanner 1943), Leo Kanner noted that 5 out of 11 of his patients had larger than normal heads. Since that report, head and brain size has been revisited well over a hundred times in the literature on autism spectrum disorder (ASD) (Sacco et al. 2015). Studies have examined both head circumference and brain volume, and findings generally suggest that they are enlarged in ASD. However, findings are inconsistent, making it difficult to draw clear conclusions about the course of brain development across the life span. This chapter aims to provide some clarity on head and brain size alterations in ASD, and discusses areas for future investigation.

10.2 Studies of macrocephaly

Macrocephaly refers to having enlarged cranial or head circumference (typically greater than the 97th percentile). Studies of macrocephaly are conducted by measuring across the supraorbital rims (or eyebrows) and around the head over the most posterior protuberance of the occiput (Cameron 1978; Deutsch and Farkas 1994). The earliest medical studies of ASD sought to find clinical markers for the disorder through physical examinations that included measures of head circumference. While these studies reported cases of macrocephaly in children with ASD (Schain and Yannet 1960; Gubbay et al. 1970; Steg and Rapoport 1975; Walker 1977), the findings were based on populations that were made up entirely of children with profound intellectual disability, who often resided in psychiatric wards (Schain and Yannet 1960; Steg and Rapoport 1975). In one study, the residential treatment group that was reported to have significantly greater head circumference was not homogeneous for ASD, with 9 of the 28 boys having other psychiatric diagnoses (Steg and Rapoport 1975). More recent studies have focused on larger samples of individuals across the spectrum of ASD and generally report a greater incidence of macrocephaly, when compared to either typically developing (TD) individuals or population norms (Bolton et al. 1994; Bailey et al. 1995; Davidovitch et al. 1996; Woodhouse et al. 1996; Lainhart et al. 1997, 2006; Stevenson et al. 1997; Skjeldal et al. 1998; Fombonne et al. 1999; Fidler et al. 2000; Miles et al. 2000, 2008; Aylward et al. 2002; Gillberg and De Souza 2002; Courchesne et al. 2003; Deutsch and Joseph 2003; Mraz et al. 2007; Webb et al. 2007; Fukumoto et al. 2011; Nordahl et al. 2011; Ververi et al. 2012; Froehlich et al. 2013; Grandgeorge et al. 2013; Shen et al. 2013). Fombonne and colleagues (1999) carried out an early meta-analysis of this topic and came to the conclusion that macrocephaly is found in about 20% of individuals with ASD (Fombonne et al. 1999). A more recent, comprehensive meta-analysis of the head and brain size literature on ASD (Sacco et al. 2015) concluded that 15.7% of individuals with ASD have macrocephaly. However, it is important to point out that the ASD literature is peppered with reports that claim no greater incidence of macrocephaly in individuals with ASD (Walker 1977; Rodier et al. 1997; Torrey et al. 2004; Tate et al. 2007; Cederlund et al. 2014; Zwaigenbaum et al. 2014).

It has been proposed that some of the inconsistencies in the head circumference literature stem from studies that utilize population norms as a reference group rather than recruiting TD control samples (Raznahan et al. 2013b). In a systematic review of head circumference studies, Raznahan and colleagues found that studies that utilized a norm-based reference group were more likely to report evidence of early brain overgrowth than did studies that utilized a locally recruited TD group. They suggested that the evidence for macrocephaly in ASD may be more of an artifact of biases related to utilizing norm-based reference groups rather than a specific biomarker for ASD.

One of the problems in using norm-based reference groups is that many published norms have differing distributions. To illustrate this point, consider a male infant born with a head circumference of 37.2 cm. Based on the National Center for Health Statistics (NCHS) growth charts published in 1977, he would be classified as normocephalic at the 95th percentile for head circumference (Hamill et al. 1979). Similarly, if growth charts published by the Centers for Disease Control and Prevention in 2000 were utilized, this male infant would also be classified as normocephalic, at the 78.5th percentile (Centers for Disease Control and Prevention 2000). However, growth charts published by the World Health Organization (WHO) in 2006 would classify this male infant as having macrocephaly, with his head circumference corresponding to the 98.5th percentile (De Onis 2006). These differing distributions across the published norms reflect differences in the study design and sample characteristics used to develop each set of norm tables (de Onis et al. 2007). Variation across norms used in studies of ASD may be one contribution to the inconsistencies in the reported literature on macrocephaly. Rather than relying on potentially biased references, comparing patient participants to locally recruited, TD controls of the same age may ultimately be the best way to identify individuals with ASD and macrocephaly.

10.3 Studies of megalencephaly

Whereas macrocephaly is defined as enlarged head size, megalencephaly specifically refers to having enlarged brain size. Despite the fact that head circumference is highly correlated with brain size early in development, it becomes less so in older individuals (Bartholomeusz et al. 2002). Studies investigating megalencephaly are conducted using structural magnetic resonance imaging (MRI) and manual or automated segmentation to calculate total brain volume. Several studies have examined total brain volume in participants with ASD and found enlargement when compared to TD controls (Filipek et al. 1992; Piven et al. 1995; Courchesne et al. 2001; Sparks et al. 2002; Palmen et al. 2005; Hazlett et al. 2006; Bloss and Courchesne 2007; Freitag et al. 2009; Schumann et al. 2010; Hazlett et al. 2011; Nordahl et al. 2011; Calderoni et al. 2012; Nordahl et al. 2013; Shen et al. 2013). However, a larger number of studies have reported no significant differences in total brain volume between participants with ASD and those with typical development (Gaffney et al. 1987; Aylward et al. 1999; Elia et al. 2000; Haznedar et al. 2000; McAlonan et al. 2002, 2005; Hardan et al. 2003, 2006a,b, 2008, 2009; Rojas et al. 2004; Schumann et al. 2004; Vidal et al. 2006; Girgis et al. 2007; Mostofsky et al. 2007; Tate et al. 2007; Cleavinger et al. 2008; Hallahan et al. 2009; Jou et al. 2010a,b; Tamura et al. 2010; Tepest et al. 2010; Cheung et al. 2011; Hong et al. 2011; Greimel et al. 2013; Raznahan et al. 2013a; Say et al. 2014; Lange et al. 2015). Based on a meta-analysis of head circumference and brain volume studies, Redcay and Courchesne (2005) concluded that the age of the subject is an important variable. They posited that head and brain size is increased early in life in ASD followed by a normalization by adulthood. In other words, they proposed that brains were too large in the first few years of life but by adolescence or adulthood had become normal sized and more closely resemble TD individuals of similar age. This perspective has been influential on the field since it was first proposed.

Based on our own MRI studies, we suggest, however, that a number of technical issues need to be considered in addition to age, including different subject selection procedures in these cross-sectional studies, the relatively small number of subjects that they involve, and the inconsistency in sex balance across the various studies. The notion of early overgrowth followed by normalization was based largely on cross-sectional studies that generally had small numbers of subjects (the average sample size was 32 individuals). Moreover, while some studies included participants at all levels of functioning, others included only higher functioning individuals with ASD. Specifically, the studies that reported on younger subjects employed participants that were either anesthetized or scanned while sleeping. Thus, these studies were more likely to include participants that were more severely affected or had comorbid intellectual disability. For studies targeting adolescents or adults, anesthesia was typically not used and thus more compliant, higher functioning subjects were typically assessed. The other issue is that the ratio of male and female subjects varied in these cross-sectional studies. As summarized below, these factors may be an important consideration in determining whether abnormal brain size followed by normalization is a consistent feature of ASD.

10.4 Brain enlargement in a subsample of individuals with ASD

It is a misconception that all individuals with ASD have abnormally enlarged brains. This belief may stem from a historical shift in methodology used to identify alterations in brain size. Initial medical studies typically calculated the percentage of children above a specific percentile cutoff for macrocephaly (e.g., those above the 97th percentile for their age), determined either by published population norms or in comparison to a sample of TD controls. As we indicated above, these studies suggested that a subset of individuals with ASD, perhaps 20%, have macrocephaly by this criterion. When the first MRI studies were carried out, however, analyses shifted to comparisons of group means (all children with ASD compared to a sample of TD control children). This shift is likely due to the fact that population norms for brain volumes were not readily available. This led, we believe, to the mistaken conclusion that, while mean brain volume might be significantly greater in ASD than in TD controls, this inaccurately implied that all individuals with ASD have enlarged brains. If fact, our data are consistent with the idea that a subset of individuals with ASD have enlarged brains and they drive the significant total brain volume mean group difference between individuals with ASD and TD controls.

We have directly evaluated brain size in a large cohort of young subjects with ASD and age-matched TD controls who were followed longitudinally in the UC Davis MIND Institute Autism Phenome Project (APP). Families are recruited into the APP soon after diagnosis, when the child is 2 to 3-1/2 years old. Families are invited to come to the MIND Institute where the child's diagnosis is confirmed, and a variety of behavioral tests are carried out. The medical records for the child since birth are requested from family physicians. The parents also provide information through questionnaires. The child has an MRI of their brain at night during natural sleep, and they also provide a small blood sample for immune and genetic testing. The families are invited to come back 1 year and 2 years later to follow up on the development of the brain. By analyzing both head circumference and total cerebral volume of the children in the APP, we have concluded that approximately 15% of boys with ASD have megalencephaly (Figure 10.1), but it is far less common in females (Nordahl et al. 2011). Our findings are consistent with the meta-analysis of Sacco et al. (2015), who concluded that 9.1% of ASD subjects who have had an MRI have megalencephaly. The authors acknowledge that the prevalence of megalencephaly may be underestimated due to participant selection bias (e.g., using mainly patients deemed high functioning). Thus, the first conclusion of this analysis is that only 15% of boys with ASD have megalencephaly. The large majority of boys with ASD have brains that are in the normal size range (Figure 10.2). How does this compare to the prevalence of megalencephaly in girls with ASD?

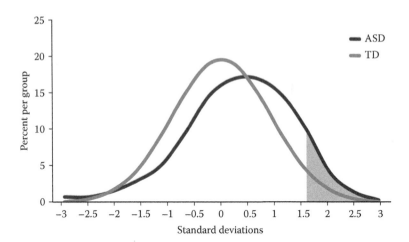

Figure 10.1 Schematic distribution of total brain volume in boys with autism spectrum disorder (ASD; red) and typical development (TD; blue). Illustrated are the percentages of boys from each group falling within each standard deviation from the mean of the normal or TD distribution. The shaded region represents the individuals with megalencephaly, or enlarged brain size. In boys with ASD, prevalence of megalencephaly is around 15%, while megalencephaly presents in only 6.7% of TD individuals.

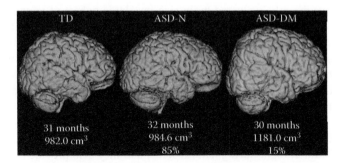

Figure 10.2 An illustration of rendered brains from a boy with typical development (TD), a boy with autism and normal brain volume (ASD-N), and a boy with autism and megalencephaly (ASD-DM). These example children are matched on age; however, the boy with autism and megalencephaly clearly has a much larger brain size than the two children of similar age but with normal brain growth. Within the male ASD population, around 85% have brain volumes within the normal range, while about 15% have megalencephaly.

10.5 Sex differences

Historically, girls have been under-represented in studies of ASD. While many studies include both male and female participants when examining head circumference and brain volume in ASD, the sex balance often reflects the male bias of ASD, and few studies have had enough females in their samples to investigate potential sex differences in brain size. The literature provides some indications that head and brain enlargement is less common in females with ASD (Davidovitch et al. 1996; Piven et al. 1996; Campbell et al. 2014) and in the APP cohort, we do not observe brain volume differences between females with ASD and sex-matched controls (Nordahl et al. 2011). There are a few studies that report abnormal brain enlargement in females with ASD (Sparks et al. 2002; Bloss and Courchesne 2007; Calderoni et al. 2012); one longitudinal study of a cohort of nine girls with ASD found pronounced brain growth in girls compared to boys with ASD (Schumann et al. 2010). Unfortunately, the majority of MRI studies do not have large enough samples of females to evaluate sex differences in the brain volume. Normative studies have shown that brain development is sexually dimorphic throughout middle childhood and adolescence. Given that females attain peak volumes in cortical and subcortical volumes 1–3 years earlier than boys during middle childhood and adolescence (Giedd et al. 1996, 1999; Sowell et al. 2007), it would not be surprising if the trajectories of altered brain development in ASD are also sex-specific. Data from the APP suggest that only 4% of the girls with ASD exhibit megalencephaly, but this finding awaits replication as the number of female subjects is increased.

10.6 Body size

Periodically the notion has been raised that while head size might be larger in individuals with ASD, the reason is because they are taller and generally larger. There is clearly a proportional relationship between brain size and height (Weinberg et al. 1974; Gould 1981; Jones and Lewis 1991; Lainhart et al. 2006). In the context of ASD, there is some evidence that children with ASD are taller than TD children (Davidovitch et al. 1996; Lainhart et al. 1997; Miles et al. 2000; Dissanayake et al. 2006; Chawarska et al. 2011). There are reports of increased body length in boys with ASD beginning by 4.8 months of age (Chawarska et al. 2011), or greater height in children with ASD by 3 years (Lainhart et al. 1997; Dissanayake et al. 2006). These studies suggest that somatic overgrowth accounts for enlargement in head circumference (Dissanayake et al. 2006; Chawarska et al. 2011). However, parallel MRI analyses of brain size were not carried out in these studies of body size. There is evidence that body size may not be the driving force of increased brain size. A few studies have reported macrocephaly (Aylward et al. 2002; Lainhart et al. 2006; Fukumoto et al. 2011; Grandgeorge et al. 2013) and megalencephaly (Piven et al. 1995) in individuals with ASD even when controlling for height. To control for the confound of body size on brain size, we have defined a cohort of boys with brain size disproportionate to body size. Inclusion in this group is based on having a ratio of brain size to height that is greater than 1.5 standard deviations above the mean of the TD boys. About 15% of boys with ASD have brain size that is disproportionate to their height. In fact, the boys that have brain enlargement tend to be of average height rather than the tallest members of the group. Thus, we have concluded that generalized somatic overgrowth cannot explain the phenomenon of megalencephaly in a subset of children with ASD.

10.7 Normalization of brain size

What about the idea (Redcay and Courchesne 2005) that the subset of children that have an enlarged brain when they are young ultimately have a normal-sized brain as they enter adolescence and adulthood? This perspective appears to be supported by a trend in findings of increased head and brain size in very young children (Piven et al. 1995, 1996; Courchesne et al. 2001; Sparks et al. 2002; Hazlett et al. 2005; Schumann et al. 2010; Courchesne et al. 2011), but no differences in adolescents and adults with ASD (Aylward et al. 1999, 2002; Herbert et al. 2004; Schumann et al. 2004; Hardan et al. 2006b). Yet, there are also several studies that have found brain volume enlargement in adolescents and adults with ASD (Piven et al. 1995; Palmen et al. 2005; Hazlett et al. 2006; Freitag et al. 2009). The only way to clarify this issue is to evaluate a cohort of children with disproportionate megalencephaly when they are younger and follow them into adulthood with periodic brain assessments. This is one of the goals of the Autism Phenome Project, which will hopefully be accomplished in due course. Thus far, we have evaluated this cohort of children when they were approximately 3, 4, and 5 years of age. Our findings indicate that the subgroup of boys with autism and disproportionate megalencephaly have enlarged brains at all ages compared to other boys with ASD and TD boys (Libero et al. 2016). In fact, they demonstrate an accelerated rate of brain growth compared to TD boys and boys with ASD that have normal brain size (Figure 10.3). At the present time, we see no indication that the abnormal brain size of these children is normalizing, although this may change in the future.

10.8 Neurobiology of brain enlargement

What could be leading to the enlarged brain size in the subset of boys with megalencephaly? The brain of an infant is about 25% of the adult size at birth and grows to 95% of the adult size by about 6 years of life (Stuart and Stevenson 1950; Giedd et al. 1999). Since virtually all neurons are generated during fetal life, the increased size of the brain is primarily due to dendrogenesis, the formation of axonal collaterals and synapses, and glial proliferation (Stiles and Jernigan 2010). Interestingly, a consistent finding is that children with ASD do not differ in head size at birth from their TD counterparts (Mason-brothers et al. 1987; Mason-Brothers et al. 1990; Courchesne et al. 2001; Hultman et al. 2002; Torrey

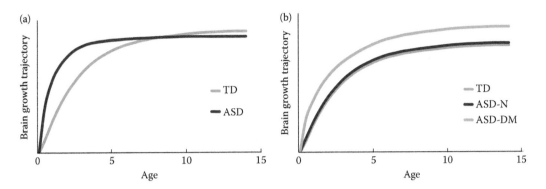

Figure 10.3 A depiction of brain volume growth across childhood and adolescence. In typical development, at birth, the brain is around 25% of the adult size (Stuart and Stevenson 1950). In the first 2 years of life, the brain grows to about 80% of adult size (Lenroot and Giedd 2006). By age 5, the brain is 90% of its adult weight, and 95% by age 6 (Dekaban and Sadowsky 1978; Giedd et al. 1999). (a) Brain growth curves represent the perspective from the literature (Redcay and Courchesne 2005) that the brains of children with ASD grow rapidly within the first year of life, then have brain volumes that normalize during childhood and into adolescence. (b) Brain growth trajectories are presented for TD boys, as well as boys with autism spectrum disorder and normal-sized brain (ASD-N) or megalencephaly (ASD-DM) based on data from the Autism Phenome Project. In this illustration, the TD and ASD-N children follow the same pattern of growth. However, the subgroup of boys with ASD-DM grow more rapidly in the first 2 years of life and maintain a greater brain volume across childhood.

et al. 2004; Hazlett et al. 2005; Chiu et al. 2007; Webb et al. 2007; Fukumoto et al. 2008; Nordahl et al. 2011; Grandgeorge et al. 2013). Thus, the abnormal brain growth could be due to dysregulation of dendritic growth, excessive production, or lack of pruning of axonal connections, or abnormal gliogenesis.

MRI studies have found that the altered brain enlargement is both of gray matter volume (Courchesne et al. 2001; Akshoomoff et al. 2004; Hazlett et al. 2005, 2006, 2011; Palmen et al. 2005; Bloss and Courchesne 2007; Freitag et al. 2009; Schumann et al. 2010; Calderoni et al. 2012) and white matter volume (Courchesne et al. 2001; Hazlett et al. 2005, 2011; Palmen et al. 2005; Freitag et al. 2009; Schumann et al. 2010; Calderoni et al. 2012). It is still unknown whether gray and white matter contribute equally or disproportionately to brain enlargement. One study including 42 children with ASD (13 with macrocephaly) and 59 TD children (12 with macrocephaly) around 14 years of age reports nonspecific (generalized) enlarged white matter in those with ASD suggesting an alternate (perhaps pathological) biological course for their brain enlargement (Bigler et al. 2010). In the APP cohort, we found both gray matter and white matter volumes are enlarged across early childhood in boys with ASD and disproportionate megalencephaly, compared to boys with ASD and brain size within the normal range and TD boys (Libero et al. 2016). We have also investigated whether the children with disproportionate megalencephaly in the Autism Phenome Project have thicker cortices, more surface area, or both. We quite clearly found that the enlarged brain was due to increased surface area (Ohta et al. 2015). It has been proposed that cortical surface expansion is due to increased radial columnar units (i.e., minicolumns) (Rakic 1995). Together, this would imply that there would be a greater number of cortical columns and perhaps an indication for minicolumnopathy (e.g., pathological organization of minicolumns) in ASD (Casanova et al. 2002, 2006; Casanova 2006). This is a possibility that will only be confirmed through future comprehensive postmortem studies of brains from individuals with the megalencephalic form of ASD.

Courchesne et al. (2011) have provided evidence that the enlarged brain may be due to an increased number of neurons in the prefrontal cortex (Courchesne et al. 2011). This study was carried out on a small number of postmortem cases. As intriguing as this finding is that its validity will depend on replication with a much larger sample of cases. In particular, it would be important to demonstrate that the megalencephalic brains have increased numbers of neurons whereas the brains from subjects with ASD and normal-sized brains do not. It should be noted that there are also studies reporting reduced neuron counts (Bauman 1991; Bailey et al. 1998; Schumann and Amaral 2006; van Kooten et al. 2008) and reduced neuron size (van Kooten et al. 2008; Jacot-Descombes et al. 2012) in the brains of older cases with ASD compared to control cases. This perhaps indicates that there is a degenerative process taking place, which, if widespread in the brain, could lead to a decrease in the size of enlarged brains. Again, this finding is not specific for ASD cases that demonstrated megalencephaly.

Another possibility is that an immune process may be contributing to brain enlargement. Studies focusing on neuroinflammation have supported this idea, with findings of microglial and astroglial activation in the neocortex, white matter, and cerebellum of cases with ASD (Vargas et al. 2005), as well as an increased density of microglia (Tetreault et al. 2012). Data from the APP cohort also support the idea of an immune process contributing to megalencephaly, as children with ASD born to mothers with 37/73 kDa IgG autoantibodies were found to have greater brain enlargement compared to TD children and the children with ASD born to mothers who were negative for the autoantibodies (Nordahl et al. 2013).

A few studies have offered some evidence for genetic alterations that could lead to macrocephaly. For example, increased head circumference was found in patients with ASD and copies of the G allele of the HOXA1 *A218G* polymorphism (vs. the A allele) (Conciatori et al. 2004). In addition, macrocephaly in ASD is linked to having a genetic mutation of *PTEN* (Butler et al. 2005) and *CHD8* (Bernier et al. 2014). Interestingly, one study using the APP cohort found differential alternative splicing in blood mRNA of boys with ASD was more related to having normal brain volume than brain enlargement (Stamova et al. 2013). So far, no clear genetic explanations have been identified to account for most of the cases of individuals with ASD and megalencephaly.

10.9 Microcephaly

While this chapter has focused on abnormal brain enlargement in ASD, it is important to note that there is also a smaller subset of children with ASD and microcephaly. Microcephaly is defined as having an abnormally small head or brain size compared to children of the same sex and age (typically below the 3rd percentile). The prevalence of microcephaly and ASD has not been consistently determined. The literature contains studies that report percentages of microcephaly in ASD ranging from 3% to 7% (Miles et al. 2000, 2008; Dementieva et al. 2005) to 15.1% (Fombonne et al. 1999) and 36% (Skjeldal et al. 1998) of children with ASD. However, the largest percentage reported comes from a study including only 25 children with ASD (Skjeldal et al. 1998), whereas the studies, including the largest number of subjects with ASD (over 200 each), reported the lowest percentages of children with ASD and microcephaly (Dementieva et al. 2005; Miles et al. 2008). In the APP cohort, around 5% of boys have microcephaly. While this subset is much smaller than the group of children with megalencephaly, they may still represent an important neurophenotype of the disorder. Children with microcephaly and ASD are more likely to have abnormal physical morphology, lower IQ, family history of seizures, and a lower sex ratio compared to children with ASD and macrocephaly or head size within the norm (Miles et al. 2000). Microcephaly in ASD is also more associated with syndromic (genetic) forms of ASD (Betancur 2011).

10.10 Conclusion

In this chapter, we have briefly described the history of head and brain size research in ASD, and the issues surrounding it. We have come to a number of conclusions: (1) about 15% of boys with ASD have brain sizes that are larger and disproportionate to their body size; (2) the enlarged brain size is not evident at birth but becomes so during the first few years of life; (3) megalencephaly in ASD does not appear to be as strongly associated with girls who have ASD; (4) data from the Autism Phenome Project indicate that boys with enlarged brains at 3 years of age maintain an enlarged brain at 5 years of age. Whether they will undergo a "normalization" of brain size as they age remains to be determined; (5) the functional consequences of having ASD and an enlarged brain are currently being evaluated. A summary of possible consequences has recently been provided (Amaral et al. in press).

References

Akshoomoff, N., C. Lord, A. J. Lincoln, R. Y. Courchesne, R. A. Carper, J. Townsend, and E. Courchesne. 2004. Outcome classification of preschool children with autism spectrum disorders using MRI brain measures. *J. Am. Acad. Child Adolesc. Psychiatry* 43:349–57.

Amaral, D., D. Li, L. Libero, M. Solomon, J. van de Water, A. Mastergeorge, L. Naigles, S. Rogers, and C. Nordahl. in press. In pursuit of neurophenotyping: The consequences of having autism and a big brain. *Autism Res.*

Aylward, N. M., K. Field, B. Sparks, and N. Singh. 2002. Effects of age on brain volume and head circumference in autism. *Neurology* 59:175–83.

Aylward, N. M., G. Goldstein, N. Honeycutt, A. Augustine, K. Yates, P. Barta, and G. Pearlson. 1999. MRI volumes of amygdala and hippocampus in non-mentally retarded autistic adolescents and adults. *Neurology* 53:2145–50.

Bailey, A., A. Le Couteur, I. Gottesman, P. Bolton, E. Simonoff, E. Yuzda, and M. Rutter. 1995. Autism as a strongly genetic disorder: Evidence from a British twin study. *Psychol. Med.* 25:63–77.

Bailey, P. L., A. Dean, B. Harding, I. Janota, M. Montgomery, M. Rutter, and P. Lantos. 1998. A clinicopathological study of autism. *Brain* 121:889–905.

Bartholomeusz, H., E. Courchesne, and C. Karns. 2002. Relationship between head circumference and brain volume in healthy normal toddlers, children, and adults. *Neuropediatrics* 33:239–41.

Bauman, M. L. 1991. Microscopic neuroanatomic abnormalities in autism. *Pediatrics* 87:791–6.

Bernier, R., C. Golzio, B. Xiong, H. A. Stessman, B. P. Coe, O. Penn, K. Witherspoon, J. Gerdts, C. Baker, and A. T. Vulto-van Silfhout. 2014. Disruptive CHD8 mutations define a subtype of autism early in development. *Cell* 158:263–76.

Betancur, C. 2011. Etiological heterogeneity in autism spectrum disorders: More than 100 genetic and genomic disorders and still counting. *Brain Res.* 1380:42–77.

Bigler, E. D., T. J. Abildskov, J. A. Petrie, M. Johnson, N. Lange, J. Chipman, J. Lu, W. McMahon, and J. E. Lainhart. 2010. Volumetric and voxel-based morphometry findings in autism subjects with and without macrocephaly. *Dev. Neuropsychol.* 35:278–95.

Bloss, C. S. and E. Courchesne. 2007. MRI neuroanatomy in young girls with autism: A preliminary study. *J. Am. Acad. Child Adolesc. Psychiatry* 46:515–23.

Bolton, P., H. Macdonald, A. Pickles, P. a. Rios, S. Goode, M. Crowson, A. Bailey, and M. Rutter. 1994. A case–control family history study of autism. *J. Child Psychol. Psychiatry* 35:877–900.

Butler, M., M. Dasouki, X. Zhou, Z. Talebizadeh, M. Brown, T. Takahashi, J. Miles, C. Wang, R. Stratton, and R. Pilarski. 2005. Subset of individuals with autism spectrum disorders and extreme macrocephaly associated with germline PTEN tumour suppressor gene mutations. *J. Med. Genet.* 42:318–21.

Calderoni, S., A. Retico, L. Biagi, R. Tancredi, F. Muratori, and M. Tosetti. 2012. Female children with autism spectrum disorder: An insight from mass-univariate and pattern classification analyses. *NeuroImage* 59:1013–22.

Cameron, N. 1978. The methods of auxological anthropometry. In *Human Growth*, 35–90. Berlin: Springer.

Campbell, D. J., J. Chang, and K. Chawarska. 2014. Early generalized overgrowth in autism spectrum disorder: Prevalence rates, gender effects, and clinical outcomes. *J. Am. Acad. Child Adolesc. Psychiatry* 53:1063–73. e5.

Casanova, M. F. 2006. Neuropathological and genetic findings in autism: The significance of a putative minicolumnopathy. *Neuroscientist* 12:435–41.

Casanova, M. F., D. P. Buxhoeveden, A. E. Switala, and E. Roy. 2002. Minicolumnar pathology in autism. *Neurology* 58:428–32.

Casanova, M. F., I. A. van Kooten, A. E. Switala, H. van Engeland, H. Heinsen, H. W. Steinbusch, P. R. Hof, J. Trippe, J. Stone, and C. Schmitz. 2006. Minicolumnar abnormalities in autism. *Acta Neuropathol.* 112:287–303.

Cederlund, M., C. Miniscalco, and C. Gillberg. 2014. Pre-schoolchildren with autism spectrum disorders are rarely macrocephalic: A population study. *Res. Dev. Disabil.* 35:992–8.

Centers for Disease Control and Prevention. 2000. *2000 CDC Growth Charts: United States*: US Department of Health and Human Services, Centers for Disease Control and Prevention, National Center for Health Statistics.

Chawarska, K., D. Campbell, L. Chen, F. Shic, A. Klin, and J. Chang. 2011. Early generalized overgrowth in boys with autism. *Arch. Gen. Psychiatry* 68:1021–31.

Cheung, C., G. M. McAlonan, Y. Y. Fung, G. Fung, K. K. Yu, K.-S. Tai, P. C. Sham, and S. E. Chua. 2011. MRI study of minor physical anomaly in childhood autism implicates aberrant neurodevelopment in infancy. *PLoS One* 6:e20246.

Chiu, S., J. A. Wegelin, J. Blank, M. Jenkins, J. Day, D. Hessl, F. Tassone, and R. Hagerman. 2007. Early acceleration of head circumference in children with fragile x syndrome and autism. *J. Dev. Behav. Pediatr.* 28:31–5.

Cleavinger, H. B., E. D. Bigler, J. L. Johnson, J. Lu, W. McMahon, and J. E. Lainhart. 2008. Quantitative magnetic resonance image analysis of the cerebellum in macrocephalic and normocephalic children and adults with autism. *J. Int. Neuropsychol. Soc.* 14:401–13.

Conciatori, M., C. J. Stodgell, S. L. Hyman, M. O'Bara, R. Militerni, C. Bravaccio, S. Trillo, F. Montecchi, C. Schneider, and R. Melmed. 2004. Association between the HOXA1 A218G polymorphism and increased head circumference in patients with autism. *Biol. Psychiatry* 55:413–9.

Courchesne, E., R. Carper, and N. Akshoomoff. 2003. Evidence of brain overgrowth in the first year of life in autism. *JAMA* 290:337–44.

Courchesne, E., C. Karns, H. Davis, R. Ziccardi, R. Carper, Z. Tigue, H. Chisum, P. Moses, K. Pierce, and C. Lord. 2001. Unusual brain growth patterns in early life in patients with autistic disorder an MRI study. *Neurology* 57:245–54.

Courchesne, E., P. R. Mouton, M. E. Calhoun, K. Semendeferi, C. Ahrens-Barbeau, M. J. Hallet, C. C. Barnes, and K. Pierce. 2011. Neuron number and size in prefrontal cortex of children with autism. *JAMA* 306:2001–10.

Davidovitch, M., B. Patterson, and P. Gartside. 1996. Head circumference measurements in children with autism. *J. Child Neurol.* 11:389–93.

De Onis, M. 2006. *WHO Child Growth Standards: Length/Height-for-Age, Weight-for-Age, Weight-for-Length, Weight-for-Height and Body Mass Index-for-Age.* Washington, DC: WHO.

de Onis, M., C. Garza, A. W. Onyango, and E. Borghi. 2007. Comparison of the WHO child growth standards and the CDC 2000 growth charts. *J. Nutrit.* 137:144–8.

Dekaban, A. S. and D. Sadowsky. 1978. Changes in brain weights during the span of human life: Relation of brain weights to body heights and body weights. *Ann. Neurol.* 4:345–56.

Dementieva, Y. A., D. D. Vance, S. L. Donnelly, L. A. Elston, C. M. Wolpert, S. A. Ravan, G. R. DeLong, R. K. Abramson, H. H. Wright, and M. L. Cuccaro. 2005. Accelerated head growth in early development of individuals with autism. *Ped. Neurol.* 32:102–8.

Deutsch, C. K. and L. G. Farkas. 1994. Quantitative methods of dysmorphology diagnosis. *Anthrop. Head Face*:151–8.

Deutsch, C. K. and R. M. Joseph. 2003. Brief report: Cognitive correlates of enlarged head circumference in children with autism. *J. Autism Dev. Disord.* 33:209–15.

Dissanayake, C., Q. M. Bui, R. Huggins, and D. Z. Loesch. 2006. Growth in stature and head circumference in high-functioning autism and Asperger disorder during the first 3 years of life. *Dev. Psychopathol.* 18:381–93.

Elia, M., R. Ferri, S. A. Musumeci, S. Panerai, M. Bottitta, and C. Scuderi. 2000. Clinical correlates of brain morphometric features of subjects with low-functioning autistic disorder. *J. Child Neurol.* 15:504–8.

Fidler, D. J., J. N. Bailey, and S. L. Smalley. 2000. Macrocephaly in autism and other pervasive developmental disorders. *Dev. Med. Child Neurol.* 42:737–40.

Filipek, P., C. Richelme, D. Kennedy, J. Rademacher, D. Pitcher, S. Zidel, and V. Caviness. 1992. Morphometric analysis of the brain in developmental language disorders and autism. *Ann. Neurol.* 32:78.153–24.

Fombonne, E., B. Rogé, J. Claverie, S. Courty, and J. Fremolle. 1999. Microcephaly and macrocephaly in autism. *J. Autism Dev. Disord.* 29:113–9.

Freitag, C. M., E. Luders, H. E. Hulst, K. L. Narr, P. M. Thompson, A. W. Toga, C. Krick, and C. Konrad. 2009. Total brain volume and corpus callosum size in medication-naive adolescents and young adults with autism spectrum disorder. *Biol. Psychiatry* 66:316–9.

Froehlich, W., S. Cleveland, A. Torres, J. Phillips, B. Cohen, T. Torigoe, J. Miller, A. Fedele, J. Collins, and K. Smith. 2013. Head circumferences in twins with and without autism spectrum disorders. *J. Autism Dev. Disord.* 43:2026–37.

Fukumoto, A., T. Hashimoto, H. Ito, M. Nishimura, Y. Tsuda, M. Miyazaki, K. Mori, K. Arisawa, and S. Kagami. 2008. Growth of head circumference in autistic infants during the first year of life. *J. Autism Dev. Disord.* 38:411–8.

Fukumoto, A., T. Hashimoto, K. Mori, Y. Tsuda, K. Arisawa, and S. Kagami. 2011. Head circumference and body growth in autism spectrum disorders. *Brain Dev.* 33:569–75.

Gaffney, G. R., S. Kuperman, L. Y. Tsai, S. Minchin, and K. M. Hassanein. 1987. Midsagittal magnetic resonance imaging of autism. *Br. J. Psychiatry* 151:831–3.

Giedd, J. N., J. Blumenthal, N. O. Jeffries, F. X. Castellanos, H. Liu, A. Zijdenbos, T. Paus, A. C. Evans, and J. L. Rapoport. 1999. Brain development during childhood and adolescence: A longitudinal MRI study. *Nat. Neurosci.* 2:861–3.

Giedd, J. N., J. W. Snell, N. Lange, J. C. Rajapakse, B. Casey, P. L. Kozuch, A. C. Vaituzis, Y. C. Vauss, S. D. Hamburger, and D. Kaysen. 1996. Quantitative magnetic resonance imaging of human brain development: Ages 4–18. *Cerebral Cortex* 6:551–9.

Gillberg, C. and L. De Souza. 2002. Head circumference in autism, Asperger syndrome, and ADHD: A comparative study. *Develop. Med. Child Neurol.* 44:296–300.

Girgis, R. R., N. J. Minshew, N. M. Melhem, J. J. Nutche, M. S. Keshavan, and A. Y. Hardan. 2007. Volumetric alterations of the orbitofrontal cortex in autism. *Prog. Neuro-Psychopharmacol. Biol. Psychiatry* 31:41–5.

Gould, S. J. 1981. Measuring heads. *Mismeasure Man* 73–112.

Grandgeorge, M., E. Lemonnier, and N. Jallot. 2013. Autism spectrum disorders: Head circumference and body length at birth are both relative. *Acta Paed.* 102:901–7.

Greimel, E., B. Nehrkorn, M. Schulte-Rüther, G. R. Fink, T. Nickl-Jockschat, B. Herpertz-Dahlmann, K. Konrad, and S. B. Eickhoff. 2013. Changes in grey matter development in autism spectrum disorder. *Brain Struct. Funct.* 218:929–42.

Gubbay, S., M. Lobascher, and P. Kingerlee. 1970. A neurological appraisal of autistic children: Results of a Western Australian survey. *Dev. Med. Child Neurol.* 12:422–9.

Hallahan, B., E. Daly, G. McAlonan, E. Loth, F. Toal, F. O'brien, D. Robertson, S. Hales, C. Murphy, and K. Murphy. 2009. Brain morphometry volume in autistic spectrum disorder: A magnetic resonance imaging study of adults. *Psychol. Med.* 39:337.

Hamill, P., T. A. Drizd, C. L. Johnson, R. B. Reed, A. F. Roche, and W. M. Moore. 1979. Physical growth: National Center for Health Statistics percentiles. *Am. J. Clin. Nutr.* 32:607–29.

Hardan, A. Y., R. A. Libove, M. S. Keshavan, N. M. Melhem, and N. J. Minshew. 2009. A preliminary longitudinal magnetic resonance imaging study of brain volume and cortical thickness in autism. *Biol. Psychiatry* 66:320–6.

Hardan, A. Y., N. J. Minshew, N. M. Melhem, S. Srihari, B. Jo, R. Bansal, M. S. Keshavan, and J. A. Stanley. 2008. An MRI and proton spectroscopy study of the thalamus in children with autism. *Psychiatry Res.: Neuroimaging* 163:97–105.

Hardan, M. K., M. S. Keshavan, and N. J. Minshew. 2003. Motor performance and anatomic magnetic resonance imaging (MRI) of the basal ganglia in autism. *J. Child Neurol.* 18:317–24.

Hardan, A. Y., R. R. Girgis, J. Adams, A. R. Gilbert, M. S. Keshavan, and N. J. Minshew. 2006a. Abnormal brain size effect on the thalamus in autism. *Psychiatry Res.: Neuroimaging* 147:145–51.

Hardan, S. Muddasani, M. Vemulapalli, M. S. Keshavan, and N. J. Minshew. 2006b. An MRI study of increased cortical thickness in autism. *Am. J. Psychiatry* 163:1290–2.

Hazlett, H. C., M. D. Poe, G. Gerig, R. G. Smith, and J. Piven. 2006. Cortical gray and white brain tissue volume in adolescents and adults with autism. *Biol. Psychiatry* 59:1–6.

Hazlett, H. C., M. Poe, G. Gerig, R. G. Smith, J. Provenzale, A. Ross, J. Gilmore, and J. Piven. 2005. Magnetic resonance imaging and head circumference study of brain size in autism: Birth through age 2 years. *Arch. Gen. Psychiatry* 62:1366–76.

Hazlett, H. C., M. D. Poe, G. Gerig, M. Styner, C. Chappell, R. G. Smith, C. Vachet, and J. Piven. 2011. Early brain overgrowth in autism associated with an increase in cortical surface area before age 2 years. *Arch. Gen. Psychiatry* 68:467–76.

Haznedar, M. M., M. S. Buchsbaum, T.-C. Wei, P. R. Hof, C. Cartwright, C. A. Bienstock, and E. Hollander. 2000. Limbic circuitry in patients with autism spectrum disorders studied with positron emission tomography and magnetic resonance imaging. *Am. J. Psychiatry* 157:1994–2001.

Herbert, M. R., D. A. Ziegler, N. Makris, P. A. Filipek, T. L. Kemper, J. J. Normandin, H. A. Sanders, D. N. Kennedy, and V. S. Caviness. 2004. Localization of white matter volume increase in autism and developmental language disorder. *Ann. Neurol.* 55:530–40.

Hong, S., X. Ke, T. Tang, Y. Hang, K. Chu, H. Huang, Z. Ruan, Z. Lu, G. Tao, and Y. Liu. 2011. Detecting abnormalities of corpus callosum connectivity in autism using magnetic resonance imaging and diffusion tensor tractography. *Psychiatry Res.: Neuroimaging* 194:333–9.

Hultman, C. M., P. Sparén, and S. Cnattingius. 2002. Perinatal risk factors for infantile autism. *Epidemiology* 13:417–23.

Jacot-Descombes, S., N. Uppal, B. Wicinski, M. Santos, J. Schmeidler, P. Giannakopoulos, H. Heinsein, C. Schmitz, and P. R. Hof. 2012. Decreased pyramidal neuron size in Brodmann areas 44 and 45 in patients with autism. *Acta Neuropathol.* 124:67–79.

Jones, G. H. and J. E. Lewis. 1991. Head circumference in elderly long-stay patients with schizophrenia. *Br. J. Psychiatry* 159:435–8.

Jou, R. J., N. J. Minshew, M. S. Keshavan, and A. Y. Hardan. 2010a. Cortical gyrification in autistic and Asperger disorders: A preliminary magnetic resonance imaging study. *J. Child Neurol.* 25:1462–7.

Jou, R. J., N. J. Minshew, M. S. Keshavan, M. P. Vitale, and A. Y. Hardan. 2010b. Enlarged right superior temporal gyrus in children and adolescents with autism. *Brain Res.* 1360:205–12.

Kanner, L. 1943. *Autistic Disturbances of Affective Contact.* Publisher not known.

Lainhart, J. E., E. D. Bigler, M. Bocian, H. Coon, E. Dinh, G. Dawson, C. K. Deutsch, M. Dunn, A. Estes, and H. Tager-Flusberg. 2006. Head circumference and height in autism: A study by the Collaborative Program of Excellence in Autism. *Am. J. Med. Genetics Part A* 140:2257–74.

Lainhart, J. E., J. Piven, M. Wzorek, R. Landa, S. L. Santangelo, H. Coon, and S. E. Folstein. 1997. Macrocephaly in children and adults with autism. *J. Am. Acad. Child Adolesc. Psychiatry* 36:282–90.

Lange, N., B. G. Travers, E. D. Bigler, M. B. Prigge, A. L. Froehlich, J. A. Nielsen, A. N. Cariello, B. A. Zielinski, J. S. Anderson, and P. T. Fletcher. 2015. Longitudinal volumetric brain changes in autism spectrum disorder ages 6–35 years. *Autism Res.* 8:82–93.

Lenroot, R. K. and J. N. Giedd. 2006. Brain development in children and adolescents: Insights from anatomical magnetic resonance imaging. *Neurosci. Biobehav. Rev.* 30:718–29.

Libero, L. E., C. W. Nordahl, D. D. Li, E. Ferrer, S. J. Rogers, and D. G. Amaral. 2016. Persistence of megalencephaly in a subgroup of young boys with autism spectrum disorder. *Autism Res.* doi: 10.1002/aur.1643.

Mason-brothers, A., E. R. Ritvo, B. Guze, A. Mo, B. Freeman, S. J. Funderburk, and P. C. Schroth. 1987. Pre-, peri-, and postnatal factors in 181 autistic patients from single and multiple incidence families. *J. Am. Acad. Child Adolesc. Psychiatry* 26:39–42.

Mason-Brothers, A., E. R. Ritvo, C. Pingree, P. B. Petersen, W. R. Jenson, W. M. McMahon, B. Freeman, L. B. Jorde, M. J. Spencer, and A. Mo. 1990. The UCLA–University of Utah epidemiologic survey of autism: Prenatal, perinatal, and postnatal factors. *Pediatrics* 86:514–9.

McAlonan, E. D., V. Kumari, H. D. Critchley, T. van Amelsvoort, J. Suckling, A. Simmons, T. Sigmundsson, K. Greenwood, and A. Russell. 2002. Brain anatomy and sensorimotor gating in Asperger's syndrome. *Brain* 125:1594–606.

McAlonan, V. C., C. Cheung, J. Suckling, G. Y. Lam, K. Tai, L. Yip, D. G. Murphy, and S. E. Chua. 2005. Mapping the brain in autism. A voxel-based MRI study of volumetric differences and intercorrelations in autism. *Brain* 128:268–76.

Miles, L. H., T. Takahashi, and R. Hillman. 2000. Head circumference is an independent clinical finding associated with autism. *Am. J. Med. Genet.* 95:339–50.

Miles, T. N. T., J. Hong, N. Munden, N. Flournoy, S. R. Braddock, R. A. Martin, M. A. Spence, R. E. Hillman, and J. E. Farmer. 2008. Development and validation of a measure of dysmorphology: Useful for autism subgroup classification. *Am. J. Med. Genet. Part A* 146:1101–16.

Mostofsky, S. H., M. P. Burgess, and J. C. G. Larson. 2007. Increased motor cortex white matter volume predicts motor impairment in autism. *Brain* 130:2117–22.

Mraz, K. D., J. Green, T. Dumont-Mathieu, S. Makin, and D. Fein. 2007. Correlates of head circumference growth in infants later diagnosed with autism spectrum disorders. *J. Child Neurol.* 22:700–13.

Nordahl, C. W., D. Braunschweig, A.-M. Iosif, A. Lee, S. Rogers, P. Ashwood, D. G. Amaral, and J. Van de Water. 2013. Maternal autoantibodies are associated with abnormal brain enlargement in a subgroup of children with autism spectrum disorder. *Brain Behav. Immunity* 30:61–5.

Nordahl, C. W., N. Lange, D. D. Li, L. A. Barnett, A. Lee, M. H. Buonocore, T. J. Simon, S. Rogers, S. Ozonoff, and D. G. Amaral. 2011. Brain enlargement is associated with regression in preschool-age boys with autism spectrum disorders. *Proc. Natl. Acad. Sci.* 108:20195–200.

Ohta, H., C. W. Nordahl, A. M. Iosif, A. Lee, S. Rogers, and D. G. Amaral. 2015. Increased surface area, but not cortical thickness, in a subset of young boys with autism spectrum disorder. *Autism Res.* 9:232–48.

Palmen, S. J., H. E. Hulshoff Pol, C. Kemner, H. G. Schnack, S. Durston, B. E. Lahuis, R. S. Kahn, and H. Van Engeland. 2005. Increased gray-matter volume in medication-naive high-functioning children with autism spectrum disorder. *Psychol. Med.* 35:561–70.

Piven, J., S. Arndt, J. Bailey, and N. Andreasen. 1996. Regional brain enlargement in autism: A magnetic resonance imaging study. *J. Am. Acad. Child Adolesc. Psychiatry* 35:530–6.

Piven, J., S. Arndt, J. Bailey, S. Havercamp, N. C. Andreasen, and P. Palmer. 1995. An MRI study of brain size in autism. *Am. J. Psychiatry* 152:1145–9.

Rakic, P. 1995. A small step for the cell, a giant leap for mankind: A hypothesis of neocortical expansion during evolution. *Trends Neurosci.* 18:383–8.

Raznahan, A., R. Lenroot, A. Thurm, M. Gozzi, A. Hanley, S. J. Spence, S. E. Swedo, and J. N. Giedd. 2013a. Mapping cortical anatomy in preschool aged children with autism using surface-based morphometry. *NeuroImage: Clin.* 2:111–9.

Raznahan, A., G. L. Wallace, L. Antezana, D. Greenstein, R. Lenroot, A. Thurm, M. Gozzi, S. Spence, A. Martin, and S. E. Swedo. 2013b. Compared to what? Early brain overgrowth in autism and the perils of population norms. *Biol. Psychiatry* 74:563–75.

Redcay, E. and E. Courchesne. 2005. When is the brain enlarged in autism? A meta-analysis of all brain size reports. *Biol. Psychiatry* 58:1–9.

Rodier, P. M., S. E. Bryson, and J. P. Welch. 1997. Minor malformations and physical measurements in autism: Data from Nova Scotia. *Teratology* 55:319–25.

Rojas, D. C., J. A. Smith, T. L. Benkers, S. L. Camou, M. L. Reite, and S. J. Rogers. 2004. Hippocampus and amygdala volumes in parents of children with autistic disorder. *Am. J. Psychiatry* 161:2038–44.

Sacco, R., S. Gabriele, and A. M. Persico. 2015. Head circumference and brain size in autism spectrum disorder: A systematic review and meta-analysis. *Psychiatry Res.* 234:239–51.

Say, G. N., B. Şahin, K. Aslan, S. Akbaş, and M. Ceyhan. 2014. Increased laterality of the thalamus in children and adolescents with Asperger's disorder: An MRI and proton spectroscopy study. *Psychiatry Investig.* 11:237–42.

Schain, R. J. and H. Yannet. 1960. Infantile autism: An analysis of 50 cases and a consideration of certain relevant neurophysiologic concepts. *J. Pediatr.* 57:560–7.

Schumann, C., S. Bloss, C. C. Barnes, G. M. Wideman, R. A. Carper, N. Akshoomoff, K. Pierce, D. Hagler, N. Schork, and C. Lord. 2010. Longitudinal magnetic resonance imaging study of cortical development through early childhood in autism. *J. Neurosci.* 30:4419–27.

Schumann, J. H., B. L. Goodlin-Jones, L. J. Lotspeich, H. Kwon, M. H. Buonocore, C. R. Lammers, A. L. Reiss, and D. G. Amaral. 2004. The amygdala is enlarged in children but not adolescents with autism; the hippocampus is enlarged at all ages. *J. Neurosci.* 24:6392–401.

Schumann, C. and D. G. Amaral. 2006. Stereological analysis of amygdala neuron number in autism. *J. Neurosci.* 26:7674–9.

Shen, M. D., C. W. Nordahl, G. S. Young, S. L. Wootton-Gorges, A. Lee, S. E. Liston, K. R. Harrington, S. Ozonoff, and D. G. Amaral. 2013. Early brain enlargement and elevated extra-axial fluid in infants who develop autism spectrum disorder. *Brain* 136:2825–35.

Skjeldal, O. H., E. Sponheim, T. Ganes, E. Jellum, and S. Bakke. 1998. Childhood autism: The need for physical investigations. *Brain Dev.* 20:227–33.

Sowell, E. R., P. M. Thompson, and A. W. Toga. 2007. Mapping adolescent brain maturation using structural magnetic resonance imaging. In Romer, D. and Walker, E., (Eds.), *Adolesc. Psychopathol. Dev. Brain*, pp. 55–84.

Sparks, B., S. Friedman, D. Shaw, E. Aylward, D. Echelard, A. Artru, K. Maravilla, J. Giedd, J. Munson, and G. Dawson. 2002. Brain structural abnormalities in young children with autism spectrum disorder. *Neurology* 59:184–92.

Stamova, B. S., Y. Tian, C. W. Nordahl, M. D. Shen, S. Rogers, D. G. Amaral, and F. R. Sharp. 2013. Evidence for differential alternative splicing in blood of young boys with autism spectrum disorders. *Mol. Autism* 4:1.

Steg, J. P. and J. L. Rapoport. 1975. Minor physical anomalies in normal, neurotic, learning disabled, and severely disturbed children. *J. Autism Childhood Schizophrenia* 5:299–307.

Stevenson, R. E., R. J. Schroer, C. Skinner, D. Fender, and R. J. Simensen. 1997. Autism and macrocephaly. *The Lancet* 349:1744–5.

Stiles, J. and T. L. Jernigan. 2010. The basics of brain development. *Neuropsychol. Rev.* 20:327–48.

Stuart, H. and S. Stevenson. 1950. Physical growth and development. In Nelson, W. E. (Ed.0), *Textbook of Pediatrics*, ed. 5, Saunders, Philadelphia, pp. 14–73.

Tamura, R., H. Kitamura, T. Endo, N. Hasegawa, and T. Someya. 2010. Reduced thalamic volume observed across different subgroups of autism spectrum disorders. *Psychiatry Res.: Neuroimaging* 184:186–8.

Tate, D., E. Bigler, W. McMahon, and J. Lainhart. 2007. The relative contributions of brain, cerebrospinal fluid-filled structures and non-neural tissue volumes to occipital-frontal head circumference in subjects with autism. *Neuropediatrics* 38:18–24.

Tepest, R., E. Jacobi, A. Gawronski, B. Krug, W. Möller-Hartmann, F. G. Lehnhardt, and K. Vogeley. 2010. Corpus callosum size in adults with high-functioning autism and the relevance of gender. *Psychiatry Res.: Neuroimaging* 183:38–43.

Tetreault, N. A., A. Y. Hakeem, S. Jiang, B. A. Williams, E. Allman, B. J. Wold, and J. M. Allman. 2012. Microglia in the cerebral cortex in autism. *J. Autism Dev. Disord.* 42:2569–84.

Torrey, E. F., D. Dhavale, J. P. Lawlor, and R. H. Yolken. 2004. Autism and head circumference in the first year of life. *Biol. Psychiatry* 56:892–4.

van Kooten, I. A., S. J. Palmen, P. von Cappeln, H. W. Steinbusch, H. Korr, H. Heinsen, P. R. Hof, H. van Engeland, and C. Schmitz. 2008. Neurons in the fusiform gyrus are fewer and smaller in autism. *Brain* 131:987–99.

Vargas, D. L., C. Nascimbene, C. Krishnan, A. W. Zimmerman, and C. A. Pardo. 2005. Neuroglial activation and neuroinflammation in the brain of patients with autism. *Ann. Neurol.* 57:67–81.

Ververi, A., E. Vargiami, V. Papadopoulou, D. Tryfonas, and D. I. Zafeiriou. 2012. Clinical and laboratory data in a sample of Greek children with autism spectrum disorders. *J. Autism Dev. Disord.* 42:1470–6.

Vidal, C. N., R. Nicolson, T. J. DeVito, K. M. Hayashi, J. A. Geaga, D. J. Drost, P. C. Williamson, N. Rajakumar, Y. Sui, and R. A. Dutton. 2006. Mapping corpus callosum deficits in autism: An index of aberrant cortical connectivity. *Biol. Psychiatry* 60:218–25.

Walker, H. A. 1977. Incidence of minor physical anomaly in autism. *J. Autism Childhood Schizophrenia* 7:165–76.

Webb, S. J., T. Nalty, J. Munson, C. Brock, R. Abbott, and G. Dawson. 2007. Rate of head circumference growth as a function of autism diagnosis and history of autistic regression. *J. Child Neurol.* 22:1182–90.

Weinberg, W. A., S. G. Dietz, E. C. Penick, and W. H. McAlister. 1974. Intelligence, reading achievement, physical size, and social class: A study of St. Louis Caucasian boys aged 8–0 to 9–6 years, attending regular schools. *J. Pediatr.* 85:482–9.

Woodhouse, W., A. Bailey, M. Rutter, P. Bolton, G. Baird, and A. Couteur. 1996. Head circumference in autism and other pervasive developmental disorders. *J. Child Psychol. Psychiatry* 37:665–71.

Zwaigenbaum, L., G. S. Young, W. L. Stone, K. Dobkins, S. Ozonoff, J. Brian, S. E. Bryson, L. J. Carver, T. Hutman, and J. M. Iverson. 2014. Early head growth in infants at risk of autism: A baby siblings research consortium study. *J. Am. Acad. Child Adolesc. Psychiatry* 53:1053–62.

Chapter 11 Imaging the striatum in autism spectrum disorder

Adriana Di Martino, Eun
Young Choi, Rebecca M.
Jones, F. Xavier Castellanos,
and Ayman Mukerji

Contents

Abstract 189
11.1 Introduction 190
    11.1.1 Striatal anatomy and neurochemistry. 191
    11.1.2 Corticostriatal connectivity 191
        11.1.2.1 Specific circuits 192
    11.1.3 Studying striatum in humans 194
    11.1.4 Typical striatal development. 196
11.2 Striatal imaging in ASD. 197
    11.2.1 Regional striatal studies 198
        11.2.1.1 Structural imaging. 198
        11.2.1.2 Functional imaging 200
11.3 ASD striatal connectivity 203
    11.3.1 Structural connectivity 203
    11.3.2 Functional connectivity 203
11.4. Summary and conclusions 205
Acknowledgments 207
References 207

Abstract

The striatum represents the main input station for cortical afferent connections within cortico-basal ganglia–thalamic circuits. These have been detailed in non-human primates and begun to be characterized with noninvasive brain imaging in humans. This chapter focuses on brain imaging research of striatal circuitry in autism. This research has been motivated by the role of striatal circuitry in a wide range of motor, cognitive and emotional processes also found to be abnormal in autism. Results from morphological and functional magnetic resonance imaging suggest that striatal abnormalities are implicated in restricted behaviors/interests, executive and reward dysfunctions in this population. Yet, the specific nature of striatal abnormalities in autism remains unclear. Building on the first generation of studies summarized here, greater insights is likely to be attained with the advancements of imaging acquisition technologies and emerging analytical approaches able to capture fine-grained properties of striatal-based networks in large-scale studies able to account for the striking heterogeneity of autism.

11.1 Introduction

Basal ganglia (*Lt*: collection of cells) are subcortical structures located above the brainstem at the base of each cortical hemisphere. They consist of striatum, pallidum (globus pallidus and ventral pallidum), substantia nigra in the brainstem, and subthalamic nucleus. The basal ganglia receive topographic input from all cortical regions, except for primary visual cortex, as well as from subcortical regions, including thalamus, amygdala, hippocampus, and brainstem. The basal ganglia send output primarily to thalamus, from which connections return to cerebral cortex and brainstem. The functions of these connections are not completely understood, but basal ganglia appear to integrate information received by association, motor, and limbic cortex to form associations between features, actions, and outcomes to influence neural processing or trigger actions (Haber 2003; Haber et al. 2011).

The striatum (*Lt*: striped, from its appearance due to passing fibers) is the largest basal ganglia structure and main input station for cortical afferent connections within corticobasal ganglia-thalamic circuits. Although historically characterized as motor connections (Nauta and Mehler 1966), investigations in monkeys and humans have shown that multiple, additional nonmotor corticobasal ganglia-thalamic circuits exist (Heimer and Wilson 1975). These circuits subserve executive/cognitive control and reward-related/motivational processes, including verbal and spatial working memory, response inhibition, task-switching, reasoning as well as processing prediction errors, reinforcement learning, reward anticipation, and incentive salience for primary, secondary, or social rewards. This list highlights the functional diversity of the processes underlined by striatal circuits. Many of these processes have been implicated in the clinical presentation of autism spectrum disorder (ASD; American Psychiatric Association 2013). Several behavioral cognitive anomalies associated with ASD are consistent with abnormal striatal functions (i.e., motor stereotypies, reduced social motivation, difficulties with response inhibition). Thus, the past decade has seen a dramatic increase in the number of studies examining the striatum in individuals with ASD, particularly with noninvasive *in vivo* brain imaging approaches.

This chapter begins with an overview of the structural and functional organization of the striatum in nonhuman primates as a benchmark for translational research. Second, we summarize the brain imaging approaches commonly utilized to examine human striatum noninvasively. Third, to provide a framework for an early-onset disorder such as ASD, we summarize the developmental changes described in typical children. We conclude with a critical review of the ASD striatal imaging literature.

11.1.1 Striatal anatomy and neurochemistry

The striatum is composed of three nuclei—caudate (*Lt*: tail), putamen (*Lt*: husk), and nucleus accumbens (short for *nucleus accumbens septi*, *Lt*: nucleus against wall)—and the olfactory tubercle. The caudate and putamen are parallel longitudinal structures with the caudate located medially. The C-shaped caudate is divided into a rostrally located head, a body, and a caudally located tail. The nucleus accumbens and olfactory tubercle, located below caudate and putamen, span the rostral half of the striatum, ending approximately where the anterior commissure intercepts the striatum. The caudate and putamen are almost completely separated by the internal capsule, a large white-matter bundle, except for cell bridges connecting the two sides (Haber et al. 2011). Nearly all striatal neurons are medium spiny GABAergic projection neurons. Nonetheless, the striatum has a heterogeneous cytoarchitecture. Dorsal striatum has clusters (called patches or striosomes) of neurons initially identified as acetylcholinesterase-poor regions (Graybiel and Ragsdale 1978). These clusters also express a variety of other substances, such as dopamine receptors, opioid receptors, substance P, enkephalin, and calbindin. The ventral striatum lacks clear cluster boundaries (Graybiel 1990; Holt et al. 1997). The functional significance of this fractionated cytoarchitecture is not well understood.

11.1.2 Corticostriatal connectivity

Using tract-tracing techniques in monkeys, investigators have detailed connections from cortex to striatum (Künzle 1975; Goldman and Nauta 1977; Künzle and Akert 1977; Selemon and Goldman-Rakic 1985; Haber et al. 2006). Although the circuitry linking cortex, basal ganglia, and thalamus was initially characterized only in terms of motor connections (Nauta et al. 1966), multiple, nonmotor, associative corticobasal ganglia-thalamic circuits have since been identified (Heimer and Wilson 1975; Heimer 1978; DeLong and Georgopoulos 1981; DeLong et al. 1984). In aggregate, these studies have shown that corticostriatal projections form form a broad circuitry connecting sensorimotor, association and limbic functional territories (see Parent 1990; Haber 2003), organized on a dorsolateral-to-ventromedial axis (Voorn et al. 2004). This topography is broadly maintained throughout the basal ganglia (Szabo 1967, 1970;

Lynd-Balta and Haber 1994; Haynes and Haber 2013), and connections remain segregated in the thalamic nuclei (Carpenter et al. 1976; Kim et al. 1976), which in turn send outputs to cortex. On the basis of the maintained topography of connections through cortex, basal ganglia, and thalamus, Alexander et al. (1986) identified at least five parallel segregated circuits differing in functionality. Distinct association and motor circuits were confirmed by Strick and colleagues, using transsynaptic viral tracing (Middleton and Strick 1994, 2000, 2002; Kelly and Strick 2004).

Intriguingly, although the general functional topography of parallel corticobasal ganglia-thalamic circuits is preserved, these circuits are also highly integrated (Mogenson et al. 1980; Percheron and Filion 1991; Haber 2003) (Figure 11.1). This involves convergence of projections from different functional cortical territories onto the same neurons (Smith and Bolam 1991; Bevan et al. 1996, 1997), dendrites, and axons crossing topographical boundaries (Yelnik et al. 1996, 1997), and closed and open connectional loops between structures (Heimer et al. 1982; Joel and Weiner 1997; Haber et al. 2000; McFarland and Haber 2000). Within striatum in particular, Haber and colleagues (Haber et al. 2006; Calzavara et al. 2007; Averbeck et al. 2014; Choi et al. 2016) showed that dense focal projection fields from different prefrontal regions overlap with one another, in addition to broad overlaps in diffuse projection fields. Haber et al. (2000) also discovered a set of spiraling pathways between striatum and substantia nigra pars compacta suggesting a flow of information from limbic to association to sensorimotor striatum. In short, converging lines of evidence support the existence of a combination of parallel and integrated circuits, which likely support the complex, integrated behaviors underpinned by striatum.

11.1.2.1 Specific circuits   Caudal putamen mostly receives motor cortical projections with an inverted somatotopy (Kunzle 1975; Flaherty and Graybiel 1991) as well as a second, more medially located, inverted somatotopy from the supplementary motor area (SMA; Inase et al. 1996; Takada et al. 1998). By contrast, rostral putamen and caudate are dominated by association and limbic projections, many spanning caudate and putamen via cell bridges across the internal capsule. Prefrontal cortex sends the strongest projections to rostral striatum with broadly different functional regions sending distinct, but overlapping, corticostriatal projections (Haber et al. 2006; Averbeck et al. 2014). Premotor cortex (area 6, SMA, pre-SMA) and frontal and supplementary eye fields (FEF, SEF) project to dorsal-most caudate, the dorsal half of putamen, and regions around the internal capsule. Slightly ventral to and overlapping these are projections from dorsolateral prefrontal cortex (DLPFC; areas 9, 46, 9/46), which also span the caudate, internal capsule, and a portion of adjacent medial putamen. Projections from anterior cingulate cortex (ACC; area 24) and orbitofrontal cortex (OFC; areas 11, 13) are broad, spanning most ventral caudate and medial ventral putamen as well as

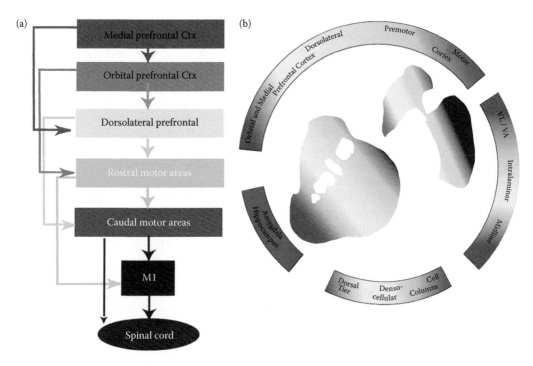

Figure 11.1 Schematic illustration of the functional organization of the frontal cortex (a) and the striatum (b), highlighting cortical and subcortical projections to striatum. The functional processes underpinned by each frontal cortex territory and their striatal projections are color-coded as follows: blue: motor cortex, execution of motor actions; green: *premotor cortex*, planning of movements; yellow: dorsolateral prefrontal cortex, cognitive and executive functions; orange: orbitofrontal cortex, goal-directed behaviors and motivation; and red: medial prefrontal cortex, goal-directed behaviors and emotional processing. (Reprinted by permission from Haber, S. N. 2003. *J. Chem. Neuroanat.* 26:317–30.)

part of the projections from dorsolateral and motor-related cortex in dorsal striatum. Projections from ventromedial prefrontal cortex (vmPFC; areas 14, 25) lie along the medial wall of caudate and overlap those from ACC and OFC in ventral caudate. Each of these projections continue caudally in striatum, although their patterns become less distinct as caudate and putamen taper. In addition to these frontal projections, amygdala sends strong projections to ventral striatum, overlapping with those from vmPFC, ACC, and OFC (Russchen et al. 1985; Fudge et al. 2002, 2004). Although a rough one-to-one mapping of frontal regions to striatum exists (Averbeck et al. 2014), corticostriatal projections are not evenly distributed across striatum. Rather, certain striatal regions receive greater proportions of converging projections, that is, regions in rostral dorsal caudate (Calzavara et al. 2007; Choi et al. 2016), rostral ventral caudate (Averbeck et al. 2014), and medial putamen (Calzavara et al. 2007). These convergence regions may be critical hubs of integration that are both particularly susceptible to disease and efficacious treatment targets (Haber et al. 2006; Choi et al. 2016).

193

Less is known of projections from parietal, temporal, posterior cingulate, and visual cortex. Parietal projections together cover dorsal caudate and medial dorsal putamen (Cavada and Goldman-Rakic 1991; Yeterian and Pandya 1993), likely overlapping with dorsally terminating frontal projections (e.g., from SEF, FEF, premotor cortex, DLPFC; Choi et al. 2016). Caudal superior temporal projections, including from auditory cortex, also generally project to dorsal striatum (Yeterian and Pandya 1998). Rostral superior and inferior temporal projections, including those from hippocampus, terminate primarily in ventral striatum, potentially overlapping with projections from vmPFC, ACC, OFC, and amygdala (Van Hoesen et al. 1981; Yeterian and Pandya 1998; Friedman et al. 2002). Temporal polar projections target the caudate medial wall, similar to vmPFC projections (Van Hoesen et al. 1981; Yeterian and Pandya 1998). The few posterior cingulate cases available indicate that projections terminate in dorsal caudate (Powell 1978; Baleydier and Mauguiere 1980; Parvizi et al. 2006), potentially overlapping with projections from vmPFC and temporal pole. Visual cortical projections are weakest, terminating in posterior striatum (Maunsell and Van Essen 1983; Ungerleider et al. 1984; Saint-Cyr et al. 1990; Boussaoud et al. 1992).

In summary, striatum receives projections from nearly the entire cerebral cortex (except V1), as well as from subcortical structures. However, rather than simply being a funnel for distributing incoming projections into three broad functional territories, there is evidence of a more complex organization of cortical inputs. Noninvasive neuroimaging studies in typically developing humans have confirmed striatum motor, associative, and limbic organization. In what follows, we briefly review the *in vivo* neuroimaging approaches utilized to examine the striatal structural and functional organization and identify their advantages and limitations.

11.1.3 Studying striatum in humans

High-resolution human neuroimaging studies first became feasible with the widespread availability of magnetic resonance imaging (MRI) scanners in the early 1990s. First-generation MRI studies provided quantitative morphometric indices, based on T1-weighted sequences, such as volumes of caudate and putamen obtained by hand-tracing. Hand-tracings represent the gold standard for quantitative indices, but reliability of operator-based measurements is inevitably limited, besides being time consuming. Accordingly, investigators have increasingly adopted fully or nearly fully automated methods. These include voxel-based morphometry (VBM), automatically comparing spatially normalized estimates of gray or white matter volume across subjects in the whole brain using a standard template space (Wilke et al. 2008). Algorithmic T1-based methods have also been devised to delineate surfaces of subcortical structures to reveal structural deviations that can be missed by volumetric studies. For example, both expansions and contractions can occur in separate subregions of the same structure, which could cancel out in volumetric analyses.

Diffusion tensor imaging (DTI) tractography studies mapping fibers originating in frontal cortex and projecting to striatum have revealed the rostrocaudal topographical organization of parallel and integrated corticostriatal loops (Lehericy et al. 2004; Draganski et al. 2008; Verstynen et al. 2012). An alternative approach entails quantifying covariance of cortical thickness or gray matter volume across subjects. Although it does not directly examine anatomical connections, structural covariance has been shown to relate to functional connectivity (Alexander-Bloch et al. 2013). Functional connectivity can be examined based on patterns of coactivation during task-based fMRI (referred to as extrinsic functional connectivity) or derived from resting-state fMRI (referred to as intrinsic functional connectivity; iFC).

Task-based fMRI allows focused testing of specific hypotheses within the constraints of specific tasks and has been the workhorse of cognitive and affective neuroscience. However, designing tasks that are relevant for multiple developmental periods and varying levels of ability represents a major challenge. A complementary method, task-free functional imaging (also known as resting-state fMRI; R-fMRI), can be obtained across wide age ranges and abilities and allows testing of innumerable questions within a single data set. The field of R-fMRI is based on the seminal observation that spontaneous or intrinsic brain activity includes large-amplitude low-frequency fluctuations synchronized across widespread regions underpinning similar processes (Biswal et al. 1995; for reviews see Raichle and Snyder 2007; Craddock et al. 2013). Patterns of synchrony are quantified by their temporal correlations that are interpreted as reflecting functional connectivity (Raichle and Snyder 2007; Craddock et al. 2013; Matthews and Fair 2015). The finding that such patterns recapitulate coactivation patterns revealed in task-based fMRI (Smith et al. 2009) has supported its increasing application in clinical neuroscience (Fox and Greicius 2010; Castellanos et al. 2013; Di Martino et al. 2014a). The field of R-fMRI is still rapidly developing, with investigators addressing troublesome confounds such as micromotion, which produces artifacts that cannot be eliminated by increasing sample size or lengthening scan duration (Yan et al. 2013; Power et al. 2015). Nevertheless, R-fMRI has recapitulated many of the striatal findings from basic neuroscience as well as from coactivation patterns revealed by a meta-analysis of 126 human imaging studies (Postuma and Dagher 2006). These corticostriatal patterns have been directly discerned in single-sample R-fMRI studies (e.g., Di Martino et al. 2008; Choi et al. 2012). The replicability of this approach has motivated the examination of striatum in clinical populations, including ASD.

11.1.4 Typical striatal development

Human imaging research starting in infancy and extending into early adulthood has begun to provide critical information on brain developmental trajectories. With a few notable exceptions (e.g., Giedd et al. 1999), most studies have utilized cross-sectional rather than longitudinal designs, have focused on the time shift from school age to adulthood, and have generally focused on volumes at the macroscale resolution. Despite these understandable limitations, the field has begun to delineate fundamental principles. Human brain imaging studies have revealed regionally specific nonlinear developmental trajectories presumably reflecting behavioral developmental milestones (Gogtay et al. 2004; Brain Development Cooperative 2012).

Similarly, longitudinal volumetric studies have shown that nonlinear developmental trajectories occur in the striatum (Raznahan et al. 2014; Shaw et al. 2014). Striatal volume increases in childhood, reaches a peak in mid-adolescence, and decreases thereafter (Shaw et al. 2014). Although results are preliminary, distinct striatal regions manifest distinct trajectories (cubic vs. quadratic) and magnitude of change (Goddings et al. 2014). For example, a longitudinal study of more than 100 typical children followed to young adulthood reported greater pubertal changes in nucleus accumbens (more than 9%) in contrast with more modest changes in caudate volumes (Goddings et al. 2014). Heterochronicity has also been shown in studies of striatum shape (Raznahan et al. 2014). Specifically, caudate tail and caudal lateral putamen showed greater expansion with age, in contrast with rostroventral striatal regions showing shape contraction. The pattern of striatal contractions and expansions mapped to regions of pallidum and thalamus preferentially connected with specifically contracting or expanding striatal regions. The striato-pallido-thalamic tract connected to more rostral prefrontal and superior parietal cortex contracted with increasing age, whereas areas more strongly associated to caudolateral prefrontal and primary sensorimotor cortex expanded (Raznahan et al. 2014). Although it is unknown whether local shape changes stem from changes in parenchyma or reflect related white matter processes, these results suggest that examining developmental striatal changes in the context of cortical connections can be fruitful.

In this context, fMRI studies have captured the functional role of striatal developmental changes and its cortical relationships both indirectly, by examining activations in striatum and cortex in parallel, and directly, by measuring functional connectivity. A large body of work has examined how motivational tasks modulate striatal circuitry at different ages during typical development (summarized in Casey 2015). For example, increased activity in ventral striatum to reward cues has been observed in multiple studies in adolescents compared to children and adults (Galvan et al. 2006; Cohen et al. 2010; Geier et al. 2010; van Leijenhorst et al.

2010). Other studies, however, have shown decreased nucleus accumbens activation in anticipation of rewards in adolescents relative to children and adults (Bjork et al. 2004). Despite apparent contradictions, this work demonstrates that adolescence is a period of increased sensitivity to motivational or rewarding cues with different functional activity in frontostriatal circuitry compared to children and adults. Examining this circuitry directly during reward learning, van den Bos et al. (2012) found no age-related differences in ventral striatum or prefrontal cortex activation per se but found age-related differences in functional connectivity between these regions. Together, these task-based fMRI studies demonstrate age-dependent influences on striatal circuits in the typically developing brain.

More recently, typical development of corticostriatal connectivity has been characterized in cross-sectional R-fMRI studies. One study examining whole-brain properties of the connectome suggested that iFC of striatum and other subcortical regions tends to decrease from childhood to young adulthood, while corticocortical iFC increases (Supekar et al. 2009). An emerging literature is increasingly focusing on typical development of specific striatal iFC patterns. Results are preliminary but overall support the notion of developmental regional variation (Bo et al. 2014; Greene et al. 2014; Fareri et al. 2015; Padmanabhan et al. 2015; Porter et al. 2015). For example, a recent cross-sectional study of the life span (10–74 years) suggested an inverted-U trajectory characterizes several motor and cognitive striatal circuits (Bo et al. 2014). Similarly, recent work suggests that ventral and dorsal striatum differ in age trajectories (Porter et al. 2015), and Fareri et al. (2015) demonstrated both nonlinear patterns (adolescent-specific) and linear patterns (increasing with age) of differences in ventral striatal iFC. Findings of developmental changes of striatum provide the context to interpret the role of striatum in individuals with ASD differing for chronological age. They also motivate age-related investigations in this population.

11.2 Striatal imaging in ASD

Initial striatal studies in ASD have been motivated by the similarities of repetitive restricted behaviors/interest (RRB) observed in ASD and other neuropsychiatric disorders characterized by striatal abnormalities such as obsessive-compulsive or Tourette's disorders (Langen et al. 2011). Based on the increased appreciation that striatum circuitry subserves not only sensorimotor but also cognitive and emotional processes, later investigations of striatum in ASD have extended beyond RRB. Whereas initial efforts have examined striatal morphometry in relation to measures of RRB, subsequent structural studies have included other symptom domains such as executive dysfunctions (Voelbel et al. 2006) and impairment in social communicative skills (Rojas et al. 2006). Task-based fMRI studies have expanded understanding of the scope of striatal involvement in ASD. Abnormal activation patterns in ASD have been revealed during paradigms probing a range of social and nonsocial processes (Section 11.3). More recently, given the increased understanding of ASD as a disconnection syndrome (Geschwind and Levitt 2007; Minshew and Williams 2007), the field has shifted from a focus on specific regional abnormalities to brain network models of ASD. Accordingly, first we review the structural and functional imaging literature on striatum in ASD by focusing on regional studies, followed by studies of quantitative measures of striatal connectivity.

11.2.1 Regional striatal studies

11.2.1.1 Structural imaging Structural regional imaging studies implicating striatal physiopathology in ASD include volumetric examinations of regions of interest and whole-brain voxel-based morphometric studies. Only one investigation of striatal shape has been published to date (Qiu et al. 2010).

11.2.1.1.1 Volumetrics Volumetric studies have targeted striatal regions selected *a priori*, based on hand-tracing or automated segmentation algorithms. Most studies include caudate and putamen with nucleus accumbens rarely distinguished. Comparisons of individuals with ASD relative to typically developing controls (TDC) have most consistently reported enlarged caudate volume in samples of children (Herbert et al. 2003; Langen et al. 2007; Estes et al. 2011) and adolescents or young adults (Sears et al. 1999; Hollander et al. 2005; Haznedar et al. 2006; Rojas et al. 2006; Langen et al. 2007). However, it is unclear whether caudate enlargement is proportional to total brain volume (TBV) or not. Some studies report volume increases after correcting for TBV (Hollander et al. 2005; Haznedar et al. 2006; Rojas et al. 2006; Voelbel et al. 2006; Langen et al. 2009, 2014), and others identify larger caudate size only before correcting for TBV (Sears et al. 1999; Herbert et al. 2003; Estes et al. 2011). Regardless of TBV correction, some studies have not found significant diagnostic differences in striatum volume in young adults (Gaffney et al. 1989; Hardan et al. 2003; Qiu et al. 2010), children (Sussman et al. 2015), or both (Haar et al. 2016). In interpreting these mixed results, several authors have highlighted the role of age effects in regard to TBV and striatal volumes. We note, however, that the literature is just beginning to include longitudinal studies, the gold standard to reach definitive conclusions on developmental trajectories (Kraemer et al. 2000). Only two longitudinal studies have included striatum in statistical analyses and they reached different conclusions. A study of 49 children with ASD and 37 TDC (mean age 9.9 years), scanned twice (mean interval 2.4 years, covering ages 7–17), found a significant increase in caudate size in ASD relative to TDC (Langen et al. 2014). A larger study ($n = 100$, ASD; $n = 56$, TDC) of individuals in the age range of 3–35 years scanned up to three times, examined TBV, total gray matter (GM), and 10 brain regions, including the caudate. Unlike other cortical and subcortical regions showing ASD-specific trajectories, caudate volume variation with age did not differ between groups across this wider age range (Lange et al. 2015).

Methodological and ASD-intrinsic factors may also account for contrasting volumetric results. A complex issue is the role of intelligence quotient (IQ) and its relationship with TBV. In large samples selected from the open multisite repository, Autism Brain Imaging Data Exchange (ABIDE; Di Martino et al. 2014b) IQ and TBV were significantly correlated in TDC but to a lesser extent in individuals with ASD (Lefebvre et al. 2015; Riddle et al. 2016). Both of these factors have been differently accounted for in volumetric research. Studies vary in regard to group-matching samples for IQ, which in turn can introduce artifactual diagnostic differences in TBV. Thus, heterogeneity across studies in regard to IQ, TBV, as well as sample matching for IQ and TBV may lead to contrasting volumetric findings. To systematically discern the role of these factors, future work will need to include sufficiently large independent samples that include a broad range of the relevant variables.

11.2.1.1.2 Voxel-based morphometry Volumetric analyses of regions of interest are relatively coarse measures and are likely to miss localized structural characteristics. For this reason, VBM has been increasingly applied in individuals with ASD versus TDC. Using anatomic likelihood estimation, a meta-analysis of 16 whole-brain VBM studies published before 2010 revealed consistent ASD-related gray and white matter abnormalities. Analyses combining all foci reported revealed six clusters of significant group differences. One was localized in right caudate, another in left putamen (Nickl-Jockschat et al. 2012). Secondary analyses investigating gray and white matter decreases or increases found a significant probability for GM decreases in left putamen; the nature of caudate ASD-related differences could not be discerned significantly (Nickl-Jockschat et al. 2012). The five VBM studies directly revealing striatal abnormalities in ASD (McAlonan et al. 2008, 2009, 2010; Langen et al. 2009; Ecker et al. 2012) report inconsistent findings. Increases in white matter surrounding the basal ganglia and the thalamus were reported in two studies (McAlonan et al. 2002, 2009), whereas another study found decreases in white matter of the internal capsule hosting frontostriatal and thalamocortical projections (Ecker et al. 2012). ASD-related increased striatal GM density has been reported in the right caudate head (Langen et al. 2009) and left caudate and putamen (Ecker et al. 2012). In contrast, decreased striatal GM was only found in 17 individuals with Asperger's syndrome but not in 16 with *DSM-IV* Autistic Disorder (McAlonan et al. 2008). This suggests that inconsistent results may relate to the clinical and biological heterogeneity of ASD that cannot be easily captured in small-to-moderate samples. We note, however, that a recent VBM study examining two large overlapping multisite samples (total sample, $N = 800$; age-matched sample, $n = 600$) of individuals with ASD and TDC selected from ABIDE showed minimal group differences in GM density. These were localized in the anterior portions of superior temporal gyrus (STG); none were found in striatum (Riddle et al. 2016). Minimal regional differences in ASD in regard to other structural metrics such as cortical thickness and surface as well as cortical and subcortical volumes have also been reported in another study using overlapping samples selected from ABIDE ($N = 906$; $n = 590$) (Haar et al. 2016). Since ABIDE comprises retrospectively aggregated data, these findings may be confounded by intersite variation. At the same time, given the sample sizes of pre-ABIDE morphometric studies (ranging from $n = 8$ to $n = 100$ per group; mean $n = 39 \pm 30$/group), the possibility that earlier findings are false-positives cannot be excluded. Alternatively, if the core physiopathology of ASD is related to disconnections, other imaging approaches may be more robust for capturing ASD abnormalities.

11.2.1.1.3 Correlation with RRB Inconsistencies have also been reported in regard to the relationship between striatal morphometry and RRB severity. RRB have been indexed using various clinical measures, albeit most frequently with the Autism Diagnostic Interview–Revised (Rutter et al. 2003). Specifically, investigators focused on lower-order RRB, such as repetitive motor behaviors and unusual sensory interests, and/or higher-order RRB, such as restricted interests, and adherence to routines. Of the volumetric studies exploring relationships between striatal volume and RRB indices, seven did not find any statistically significant correlations (Hollander et al. 2005; Voelbel et al. 2006; Langen et al. 2007; Qiu et al. 2010; Ecker et al. 2012). Others have reported significant correlations but results varied in terms of directionality. Some investigators reported increased RRB severity with larger striatal volumes (Hardan et al. 2003; Rojas et al. 2006; Wolff et al. 2013; Langen et al. 2014; Staal et al. 2015); others found the opposite relationship (Sears et al. 1999; Langen et al. 2009; Estes et al. 2011). These mixed results suggest that caudate volumetric measures are not optimal correlates of RRB severity. Limitations are also introduced by RRB clinical measures, which were designed to be specific for ASD. Their narrow ranges limit the power to detect correlations, particularly when applied within patient groups.

11.2.1.2 Functional imaging Task-based fMRI in ASD has examined striatal involvement for a broad range of social and nonsocial processes with variation in the specific domains examined and the tasks carried out. Although only in their nascent stage, studies have most frequently examined reward processes (Scott-Van Zeeland et al. 2010a; Delmonte et al. 2012; Dichter et al. 2012a; Kohls et al. 2013, 2014; Chantiluke et al. 2014; Damiano et al. 2015) and inhibitory control

(Lee et al. 2009; Vaidya et al. 2011; Daly et al. 2012; Chantiluke et al. 2015; Padmanabhan et al. 2015; Shafritz et al. 2015). Other domains examined include visual-spatial skills (Silk et al. 2006; McGrath et al. 2012), sensorimotor processes (Takarae et al. 2007), executive functions (Luna et al. 2002; Murphy et al. 2014), language (Kenworthy et al. 2013; Radulescu et al. 2013; Murdaugh et al. 2016), learning (Scott-Van Zeeland et al. 2010b; Solomon et al. 2015; Travers et al. 2015), face perception (Weng et al. 2011; Sims et al. 2014), and other social processes (Greene et al. 2011; Masten et al. 2011; Gordon et al. 2013; Ventola et al. 2015). These studies have typically recruited moderate samples of adolescents or young adults (mean sample size, $n = 19 \pm 7/$ group; mean group age $=17.4 \pm 7.1$ years). The majority of these studies have focused on regional activations based on whole-brain contrasts or regions-of-interest analyses; some ($n = 6$) have also explored striatal functional connectivity modulated by task (Lee et al. 2009; McGrath et al. 2012; Radulescu et al. 2013; Sims et al. 2014; Solomon et al. 2015; Ventola et al. 2015). For most of the domains examined, sufficient depth of coverage has yet to emerge. For example, a voxel-wise meta-analysis of 13 studies of face emotion recognition in ASD identified caudate as a locus of ASD-related hyperactivation for emotional faces versus non-faces—a pattern that could only be discerned by pooling multiple studies together (Aoki et al. 2015). In what follows, we detail the domains examined by more than five studies.

11.2.1.2.1 Reward The social motivation hypothesis suggests that individuals with ASD do not find social interactions as rewarding as TDC and have reduced motivation to engage socially (Grelotti et al. 2002; Dawson 2008; Kohls et al. 2012). This theory has motivated recent studies of reward processing in adults (Schmitz et al. 2008) and adolescents with ASD relative to TDC (Delmonte et al. 2012; Dichter et al. 2012a; Kohls et al. 2013, 2014; Damiano et al. 2015). Studies in adolescents have demonstrated consistent reduced striatal activation during reward processing in conjunction with behavioral differences in task performance (e.g., Scott-Van Zeeland et al. 2010a; Kohls et al. 2013; Damiano et al. 2015). Often these tasks use monetary rewards versus social rewards (e.g., happy faces). Along with striatum, ASD-related abnormal activity was also revealed in cortical regions known to be involved in frontostriatal reward circuitry such as OFC and ACC (e.g., Dichter et al. 2012b; Kohls et al. 2013). In an intriguing work comparing teens with ASD to attention deficit hyperactivity disorder (ADHD) and TDC, overlapping and distinct patterns of ventral striatal and fronto-striato-parietal regions emerged in response to social versus monetary rewards. Adolescents with ASD showed reduced activation in the ventral striatum to both social and monetary rewards compared to those with ADHD and TD. By contrast, children with ADHD responded more strongly to both types of rewards and TD children responded more strongly to monetary rewards (Kohls et al. 2014). Together these fMRI studies implicate abnormal reward processing in ASD. However, one concern is that the stimuli used in previous studies might be inherently less rewarding to individuals with ASD and, therefore, less likely to engage striatal reward circuitry (Sasson et al. 2012). Using stimuli based on an individual's special interest, Dichter et al. (2012b) found that ventral striatum and ventral medial prefrontal cortex were engaged in ASD similarly to TDC as compared to monetary rewards. These findings suggest stimulus type may be critical when studying reward processing in ASD and must be considered when interpreting fMRI task results.

Nevertheless, clarifying the nature of reward dysfunction in ASD is not only important for understanding the mechanisms leading to ASD impairments in social communication but also due to its implications in treatment. Behavioral intervention is the most common form of treatment in ASD and is the most successful. Yet, approximately 50% of children do not respond to classic behavioral interventions (Lovaas 1987; Rogers et al. 2012). Reward-learning abilities may be intact in some children with ASD but not in others. Differences in how children learn from rewards may be important for predicting treatment response. Tantalizing results from a recent imaging study of preschoolers with ASD ($N = 10$) scanned before and after pivotal response treatment support this hypothesis. Specifically, children with ASD completing a biological motion passive-viewing task showing baseline hypoactivation of the superior temporal gyrus (STG) relative to typical children ($n = 5$) showed increased STG and ventral striatum activation after treatment. By contrast, children with baseline STG hyperactivation displayed decreased activity in amygdala, thalamus, and hippocampus after treatment (Ventola et al. 2015). This pilot study illustrates the opportunity for imaging to contribute to stratified medicine (Kapur et al. 2012).

11.2.1.2.2 Inhibitory control   Across the studies of inhibitory control that involve striatum, there is limited consistency in the paradigms used as well as in the direction of the striatal activation patterns identified in ASD versus TDC (hyper- vs. hypo-activation). For example, one study used a Stroop-like paradigm with and without social cues (eye gaze vs. arrows; Vaidya et al. 2011), another used an antisaccade task (Padmanabhan et al. 2015), and only two used a Go/No-go design (Daly et al. 2012; Langen et al. 2012). Although the directionality of striatal effects varies, an emerging theme is that frontal cortex areas associated with striatal circuits (e.g., ACC, DLPFC) and implicated in cognitive control often present abnormal activation. Abnormal coactivation of cortical and subcortical regions known to constitute striatal circuits has characterized other ASD studies, beyond inhibitory control (e.g., Greene et al. 2011; Weng et al. 2011; Kohls et al. 2013). This highlights the utility of connectivity studies investigating interregional relationships.

11.3 ASD striatal connectivity

11.3.1 Structural connectivity

As discussed in Section 11.1.3, structural connectivity can be examined with diffusion imaging or structural covariance analyses of T1 morphometric images. Both approaches have been applied in ASD (Aoki et al. 2013; Bernhardt et al. 2016) but with a primary focus on corticocortical interactions. Thus, little is known about striatal structural connectivity in ASD.

For example, to date, only one group (Eisenberg et al. 2015) has explicitly interrogated both cortical and subcortical relationships. Specifically, the authors examined interregional covariance in relationship to interindividual differences in ratings of insistence on sameness in 55 young adults with ASD. Increased covariance between amygdala, nucleus accumbens, and pallidum was associated to increased insistence on sameness but not to other RRB metrics. Although preliminary, these results support the feasibility of using connectivity indices to investigate brain–behavior relationships in ASD.

In the diffusion imaging ASD literature, just a few studies have explicitly focused on striatal connectivity (Brito et al. 2009; Langen et al. 2012; Delmonte et al. 2013; McGrath et al. 2013a; Roine et al. 2015). These studies have varied in acquisition parameters and analytical approaches used to select regions or tracts of interest. Results also vary, albeit three of these five studies reveal decreased fractional anisotropy in corticostriatal tracts. Notably, two tractography studies have investigated the relationship between functional and structural connectivity in striatal and cortical nodes (Delmonte et al. 2013; McGrath et al. 2013b). Both studies reported nonsignificant relationships within groups for each of the tracts examined. One group used an advanced diffusion imaging approach (constrained spherical deconvolution) to reliably identify tracts among 10 regions of interest displaying group differences in functional connectivity during a mental rotation task (McGrath et al. 2012, 2013b). More important, regardless of diagnosis, not all region pairs displayed direct white matter tracts, supporting the notion that functional and structural connectivity do not have a one-to-one relationship (Honey et al. 2009). In fact, functional connectivity may exist even when white matter connections are indirect (Behrens and Sporns 2012). Improvements in spatial resolution heralded by the Human Connectome Project and related projects promise to provide increasing ability to delineate both structural and functional connectomics (Van Essen et al. 2013).

11.3.2 Functional connectivity

The striatal functional connectivity literature is still in its infancy. To date, six studies have examined striatal functional connectivity mediated by a task (Lee et al. 2009; McGrath et al. 2012; Radulescu et al. 2013; Sims et al. 2014; Solomon et al. 2015; Ventola et al. 2015), and six have focused on R-fMRI data (Di Martino et al. 2011, 2013; Delmonte et al. 2013; Padmanabhan et al. 2013; Zhou et al. 2014; Mitra et al. 2016). Although task-based functional studies suggest the utility of examining the role played by striatal circuitry in specific cognitive and affective processes in ASD, results are as variable as the heterogeneous range of paradigms investigated to date (see Section 11.2.1.2). Thus, current results do not allow the identification of specific striatal patterns of task-based striatal functional connectivity in ASD. Still, this literature and the broader body of work encompassing task-based fMRI, taken together, support the notion that ASD reflects disconnections in distributed brain networks.

Striatal findings from R-fMRI studies are similarly preliminary and generally supportive of the disconnection model of ASD, with somewhat greater consistency. Specifically, two independent investigations in school-age children (Di Martino et al. 2011) and adolescents (Delmonte et al. 2013) showed increased striatal connectivity with cortical regions in ASD relative to age-matched TDC. Intriguingly, by examining whole-brain striatal iFC, Di Martino et al. (2011) also revealed greater striatal iFC with the pons, suggesting that "lower-level" fundamental processes should be investigated in ASD. Given the earlier findings that striatocortical iFC decreases from childhood to adulthood (Supekar et al. 2009; Padmanabhan et al. 2013), findings of increased iFC in youth with ASD could be interpreted as suggesting delayed maturation. However, both indirect and direct evidence paint a more complex picture of age-related differences in ASD (Di Martino et al. 2011; Padmanabhan et al. 2013). Specifically, distinct age-related patterns seem to characterize different striatal circuits. This was suggested indirectly by comparing striatal iFC patterns in typical children and adults with those of children with ASD (Di Martino et al. 2011). Only iFC between ventral striatum and STG was consistent with delayed maturation in ASD (i.e., increased relative to children and adult controls). Other striatal circuits did not show a pattern consistent with immaturity. In fact, increased iFC in ASD largely localized in areas that did not exhibit significant iFC in either children or adult TDC. Thus, these intrinsic functional connections in ASD were interpreted as "ectopic." Their underlying mechanisms are unclear, but if replicated, an intriguing hypothesis would be that they may relate to gray matter heterotopias observed in ASD (Blackmon et al. 2016). Findings of distinct age-related patterns varying across striatal circuits were also reported in a cross-sectional sample of individuals with ASD versus TDC (age range 8–36 years; Padmanabhan et al. 2013). For example, dorsal putamen iFC did not show ASD-specific differences with age, in contrast with dorsal caudate (iFC was greater at older ages in ASD, and of lower magnitude in TDC). Collectively, these intriguing results should be considered preliminary pending confirmation in longitudinal studies.

Increased striatal iFC is likely consistent with increased striatal degree centrality (DC)—a graph theory measure indexing the number of direct connections of a node within the connectome (Bullmore and Bassett 2011). In a study comparing children with ASD to children with ADHD and TDC, increased DC of the right caudate head, right putamen, and pallidum characterized children with ADHD as well as those with ASD with comorbid ADHD but not those with ASD only (Di Martino et al. 2013). These findings might have been missed if ASD had not been stratified based on comorbidity, an important source of heterogeneity in ASD. Several clinical studies have shown that individuals with ASD present a higher prevalence of psychiatric comorbidities relative to the general population (Simonoff et al. 2008). Approximately 29% of children with ASD also meet diagnostic criteria for ADHD and 30% have a comorbid anxiety disorder. These and other comorbidities may contribute to variation in striatal anatomical and functional organization within ASD. Unfortunately, with a few exceptions (e.g., Di Martino et al. 2013; Chantiluke et al. 2014), the current imaging literature does not account for these comorbidities, both when sample characteristics are reported and in analyses.

Greater specificity is still required in regard to the impact of ASD and its various sources of heterogeneity on distinct striatal circuits. This and other questions, such as the nature of the temporal dynamics of iFC, remain largely unanswered. Intriguingly, recent work has investigated the time-lag structure of the R-fMRI signal (Mitra et al. 2015) of young adults with ASD and TDC ($n = 23$/group). Results showed time-lag diagnostic group differences in putamen bilaterally as well as in right frontal pole and occipital cortex. In regard to the putamen findings, time lag was near zero in TDC but significantly negative (early) in ASD; this measure was significantly and positively related to RRB severity in ASD (Mitra et al. 2016).

In sum, albeit preliminary, both task and R-fMRI studies have reported striatal functional connectivity abnormalities in ASD. While the field is rapidly progressing to address methodological challenges, greater insight in regard to the relationship between task-based and intrinsic functional connectivity will be likely attained.

11.4 Summary and conclusions

The striatum is the main input station for cortical afferent connections within corticobasal ganglia-thalamic circuits. The ability of MRI to translate the striatal organization identified in monkeys into human physiology has motivated clinical applications *in vivo*. Propositions that many of the social, cognitive, and motor impairments characteristics of ASD may be related to striatal disruptions drove investigations in this population. Earlier volumetric studies and more recent fMRI and connectivity examinations suggest a role of striatal circuitry in the physiopathology of ASD, with emerging convergence in regard to its relationship with RRB and social motivation. However, the literature is limited by modest reproducibility, particularly when the investigative resolution increases (e.g., specificity of the spatial extent of affected circuits, directionality of effects, and relevance for specific features). Limited reproducibility is not proprietary to the striatal ASD literature as it is an issue for the entire field of biological psychiatry (Kapur et al. 2012). Several methodological and ASD intrinsic factors come into play when considering limited reproducibility, as noted elsewhere (Amaral 2011; Kapur et al. 2012; Di Martino et al. 2014a; Bernhardt et al. 2016; Vasa et al. 2016). An obvious one is the small study samples that characterize most studies. Beyond statistical power considerations (Button et al. 2013), limited sample size is problematic when facing the striking heterogeneity of ASD. Collaborative multisite efforts have shown the feasibility of aggregating and analyzing unprecedentedly large ASD samples such as the ABIDE repository (e.g., Di Martino et al. 2014b; Chen et al. 2015; Valk et al. 2015), although concerns regarding site heterogeneity remain. One strategy would be to use independent discovery and replication samples, selected at random from an aggregated or large-scale sample. More efforts are needed to provide larger as well as more deeply phenotyped samples that will allow stratification of ASD based on known sources of heterogeneity (e.g., severity of core ASD symptoms and comorbid psychopathology, sex, intelligence, language abilities, and age). Likely many additional unknown sources of heterogeneity exist; thus, an alternative approach would be to subtype ASD starting from the imaging data and investigate the phenotypic characteristics of the imaging subtypes. Encouraging results from similar multivariate data-driven approaches are emerging in other fields (e.g., Yang et al. 2012; Karalunas et al. 2014). To facilitate data-driven strategies (Zhao and Castellanos 2016), an enhanced version of ABIDE (ABIDE-2) is currently being aggregated with the goal of establishing a larger and more deeply phenotyped sample of individuals with ASD and TDC for open science data sharing (Milham 2012).

The next generation of studies will also need to shift from systematic characterizations of striatal involvement in ASD to the identification of potential causative mechanisms. Initiatives combining genetic and imaging data can guide such efforts. For example, a recent study combining imaging anatomical data from 26 genetic mice models of ASD consistently found neuroanatomical abnormalities in three circuits, including corticostriatal loops. The mouse models contributing to this finding include mutations in Mecp2, XO, and 16p11 (Ellegood et al. 2015). In humans, the 16p11 locus has been a focus of study by the Simons Foundation Variation in Individual Project (VIP) aggregating a data repository from individuals with a deletion or duplication in 16p11 (Simons VIP Consortium 2012). Examination of striatal connectivity in the context of well-defined genetic mutations or variations should provide an additional fruitful way of addressing the profound heterogeneity of ASD.

Another lacuna in the ASD imaging literature involves the scarcity of functional data obtained in children below age 7. Investigators are beginning to conduct R-fMRI studies during natural sleep, which can expand the age range of children who can be studied (Di Martino et al. 2014a; Lombardo et al. 2015). Finally, we note that most of the literature reviewed in this chapter has focused on exclusively or predominantly male samples, reflecting the higher male prevalence of ASD as well as probable recruitment and diagnostic biases. Thus, little is known about striatal organization in females with ASD and whether it differs from that of males. Indeed in typical development, striatal structural trajectories differ between the sexes (e.g., Raznahan et al. 2014). Greater inclusion of females with ASD and attention to sex differences in analyses is long overdue (Halladay et al. 2015; Lai et al. 2015).

Acknowledgments

The authors are grateful to Suzanne N. Haber, PhD, for her input regarding basal ganglia anatomy, and to Yuta Aoki, MD, PhD, for his editorial suggestions.

References

Alexander, G. E., M. R. Delong, and P. L. Strick. 1986. Parallel organization of functionally segregated circuits linking basal ganglia and cortex. *Annu. Rev. Neurosci.* 9:357–81.

Alexander-Bloch, A., J. N. Giedd, and E. Bullmore. 2013. Imaging structural covariance between human brain regions. *Nat. Rev. Neurosci.* 14:322–36.

Amaral, D. G. 2011. The promise and the pitfalls of autism research: An introductory note for new autism researchers. *Brain Res.* 1380:3–9.

American Psychiatric Association. 2013. *Diagnostic and Statistical Manual of Mental Disorder*, 5th edn. Washington, DC: American Psychiatric Association.

Aoki, Y., O. Abe, Y. Nippashi, and H. Yamasu. 2013. Comparison of white matter integrity between autism spectrum disorder subjects and typically developing individuals: A meta-analysis of diffusion tensor imaging tractography studies. *Mol. Autism* 4:25.

Aoki, Y., S. Cortese, and M. Tansella. 2015. Neural bases of atypical emotional face processing in autism: A meta-analysis of fMRI studies. *World J. Biol. Psychiatry* 16:291–300.

Averbeck, B. B., J. Lehman, M. Jacobson, and S. N. Haber. 2014. Estimates of projection overlap and zones of convergence within frontal-striatal circuits. *J. Neurosci.* 34:9497–505.

Baleydier, C. and F. Mauguiere. 1980. The duality of the cingulate gyrus in monkey. Neuroanatomical study and functional hypothesis. *Brain* 103:525–54.

Behrens, T. E. and O. Sporns. 2012. Human connectomics. *Curr. Opin. Neurobiol.* 22:144–53.

Bernhardt, B. C., A. Di Martino, S. L. Valk, and G. L. Wallace. 2016. Neuroimaging-based phenotyping of the autism spectrum. *Curr. Top. Behav. Neurosci.* PubMed PMID: 26946501.

Bevan, M. D., N. P. Clarke, and J. P. Bolam. 1997. Synaptic integration of functionally diverse pallidal information in the entopeduncular nucleus and subthalamic nucleus in the rat. *J. Neurosci.* 17:308–24.

Bevan, M. D., A. D. Smith, and J. P. Bolam. 1996. The substantia nigra as a site of synaptic integration of functionally diverse information arising from the ventral pallidum and the globus pallidus in the rat. *Neuroscience* 75:5–12.

Biswal, B., F. Z. Yetkin, V. M. Haughton, and J. S. Hyde. 1995. Functional connectivity in the motor cortex of resting human brain using echo-planar MRI. *Magn. Reson. Med.* 34:537–41.

Bjork, J. M., B. Knutson, G. W. Fong, D. M. Caggiano, S. M. Bennett, and D. W. Hommer. 2004. Incentive-elicited brain activation in adolescents: Similarities and differences from young adults. *J. Neurosci.* 24:1793–802.

Blackmon, K., E. Ben-Avi, X. Wang, H. R. Pardoe, A. Di Martino, E. Halgren, O. Devinsky, T. Thesen, and R. Kuzniecky. 2016. Periventricular white matter abnormalities and restricted repetitive behavior in autism spectrum disorder. *Neuroimage Clin.* 10:36–45.

Bo, J., C. M. Lee, Y. Kwak, S. J. Peltier, J. A. Bernard, M. Buschkuehl, et al. 2014. Lifespan differences in cortico-striatal resting state connectivity. *Brain Connect* 4:166–80.

Boussaoud, D., R. Desimone, and L. G. Ungerleider. 1992. Subcortical connections of visual areas MST and FST in macaques. *Vis. Neurosci.* 9:291–302.

Brain Development Cooperative Group. 2012. Total and regional brain volumes in a population-based normative sample from 4 to 18 years: The NIH MRI Study of Normal Brain Development. *Cereb. Cortex* 22:1–12.

Brito, A. R., M. M. Vasconcelos, R. C. Domingues, L. C. Hygino Da Cruz Jr., L. de S. Rodrigues, E. L. Gasparetto, and C. A. B. P. Calçada. 2009. Diffusion tensor imaging findings in school-aged autistic children. *J. Neuroimaging* 19:337–43.

Bullmore, E. T. and D. S. Bassett. 2011. Brain graphs: Graphical models of the human brain connectome. *Annu. Rev. Clin. Psychol.* 7:113–40.

Button, K. S., J. P. Ioannidis, C. Mokrysz, B. A. Nosek, J. Flint, E. S. Robinson, and M. R. Munafo. 2013. Power failure: Why small sample size undermines the reliability of neuroscience. *Nat. Rev. Neurosci.* 14:365–76.

Calzavara, R., P. Mailly, and S. N. Haber. 2007. Relationship between the cortico-striatal terminals from areas 9 and 46, and those from area 8A, dorsal and rostral premotor cortex and area 24c: An anatomical substrate for cognition to action. *Eur. J. Neurosci.* 26:2005–24.

Carpenter, M. B., K. Nakano, and R. Kim. 1976. Nigrothalamic projections in the monkey demonstrated by autoradiographic technics. *J. Comp. Neurol.* 165:401–15.

Casey, B. J. 2015. Beyond simple models of self-control to circuit-based accounts of adolescent behavior. *Annu. Rev. Psychol.* 66:295–319.

Castellanos, F. X., A. Di Martino, R. C. Craddock, A. D. Mehta, and M. P. Milham. 2013. Clinical applications of the functional connectome. *Neuroimage* 80:527–40.

Cavada, C. and P. S. Goldman-Rakic. 1991. Topographic segregation of corticostriatal projections from posterior parietal subdivisions in the macaque monkey. *Neuroscience* 42:683–96.

Chantiluke, K., N. Barrett, V. Giampietro, P. Santosh, M. Brammer, A. Simmons, D. G. Murphy, and K. Rubia. 2015. Inverse fluoxetine effects on inhibitory brain activation in non-comorbid boys with ADHD and with ASD. *Psychopharmacology (Berl)* 232:2071–82.

Chantiluke, K., A. Christakou, C. M. Murphy, V. Giampietro, E. M. Daly, C. Ecker, M. Brammer, D. G. Murphy, the MRC AIMS Consortium, and K. Rubia. 2014. Disorder-specific functional abnormalities during temporal discounting in youth with Attention Deficit Hyperactivity Disorder (ADHD), Autism and comorbid ADHD and Autism. *Psychiatry Res.* 223:113–20.

Chen, C. P., C. L. Keown, A. Jahedi, A. Nair, M. E. Pflieger, B. A. Bailey, and R. A. Muller. 2015. Diagnostic classification of intrinsic functional connectivity highlights somatosensory, default mode, and visual regions in autism. *Neuroimage Clin.* 8:238–45.

Choi, E. Y., B. T. Yeo, and R. L. Buckner. 2012. The organization of the human striatum estimated by intrinsic functional connectivity. *J. Neurophysiol.* 108:2242–63.

Choi, E. Y., Y. Tanimura, P. R. Vage, E. Yates, and S. N. Haber. 2016. Convergence of prefrontal and parietal anatomical projections in a connectional hub in the striatum. In press. http://dx.doi.org/10.1016/j.neuroimage.2016.09.037

Cohen, J. R., R. F. Asarnow, F. W. Sabb, R. M. Bilder, S. Y. Bookheimer, B. J. Knowlton, and R. A. Poldrack. 2010. A unique adolescent response to reward prediction errors. *Nat. Neurosci.* 13:669–71.

Craddock, R. C., S. Jbabdi, C. G. Yan, J. T. Vogelstein, F. X. Castellanos, A. Di Martino, C. Kelly, K. Heberlein, S. Colcombe, and M. P. Milham. 2013. Imaging human connectomes at the macroscale. *Nat. Methods* 10:524–39.

Daly, E. M., Q. Deeley, C. Ecker et al. 2012. Serotonin and the neural processing of facial emotions in adults with autism: An fMRI study using acute tryptophan depletion facial emotion processing in adults with autism. *Arch. Gen. Psychiatry* 69(10):1–11.

Damiano, C. R., D. C. Cockrell, K. Dunlap et al. 2015. Neural mechanisms of negative reinforcement in children and adolescents with autism spectrum disorders. *J. Neurodev. Disord.* 7:12.

Dawson, G. 2008. Early behavioral intervention, brain plasticity, and the prevention of autism spectrum disorder. *Dev. Psychopathol.* 20:775–803.

Delmonte, S., J. H. Balsters, J. McGrath, J. Fitzgerald, S. Brennan, A. J. Fagan, L. Gallagher. 2012. Social and monetary reward processing in autism spectrum disorders. *Mol. Autism* 3:7.

Delmonte, S., L. Gallagher, E. O'Hanlon, J. McGrath, and J. H. Balsters. 2013. Functional and structural connectivity of frontostriatal circuitry in Autism Spectrum Disorder. *Front Hum. Neurosci.* 7:430.

Delong, M. R. and A. Georgopoulos. 1981. Motor functions of the basal ganglia. In *The Nervous System: Motor Control*, eds. J. M. Brookhart, V. B. Mountcastle, V. B. Brooks, and S. R. Geiger, 1017–61. Bethesda: American Physiological Society.

Delong, M. R., A. P. Georgopoulos, M. D. Crutcher, S. J. Mitchell, R. T. Richardson, and G. E. Alexander. 1984. Functional organization of the basal ganglia: Contributions of single-cell recording studies. *Ciba Found. Symp.* 107:64–82.

Di Martino, A., D. A. Fair, C. Kelly et al. 2014a. Unraveling the miswired connectome: A developmental perspective. *Neuron* 83:1335–53.

Di Martino, A., C. Kelly, R. Grzadzinski, X. N. Zuo, M. Mennes, M. A. Mairena, C. Lord, F. X. Castellanos, and M. P. Milham. 2011. Aberrant striatal functional connectivity in children with autism. *Biol. Psychiatry* 69:847–56.

Di Martino, A., A. Scheres, D. S. Margulies, A. M. Kelly, L. Q. Uddin, Z. Shehzad, B. Biswal, J. R. Walters, F. X. Castellanos, and M. P. Milham. 2008. Functional connectivity of human striatum: A resting state FMRI study. *Cereb. Cortex* 18:2735–47.

Di Martino, A., C. G. Yan, Q. Li, E. Denio et al. 2014b. The autism brain imaging data exchange: Towards a large-scale evaluation of the intrinsic brain architecture in autism. *Mol. Psychiatry* 19:659–67.

Di Martino, A., X. N. Zuo, C. Kelly, R. Grzadzinski, M. Mennes, A. Schvarcz, J. Rodman, C. Lord, F. X. Castellanos, and M. P. Milham. 2013. Shared and distinct intrinsic functional network centrality in autism and attention-deficit/hyperactivity disorder. *Biol. Psychiatry* 74:623–32.

Dichter, G. S., J. N. Felder, S. R. Green, A. M. Rittenberg, N. J. Sasson, and J. W. Bodfish. 2012a. Reward circuitry function in autism spectrum disorders. *Soc. Cogn. Affect Neurosci.* 7:160–72.

Dichter, G. S., J. A. Richey, A. M. Rittenberg, A. Sabatino, and J. W. Bodfish. 2012b. Reward circuitry function in autism during face anticipation and outcomes. *J. Autism Dev. Disord.* 42:147–60.

Draganski, B., F. Kherif, S. Kloppel, P. A. Cook, D. C. Alexander, G. J. Parker, R. Deichmann, J. Ashburner, and R. S. Frackowiak 2008. Evidence for segregated and integrative connectivity patterns in the human basal ganglia. *J. Neurosci.* 28:7143–52.

Ecker, C., J. Suckling, S. C. Deoni et al. 2012. Brain anatomy and its relationship to behavior in adults with autism spectrum disorder: A multicenter magnetic resonance imaging study. *Arch. Gen. Psychiatry* 69:195–209.

Eisenberg, I. W., G. L. Wallace, L. Kenworthy, S. J. Gotts, and A. Martin. 2015. Insistence on sameness relates to increased covariance of gray matter structure in autism spectrum disorder. *Mol. Autism* 6:54.

Ellegood, J., E. Anagnostou, B. A. Babineau, J. N. Crawley, L. Lin, M. Genestine, et al. 2015. Clustering autism: Using neuroanatomical differences in 26 mouse models to gain insight into the heterogeneity. *Mol. Psychiatry* 20:118–25.

Estes, A., D. W. Shaw, B. F. Sparks, S. Friedman, J. N. Giedd, G. Dawson, M. Bryan, and S. R. Dager. 2011. Basal ganglia morphometry and repetitive behavior in young children with autism spectrum disorder. *Autism Res.* 4:212–20.

Fareri, D. S., L. Gabard-Durnam, B. Goff, J. Flannery, D. G. Gee, D. S. Lumian, C. Caldera, and N. Tottenham. 2015. Normative development of ventral striatal resting state connectivity in humans. *Neuroimage* 118:422–37.

Flaherty, A. W. and A. M. Graybiel. 1991. Corticostriatal transformations in the primate somatosensory system. Projections from physiologically mapped body-part representations. *J. Neurophysiol.* 66:1249–63.

Fox, M. D. and M. Greicius. 2010. Clinical applications of resting state functional connectivity. *Front Syst. Neurosci.* 4:19.

Friedman, D. P., J. P. Aggleton, and R. C. Saunders. 2002. Comparison of hippocampal, amygdala, and perirhinal projections to the nucleus accumbens: Combined anterograde and retrograde tracing study in the Macaque brain. *J. Comp. Neurol.* 450:345–65.

Fudge, J. L., M. A. Breitbart, and C. McClain. 2004. Amygdaloid inputs define a caudal component of the ventral striatum in primates. *J. Comp. Neurol.* 476:330–47.

Fudge, J. L., K. Kunishio, P. Walsh, C. Richard, and S. N. Haber. 2002. Amygdaloid projections to ventromedial striatal subterritories in the primate. *Neuroscience* 110:257–75.

Gaffney, G. R., S. Kuperman, L. Y. Tsai, and S. Minchin. 1989. Forebrain structure in infantile autism. *J. Am. Acad. Child Adolesc. Psychiatry* 28:534–7.

Galvan, A., T. A. Hare, C. E. Parra, J. Penn, H. Voss, G. Glover, and B. J. Casey. 2006. Earlier development of the accumbens relative to orbitofrontal cortex might underlie risk-taking behavior in adolescents. *J. Neurosci.* 26:6885–92.

Geier, C. F., R. Terwilliger, T. Teslovich, K. Velanova, and B. Luna. 2010. Immaturities in reward processing and its influence on inhibitory control in adolescence. *Cereb. Cortex* 20:1613–29.

Geschwind, D. H. and P. Levitt. 2007. Autism spectrum disorders: Developmental disconnection syndromes. *Curr. Opin. Neurobiol.* 17:103–11.

Giedd, J. N., J. Blumenthal, N. O. Jeffries, F. X. Castellanos, H. Liu, A. Zijdenbos, T. Paus, A. C. Evans, and J. L. Rapoport. 1999. Brain development during childhood and adolescence: A longitudinal MRI study. *Nat. Neurosci.* 2:861–3.

Goddings, A. L., K. L. Mills, L. S. Clasen, J. N. Giedd, R. M. Viner, and S. J. Blakemore. 2014. The influence of puberty on subcortical brain development. *Neuroimage* 88:242–51.

Gogtay, N., J. N. Giedd, L. Lusk et al. 2004. Dynamic mapping of human cortical development during childhood through early adulthood. *Proc. Natl. Acad. Sci. USA* 101:8174–9.

Goldman, P. S. and W. J. Nauta. 1977. An intricately patterned prefronto-caudate projection in the rhesus monkey. *J. Comp. Neurol.* 72:369–86.

Gordon, I., B. C. Vander Wyk, R. H. Bennett, C. Cordeaux, M. V. Lucas, J. A. Eilbott, O. Zagoory-Sharon, J. F. Leckman, R. Feldman, and K. A. Pelphrey. 2013. Oxytocin enhances brain function in children with autism. *Proc. Natl. Acad. Sci. USA* 110:20953–8.

Graybiel, A. M. 1990. Neurotransmitters and neuromodulators in the basal ganglia. *Trends Neurosci.* 13:244–54.

Graybiel, A. M. and C. W. Ragsdale Jr. 1978. Histochemically distinct compartments in the striatum of human, monkeys, and cat demonstrated by acetylthiocholinesterase staining. *Proc. Natl. Acad. Sci. USA* 75:5723–6.

Greene, D. J., N. Colich, M. Iacoboni, E. Zaidel, S. Y. Bookheimer, and M. Dapretto. 2011. Atypical neural networks for social orienting in autism spectrum disorders. *Neuroimage* 56:354–62.

Greene, D. J., T. O. Laumann, J. W. Dubis, S. K. Ihnen, M. Neta, J. D. Power, J. R. Pruett Jr., K. J. Black, and B. L. Schlaggar. 2014. Developmental changes in the organization of functional connections between the basal ganglia and cerebral cortex. *J. Neurosci.* 34:5842–54.

Grelotti, D. J., I. Gauthier, and R. T. Schultz. 2002. Social interest and the development of cortical face specialization: What autism teaches us about face processing. *Dev. Psychobiol.* 40:213–25.

Haar, S., S. Berman, M. Behrmann, and I. Dinstein. 2016. Anatomical abnormalities in autism? *Cereb. Cortex* 26:1440–52.

Haber, S. N. 2003. The primate basal ganglia: Parallel and integrative networks. *J. Chem. Neuroanat.* 26:317–30.

Haber, S. N., A. Adler, and H. Bergman. 2011. The basal ganglia. In *The Human Nervous System*, 3rd ed., eds. J. K. Mai and G. Paxinos, 678–738. Amsterdam: Elsevier Academic.

Haber, S. N., J. L. Fudge, and N. R. McFarland. 2000. Striatonigrostriatal pathways in primates form an ascending spiral from the shell to the dorsolateral striatum. *J. Neurosci.* 20:2369–82.

Haber, S. N., K. S. Kim, P. Mailly, and R. Calzavara. 2006. Reward-related cortical inputs define a large striatal region in primates that interface with associative cortical connections, providing a substrate for incentive-based learning. *J. Neurosci.* 26:8368–76.

Halladay, A. K., S. Bishop, J. N. Constantino et al. 2015. Sex and gender differences in autism spectrum disorder: Summarizing evidence gaps and identifying emerging areas of priority. *Mol. Autism* 6:36.

Hardan, A. Y., M. Kilpatrick, M. S. Keshavan, and N. J. Minshew. 2003. Motor performance and anatomic magnetic resonance imaging (MRI) of the basal ganglia in autism. *J. Child Neurol.* 18:317–24.

Haynes, W. I. and S. N. Haber. 2013. The organization of prefrontal-subthalamic inputs in primates provides an anatomical substrate for both functional specificity and integration: Implications for basal ganglia models and deep brain stimulation. *J. Neurosci.* 33:4804–14.

Haznedar, M. M., M. S. Buchsbaum, E. A. Hazlett, E. M. Licalzi, C. Cartwright, and E. Hollander. 2006. Volumetric analysis and three-dimensional glucose metabolic mapping of the striatum and thalamus in patients with autism spectrum disorders. *Am. J. Psychiatry* 163:1252–63.

Heimer, L. 1978. The olfactory cortex and the ventral striatum. In *Limbic Mechanisms: The Continuing Evolution of the Limbic System Concept*, eds. K. E. Livingston and O. Hornykiewicz, 95–187. New York: Plenum.

Heimer, L. and R. Wilson. 1975. The subcortical projections of the allocortex: Similarities in the neural associations of the hippocampus, the piriform cortex, and the neocortex. In *Golgi Centennial Symposium: Perspectives in Neurobiology*, ed. M. Santini, 177–93. New York: Raven Press.

Heimer, L., R. D. Switzer, and G. W. Vanhoesen. 1982. Ventral striatum and ventral pallidum—Components of the motor system. *Trends Neurosci.* 5:83–7.

211

Herbert, M. R., D. A. Ziegler, C. K. Deutsch et al. 2003. Dissociations of cerebral cortex, subcortical and cerebral white matter volumes in autistic boys. *Brain* 126 (Pt 5):1182–92.

Hollander, E., E. Anagnostou, W. Chaplin, K. Esposito, M. M. Haznedar, E. Licalzi, S. Wasserman, L. Soorya, and M. Buchsbaum. 2005. Striatal volume on magnetic resonance imaging and repetitive behaviors in autism. *Biol. Psychiatry* 58:226–32.

Holt, D. J., A. M. Graybiel, and C. B. Saper. 1997. Neurochemical architecture of the human striatum. *J. Comp. Neurol.* 384:1–25.

Honey, C. J., O. Sporns, L. Cammoun, X. Gigandet, J. P. Thiran, R. Meuli, and P. Hagmann. 2009. Predicting human resting-state functional connectivity from structural connectivity. *Proc. Natl. Acad. Sci. USA* 106:2035–40.

Inase, M., S. T. Sakai, and J. Tanji. 1996. Overlapping corticostriatal projections from the supplementary motor area and the primary motor cortex in the macaque monkey: An anterograde double labeling study. *J. Comp. Neurol.* 373:283–96.

Joel, D. and I. Weiner. 1997. The connections of the primate subthalamic nucleus: Indirect pathways and the open-interconnected scheme of basal ganglia-thalamocortical circuitry. *Brain Res. Brain Res. Rev.* 23 (1–2):62–78.

Kapur, S., A. G. Phillips, and T. R. Insel. 2012. Why has it taken so long for biological psychiatry to develop clinical tests and what to do about it? *Mol. Psychiatry* 17:1174–9.

Karalunas, S. L., D. Fair, E. D. Musser, K. Aykes, S. P. Iyer, and J. T. Nigg. 2014. Subtyping attention-deficit/hyperactivity disorder using temperament dimensions: Toward biologically based nosologic criteria. *JAMA Psychiatry* 71:1015–24.

Kelly, R. M. and P. L. Strick. 2004. Macro-architecture of basal ganglia loops with the cerebral cortex: Use of rabies virus to reveal multisynaptic circuits. *Prog. Brain Res.* 143:449–59.

Kenworthy, L., G. L. Wallace, R. Birn, S. C. Milleville, L. K. Case, P. A. Bandettini, and A. Martin. 2013. Aberrant neural mediation of verbal fluency in autism spectrum disorders. *Brain Cogn.* 83:218–26.

Kim, R., K. Nakano, A. Jayaraman, and M. B. Carpenter. 1976. Projections of the globus pallidus and adjacent structures: An autoradiographic study in the monkey. *J. Comp. Neurol.* 169:263–90.

Kohls, G., C. Chevallier, V. Troiani, and R. T. Schultz. 2012. Social "wanting" dysfunction in autism: Neurobiological underpinnings and treatment implications. *J. Neurodev. Disord.* 4:10.

Kohls, G., M. Schulte-Rüther, B. Nehrkorn, K. Müller, G. R. Fink, I. Kamp-Becker, B. Herpertz-Dahlmann, R. T. Schultz, and K. Konrad. 2013. Reward system dysfunction in autism spectrum disorders. *Soc. Cogn. Affect. Neurosci.* 8:565–72.

Kohls, G., H. Thonessen, G. K. Bartley, N. Grossheinrich, G. R. Fink, B. Herpertz-Dahlmann, and K. Konrad. 2014. Differentiating neural reward responsiveness in autism versus ADHD. *Dev. Cogn. Neurosci.* 10:104–16.

Kraemer, H. C., J. A. Yesavage, J. L. Taylor, and D. Kupfer. 2000. How can we learn about developmental processes from cross-sectional studies, or can we? *Am. J. Psychiatry* 157:163–71.

Künzle, H. 1975. Bilateral projections from precentral motor cortex to the putamen and other parts of the basal ganglia: An autoradiographic study in *Macaca fascicularis*. *Brain Res.* 88:195–209.

Künzle, H. and K. Akert. 1977. Efferent connections of cortical, area 8 (frontal eye field) in *Macaca fascicularis*: A reinvestigation using the autoradiographic technique. *J. Comp. Neurol.* 173:147–64.

Lai, M. C., M. V. Lombardo, B. Auyeung, B. Chakrabarti, and S. Baron-Cohen. 2015. Sex/gender differences and autism: Setting the scene for future research. *J. Am. Acad. Child Adolesc. Psychiatry* 54:11–24.

Lange, N., B. G. Travers, E. D. Bigler et al. 2015. Longitudinal volumetric brain changes in autism spectrum disorder ages 6–35 years. *Autism Res.* 8:82–93.

Langen, M., D. Bos, S. D. Noordermeer, H. Nederveen, H. van Engeland, and S. Durston. 2014. Changes in the development of striatum are involved in repetitive behavior in autism. *Biol. Psychiatry* 76:405–11.

Langen, M., S. Durston, W. G. Staal, S. J. M. C. Palmen, and H. van Engeland. 2007. Caudate nucleus is enlarged in high-functioning medication-naive subjects with autism. *Biol. Psychiatry* 62:262–6.

Langen, M., S. Durston, M. J. Kas, H. van Engeland, and W. G. Staal. 2011. The neurobiology of repetitive behavior: …and men. *Neurosci. Biobehav. Rev.* 35:356–65.

Langen, M., A. Leemans, P. Johnston, C. Ecker, E. Daly, C. M. Murphy, F. Dell'acqua, S. Durston, and D. G. Murphy. 2012. Fronto-striatal circuitry and inhibitory control in autism: Findings from diffusion tensor imaging tractography. *Cortex* 48:183–93.

Langen, M., H. G. Schnack, H. Nederveen, D. Bos, B. E. Lahuis, M. V. De Jonge, H. van Engeland, and S. Durston. 2009. Changes in the developmental trajectories of striatum in autism. *Biol. Psychiatry* 66:327–33.

Lee, P. S., B. E. Yerys, A. Della Rosa, J. Foss-Feig, K. A. Barnes, J. D. James, J. Vanmeter, C. J. Vaidya, W. D. Gaillard, and L. E. Kenworthy. 2009. Functional connectivity of the inferior frontal cortex changes with age in children with autism spectrum disorders: A fcMRI study of response inhibition. *Cereb. Cortex* 19:1787–94.

Lefebvre, A., A. Beggiato, T. Bourgeron, and R. Toro. 2015. Neuroanatomical diversity of corpus callosum and brain volume in autism: Meta-analysis, analysis of the Autism Brain Imaging Data Exchange Project, and simulation. *Biol. Psychiatry* 78:126–34.

Lehericy, S., M. Ducros, P. F. Van De Moortele, C. Francois, L. Thivard, C. Poupon, N. Swindale, K. Ugurbil, and D. S. Kim. 2004. Diffusion tensor fiber tracking shows distinct corticostriatal circuits in humans. *Ann. Neurol.* 55:522–9.

Lombardo, M. V., K. Pierce, L. T. Eyler, C. Carter Barnes, C. Ahrens-Barbeau, S. Solso, K. Campbell, and E. Courchesne. 2015. Different functional neural substrates for good and poor language outcome in autism. *Neuron* 86:567–77.

Lovaas, O. I. 1987. Behavioral treatment and normal educational and intellectual functioning in young autistic children. *J. Consult Clin. Psychol.* 55:3–9.

Luna, B., N. J. Minshew, K. E. Garver, N. A. Lazar, K. R. Thulborn, W. F. Eddy, and J. A. Sweeney. 2002. Neocortical system abnormalities in autism: An fMRI study of spatial working memory. *Neurology* 59:834–40.

Lynd-Balta, E. and S. N. Haber. 1994. The organization of midbrain projections to the striatum in the primate: Sensorimotor-related striatum versus ventral striatum. *Neuroscience* 59:625–40.

Masten, C. L., N. L. Colich, J. D. Rudie, S. Y. Bookheimer, N. I. Eisenberger, and M. Dapretto. 2011. An fMRI investigation of responses to peer rejection in adolescents with autism spectrum disorders. *Dev. Cogn. Neurosci.* 1:260–70.

Matthews, M. and D. A. Fair. 2015. Research review: Functional brain connectivity and child psychopathology—Overview and methodological considerations for investigators new to the field. *J. Child Psychol. Psychiatry* 56:400–14.

Maunsell, J. H. R. and D. C. Van Essen. 1983. The connections of the middle temporal visual area (Mt) and their relationship to a cortical hierarchy in the macaque monkey. *J. Neurosci.* 3:2563–86.

McAlonan, G. M., C. Cheung, V. Cheung, N. Wong, J. Suckling, and S. E. Chua. 2009. Differential effects on white-matter systems in high-functioning autism and Asperger's syndrome. *Psychol. Med.* 39:1885–93.

McAlonan, G. M., E. Daly, V. Kumari et al. 2002. Brain anatomy and sensorimotor gating in Asperger's syndrome. *Brain* 125:1594–606.

McAlonan, G. M., Q. Li, and C. Cheung. 2010. The timing and specificity of prenatal immune risk factors for autism modeled in the mouse and relevance to schizophrenia. *Neurosignals* 18:129–39.

McAlonan, G. M., J. Suckling, N. Wong, V. Cheung, N. Lienenkaemper, C. Cheung, and S. E. Chua. 2008. Distinct patterns of grey matter abnormality in high-functioning autism and Asperger's syndrome. *J. Child Psychol. Psychiatry* 49:1287–95.

McFarland N. R. and S. N. Haber. 2000. Convergent inputs from thalamic motor nuclei and frontal cortical areas to the dorsal striatum in the primate. *J. Neurosci.* 20:3798–813.

McGrath, J., K. Johnson, C. Ecker, E. O'Hanlon, M. Gill, L. Gallagher, and H. Garavan. 2012. Atypical visuospatial processing in autism: Insights from functional connectivity analysis. *Autism Res.* 5:314–30.

McGrath, J., K. Johnson, E. O'Hanlon, H. Garavan, L. Gallagher, and A. Leemans. 2013a. White matter and visuospatial processing in autism: A constrained spherical deconvolution tractography study. *Autism Res.* 6:307–19.

McGrath, J., K. Johnson, E. O'Hanlon, H. Garavan, A. Leemans, and L. Gallagher. 2013b. Abnormal functional connectivity during visuospatial processing is associated with disrupted organisation of white matter in autism. *Front Hum. Neurosci.* 7:434.

Middleton, F. A. and P. L. Strick. 1994. Anatomical evidence for cerebellar and basal ganglia involvement in higher cognitive function. *Science* 266 (5184):458–61.

Middleton, F. A. and P. L. Strick. 2000. Basal ganglia output and cognition: Evidence from anatomical, behavioral, and clinical studies. *Brain Cogn.* 42:183–200.

Middleton, F. A. and P. L. Strick. 2002. Basal-ganglia 'projections' to the prefrontal cortex of the primate. *Cereb. Cortex* 12:926–35.

Milham, M. P. 2012. Open neuroscience solutions for the connectome-wide association era. *Neuron* 73:214–18.

Minshew, N. J. and D. L. Williams. 2007. The new neurobiology of autism: Cortex, connectivity, and neuronal organization. *Arch. Neurol,* 64:945–50.

Mitra, A., A. Z. Snyder, T. Blazey, and M. E. Raichle. 2015. Lag threads organize the brain's intrinsic activity. *Proc. Natl. Acad. Sci. USA* 112:E2235–44.

Mitra, A., A. Z. Snyder, J. N. Constantino, and M. E. Raichle. 2016. The lag structure of intrinsic activity is focally altered in high functioning adults with autism. *Cereb. Cortex* in press. doi: 10.1093/cercor/bhv294.

Mogenson, G. J., D. L. Jones, and C. Y. Yim. 1980. From motivation to action: Functional interface between the limbic system and the motor system. *Prog. Neurobiol.* 14:69–97.

Murdaugh, D. L., H. D. Deshpande, and R. K. Kana. 2016. The impact of reading intervention on brain responses underlying language in children with autism. *Autism Res.* 9:141–54.

Murphy, C. M., A. Christakou, E. M. Daly et al. 2014. Abnormal functional activation and maturation of fronto-striato-temporal and cerebellar regions during sustained attention in autism spectrum disorder. *Am. J. Psychiatry* 171:1107–16.

Nauta, W. J. and W. R. Mehler. 1966. Projections of the lentiform nucleus in the monkey. *Brain Res.* 1:3–42.

Nickl-Jockschat, T., U. Habel, T. M. Michel, J. Manning, A. R. Laird, P. T. Fox, et al. 2012. Brain structure anomalies in autism spectrum disorder—A meta-analysis of VBM studies using anatomic likelihood estimation. *Hum. Brain Mapp.* 33:1470–89.

Padmanabhan, A., K. Garver, K. O'Hearn, N. Nawarawong, R. Liu, N. Minshew, J. Sweeney, and B. Luna. 2015. Developmental changes in brain function underlying inhibitory control in autism spectrum disorders. *Autism Res.* 8:123–35.

Padmanabhan, A., A. Lynn, W. Foran, B. Luna, and K. O'Hearn. 2013. Age related changes in striatal resting state functional connectivity in autism. *Front. Hum. Neurosci.* 7:814.

Parent, A. 1990. Extrinsic connections of the basal ganglia. *Trends Neurosci.* 13:254–8.

Parvizi, J., G. W. Van Hoesen, J. Buckwalter, and A. Damasio. 2006. Neural connections of the posteromedial cortex in the macaque. *Proc. Natl. Acad. Sci. USA* 103:1563–8.

Percheron, G. and M. Filion. 1991. Parallel processing in the basal ganglia: Up to a point. *Trends Neurosci.* 14:55–9.

Porter, J. N., A. K. Roy, B. Benson, C. Carlisi, P. F. Collins, E. Leibenluft, D. S. Pine, M. Luciana, and M. Ernst. 2015. Age-related changes in the intrinsic functional connectivity of the human ventral vs. dorsal striatum from childhood to middle age. *Dev. Cogn. Neurosci.* 11:83–95.

Postuma, R. B. and A. Dagher. 2006. Basal ganglia functional connectivity based on a meta-analysis of 126 positron emission tomography and functional magnetic resonance imaging publications. *Cereb. Cortex* 16:1508–21.

Powell, E. W. 1978. The cingulate bridge between allocortex, isocortex and thalamus. *Anat. Rec.* 190:783–93.

Power, J. D., B. L. Schlaggar, and S. E. Petersen. 2015. Recent progress and outstanding issues in motion correction in resting state fMRI. *Neuroimage* 105:536–51.

Qiu, A., M. Adler, D. Crocetti, M. I. Miller, and S. H. Mostofsky. 2010. Basal ganglia shapes predict social, communication, and motor dysfunctions in boys with autism spectrum disorder. *J. Am. Acad. Child Adolesc. Psychiatry* 49:539–51.

Radulescu, E., L. Minati, B. Ganeshan, N. A. Harrison, M. A. Gray, F. D. Beacher, C. Chatwin, R. C. Young, and H. D. Critchley. 2013. Abnormalities in frontostriatal connectivity within language networks relate to differences in grey-matter heterogeneity in Asperger syndrome. *Neuroimage Clin.* 2:716–26.

Raichle, M. E. and A. Z. Snyder. 2007. A default mode of brain function: A brief history of an evolving idea. *Neuroimage* 37:1083–90.

Raznahan, A., P. W. Shaw, J. P. Lerch, L. S. Clasen, D. Greenstein, R. Berman, J. Pipitone, M. M. Chakravarty, and J. N. Giedd. 2014. Longitudinal four-dimensional mapping of subcortical anatomy in human development. *Proc. Natl. Acad. Sci. USA* 111:1592–7.

Riddle, K., C. J. Cascio, and N. D. Woodward. 2016. Brain structure in autism: A voxel-based morphometry analysis of the Autism Brain Imaging Database Exchange (ABIDE). *Brain Imaging Behav.* in press. doi: 10.1007/s11682-016-9534-5.

Rogers, S. J., A. Estes, C. Lord, L. Vismara, J. Winter, A. Fitzpatrick, M. Guo, and G. Dawson. 2012. Effects of a brief Early Start Denver model (ESDM)-based parent intervention on toddlers at risk for autism spectrum disorders: A randomized controlled trial. *J. Am. Acad. Child Adolesc. Psychiatry* 51:1052–65.

Roine, U., T. Roine, J. Salmi, T. Nieminen-Von Wendt, P. Tani, S. Leppamaki, P. Rintahaka, K. Caeyenberghs, A. Leemans, and M. Sams. 2015. Abnormal wiring of the connectome in adults with high-functioning autism spectrum disorder. *Mol. Autism* 6:65.

Rojas, D. C., E. Peterson, E. Winterrowd, M. L. Reite, S. J. Rogers, and J. R. Tregellas. 2006. Regional gray matter volumetric changes in autism associated with social and repetitive behavior symptoms. *BMC Psychiatry* 6:56.

Russchen, F. T., I. Bakst, D. G. Amaral, and J. L. Price. 1985. The amygdalostriatal projections in the monkey: An anterograde tracing study. *Brain Res.* 329:241–57.

Rutter, M., A. LeCouteur, and C. Lord. 2003. *Autism Diagnostic Interview-Revised (ADI-R) Manual.* Los Angeles: Western Psychological Services.

Saint-Cyr, J. A., L. G. Ungerleider, and R. Desimone. 1990. Organization of visual cortical inputs to the striatum and subsequent outputs to the pallido-nigral complex in the monkey. *J. Comp. Neurol.* 298:129–56.

Sasson, N. J., G. S. Dichter, and J. W. Bodfish. 2012. Affective responses by adults with autism are reduced to social images but elevated to images related to circumscribed interests. *PLoS One* 7:e42457.

Schmitz, N., K. Rubia, T. Van Amelsvoort, E. Daly, A. Smith, and D. G. Murphy. 2008. Neural correlates of reward in autism. *Br. J. Psychiatry* 192:19–24.

Scott-Van Zeeland, A. A., M. Dapretto, D. G. Ghahremani, R. A. Poldrack, and S. Y. Bookheimer. 2010a. Reward processing in autism. *Autism Res.* 3:53–67.

Scott-Van Zeeland, A. A., K. McNealy, A. T. Wang, M. Sigman, S. Y. Bookheimer, and M. Dapretto. 2010b. No neural evidence of statistical learning during exposure to artificial languages in children with autism spectrum disorders. *Biol. Psychiatry* 68:345–51.

Sears, L. L., C. Vest, S. Mohamed, J. Bailey, B. J. Ranson, and J. Piven. 1999. An MRI study of the basal ganglia in autism. *Prog. Neuropsychopharmacol Biol. Psychiatry* 23:613–24.

Selemon, L. D. and P. S. Goldman-Rakic. 1985. Longitudinal topography and inter-digitation of corticostriatal projections in the rhesus monkey. *J. Neurosci.* 5:776–94.

Shafritz, K. M., J. D. Bregman, T. Ikuta, and P. R. Szeszko. 2015. Neural systems mediating decision-making and response inhibition for social and nonsocial stimuli in autism. *Prog. Neuropsychopharmacol Biol. Psychiatry* 60:112–20.

Shaw, P., P. De Rossi, B. Watson, A. Wharton, D. Greenstein, A. Raznahan, W. Sharp, J. P. Lerch, and M. M. Chakravarty. 2014. Mapping the development of the basal ganglia in children with attention-deficit/hyperactivity disorder. *J. Am. Acad. Child Adolesc. Psychiatry* 53:780–9.e11.

Silk, T. J., N. Rinehart, J. L. Bradshaw, B. Tonge, G. Egan, M. W. O'Boyle, and R. Cunnington. 2006. Visuospatial processing and the function of prefrontal-parietal networks in autism spectrum disorders: A functional MRI study. *Am. J. Psychiatry* 163:1440–3.

Simonoff, E., A. Pickles, T. Charman, S. Chandler, T. Loucas, and G. Baird. 2008. Psychiatric disorders in children with autism spectrum disorders: Prevalence, comorbidity, and associated factors in a population-derived sample. *J. Am. Acad Child Adolesc. Psychiatry* 47:921–9.

Simons VIP Consortium. 2012. Simons Variation in Individuals Project (Simons VIP): A genetics-first approach to studying autism spectrum and related neurodevelopmental disorders. *Neuron* 73:1063–7.

Sims, T. B., J. Neufeld, T. Johnstone, and B. Chakrabarti. 2014. Autistic traits modulate frontostriatal connectivity during processing of rewarding faces. *Soc. Cogn. Affect Neurosci.* 9:2010–16.

Smith, S. M., P. T. Fox, K. L. Miller, D. C. Glahn, P. M. Fox, C. E. Mackay, et al. 2009. Correspondence of the brain's functional architecture during activation and rest. *Proc. Natl. Acad. Sci. USA* 106:13040–5.

Smith, Y. and J. P. Bolam. 1991. Convergence of synaptic inputs from the striatum and the globus pallidus onto identified nigrocollicular cells in the rat: A double anterograde labelling study. *Neuroscience* 44:45–73.

Solomon, M., J. D. Ragland, T. A. Niendam, T. A. Lesh, J. S. Beck, J. C. Matter, M. J. Frank, and C. S. Carter. 2015. Atypical learning in autism spectrum disorders: A functional magnetic resonance imaging study of transitive inference. *J. Am. Acad. Child Adolesc. Psychiatry* 54:947–55.

Staal, W. G., M. Langen, S. Van Dijk, V. T. Mensen, and S. Durston. 2015. *DRD3* gene and striatum in autism spectrum disorder. *Br. J. Psychiatry* 206:431–2.

Supekar, K., M. Musen, and V. Menon. 2009. Development of large-scale functional brain networks in children. *PLoS. Biol.* 7:e1000157.

Sussman, D., R. C. Leung, V. M. Vogan, W. Lee, S. Trelle, S. Lin, D. B. Cassel, M. M. Chakravarty, J. P. Lerch, E. Anagnostou, and M. J. Taylor. 2015. The autism puzzle: diffuse but not pervasive neuroanatomical abnormalities in children with ASD. *Neuroimage Clin.* 8:170–9.

Szabo, J. 1967. The efferent projections of the putamen in the monkey. *Exp. Neurol.* 19:463–76.

Szabo, J. 1970. Projections from the body of the caudate nucleus in the rhesus monkey. *Exp. Neurol.* 27:1–15.

Takada, M., H. Tokuno, A. Nambu, and M. Inase. 1998. Corticostriatal input zones from the supplementary motor area overlap those from the contra- rather than ipsilateral primary motor cortex. *Brain Res.* 791 (1–2):335–40.

Takarae, Y., N. J. Minshew, B. Luna, and J. A. Sweeney. 2007. Atypical involvement of frontostriatal systems during sensorimotor control in autism. *Psychiatry Res.* 156:117–27.

Travers, B. G., R. K. Kana, L. G. Klinger, C. L. Klein, and M. R. Klinger. 2015. Motor learning in individuals with autism spectrum disorder: Activation in superior parietal lobule related to learning and repetitive behaviors. *Autism Res.* 8:38–51.

Ungerleider, L. G., R. Desimone, T. W. Galkin, and M. Mishkin. 1984. Subcortical projections of area MT in the macaque. *J. Comp. Neurol.* 223:368–86.

Vaidya, C. J., J. Foss-Feig, D. Shook, L. Kaplan, L. Kenworthy, and W. D. Gaillard. 2011. Controlling attention to gaze and arrows in childhood: An fMRI study of typical development and autism spectrum disorders. *Dev. Sci.* 14:911–24.

Valk, S. L., A. Di Martino, M. P. Milham, and B. C. Bernhardt. 2015. Multicenter mapping of structural network alterations in autism. *Hum. Brain Mapp.* 36:2364–73.

Van Den Bos, W., M. X. Cohen, T. Kahnt, and E. A. Crone. 2012. Striatum-medial prefrontal cortex connectivity predicts developmental changes in reinforcement learning. *Cereb. Cortex* 22:1247–55.

Van Essen, D. C., S. M. Smith, D. M. Barch, T. E. Behrens, E. Yacoub, and K. Ugurbil. 2013. The WU-Minn Human Connectome Project: An overview. *Neuroimage* 80:62–79.

Van Hoesen, G. W., E. H. Yeterian, and R. Lavizzo-Mourey. 1981. Widespread corticostriate projections from temporal cortex of the rhesus monkey. *J. Comp. Neurol.* 199:205–19.

Van Leijenhorst, L., B. Gunther Moor, Z. A. Op De Macks, S. A. Rombouts, P. M. Westenberg, and E. A. Crone. 2010. Adolescent risky decision-making: Neurocognitive development of reward and control regions. *Neuroimage* 51:345–55.

Vasa, R. A., S. H. Mostofsky, and J. B. Ewen. 2016. The disrupted connectivity hypothesis of autism spectrum disorder: Time for the next phase of research. *Biol. Psychiatry Cogn. Neurosci. Neuroimaging* in press. doi: 10.1016/j.bpsc.2016.02.003.

Ventola, P., D. Y. Yang, H. E. Friedman, D. Oosting, J. Wolf, D. G. Sukhodolsky, and K. A. Pelphrey. 2015. Heterogeneity of neural mechanisms of response to pivotal response treatment. *Brain Imaging Behav.* 9:74–88.

Verstynen, T. D., D. Badre, K. Jarbo, and W. Schneider. 2012. Microstructural organizational patterns in the human corticostriatal system. *J. Neurophysiol.* 107:2984–95.

Voelbel, G. T., M. E. Bates, J. F. Buckman, G. Pandina, and R. L. Hendren. 2006. Caudate nucleus volume and cognitive performance: Are they related in childhood psychopathology? *Biol. Psychiatry* 60:942–50.

Voorn, P., L. J. Vanderschuren, H. J. Groenewegen, T. W. Robbins, and C. M. Pennartz. 2004. Putting a spin on the dorsal-ventral divide of the striatum. *Trends Neurosci.* 27:468–74.

Weng, S. J., M. Carrasco, J. R. Swartz, J. L. Wiggins, N. Kurapati, I. Liberzon, S. Risi, C. Lord, and C. S. Monk. 2011. Neural activation to emotional faces in adolescents with autism spectrum disorders. *J. Child Psychol. Psychiatry* 52:296–305.

Wilke, M., S. K. Holland, M. Altaye, and C. Gaser. 2008. Template-O-Matic: A toolbox for creating customized pediatric templates. *Neuroimage* 41:903–13.

Wolff, J. J., H. C. Hazlett, A. A. Lightbody, A. L. Reiss, and J. Piven. 2013. Repetitive and self-injurious behaviors: Associations with caudate volume in autism and fragile X syndrome. *J. Neurodev. Disord.* 5:12.

Yan, C. G., B. Cheung, C. Kelly, S. Colcombe, R. C. Craddock, A. Di Martino, Q. Li, X. N. Zuo, F. X. Castellanos, and M. P. Milham. 2013. A comprehensive assessment of regional variation in the impact of head micromovements on functional connectomics. *Neuroimage* 76:183–201.

Yang, Z., X. N. Zuo, P. Wang, Z. Li, S. M. Laconte, P. A. Bandettini, and X. P. Hu. 2012. Generalized RAICAR: Discover homogeneous subject (sub)groups by reproducibility of their intrinsic connectivity networks. *Neuroimage* 63:403–14.

Yelnik, J., C. Francois, and G. Percheron. 1997. Spatial relationships between striatal axonal endings and pallidal neurons in macaque monkeys. *Adv. Neurol.* 74:45–56.

Yelnik, J., C. Francois, G. Percheron, and D. Tande. 1996. A spatial and quantitative study of the striatopallidal connection in the monkey. *Neuroreport* 7:985–8.

Yeterian, E. H. and D. N. Pandya. 1993. Striatal connections of the parietal association cortices in rhesus monkeys. *J. Comp. Neurol.* 332:175–97.

Yeterian, E. H. and D. N. Pandya. 1998. Corticostriatal connections of the superior temporal region in rhesus monkeys. *J. Comp. Neurol.* 399:384–402.

Zhao, Y. and F. X. Castellanos. 2016. Annual Research Review: Discovery science strategies in studies of the pathophysiology of child and adolescent psychiatric disorders—Promises and limitations. *J. Child Psychol. Psychiatry* 57:421–39.

Zhou, Y., F. Yu, and T. Duong. 2014. Multiparametric MRI characterization and prediction in autism spectrum disorder using graph theory and machine learning. *PLoS One* 9:e90405.

Chapter 12 GABA system dysfunction in autism and related disorders
From synapse to symptoms?

Jamie Horder

Contents

Abstract 220
12.1 Introduction 220
12.2 The GABA system 220
    12.2.1 GABA metabolism, release, and recycling. 220
    12.2.2 GABA interneurons 222
    12.2.3 GABA receptors 222
    12.2.4 GABA in neuropsychiatric disorders 223
12.3 Autism spectrum disorders. 223
    12.3.1 Clinical features 223
    12.3.2 Etiology. 224
    12.3.3 ASD and GABA. 224
        12.3.3.1 Genetics 224
        12.3.3.2 Gene expression. 226
        12.3.3.3 *In vivo* human studies 227
12.4 Fragile X syndrome 229
    12.4.1 Clinical features and etiology. 229
    12.4.2 GABA and fragile X. 230
    12.4.3 Human studies of GABA in fragile X syndrome 231
12.5 Rett syndrome. 231
12.6 Fetal anticonvulsant and alcohol syndromes 232
12.7 Theoretical and clinical implications 234
    12.7.1 Minicolumns and feature discrimination 234
    12.7.2 Gamma-band activity and feature binding 234
    12.7.3 Clinical implications. 235
12.8 Conclusions. 236
Acknowledgments and conflict of interest statement. 236
References 236

Abstract

Autism spectrum disorders (ASD) are neurodevelopmental syndromes characterized by repetitive behaviors and restricted interests, impairments in social behavior and relationships, and in language and communication. Some or all of these symptoms are also observed in a number of other developmental disorders, including fragile X Syndrome, Rett syndrome, and fetal anticonvulsant syndrome (FACS). Emerging evidence suggests that ASD and ASD-associated syndromes may be linked to dysfunction in excitatory:inhibitory (E:I) balance and, in particular, to aspects of inhibitory GABAergic signaling in the brain. This chapter reviews the genetics, molecular neurobiology, and systems neuroscience evidence implicating GABA in these conditions. We conclude by discussing how these deficits could explain the specific symptoms observed.

12.1 Introduction

Autism spectrum disorders (ASD) are a group of common neurodevelopmental syndromes. ASD is diagnosed on the basis of qualitative behavioral abnormalities in three domains: social interaction, language and communication, and repetitive or restricted interests or behaviors (American Psychiatric Association 2000). The pathophysiology of ASD is unclear and is an area of active research. In recent years, however, the hypothesis that ASD symptoms result from deficits in particular aspects of inhibitory gamma-aminobutyric acid (GABA) neurotransmission has gained influence (Coghlan et al. 2012).

In this chapter, we begin by reviewing the neurobiology of the human GABA system (see Figure 12.1 for a graphical overview of the main components of this system). We then examine the evidence relating to the hypothesis that ASD is characterized by particular abnormalities in this system. We will also examine the evidence of abnormalities in GABAergic neurons and synapses in ASD and related disorders that feature ASD-like symptoms, including fragile X syndrome, Rett syndrome, and fetal anticonvulsant syndrome (FACS). We conclude by discussing the question of the mechanisms by which the hypothesized GABA deficits may give rise to the particular symptoms of these disorders.

12.2 The GABA system

12.2.1 GABA metabolism, release, and recycling

GABA is the primary inhibitory neurotransmitter in the adult brain. The process of GABA neurotransmission depends on a complex system of enzymes, receptors, and other proteins. The GABA system is therefore vulnerable to genetic perturbation at numerous points. First, the

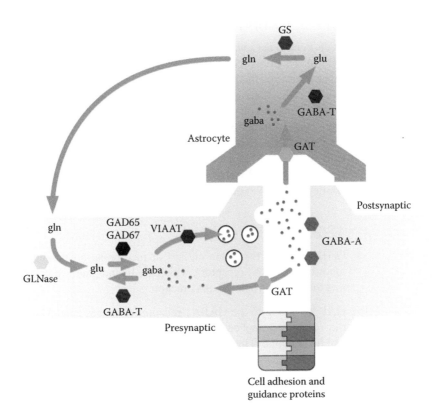

Figure 12.1 A simplified illustration of the major synaptic pathways responsible for GABA synthesis, breakdown, release, and reuptake. Abbreviations: GABA = gamma-aminobutyric acid; glu = glutamate; gln = glutamine; GLNase = glutaminase; GAD = glutamate decarboxylase; GABA-T = GABA transaminase; VIAAT = vesicular inhibitory amino acid transporter; GAT = GABA transporter; GABA-A = GABA$_A$ receptor (note: there are numerous subtypes of this receptor, but these are not shown, for simplicity); GS = glutamine synthetase. Not pictured: GABA$_B$ receptors; GABA$_A$ or GABA$_B$ autoreceptors.

formation and stabilization of GABAergic synapses depend on numerous cell adhesion and signaling molecules. Some of these are also involved in the formation of excitatory synapses, but others are uniquely involved in inhibitory synapse formation. These include neuroligin-2, neuroligin-3, neurexin-1, and SLIT and NTRK-like protein 3 (Ko et al. 2015).

GABA is synthesized from the excitatory transmitter glutamate via the action of glutamate decarboxylase (GAD) enzymes, of which there are two main isoforms, GAD$_{65}$ and GAD$_{67}$. Release of synaptic GABA depends on the loading of GABA into synaptic vesicles by the vesicular inhibitory amino acid transporter (VIAAT; Gasnier 2004). Following synaptic release, reuptake of extracellular GABA into the presynaptic interneurons is performed by the GABA transporters GAT1, GAT2, and GAT3 (Madsen et al. 2009). After reuptake, GABA is converted into glutamate by GABA transaminase (GABA-T; Madsen et al. 2008).

221

12.2.2 GABA interneurons

In the central nervous system, GABA is produced and released by inhibitory interneurons. These neurons are typically small in size, with short-range projection fields, although small populations of long-range cortical GABA projections exist (Tamamaki and Tomioka 2010). GABAergic interneurons are diverse and can be categorized on the basis of either their cytoarchitecture (e.g., basket, chandelier, stellate) or their molecular properties (e.g., as parvalbumin-expressing (PV+), calretinin+, calbindin+; De Marco Garcia et al. 2011). The cerebellum contains distinct types of GABAergic cells, including the very large Purkinje cells (Bailey et al. 1998) and others.

12.2.3 GABA receptors

GABA acts on two main classes of membrane-bound receptors—the ionotropic $GABA_A$ receptors, which are ligand-gated chloride channels, and the metabotropic $GABA_B$ receptors.

GABA binding to the $GABA_A$ receptor enhances conductance through the receptor ionophore, which conducts anions, particularly chloride and bicarbonate. The resultant increase of these negatively charged ions within the cell hyperpolarizes the membrane-resting potential, thus leading to the inhibition of cell firing under most physiological conditions. The $GABA_A$ receptor is composed of five subunits arranged around a central pore (Nutt and Malizia 2001). Subunits are derived from a family of different genes, which generates a large degree of receptor diversity, with different combinations of subunits giving rise to receptors with specific properties (Rudolph and Mohler 2004).

The $\alpha 1$ subunit of the $GABA_A$ receptor appears to be responsible for sedative effects of positive allosteric modulators of the $GABA_A$ system, such as diazepam, $\alpha 2$, and $\alpha 3$ receptors for anxiolytic effects (McKernan et al. 2000; Mohler 2006) and $\alpha 5$ receptors for cognitive and memory deficits (Collinson et al. 2006). The $\alpha 1$, $\alpha 2$, and $\alpha 3$ subtypes are located in synaptic processes, whereas the $\alpha 5$ subtype is located extrasynaptically, where they regulate tonic inhibition along with another receptor type that contains the $\alpha 4$ and δ subunits.

By contrast, $GABA_B$ receptors are involved with second messenger systems through the binding and inhibition of guanine nucleotide-binding proteins (G proteins; Bettler et al. 2004). $GABA_B$ receptors are expressed both pre- and postsynaptically (Bowery et al. 2002). The $GABA_B$ receptor comprises a homodimer with similar subunits, designated 1 and 2-t (Bowery et al. 2002).

Although GABA is an inhibitory transmitter in the adult brain, it is believed to act as an excitatory (depolarizing) neurotransmitter during neurodevelopment (Sibilla and Ballerini 2009) and in adults under certain pathological conditions (Beaumont and Maccaferri 2011). GABAergic interneurons mature relatively late, with the migration and differentiation of these cells occurring during late gestation and into early infancy in humans (Xu et al. 2011). Some of the subunits of the $GABA_A$ receptor system appear to have functional roles in neurodevelopment (Fagiolini et al. 2004).

12.2.4 GABA in neuropsychiatric disorders

GABAergic dysfunction has been implicated in anxiety (Durant et al. 2011), epilepsy (Macdonald et al. 2010), and learning impairment, among other conditions. Drugs that either act as direct agonists at the $GABA_A$ receptor or those that act as positive allosteric modulators have hypnotic, anxiolytic, anticonvulsant, and sedative effects. Other anticonvulsant drugs with antianxiety effects act by indirectly increasing $GABA_A$ transmission by promoting the synthesis of GABA or inhibiting its reuptake or breakdown (Madsen et al. 2009). Conversely, drugs that either antagonize the $GABA_A$ receptor (Fernandez et al. 2007) or inhibit GABA synthesis (Horton and Meldrum 1973) cause central nervous system stimulation, anxiety, and seizures. A detailed discussion of this topic is outside the scope of this chapter, but this is of interest given the high comorbidity of both epilepsy and anxiety disorders in ASD (see Section 12.3.1).

12.3 Autism spectrum disorders

12.3.1 Clinical features

Autism spectrum disorders are a group of neurodevelopmental disorders, with a population prevalence of approximately 1% (Baron-Cohen et al. 2009; Brugha et al. 2011; Russell et al. 2013). ASDs are more often diagnosed in males than in females, with a gender ratio of approximately 4:1 (Baron-Cohen et al. 2009).

Autism spectrum disorders are characterized by a triad of impairments in three domains: social interaction, language and communication, and repetitive and restricted interests and behaviors (Rutter 1978). For a diagnosis of ASD to be made, these symptoms must be present from before the age of 36 months (World Health Organization 1993).

Although ASD is conceptualized as a monolithic category in the current DSM-V (American Psychiatric Association 2013), the terms "autism" and "childhood autism" were previously used to refer specifically to the subset of cases characterized by delays in the acquisition of expressive language. "Asperger's Syndrome" was used to describe cases with normal language development and no intellectual disability (American Psychiatric Association 2000).

Individuals with an ASD may also have an intellectual disability. However, at least 25% of cases show normal or superior intellectual function (Rutter 1983). ASDs are described as a spectrum of disorders because the severity of these symptoms, and the associated functional impairment, vary between individuals. Epilepsy is observed in up to 25% of people with an ASD, a high rate when compared with a population prevalence of less than 1% (Bolton et al. 2011). Given the close involvement of GABA dysfunction in epilepsy, this is suggestive evidence for the presence of a GABA system deficit in ASD, in at least some cases.

12.3.2 Etiology

ASDs are highly heritable, with estimates of heritability ranging from about 0.5 to 0.9 (Constantino et al. 2013; Colvert et al. 2015). This indicates that the majority of the variability in the risk of developing ASD is due to additive genetic factors. However, most cases of ASD are idiopathic, that is, not associated with a discernable genetic or environmental cause. Symptoms of ASD are also observed in a number of genetic disorders such as fragile X syndrome and Rett syndrome, which are known to be caused by a single gene mutation. These monogenic disorders are discussed in Section 12.4 and Section 12.5, respectively.

Large genome-wide studies have implicated a number of single-nucleotide polymorphisms (SNPs) and chromosomal linkage regions in the causality of ASDs. However, thus far, known SNPs only account for a small proportion of the risk for ASD (Huguet et al. 2013). This suggests that ASDs are genetically heterogeneous with no single variant accounting for a large proportion of cases.

Evidence suggests, however, that many cases of ASD are caused by microdeletions or microduplications, collectively known as copy-number variations (CNVs). CNVs are submicroscopic chromosomal abnormalities ranging in size from a few bases up to about 500 kilobases (Feuk et al. 2006). Whole-genome CNV scans have revealed numerous candidate loci for ASD (De Rubeis et al. 2014), although in many cases ASD-associated CNVs are also associated with other neuropsychiatric disorders (Kenny et al. 2015).

12.3.3 ASD and GABA

What follows is an overview of the evidence from genetics, gene expression, and neuroimaging relevant to the role of GABA in idiopathic ASD.

12.3.3.1 Genetics One of the first chromosomal loci where microdeletion/microduplication CNVs were observed in ASD is the chromosome 15q11–q13 region. This site contains a number of genes coding for particular subunits of the $GABA_A$ receptor, namely *GABRB3*, *GABRA5*, and *GABRG3*, encoding for the β3, α5, and γ3 subunits, respectively.

Deletions spanning this region result in either Angelman's syndrome or Prader-Willi syndrome. Deletions affecting the maternally inherited copy of this region cause Angelman's, while paternal copy deletions cause Prader-Willi syndrome—an example of genomic imprinting (Knoll et al. 1989).

By contrast, duplications of the 15q11–13 locus have been observed in patients with ASD in numerous studies (Cook et al. 1998; Al Ageeli et al. 2014). Maternally derived duplications predominate, suggesting genomic imprinting, just as in the case of deletions. The prevalence of 15q11–13 duplications in the population of individuals with idiopathic ASD has been estimated at 0.5%–3%, although not everyone with the duplication meets criteria for ASD. Epilepsy, suggestive of an inhibitory signaling deficit, is also common in 15q11–13 duplication (Simon et al. 2009).

It might seem that duplication of a region containing GABA receptor subunits ought to lead to *excessive* inhibitory neurotransmission. However, *in vitro* studies of a human neuronal cell line carrying a maternal 15q duplication showed that this variant leads to reduced *GABRB3* expression via impaired homologous pairing (Meguro-Horike et al. 2011) and may also affect cell migration and maturation. Furthermore, a mutation in the *GABRB3* gene was associated with a three- to sixfold increased risk of ASD (with epilepsy in some cases), especially when maternally inherited (Delahanty et al. 2009). Other GABA$_A$ subunit variants, including GABRA4 and GABRB1, have also been linked to ASD (Ma et al. 2005).

Furthermore, although the majority of cases of idiopathic autism do not carry mutations at this locus, abnormal expression of proteins encoded by 15q11–13 genes have also been reported in autism. In the normal human brain, *GABRB3*, *GABRA5*, and *GABRG3* are biallelically expressed. However, in four out of eight cases of idiopathic ASD, expression of the maternal copies of these genes predominated, and levels of these proteins, especially *GABRB3*, were reduced (Hogart et al. 2007). This suggests that the 15q11–13 locus is commonly implicated in autism and that it can be disrupted, either directly by mutation, or indirectly, perhaps by epigenetic factors.

As discussed in the introduction, the proper development and function of GABA synapses rely on numerous signaling and scaffolding proteins. Therefore, GABAergic dysfunction could be caused by mutations in genes not directly involved in GABA transmission. Indeed, several putative ASD mutations disrupt genes known to be involved in inhibitory synaptic formation and stabilization. One example is contactin-associated protein 2 (*CNTNAP2*). Deletions of this gene have been linked to autism (Nord et al. 2011) and common variants are associated with communication and language difficulties (Stein et al. 2011; Whitehouse et al. 2011). This gene encodes a protein in the neurexin family of cell adhesion molecules required for neural development.

225

In mice, *Cntnap2* deficiency leads to specific deficits in inhibitory signaling with reduced expression of *Gad1* and of parvalbumin+ inhibitory interneurons (Penagarikano et al. 2011). Similar findings were observed in mice lacking another ASD candidate gene, *Cadps2* (Sadakata et al. 2007)—reduced cortical parvalbumin+ GABA interneurons, as well as cerebellar Purkinje cells. Likewise, mice lacking the murine homolog of *PLAUR*, another gene mutated in some ASD individuals, show epilepsy, anxiety, and impaired social behaviors, as well as reduced cortical interneurons and altered $GABA_A$ expression (Eagleson et al. 2011). This led some authors to propose a "common circuit defect of excitatory-inhibitory balance in mouse models of autism" (Gogolla et al. 2009).

Whole-exome sequencing of idiopathic ASD cases has revealed an overrepresentation of deleterious *de novo* single-nucleotide variants impacting known genes in ASD (Neale et al. 2012; O'Roak et al. 2014). These variants are widely distributed over the genome, but affected genes are overrepresented among fragile X mental retardation protein (FMR1) interaction partners (Iossifov et al. 2012). Because *Fmr1* knockout is known to create an inhibitory signaling defect in mice (see Section 12.4), it is plausible that mutations may cause ASD if they impact inhibitory signaling, whether directly or indirectly. However, this is speculative, and more work is needed.

12.3.3.2 Gene expression   The previous section discussed evidence for an association between mutations affecting GABA gene function and ASD. Other studies have reported reduced *expression* of GABAergic genes and reduced *density* of GABA-related proteins in postmortem brain samples from individuals with an ASD.

GAD_{65} and GAD_{67} proteins have been reported as reduced in the cerebellum and parietal cortex (Fatemi et al. 2002), whereas GAD_{67} messenger RNA (mRNA) was found reduced in cerebellar Purkinje cells (Yip et al. 2007), indicating reduced expression of this gene. In the hippocampus (Blatt et al. 2001) and anterior and posterior cingulate cortices, $GABA_A$ receptor binding was reduced (Oblak et al. 2009, 2010). Recent studies showed reduced *GABRB3* expression in the cingulate cortex (Thanseem et al. 2012) and the cerebellar vermis (Fatemi et al. 2011) in ASD, consistent with the genetic evidence for the involvement of this gene in ASD, as discussed in Section 12.3.3.1.

By contrast, increased expression of the excitatory glutamate receptor AMPA, and of glutamate transporter proteins, was found, most notably in the cerebellum (Purcell et al. 2001). Decreases in the number of the large GABAergic Purkinje cells in the cerebellar cortex have also been reported. In one study, 21 out of 29 ASD specimens examined showed this reduction trend (Palmen et al. 2004), although a subsequent study showed abnormalities in only three out of six specimens (Whitney et al. 2008).

Strong convergent evidence for an inhibitory deficit in ASD comes from a recent transcriptomic study (Voineagu et al. 2011). In two separate samples, they found reduced cortical expression of mRNA in "M12," a cluster of genes including *CNTNAP2*, which is highly expressed in parvalbumin+ GABA interneurons. Interestingly, one of the ASD subjects in this study was found to carry a 15q11–13 duplication, but their pattern of mRNA expression was similar to that of the other ASD cases, consistent with the view that this syndrome is a useful model of idiopathic ASD.

In summary, there is extensive evidence of abnormal patterns of expression of GABA-A receptor genes, the GABA synthesis enzymes GAD65 and GAD67, and other genes known to be expressed in GABA interneurons, in idiopathic ASD. However, little is known about the underlying molecular or epigenetic mechanisms that are responsible for these differences.

12.3.3.3 In vivo human studies   In contrast to the large number of studies using animal models and postmortem techniques, relatively few studies have attempted to measure GABA or GABA-related proteins in living ASD subjects. This is likely due to the technical difficulties in measuring GABA function *in vivo*.

For instance, proton magnetic resonance spectroscopy ([1H]MRS) is a technique widely used to quantify key neural metabolites *in vivo*, including glutamate, glutamine, and others. However, although there have been numerous [1H]MRS investigations of the brain in ASD (see Horder et al. 2013), many did not measure GABA because of the difficulties in distinguishing GABA from other similar molecules in the magnetic resonance spectrum. Advances in [1H]MRS methodology such as the MEGAPRESS technique (Rothman et al. 1993) have made it possible to measure GABA levels in humans (Edden et al. 2012).

There have been three GABA [1H]MRS studies in children with ASD. These have shown reduced GABA in the frontal cortex, motor cortex, and auditory cortex but no differences in the basal ganglia (Harada et al. 2011; Rojas et al. 2013; Gaetz et al. 2014). One study of adolescents found reduced GABA in the anterior cingulate cortex (Cochran et al. 2015). The [1H]MRS evidence is therefore consistent with a cortical GABA deficit in young people with an ASD, but no published studies have examined adults with the condition. Also, most of these studies have methodological limitations such as the use of sedatives during the scan or differences in the use of psychotropic medication between the patients and the controls. Further work using this promising technique is therefore required and in medication-free individuals.

The technique [1H]MRS can measure neurotransmitter levels, but it is not able to quantify levels of receptors or other proteins. However, using techniques such as positron emission tomography (PET) or single-photon emission computed tomography (SPECT) with selective radioligands, it is possible to quantify the density of neurotransmitter receptors in the human brain *in vivo*. For GABA, the ligands flumazenil and flunitrazepam bind $GABA_A$ receptors, and the novel Ro154513 is largely selective for the $\alpha5$ subtype of $GABA_A$ receptors (Lingford-Hughes et al. 2010).

Two *in vivo* studies investigating the $GABA_A$ receptor in ASD have recently been conducted, suggesting that $GABA_A$ is reduced in both adults and children with ASD. Mori et al. (2012) found reduced accumulation of the $GABA_A$–benzodiazepine ligand [^{123}I]iomazenil using SPECT in children with ASD. A recent pilot study from our group (Mendez et al. 2013) confirmed reduced $GABA_A$ in three adult males with ASD. Further work is called for to confirm these results.

Other researchers have attempted to indirectly probe brain GABA function. Transcranial magnetic stimulation (TMS) offers one such approach (Farzan et al. 2011). Transcranial magnetic stimulation (TMS) uses strong, pulsed, localized magnetic fields to stimulate cortical neural activity. Depending on the cortical region affected this can cause, for example, muscular contraction. When two pulses are administered in quick succession (2 ms), the effect of the second is inhibited and this is believed to reflect $GABA_A$ signaling (intracortical inhibition).

Three small studies have examined intracortical inhibition in ASD. Two showed reduced inhibition only in some subgroups of patients (Enticott et al. 2010; Oberman et al. 2011), although the most recent, and largest, study found no significant differences in ASD adults (Enticott et al. 2013). This provides mixed evidence for a cortical inhibitory deficit in some cases of ASD, but the small sample makes interpretation difficult, and the hypothesis that TMS measures of "cortical inhibition" are proxies for cortical GABA concentration has recently been questioned (Stagg et al. 2011).

Finally, it is possible to measure GABA and related molecules in blood plasma. Increased GABA in the plasma of individuals with ASD has been found in two studies (Dhossche et al. 2002; El-Ansary et al. 2011). However, decreased platelet GABA has also been observed (Rolf et al. 1993). The interpretation of such findings in terms of brain function is complicated, since neither glutamate nor GABA crosses the blood–brain barrier under normal conditions (Smith 2000).

In summary, there has been relatively little work examining the GABA system in human brains of living individuals. Those studies that have been conducted provide preliminary evidence in favor of the theory that there is a GABA defect in at least some parts of the brain of people with an ASD. However, a challenge for the future will be to relate these findings to the genetic and postmortem gene expression data, discussed previously (Sections 12.3.3.1 and 12.3.3.2), in order to understand the underlying basis of these changes.

One approach that holds great promise is the *in vitro* culture of neurons via the generation of human-induced pluripotent stem cells (iPSCs) from adult somatic cell samples. This technique has been successfully used to investigate gene expression changes in patients with schizophrenia (Brennand et al. 2011) and other neurodevelopmental disorders (Pasca et al. 2011), revealing abnormal expression of genes linked to neurotransmission and neuronal connectivity. There have been no published studies using this technique to investigate idiopathic ASD, but this approach could provide important insights into the cellular mechanisms behind neural function in ASD, including GABA system abnormalities.

12.4 Fragile X syndrome

12.4.1 Clinical features and etiology

Fragile X syndrome (FXS) is a monogenetic neurodevelopmental disorder, caused by an abnormal expansion of a CGG trinucleotide repeat within the promoter region of the gene FMR1 on the X chromosome (Wisniewski et al. 1991). Fragile X syndrome has an estimated prevalence of 1/4000 in males and 1/6000 in females (Turner et al. 1996). Common symptoms of FXS include intellectual disability, a distinctive physical phenotype, and symptoms of social and communication impairment and repetitive behaviors similar to those seen in ASD.

About 20% of those with FXS meet formal criteria for an ASD (Clifford et al. 2007; Wang et al. 2010), with others showing milder autistic symptoms. In comparison to several other monogenetic neurodevelopmental syndromes, FXS is especially associated with autistic features (Oliver et al. 2011).

Fragile X mental retardation protein (FMRP) is an mRNA-binding protein involved in the regulation of the translation of mRNA into proteins (Laggerbauer et al. 2001). Recent evidence suggests that FMRP is involved in neuronal activity-dependent trafficking of mRNA to synapses (Dictenberg et al. 2008) and that it is especially associated with transcripts involved in synapse formation and implicated in ASD (Darnell et al. 2011).

Epilepsy is observed in approximately 20%–25% of cases of FXS, suggestive of a cortical inhibitory deficit (Wisniewski et al. 1991). The most distinctive neuropathological marker of FXS is abnormal neuronal morphology, in the form of long, thin dendritic spines of pyramidal neurons (Portera-Cailliau 2012). This phenotype has been attributed to the overexpression of metabotropic glutamate receptors of the mGluR5 subtype, and it has been proposed that mGluR5 antagonists might rescue some of the deficits associated with this disorder (Wang et al. 2010; Levenga et al. 2011). However, abnormalities in the function and biology of the GABA system are also emerging as important in FXS.

12.4.2 GABA and fragile X

An early study reported regional alterations in brain tissue GABA levels in male juvenile, but not adult, mice lacking a functional copy of the *Fmr1* gene (*Fmr1* knockout mice), with both increases and decreases seen in different regions (Gruss and Braun 2001). However, it is hard to interpret differences in GABA levels without consideration of the expression of GABA receptors and other proteins.

In terms of *function*, D'Antuono et al. (2003) reported abnormal responses to the acetylcholine agonist carbachol in knockout mice. In wild-type mice, carbachol indirectly suppresses excitatory postsynaptic potentials (ePSPs) in the subiculum by promoting inhibitory GABA signaling, but in knockouts it caused potentiation of ePSPs, mimicking the effects seen in wild-type mice after administration of a $GABA_A$ antagonist. Fragile X mice also show blunted cortical inhibitory signaling in response to the administration of a glutamate agonist (Paluszkiewicz et al. 2011). This suggests a functional $GABA_A$ signaling deficit in FXS.

Direct evidence for such a deficit has come from studies of the expression of $GABA_A$ subunit proteins or mRNA in FMR1 knockout mice. $GABA_A$ β subunit immunoreactivity was decreased to 60%–70% of normal levels in several brain regions with the exception of the cerebellum, while GAD_{65} and GAD_{67} expression was increased (El Idrissi et al. 2005).

Furthermore, expressions of 8 out of the 18 known $GABA_A$ subunits was significantly reduced in the cortex, but not in the cerebellum, of Fragile X mice (D'Hulst et al. 2006, 2009; Hong et al. 2011), and in Fragile X Drosophila $GABA_A$ receptor expression levels are also impaired (D'Hulst et al. 2006), suggesting an evolutionarily conserved role for FMRP in GABA receptor function. Similarly, downregulation of $GABA_A$ α1, β2, and δ subunits, and GABA-T and SSADH were observed at different stages of postnatal development (Adusei et al. 2010).

However, FXS seems to affect the integrity of the GABA system in a region-specific fashion. As noted previously, the cerebellum seems to be spared. Furthermore, one study found a 50% decrease in the number of GABA synapses in the striatum of FMR1 knockout mice, but with a paradoxical *increase* in the level of spontaneous GABA inhibitory transmission (Centonze et al. 2008). By contrast, reduced tonic $GABA_A$ currents are seen in the subiculum of FMR1 knockouts, with normal phasic GABA currents, and reduced expression of α5 and δ subunits (Curia et al. 2009)—consistent with D'Antuono and colleagues' (2003) findings of reduced inhibitory function in the same circuits.

Profoundly reduced tonic and phasic inhibitory currents in the amygdala of FX mice have been reported, along with reduced GAD_{65} and GAD_{67} expression, reduced GABA, and a reduced number of GABAergic synapses (Olmos-Serrano et al. 2010); amygdala hyperexcitability was rescued by a $GABA_A$ δ agonist.

A marked reduction in cortical parvalbumin+ GABA interneurons together with abnormal morphology has also been observed (Selby et al. 2007). This finding is interesting, given that reduced parval-bumin+ interneuron density has been seen in other mouse models of ASD-associated genetic mutations (Gogolla et al. 2009), as previously mentioned (Section 12.3.3.1), and also in fetal anticonvulsant syndrome (see Section 12.6).

By contrast, the $GABA_B$ system has not been reported as abnormal in *Fmr1* knockout mice, although $GABA_B$ agonists such as baclofen have been shown to alleviate some of the symptoms, including seizures, in animal models (Pacey et al. 2009).

In conclusion, there is growing evidence from animal models for the involvement of GABA in FXS, alongside the established role of gluta-mate. However, abnormalities appear to be regionally and temporally specific, with the cerebellum being spared.

12.4.3 Human studies of GABA in fragile X syndrome

In contrast to the growing literature on idiopathic ASD (see Sections 12.3.3.2 and 12.3.3.3), there have been no published investigations directly measuring GABA, GABA receptors, or GABA system proteins in the brain of humans with fragile X syndrome either postmortem or *in vivo*. One small study used transcranial magnetic stimulation (TMS) to *indirectly* probe inhibitory signaling in fragile X patients, finding no differences from healthy controls (Oberman et al. 2011; see Section 12.3.3.3 for more on TMS).

Given the evidence of GABA abnormalities from rodent models of frag-ile X syndrome, the lack of human studies in this disorder is unfortunate. Future work should attempt to confirm whether the same abnormalities are seen in humans, using methods such as [1H]MRS, PET, and SPECT as this could have direct clinical applications.

12.5 Rett syndrome

Rett syndrome is a severe neurodevelopmental disorder caused by the loss of function of one copy of the methyl-CpG-binding protein 2 (*MECP2*) gene on the X chromosome. The syndrome is very rare in males, because it is lethal in those with only one X chromosome, and male fetuses with the mutation rarely survive to term (Renieri et al. 2003). Clinically, Rett syndrome presents with developmental regression usually between the ages of 6 and 18 months, with the loss of speech, social skills, and motor skills. Repetitive stereotyped movements, most notably hand flapping, subsequently emerge. Epilepsy is present in approximately 80% of cases of Rett syndrome, suggestive of an inhibitory signaling deficit (Jian et al. 2006).

MECP2 is a transcriptional regulator that is highly expressed in GABAergic neurons in the brain (Akbarian et al. 2001), but its role in the function of the GABAergic system is unclear. It appears that MECP2 may regulate the number of GABAergic synapses in the thalamus and medulla.

GABAergic abnormalities in the thalamus (Zhang et al. 2010) and medulla (Medrihan et al. 2008) develop in *Mecp2*-null mice even to the onset of symptoms. GABAergic transmission is altered in opposite directions in interconnected GABAergic and glutamatergic neurons in *Mecp2*-null mice, implying that the cellular and molecular mechanisms underlying *Mecp2*-mediated regulation of GABAergic transmission are likely to be specific to the location and cell type (Zhang et al. 2010). A reduction of the β3 subunit of the $GABA_A$ receptor has also been demonstrated in cortical samples of Rett syndrome patients and in the neocortex of *Mecp2*-deficient mice (Samaco et al. 2005).

MECP2 is critical for the normal functioning of cortical GABA-releasing neurons, which express 50% more MECP2 than non-GABAergic neurons (Chao et al. 2010). Mice with a selective MECP2 deficiency in GABAergic neurons showed abnormalities that resembled Rett syndrome and several autistic features as well as reductions in GAD_{65} and GAD_{67} mRNA levels (Chao et al. 2010).

As in the case of fragile X syndrome, there have been few studies of GABA in humans with Rett syndrome. An early study of five girls with the disorder found normal levels of GABA in the cerebrospinal fluid (Perry et al. 1988). However, reduced $GABA_A$ receptor density was observed using SPECT in three adult females *in vivo* (Yamashita et al. 1998). Postmortem studies have reported normal or *increased* GABA receptor and glutamate receptor density in girls with Rett syndrome below the age of 8 but reductions with increasing age (Blue et al. 1999a,b).

Taken together, this suggests that the GABA deficits seen in animal model of Rett syndrome may not emerge in human patients until late childhood, implying that animal models do not provide an adequate model of the pathophysiology in very young Rett patients. However, more studies are needed to confirm this possibility.

12.6 Fetal anticonvulsant and alcohol syndromes

Fetal exposure to anticonvulsant medication is linked to an increased rate of developmental defects (Holmes et al. 2001). What has been dubbed the "fetal anticonvulsant syndrome" (FACS) has varied manifestations, including a pattern of physical dysmorphic features, intellectual disability, and behavioral abnormalities, including ASD symptoms (Rasalam et al. 2005). In one study, approximately 60% of children with FACS displaying at least two autistic features and 10% had a diagnosis of an ASD, around 10 times the population prevalence (Moore et al. 2000).

The mechanism by which fetal anticonvulsants cause developmental disorders is unclear. Given that GABA is a key neurodevelopmental signaling molecule, and since the majority of anticonvulsants work by increasing GABA transmission (Vellucci and Webster 1984), one possibility is that excess GABA exerts some developmentally neurotoxic effects. However, other mechanisms such as anoxia, secondary to fetal cardiac effects, have also been suggested (Danielsson et al. 2001).

Prenatal valproate exposure has been used in rats and mice as a model for FACS and also idiopathic ASD (Dufour-Rainfray et al. 2011). A single, high-dose injection of valproate given to the pregnant female at the period of embryonic neural tube closure, that is, Embryonic Day 12 in rats, produces the most consistent behavioral effects (Kim et al. 2011).

Prenatal valproate exposure causes characteristic behavioral and neurobiological abnormalities in rodents. Behaviorally, exposed rats show fewer social behaviors from early life, along with motor incoordination, repetitive, stereotyped locomotor hyperactivity, and a reduced tendency to explore (Schneider and Przewlocki 2005). These symptoms are similar to those seen in individuals with an ASD.

Neurobiologically, prenatal valproate-exposed rats have a marked reduction in the number of cortical GABA interneurons of the parvalbumin+ type (Gogolla et al. 2009), and characteristic electro-encephalography (EEG) abnormalities, which are also seen in humans with ASD (Gandal et al. 2010). Reduced cerebellar Purkinje GABA cells are also seen, consistent with neuropathological evidence in humans with idiopathic ASD, as discussed previously (Ingram et al. 2000). In summary, prenatal exposure to anticonvulsants is a major risk factor for ASD symptoms. Although the teratogenic mechanism is unclear, there is emerging evidence that deficits in inhibitory interneuron development are a pathophysiological mechanism.

Fetal alcohol exposure is another major risk factor for neurodevelopmental problems and has been called the largest preventable cause of these disorders. In severe cases, alcohol exposure causes fetal alcohol syndrome, which is characterized by growth deficiency (below-normal weight and height), physically dysmorphic features, below-normal IQ, and behavioral disorders (Riley and McGee 2005). However, the condition exists on a spectrum of severity with the term "fetal alcohol spectrum disorders" used to cover the milder manifestations (Chudley et al. 2005).

It has been suggested that rates of ASD symptoms are higher in those with fetal alcohol syndrome (Dufour-Rainfray et al. 2011; Landgren et al. 2011). However, other studies suggest that there are key differences in the manifestations of the two disorders. Although children with fetal alcohol syndrome commonly show impairments in social skills and behavior, they do not show symptoms such as restrictive interests, lack of eye-contact, and lack of shared enjoyment in social activities (Riley and McGee 2005; Bishop et al. 2007).

The paucity of research focused on the role of GABA in fetal alcohol spectrum disorders is unfortunate, given that alcohol is known to act on GABA (Kumar et al. 2009). More work is required to investigate possible links between alcohol exposure and ASD.

12.7 Theoretical and clinical implications

We have discussed evidence supporting a role of GABA abnormalities in a number of neurodevelopmental disorders characterized by autistic features, including impaired social interaction and repetitive and restricted behaviors, and intellectual disability. However, this raises the question: Why does this neurobiology lead to these particular symptoms?

12.7.1 Minicolumns and feature discrimination

A number of theoretical frameworks for understanding the development of ASDs and related neurodevelopmental disorders have been proposed. One influential theory, proposed on the basis of neuropathological data by Casanova et al. (2003), is that inhibitory GABA signaling within and between cortical minicolumns is altered due to reductions in the neuropil that separates adjacent minicolumns. This, it is argued, leads to information processing that tends to display stronger-than-normal discrimination between related stimuli rather than generalization across them. This may explain why individuals with ASD show a preference for exact sameness (e.g., the same daily routines, the same behaviors and interests), since only exactly the same stimuli would be recognized as similar. It might also explain sensory hypersensitivities and the occasional presence of superior "savant" skills in a narrow domain.

12.7.2 Gamma-band activity and feature binding

Another model focuses on gamma activity. Evoked gamma band electrical activity (i.e., high frequency >40 Hz) has been extensively studied using EEG and magneto-encephalography (MEG). Theory suggests that these oscillations are produced within the cortex (as opposed to slower waves that likely originate subcortically) and crucially depend on GABA, specifically on fast-spiking parvalbumin-expressing (PV+) cells (Gulyas et al. 2010; Carlen et al. 2011), which act to coordinate the firing of excitatory cortical pyramidal cells. Consistent with this view, a recent study using magnetoencephalography found that occipital cortex GABA levels measured with [1H]MRS correlated with the peak frequency of the visually evoked gamma response in the visual cortex (Muthukumaraswamy et al. 2009)—increased GABA indicates a higher gamma frequency. Another recent MEG study found a similar picture in the motor cortex (Gaetz et al. 2011).

Gamma waves have been proposed as the "temporal solution to the binding problem" (Singer 2001; Brock et al. 2002). The "binding problem" in cognitive neuroscience refers to the question as to how the brain is able to represent conjunctions of features, for example, AB CD, but how does the brain represent the fact that A is paired with B, and C with D, if all are active? The proposed temporal solution is that conjunctions are represented by simultaneous activity over very short timescales, and gamma-band activity is a leading candidate for the "synchronization wave" that does this.

According to some theorists, this temporal binding is impaired in ASD, leading to weak central coherence, that is, impaired gestalt perception of "wholes" as opposed to parts (Brock et al. 2002). While hypothetical at present, this account does offer a possible explanation for how genetic or environmental effects converging on impairments in certain GABA subtypes (particularly parvalbumin+ cells) could precipitate the symptoms of this disorder.

12.7.3 Clinical implications

At present, there are no medications licensed for the *specific* treatment of ASD, fragile X syndrome, or related disorders. A number of psychoactive medications are used for symptomatic relief, for example, antidepressants for obsessive and compulsive symptoms, and atypical antipsychotics for irritability and challenging behaviors (Murray et al. 2014). However, the efficacy and tolerability of such treatments is questionable (Carrasco et al. 2012; Sharma and Shaw 2012) so there is a need for more selective treatments targeted at the pathophysiology of these conditions.

The evidence reviewed here suggests that the GABA system offers a key therapeutic target. Although a full discussion of this issue is outside the scope of this review, the $GABA_B$ agonist arbaclofen (STX209) was shown to help relieve symptoms of fragile X syndrome in a preliminary placebo-controlled trial and also showed benefits in an uncontrolled open-label trial in idiopathic ASD (Erickson et al. 2014). Another drug, acamprosate, acts as a $GABA_A$ agonist and excitatory glutamate antagonist and has similarly been shown to be tolerated and effective in open-label studies (Erickson et al. 2012, 2013). These promising results seem consistent with a GABA hypothesis of ASD symptoms but should be interpreted with caution because of the lack of double-blind, placebo-controlled trials.

12.8 Conclusions

In this review, we have discussed the evidence that autism and related neurodevelopmental disorders are characterized by abnormalities in GABA function. Several converging lines of evidence—from genetics, epigenetics, animal models, and postmortem studies of humans—point to a GABA deficit in autism, fragile X syndrome, and Rett syndrome. Theoretical perspectives that may explain how these neurobiological abnormalities relate to the specific symptoms of these disorders were also discussed.

However, despite the growing interest in the GABA hypothesis of autism and related disorders, there have been very few studies to directly examine the GABA system in the brain of living human patients. Such studies are urgently warranted as, if these abnormalities are present and measurable in humans, this would have important implications both from a purely scientific perspective and also for future drug development.

Other key challenges for the future include understanding how environmental, epigenetic, and genetic factors interact to produce the complex features observed in neurodevelopmental disorders.

Acknowledgments and conflict of interest statement

The author declares no financial conflict of interest. There was no specific source of funding for this work. This chapter is an update of a review paper published in *Neuroscience and Biobehavioral Reviews* (Coghlan et al. 2012). Many thanks to my coauthors on that paper (Suzanne Coghlan, Becky Inkster, M. Andreina Mendez, Declan Murphy, and David Nutt).

References

Adusei, D. C., L. K. Pacey, D. Chen, and D. R. Hampson. 2010. Early developmental alterations in GABAergic protein expression in fragile X knockout mice. *Neuropharmacology* 59:167–71.

Akbarian, S., R. Z. Chen, J. Gribnau, T. P. Rasmussen, H. Fong, R. Jaenisch, and E. G. Jones. 2001. Expression pattern of the Rett syndrome gene MeCP2 in primate prefrontal cortex. *Neurobiol. Dis.* 8:784–91.

Al Ageeli, E., S. Drunat, C. Delanoe et al. 2014. Duplication of the 15q11–q13 region: Clinical and genetic study of 30 new cases. *Eur. J. Med. Genet.* 57:5–14.

American Psychiatric Association. 2000. *Diagnostic and Statistical Manual of Mental Disorders: DSM-IV-TR*. Washington, DC: American Psychiatric Association.

American Psychiatric Association. 2013. *Diagnostic and Statistical Manual of Mental Disorders (DSM-V)*. Washington, DC: American Psychiatric Association.

Bailey, A., P. Luthert, A. Dean, B. Harding, I. Janota, M. Montgomery, M. Rutter, and P. Lantos. 1998. A clinicopathological study of autism. *Brain* 121:889–905.

Baron-Cohen, S., F. J. Scott, C. Allison, J. Williams, P. Bolton, F. E. Matthews, and C. Brayne. 2009. Prevalence of autism-spectrum conditions: UK school-based population study. *Br. J. Psychiatry* 194:500–9.

Beaumont, M. and G. Maccaferri. 2011. Is connexin36 critical for GABAergic hyper-synchronization in the hippocampus? *J. Physiol.* 589:1663–80.

Bettler, B., K. Kaupmann, J. Mosbacher, and M. Gassmann. 2004. Molecular structure and physiological functions of GABA(B) receptors. *Physiol. Rev.* 84:835–67.

Bishop, S., S. Gahagan, and C. Lord. 2007. Re-examining the core features of autism: A comparison of autism spectrum disorder and fetal alcohol spectrum disorder. *J. Child Psychol. Psychiatry* 48:1111–21.

Blatt, G. J., C. M. Fitzgerald, J. T. Guptill, A. B. Booker, T. L. Kemper, and M. L. Bauman. 2001. Density and distribution of hippocampal neurotransmitter receptors in autism: An autoradiographic study. *J. Autism Dev. Disord.* 31:537–43.

Blue, M. E., S. Naidu, and M. V. Johnston. 1999a. Altered development of glutamate and GABA receptors in the basal ganglia of girls with Rett syndrome. *Exp. Neurol.* 156:345–52.

Blue, M. E., S. Naidu, and M. V. Johnston. 1999b. Development of amino acid receptors in frontal cortex from girls with Rett syndrome. *Ann. Neurol.* 45:541–5.

Bolton, P. F., I. Carcani-Rathwell, J. Hutton, S. Goode, P. Howlin, and M. Rutter. 2011. Epilepsy in autism: Features and correlates. *Br. J. Psychiatry* 198:289–94.

Bowery, N. G., B. Bettler, W. Froestl, J. P. Gallagher, F. Marshall, M. Raiteri, T. I. Bonner, and S. J. Enna. 2002. International Union of Pharmacology. XXXIII. Mammalian gamma-aminobutyric acid(B) receptors: Structure and function. *Pharmacol. Rev.* 54:247–64.

Brennand, K. J., A. Simone, J. Jou et al. 2011. Modelling schizophrenia using human induced pluripotent stem cells. *Nature* 473:221–5.

Brock, J., C. C. Brown, J. Boucher, and G. Rippon. 2002. The temporal binding deficit hypothesis of autism. *Dev. Psychopathol.* 14:209–24.

Brugha, T. S., S. McManus, J. Bankart, F. Scott, S. Purdon, J. Smith, P. Bebbington, R. Jenkins, and H. Meltzer. 2011. Epidemiology of autism spectrum disorders in adults in the community in England. *Arch. Gen. Psychiatry* 68:459–65.

Carlen, M., K. Meletis, J. H. Siegle et al. 2011. A critical role for NMDA receptors in parvalbumin interneurons for gamma rhythm induction and behavior. *Mol. Psychiatry* 17:537–48.

Carrasco, M., F. R. Volkmar, and M. H. Bloch. 2012. Pharmacologic treatment of repetitive behaviors in autism spectrum disorders: Evidence of publication bias. *Pediatrics* 129:e1301–10.

Casanova, M. F., D. Buxhoeveden, and J. Gomez. 2003. Disruption in the inhibitory architecture of the cell minicolumn: Implications for autism. *Neuroscientist* 9:496–507.

Centonze, D., S. Rossi, V. Mercaldo et al. 2008. Abnormal striatal GABA transmission in the mouse model for the fragile X syndrome. *Biol. Psychiatry* 63:963–73.

Chao, H. T., H. Chen, R. C. Samaco et al. 2010. Dysfunction in GABA signalling mediates autism-like stereotypies and Rett syndrome phenotypes. *Nature* 468:263–9.

Chudley, A. E., J. Conry, J. L. Cook, C. Loock, T. Rosales, and N. LeBlanc. 2005. Fetal alcohol spectrum disorder: Canadian guidelines for diagnosis. *CMAJ* 172:S1–S21.

Clifford, S., C. Dissanayake, Q. M. Bui, R. Huggins, A. K. Taylor, and D. Z. Loesch. 2007. Autism spectrum phenotype in males and females with fragile X full mutation and premutation. *J. Autism Dev. Disord.* 37:738–47.

Cochran, D. M., E. M. Sikoglu, S. M. Hodge, R. A. Edden, A. Foley, D. N. Kennedy, C. M. Moore, and J. A. Frazier. 2015. Relationship among glutamine, gamma-aminobutyric acid, and social cognition in autism spectrum disorders. *J. Child Adolesc. Psychopharmacol.* 25:314–22.

Coghlan, S., J. Horder, B. Inkster, M. A. Mendez, D. G. Murphy, and D. J. Nutt. 2012. GABA system dysfunction in autism and related disorders: From synapse to symptoms. *Neurosci. Biobehav. Rev.* 36:2044–55.

Collinson, N., J. R. Atack, P. Laughton, G. R. Dawson, and D. N. Stephens. 2006. An inverse agonist selective for alpha5 subunit-containing GABAA receptors improves encoding and recall but not consolidation in the Morris water maze. *Psychopharmacology (Berl).* 188:619–28.

Colvert, E., B. Tick, F. McEwen et al. 2015. Heritability of autism spectrum disorder in a UK population-based twin sample. *JAMA Psychiatry* 72:415–23.

Constantino, J. N., A. Todorov, C. Hilton, P. Law, Y. Zhang, E. Molloy, R. Fitzgerald, and D. Geschwind. 2013. Autism recurrence in half siblings: Strong support for genetic mechanisms of transmission in ASD. *Mol Psychiatry* 18:137–8.

Cook, E. H., Jr., R. Y. Courchesne, N. J. Cox et al. 1998. Linkage-disequilibrium mapping of autistic disorder, with 15q11–13 markers. *Am. J. Hum. Genet.* 62:1077–83.

Curia, G., T. Papouin, P. Seguela, and M. Avoli. 2009. Downregulation of tonic GABAergic inhibition in a mouse model of fragile X syndrome. *Cereb. Cortex* 19:1515–20.

D'Antuono, M., D. Merlo, and M. Avoli. 2003. Involvement of cholinergic and GABAergic systems in the fragile X knockout mice. *Neuroscience* 119:9–13.

D'Hulst, C., N. De Geest, S. P. Reeve, D. Van Dam, P. P. De Deyn, B. A. Hassan, and R. F. Kooy. 2006. Decreased expression of the GABAA receptor in fragile X syndrome. *Brain Res.* 1121:238–45.

D'Hulst, C., I. Heulens, J. R. Brouwer, R. Willemsen, N. De Geest, S. P. Reeve, P. P. De Deyn, B. A. Hassan, and R. F. Kooy. 2009. Expression of the GABAergic system in animal models for fragile X syndrome and fragile X associated tremor/ataxia syndrome (FXTAS). *Brain Res.* 1253:176–83.

Danielsson, B. R., A. C. Skold, and F. Azarbayjani. 2001. Class III antiarrhythmics and phenytoin: Teratogenicity due to embryonic cardiac dysrhythmia and reoxygenation damage. *Curr. Pharm. Des.* 7:787–802.

Darnell, J. C., S. J. Van Driesche, C. Zhang et al. 2011. FMRP stalls ribosomal translocation on mRNAs linked to synaptic function and autism. *Cell* 146:247–61.

De Marco Garcia, N. V., T. Karayannis, and G. Fishell. 2011. Neuronal activity is required for the development of specific cortical interneuron subtypes. *Nature.* 472:351–5.

De Rubeis, S., X. He, A. P. Goldberg et al. 2014. Synaptic, transcriptional and chromatin genes disrupted in autism. *Nature* 515:209–15.

Delahanty, R. J., J. Q. Kang, C. W. Brune, E. O. Kistner, E. Courchesne, N. J. Cox, E. H. Cook, Jr., R. L. Macdonald, and J. S. Sutcliffe. 2009. Maternal transmission of a rare GABRB3 signal peptide variant is associated with autism. *Mol. Psychiatry* 16:89–96.

Dhossche, D., H. Applegate, A. Abraham, P. Maertens, L. Bland, A. Bencsath, and J. Martinez. 2002. Elevated plasma gamma-aminobutyric acid (GABA) levels in autistic youngsters: Stimulus for a GABA hypothesis of autism. *Med. Sci. Monit.* 8:PR1–6.

Dictenberg, J. B., S. A. Swanger, L. N. Antar, R. H. Singer, and G. J. Bassell. 2008. A direct role for FMRP in activity-dependent dendritic mRNA transport links filopodial-spine morphogenesis to fragile X syndrome. *Dev. Cell* 14:926–39.

Dufour-Rainfray, D., P. Vourc'h, S. Tourlet, D. Guilloteau, S. Chalon, and C. R. Andres. 2011. Fetal exposure to teratogens: Evidence of genes involved in autism. *Neurosci. Biobehav. Rev.* 35:1254–65.

Durant, C., D. Christmas, and D. Nutt. 2011. The pharmacology of anxiety. *Curr. Top. Behav. Neurosci.* 2:303–30.

Eagleson, K. L., M. C. Gravielle, L. J. Schlueter McFadyen-Ketchum, S. J. Russek, D. H. Farb, and P. Levitt. 2011. Genetic disruption of the autism spectrum disorder risk gene PLAUR induces GABAA receptor subunit changes. *Neuroscience* 168:797–810.

Edden, R. A., N. A. Puts, and P. B. Barker. 2012. Macromolecule-suppressed GABA-edited magnetic resonance spectroscopy at 3 T. *Magn. Reson. Med.* 68:657–61.

El Idrissi, A., X. H. Ding, J. Scalia, E. Trenkner, W. T. Brown, and C. Dobkin. 2005. Decreased GABA(A) receptor expression in the seizure-prone fragile X mouse. *Neurosci. Lett.* 377:141–6.

El-Ansary, A. K., A. B. Bacha, and L. Y. Ayahdi. 2011. Relationship between chronic lead toxicity and plasma neurotransmitters in autistic patients from Saudi Arabia. *Clin. Biochem.* 44:1116–20.

Enticott, P. G., H. A. Kennedy, N. J. Rinehart, B. J. Tonge, J. L. Bradshaw, and P. B. Fitzgerald. 2013. GABAergic activity in autism spectrum disorders: An investigation of cortical inhibition via transcranial magnetic stimulation. *Neuropharmacology* 68:202–9.

Enticott, P. G., N. J. Rinehart, B. J. Tonge, J. L. Bradshaw, and P. B. Fitzgerald. 2010. A preliminary transcranial magnetic stimulation study of cortical inhibition and excitability in high-functioning autism and Asperger disorder. *Dev. Med. Child Neurol.* 52:e179–83.

Erickson, C. A., M. Early, K. A. Stigler, L. K. Wink, J. E. Mullett, and C. J. McDougle. 2012. An open-label naturalistic pilot study of acamprosate in youth with autistic disorder. *J. Child Adolesc. Psychopharmacol.* 21:565–9.

Erickson, C. A., J. M. Veenstra-Vanderweele, R. D. Melmed et al. 2014. STX209 (arbaclofen) for autism spectrum disorders: An 8-week open-label study. *J. Autism Dev. Disord.* 44:958–64.

Erickson, C. A., L. K. Wink, B. Ray, M. C. Early, E. Stiegelmeyer, L. Mathieu-Frasier, V. Patrick, D. K. Lahiri, and C. J. McDougle. 2013. Impact of acamprosate on behavior and brain-derived neurotrophic factor: An open-label study in youth with fragile X syndrome. *Psychopharmacology (Berl).* 228:75–84.

Fagiolini, M., J. M. Fritschy, K. Low, H. Mohler, U. Rudolph, and T. K. Hensch. 2004. Specific GABAA circuits for visual cortical plasticity. *Science* 303:1681–3.

Farzan, F., M. S. Barr, A. J. Levinson, R. Chen, W. Wong, P. B. Fitzgerald, and Z. J. Daskalakis. 2011. Reliability of long-interval cortical inhibition in healthy human subjects: A TMS-EEG study. *J. Neurophysiol.* 104:1339–46.

Fatemi, S. H., T. D. Folsom, R. E. Kneeland, and S. B. Liesch. 2011. Metabotropic glutamate receptor 5 upregulation in children with autism is associated with underexpression of both fragile X mental retardation protein and GABAA receptor beta 3 in adults with autism. *Anat. Rec. (Hoboken)* 294:1635–45.

Fatemi, S. H., A. R. Halt, J. M. Stary, R. Kanodia, S. C. Schulz, and G. R. Realmuto. 2002. Glutamic acid decarboxylase 65 and 67 kDa proteins are reduced in autistic parietal and cerebellar cortices. *Biol. Psychiatry* 52:805–10.

Fernandez, F., W. Morishita, E. Zuniga, J. Nguyen, M. Blank, R. C. Malenka, and C. C. Garner. 2007. Pharmacotherapy for cognitive impairment in a mouse model of Down syndrome. *Nat. Neurosci.* 10:411–3.

Feuk, L., A. R. Carson, and S. W. Scherer. 2006. Structural variation in the human genome. *Nat. Rev. Genet.* 7:85–97.

Gaetz, W., L. Bloy, D. J. Wang, R. G. Port, L. Blaskey, S. E. Levy, and T. P. Roberts. 2014. GABA estimation in the brains of children on the autism spectrum: Measurement precision and regional cortical variation. *Neuroimage* 86:1–9.

Gaetz, W., J. C. Edgar, D. J. Wang, and T. P. Roberts. 2011. Relating MEG measured motor cortical oscillations to resting γ-aminobutyric acid (GABA) concentration. *Neuroimage* 55:616–21.

Gandal, M. J., J. C. Edgar, R. S. Ehrlichman, M. Mehta, T. P. Roberts, and S. J. Siegel. 2010. Validating γ oscillations and delayed auditory responses as translational biomarkers of autism. *Biol. Psychiatry* 68:1100–6.

Gasnier, B. 2004. The SLC32 transporter, a key protein for the synaptic release of inhibitory amino acids. *Pflugers. Arch.* 447:756–9.

Gogolla, N., J. J. Leblanc, K. B. Quast, T. Sudhof, M. Fagiolini, and T. K. Hensch. 2009. Common circuit defect of excitatory-inhibitory balance in mouse models of autism. *J. Neurodev. Disord.* 1:172–81.

Gruss, M. and K. Braun. 2001. Alterations of amino acids and monoamine metabolism in male Fmr1 knockout mice: A putative animal model of the human fragile X mental retardation syndrome. *Neural. Plast.* 8:285–98.

Gulyas, A. I., G. G. Szabo, I. Ulbert, N. Holderith, H. Monyer, G. Erdelyi, G. Szabo, T. F. Freund, and N. Hajos. 2010. Parvalbumin-containing fast-spiking basket cells generate the field potential oscillations induced by cholinergic receptor activation in the hippocampus. *J. Neurosci.* 30:15134–45.

Harada, M., M. M. Taki, A. Nose, H. Kubo, K. Mori, H. Nishitani, and T. Matsuda. 2011. Non-invasive evaluation of the GABAergic/glutamatergic system in autistic patients observed by MEGA-editing proton MR spectroscopy using a clinical 3 tesla instrument. *J. Autism. Dev. Disord.* 41:447–54.

Hogart, A., R. P. Nagarajan, K. A. Patzel, D. H. Yasui, and J. M. Lasalle. 2007. 15q11–13 GABA$_A$ receptor genes are normally biallelically expressed in brain yet are subject to epigenetic dysregulation in autism-spectrum disorders. *Hum. Mol. Genet.* 16:691–703.

Holmes, L. B., E. A. Harvey, B. A. Coull, K. B. Huntington, S. Khoshbin, A. M. Hayes, and L. M. Ryan. 2001. The teratogenicity of anticonvulsant drugs. *N. Engl. J. Med.* 344:1132–8.

Hong, A., A. Zhang, Y. Ke, A. El Idrissi, and C. H. Shen. 2011. Downregulation of GABA$_A$ β subunits is transcriptionally controlled by Fmr1p. *J. Mol. Neurosci.* 46:272–5.

Horder, J., T. Lavender, M. A. Mendez, R. O'Gorman, E. Daly, M. C. Craig, D. J. Lythgoe, G. J. Barker, and D. G. Murphy. 2013. Reduced subcortical glutamate/glutamine in adults with autism spectrum disorders: A [(1)H]MRS study. *Transl. Psychiatry* 3:e279.

Horton, R. W. and B. S. Meldrum. 1973. Seizures induced by allylglycine, 3-mercaptopropionic acid and 4-deoxypyridoxine in mice and photosensitive baboons, and different modes of inhibition of cerebral glutamic acid decarboxylase. *Br. J. Pharmacol.* 49:52–63.

Huguet, G., E. Ey, and T. Bourgeron. 2013. The genetic landscapes of autism spectrum disorders. *Annu. Rev. Genomics. Hum. Genet.* 14:191–213.

Ingram, J. L., S. M. Peckham, B. Tisdale, and P. M. Rodier. 2000. Prenatal exposure of rats to valproic acid reproduces the cerebellar anomalies associated with autism. *Neurotoxicol. Teratol.* 22:319–24.

Iossifov, I., M. Ronemus, D. Levy et al. 2012. De novo gene disruptions in children on the autistic spectrum. *Neuron* 74:285–99.

Jian, L., L. Nagarajan, N. de Klerk, D. Ravine, C. Bower, A. Anderson, S. Williamson, J. Christodoulou, and H. Leonard. 2006. Predictors of seizure onset in Rett syndrome. *J. Pediatr.* 149:542–7.

Kenny, E. M., P. Cormican, S. Furlong et al. 2015. Excess of rare novel loss-of-function variants in synaptic genes in schizophrenia and autism spectrum disorders. *Mol. Psychiatry* 19:872–9.

Kim, K. C., P. Kim, H. S. Go, C. S. Choi, S. I. Yang, J. H. Cheong, C. Y. Shin, and K. H. Ko. 2011. The critical period of valproate exposure to induce autistic symptoms in Sprague-Dawley rats. *Toxicol. Lett.* 201:137–42.

Knoll, J. H., R. D. Nicholls, R. E. Magenis, J. M. Graham, Jr., M. Lalande, and S. A. Latt. 1989. Angelman and Prader-Willi syndromes share a common chromosome 15 deletion but differ in parental origin of the deletion. *Am. J. Med. Genet.* 32:285–90.

Ko, J., G. Choii, and J. W. Um. 2015. The balancing act of GABAergic synapse organizers. *Trends Mol. Med.* 21:256–68.

Kumar, S., P. Porcu, D. F. Werner, D. B. Matthews, J. L. Diaz-Granados, R. S. Helfand, and A. L. Morrow. 2009. The role of GABA(A) receptors in the acute and chronic effects of ethanol: A decade of progress. *Psychopharmacology (Berl).* 205:529–64.

Laggerbauer, B., D. Ostareck, E. M. Keidel, A. Ostareck-Lederer, and U. Fischer. 2001. Evidence that fragile X mental retardation protein is a negative regulator of translation. *Hum. Mol. Genet.* 10:329–38.

Landgren, M., L. Svensson, K. Stromland, and M. Andersson Gronlund. 2011. Prenatal alcohol exposure and neurodevelopmental disorders in children adopted from Eastern Europe. *Pediatrics* 125:e1178–85.

Levenga, J., S. Hayashi, F. M. de Vrij et al. 2011. AFQ056, a new mGluR5 antagonist for treatment of fragile X syndrome. *Neurobiol. Dis.* 42:311–7.

Lingford-Hughes, A., A. G. Reid, J. Myers et al. 2010. A [11C]Ro15 4513 PET study suggests that alcohol dependence in man is associated with reduced {alpha}5 benzodiazepine receptors in limbic regions. *J. Psychopharmacol.* 26:273–81.

Ma, D. Q., P. L. Whitehead, M. M. Menold et al. 2005. Identification of significant association and gene-gene interaction of GABA receptor subunit genes in autism. *Am. J. Hum. Genet.* 77:377–88.

Macdonald, R. L., J. Q. Kang, and M. J. Gallagher. 2010. Mutations in GABAA receptor subunits associated with genetic epilepsies. *J. Physiol.* 588:1861–9.

Madsen, K. K., R. P. Clausen, O. M. Larsson, P. Krogsgaard-Larsen, A. Schousboe, and H. S. White. 2009. Synaptic and extrasynaptic GABA transporters as targets for anti-epileptic drugs. *J. Neurochem.* 109(Suppl. 1):139–44.

Madsen, K. K., O. M. Larsson, and A. Schousboe. 2008. Regulation of excitation by GABA neurotransmission: Focus on metabolism and transport. *Results Probl. Cell. Differ.* 44:201–21.

McKernan, R. M., T. W. Rosahl, D. S. Reynolds et al. 2000. Sedative but not anxiolytic properties of benzodiazepines are mediated by the GABA(A) receptor alpha1 subtype. *Nat. Neurosci.* 3:587–92.

Medrihan, L., E. Tantalaki, G. Aramuni, V. Sargsyan, I. Dudanova, M. Missler, and W. Zhang. 2008. Early defects of GABAergic synapses in the brain stem of a MeCP2 mouse model of Rett syndrome. *J. Neurophysiol.* 99:112–21.

Meguro-Horike, M., D. H. Yasui, W. Powell, D. I. Schroeder, M. Oshimura, J. M. Lasalle, and S. I. Horike. 2011. Neuron-specific impairment of inter-chromosomal pairing and transcription in a novel model of human 15q-duplication syndrome. *Hum. Mol. Genet.* 20:3798–810.

Mendez, M. A., J. Horder, J. Myers, S. Coghlan, P. Stokes, D. Erritzoe, O. D. Howes, A. Lingford-Hughes, D. G. Murphy, and D. J. Nutt. 2013. The brain GABA-benzodiazepine receptor alpha-5 subtype in autism spectrum disorder: A pilot [11C]Ro15-4513 positron emission tomography study. *Neuropharmacology* 68:195–201.

Mohler, H. 2006. GABA(A) receptor diversity and pharmacology. *Cell Tissue Res.* 326:505–16.

Moore, S. J., P. Turnpenny, A. Quinn, S. Glover, D. J. Lloyd, T. Montgomery, and J. C. Dean. 2000. A clinical study of 57 children with fetal anticonvulsant syndromes. *J. Med. Genet.* 37:489–97.

Mori, T., K. Mori, E. Fujii, Y. Toda, M. Miyazaki, M. Harada, T. Hashimoto, and S. Kagami. 2012. Evaluation of the GABAergic nervous system in autistic brain: 123I-iomazenil SPECT study. *Brain Dev.* 34:648–54.

Murray, M. L., Y. Hsia, K. Glaser, E. Simonoff, D. G. Murphy, P. J. Asherson, H. Eklund, and I. C. Wong. 2014. Pharmacological treatments prescribed to people with autism spectrum disorder (ASD) in primary health care. *Psychopharmacology (Berl).* 231:1011–21.

Muthukumaraswamy, S. D., R. A. Edden, D. K. Jones, J. B. Swettenham, and K. D. Singh. 2009. Resting GABA concentration predicts peak gamma frequency and fMRI amplitude in response to visual stimulation in humans. *Proc. Natl. Acad. Sci. USA* 106:8356–61.

Neale, B. M., Y. Kou, L. Liu et al. 2012. Patterns and rates of exonic *de novo* mutations in autism spectrum disorders. *Nature* 485:242–5.

Nord, A. S., W. Roeb, D. E. Dickel et al. 2011. Reduced transcript expression of genes affected by inherited and *de novo* CNVs in autism. *Eur. J. Hum. Genet.* 19:727–31.

Nutt, D. J. and A. L. Malizia. 2001. New insights into the role of the GABA(A)-benzodiazepine receptor in psychiatric disorder. *Br. J. Psychiatry* 179: 390–6.

O'Roak, B. J., H. A. Stessman, E. A. Boyle et al. 2014. Recurrent *de novo* mutations implicate novel genes underlying simplex autism risk. *Nat. Commun.* 5:5595.

Oberman, L., F. Ifert-Miller, U. Najib, S. Bashir, I. Woollacott, J. Gonzalez-Heydrich, J. Picker, A. Rotenberg, and A. Pascual-Leone. 2011. Transcranial magnetic stimulation provides means to assess cortical plasticity and excitability in humans with fragile x syndrome and autism spectrum disorder. *Front Synaptic. Neurosci.* 2:26.

Oblak, A., T. T. Gibbs, and G. J. Blatt. 2009. Decreased GABAA receptors and benzodiazepine binding sites in the anterior cingulate cortex in autism. *Autism Res.* 2:205–19.

Oblak, A. L., T. T. Gibbs, and G. J. Blatt. 2010. Reduced GABA(A) receptors and benzodiazepine binding sites in the posterior cingulate cortex and fusiform gyrus in autism. *Brain Res.* 1380:218–28.

Oliver, C., K. Berg, J. Moss, K. Arron, and C. Burbidge. 2011. Delineation of behavioral phenotypes in genetic syndromes: Characteristics of autism spectrum disorder, affect and hyperactivity. *J. Autism Dev. Disord.* 41:1019–32.

Olmos-Serrano, J. L., S. M. Paluszkiewicz, B. S. Martin, W. E. Kaufmann, J. G. Corbin, and M. M. Huntsman. 2010. Defective GABAergic neurotransmission and pharmacological rescue of neuronal hyperexcitability in the amygdala in a mouse model of fragile X syndrome. *J. Neurosci.* 30:9929–38.

Pacey, L. K., S. P. Heximer, and D. R. Hampson. 2009. Increased GABA(B) receptor-mediated signaling reduces the susceptibility of fragile X knockout mice to audiogenic seizures. *Mol. Pharmacol.* 76:18–24.

Palmen, S. J., H. van Engeland, P. R. Hof, and C. Schmitz. 2004. Neuropathological findings in autism. *Brain* 127:2572–83.

Paluszkiewicz, S. M., J. L. Olmos-Serrano, J. G. Corbin, and M. M. Huntsman. 2011. Impaired inhibitory control of cortical synchronization in fragile X syndrome. *J. Neurophysiol.* 106:2264–72.

Pasca, S. P., T. Portmann, I. Voineagu et al. 2011. Using iPSC-derived neurons to uncover cellular phenotypes associated with Timothy syndrome. *Nat. Med.* 17:1657–62.

Penagarikano, O., B. S. Abrahams, E. I. Herman et al. 2011. Absence of CNTNAP2 leads to epilepsy, neuronal migration abnormalities, and core autism-related deficits. *Cell* 147:235–46.

Perry, T. L., H. G. Dunn, H. H. Ho, and J. U. Crichton. 1988. Cerebrospinal fluid values for monoamine metabolites, gamma-aminobutyric acid, and other amino compounds in Rett syndrome. *J. Pediatr.* 112:234–8.

Portera-Cailliau, C. 2012. Which comes first in fragile X syndrome, dendritic spine dysgenesis or defects in circuit plasticity? *Neuroscientist* 18:28–44.

Purcell, A. E., O. H. Jeon, A. W. Zimmerman, M. E. Blue, and J. Pevsner. 2001. Postmortem brain abnormalities of the glutamate neurotransmitter system in autism. *Neurology* 57:1618–28.

Rasalam, A. D., H. Hailey, J. H. Williams, S. J. Moore, P. D. Turnpenny, D. J. Lloyd, and J. C. Dean. 2005. Characteristics of fetal anticonvulsant syndrome associated autistic disorder. *Dev. Med. Child Neurol.* 47:551–5.

Renieri, A., I. Meloni, I. Longo, F. Ariani, C. Mari, C. Pescucci, and F. Cambi. 2003. Rett syndrome: The complex nature of a monogenic disease. *J. Mol. Med.* 81:346–54.

Riley, E. P. and C. L. McGee. 2005. Fetal alcohol spectrum disorders: An overview with emphasis on changes in brain and behavior. *Exp. Biol. Med. (Maywood)* 230:357–65.

Rojas, D. C., D. Singel, S. Steinmetz, S. Hepburn, and M. S. Brown. 2013. Decreased left perisylvian GABA concentration in children with autism and unaffected siblings. *Neuroimage* 86:28–34.

Rolf, L. H., F. Y. Haarmann, K. H. Grotemeyer, and H. Kehrer. 1993. Serotonin and amino acid content in platelets of autistic children. *Acta. Psychiatr. Scand.* 87:312–6.

Rothman, D. L., O. A. Petroff, K. L. Behar, and R. H. Mattson. 1993. Localized 1H NMR measurements of gamma-aminobutyric acid in human brain *in vivo*. *Proc. Natl. Acad. Sci. USA* 90:5662–6.

Rudolph, U. and H. Mohler. 2004. Analysis of GABAA receptor function and dissection of the pharmacology of benzodiazepines and general anesthetics through mouse genetics. *Annu. Rev. Pharmacol. Toxicol.* 44:475–98.

Russell, G., L. R. Rodgers, O. C. Ukoumunne, and T. Ford. 2013. Prevalence of parent-reported ASD and ADHD in the UK: Findings from the millennium cohort study. *J. Autism. Dev. Disord.* 44(1):31–40.

Rutter, M. 1978. Diagnosis and definition of childhood autism. *J. Autism. Child Schizophr.* 8:139–61.

Rutter, M. 1983. Cognitive deficits in the pathogenesis of autism. *J. Child Psychol. Psychiatry* 24:513–31.

Sadakata, T., M. Washida, Y. Iwayama et al. 2007. Autistic-like phenotypes in Cadps2-knockout mice and aberrant CADPS2 splicing in autistic patients. *J. Clin. Invest.* 117:931–43.

Samaco, R. C., A. Hogart, and J. M. LaSalle. 2005. Epigenetic overlap in autism-spectrum neurodevelopmental disorders: MECP2 deficiency causes reduced expression of UBE3A and GABRB3. *Hum. Mol. Genet.* 14:483–92.

Schneider, T. and R. Przewlocki. 2005. Behavioral alterations in rats prenatally exposed to valproic acid: Animal model of autism. *Neuropsychopharmacology* 30:80–9.

Selby, L., C. Zhang, and Q. Q. Sun. 2007. Major defects in neocortical GABAergic inhibitory circuits in mice lacking the fragile X mental retardation protein. *Neurosci. Lett.* 412:227–32.

Sharma, A. and S. R. Shaw. 2012. Efficacy of risperidone in managing maladaptive behaviors for children with autistic spectrum disorder: A meta-analysis. *J. Pediatr. Health Care* 26:291–9.

Sibilla, S. and L. Ballerini. 2009. GABAergic and glycinergic interneuron expression during spinal cord development: Dynamic interplay between inhibition and excitation in the control of ventral network outputs. *Prog. Neurobiol.* 89:46–60.

Simon, E. W., B. Haas-Givler, and B. Finucane. 2009. A longitudinal follow-up study of autistic symptoms in children and adults with duplications of 15q11-13. *Am. J. Med. Genet. B. Neuropsychiatr. Genet.* 153B:463–7.

Singer, W. 2001. Consciousness and the binding problem. *Ann. NY Acad. Sci.* 929:123–46.

Smith, Q. R. 2000. Transport of glutamate and other amino acids at the blood-brain barrier. *J. Nutr.* 130:1016S-22S.

Stagg, C. J., S. Bestmann, A. O. Constantinescu, L. Moreno Moreno, C. Allman, R. Mekle, M. Woolrich, J. Near, H. Johansen-Berg, and J. C. Rothwell. 2011. Relationship between physiological measures of excitability and levels of glutamate and GABA in the human motor cortex. *J. Physiol.* 589:5845–55.

Stein, M. B., B. Z. Yang, D. A. Chavira, C. A. Hitchcock, S. C. Sung, E. Shipon-Blum, and J. Gelernter. 2011. A common genetic variant in the neurexin superfamily member *CNTNAP2* is associated with increased risk for selective mutism and social anxiety-related traits. *Biol. Psychiatry* 69:825–31.

Tamamaki, N. and R. Tomioka. 2010. Long-range GABAergic connections distributed throughout the neocortex and their possible function. *Front. Neurosci.* 4:202.

Thanseem, I., A. Anitha, K. Nakamura et al. 2012. Elevated transcription factor specificity protein 1 in autistic brains alters the expression of autism candidate genes. *Biol. Psychiatry* 71:410–8.

Turner, G., T. Webb, S. Wake, and H. Robinson. 1996. Prevalence of fragile X syndrome. *Am. J Med. Genet.* 64:196–7.

Vellucci, S. V. and R. A. Webster. 1984. The role of GABA in the anticonflict action of sodium valproate and chlordiazepoxide. *Pharmacol. Biochem. Behav.* 21:845–51.

Voineagu, I., X. Wang, P. Johnston, J. K. Lowe, Y. Tian, S. Horvath, J. Mill, R. M. Cantor, B. J. Blencowe, and D. H. Geschwind. 2011. Transcriptomic analysis of autistic brain reveals convergent molecular pathology. *Nature* 474:380–4.

Wang, L. W., E. Berry-Kravis, and R. J. Hagerman. 2010. Fragile X: Leading the way for targeted treatments in autism. *Neurotherapeutics* 7:264–74.

Whitehouse, A. J. O., D. V. M. Bishop, Q. W. Ang, C. E. Pennell, and S. E. Fisher. 2011. *CNTNAP2* variants affect early language development in the general population. *Genes Brain Behav.* 10:451–6.

Whitney, E. R., T. L. Kemper, M. L. Bauman, D. L. Rosene, and G. J. Blatt. 2008. Cerebellar Purkinje cells are reduced in a subpopulation of autistic brains: A stereological experiment using calbindin-D28k. *Cerebellum* 7:406–16.

Wisniewski, K. E., S. M. Segan, C. M. Miezejeski, E. A. Sersen, and R. D. Rudelli. 1991. The Fra(X) syndrome: Neurological, electrophysiological, and neuropathological abnormalities. *Am. J. Med. Genet.* 38:476–80.

World Health Organization. 1993. *ICD-10 International Statistical Classification of Diseases and Related Health Problems.* Geneva: World Health Organization.

Xu, G., K. G. Broadbelt, R. L. Haynes, R. D. Folkerth, N. S. Borenstein, R. A. Belliveau, F. L. Trachtenberg, J. J. Volpe, and H. C. Kinney. 2011. Late development of the GABAergic system in the human cerebral cortex and white matter. *J. Neuropathol. Exp. Neurol.* 70:841–58.

Yamashita, Y., T. Matsuishi, M. Ishibashi, A. Kimura, Y. Onishi, Y. Yonekura, and H. Kato. 1998. Decrease in benzodiazepine receptor binding in the brains of adult patients with Rett syndrome. *J. Neurol. Sci.* 154:146–50.

Yip, J., J. J. Soghomonian, and G. J. Blatt. 2007. Decreased GAD67 mRNA levels in cerebellar Purkinje cells in autism: Pathophysiological implications. *Acta. Neuropathol.* 113:559–68.

Zhang, Z. W., J. D. Zak, and H. Liu. 2010. MeCP2 is required for normal development of GABAergic circuits in the thalamus. *J. Neurophysiol.* 103:2470–81.

Chapter 13 Imaging brain connectivity in autism spectrum disorder

Robert Coben, Iman Mohammad-Rezazadeh, Joel Frohlich, Joseph Jurgiel, and Giorgia Michelini

Contents

Abstract 246
13.1 Autism and the importance of brain connectivity 246
13.2 Review of findings in brain connectivity and autism 249
    13.2.1 Structural connectivity studies 249
    13.2.2 Functional and effective connectivity studies 251
        13.2.2.1 Resting-state studies 252
        13.2.2.2 Task-based studies 253
13.3 How to characterize brain networks 255
13.4 Connectivity explanation 258
13.5 Measuring functional or effective connectivity with
    graph theory methods 259
13.6 Measuring effective connectivity with Granger causality 263
    13.6.1 Definition 264
    13.6.2 Mathematical form of GC 265
    13.6.3 Conditional Granger causality 265
    13.6.4 Granger causality limitations 266
13.7 Imaging GC connectivity in cases with autism spectrum
    disorder 266
    13.7.1 Results 267
        13.7.1.1 Case 1 267
        13.7.1.2 Case 2 270
        13.7.1.3 Discussion 272
13.8 Clinical applications 273
    13.8.1 Treatment case 274
13.9 Future directions 276
References 277

Abstract

Autism spectrum disorder (ASD) has a strongly neurobiological component. While the search for single brain structures to explain the symptoms of ASD has been ineffective, research over the past decade has shown that there are strong indicators for neural connectivity anomalies that do relate to the challenges that these persons face. Information is presented regarding types of connectivity with effective connectivity being the goal in the assessment of ASD-related difficulties. Using a graph theory model, we explore aspects of connectivity and its assessment related to ASD. The measure of effective connectivity with EEG technology along with the use of Granger causality is presented as a means of producing connectivity estimates that are auto-regressive, predictive and demonstrate causal and reciprocal influences across multiple brain regions. Several case studies are presented with their graphical findings to demonstrate the use and utility of this approach in the understanding of brain mechanisms impacting ASD.

13.1 Autism and the importance of brain connectivity

Autism spectrum disorders are highly heritable neurodevelopmental disorders characterized by a strong neurobiological component (Willsey and State 2015; Tick et al. 2016). Much research has sought to understand the neurobiological underpinnings of ASD through the identification of biological markers (biomarkers), representing objective measures which may lead to a more refined diagnosis and targeted treatment (Kapur et al. 2012; Loo et al. 2015). The predominant role of neurobiological factors in the etiopathogenesis of ASD is indicated by evidence of associations between ASD and genetic variants expressed in the brain (Sanders 2015; Warrier et al. 2015) and abnormalities in brain activity in individuals with ASD compared to typically developing (TD) persons (Di Martino et al. 2009; Jeste 2011; Lefebvre et al. 2015). Importantly, many of the genes that have been implicated in ASD influence synaptic pathways and synaptic connectivity (Bourgeron 2015; D'Gama et al. 2015). This atypical microscopic connectivity may further disrupt the formation of integrated networks between regions of the brain, and lead to abnormalities in macroscopic connectivity within and between brain regions in ASD (Bourgeron 2015). In addition, some 30% of individuals or more with ASD are also affected by epilepsy or show some epileptiform discharges in their brain activity, which may suggest the presence of common neurobiological mechanisms underlying both ASD and epilepsy (Amiet et al. 2008; Viscidi et al. 2013). Since epileptic discharges are thought to result from hypersyncronized brain activity in focal areas, the presence of some epileptic features in ASD may further suggest the association of atypical brain connectivity patterns with the disorder.

Brain connectivity measures investigate how brain regions are connected and communicate with each other to form brain networks that underlie both brain resting state and cognitive task performance (Coben et al. 2014; Sporns 2014). A rapidly growing body of studies over the last two decades has investigated the connectivity and brain networks in ASD, and has aided in the delineation of brain connectivity as a candidate biomarker for the disorder. Several studies using postmortem and *in vivo* neuroimaging and neurophysiological modalities indicate a significant role of aberrant brain connectivity in the etiopathogenesis of ASD (Zikopoulos and Barbas 2010; Courchesne et al. 2011). Moreover, recent advances in neuroimaging and neurophysiological methods further enable a deep and multimodal characterization of brain connections and networks, both anatomically and functionally.

Brain connectivity approaches can be divided into three categories: structural, functional, and effective connectivity.

1. Structural connectivity approaches examine how regions of the brain are physically connected via anatomical tracts of white matter fibers (Ameis and Catani 2015). White matter tracts link and are responsible for the speed of information processing between areas of gray matter; as such, white matter represents the structural basis of brain connectivity. Methods for studying structural connectivity are mainly based on magnetic resonance imaging (MRI)-based diffusion tensor imaging (DTI) acquisitions. Such methods include measurements of global or regional white matter volume, by employing whole-brain or region-of-interest (ROI) techniques, and tractography, which measures the density of specific white matter fibers within association, projection, and commissural white matter tracts (Catani 2006). These techniques map anatomical white matter tracts connecting brain areas and analyze properties of white matter microstructure by measuring the diffusion of water molecules along white matter fibers.

2. Functional connectivity approaches examine the interdependency and similarity of activities of different brain regions (Uddin et al. 2013a; Hernandez et al. 2015). By measuring the strength of the relationship and orchestration between brain activity at different areas of the brain, such methods are able to characterize the integration and segregation of brain networks activated during both rest and task performance. Functional connectivity networks are typically mapped using statistical methods (e.g., correlation, coherence) to brain signals measured using functional MRI (fMRI), electroencephalography (EEG), and magnetoencephalography (MEG).

3. Effective connectivity can be considered a subcategory of functional connectivity. Compared to other functional connectivity approaches, it not only examines the interdependency of brain

signals, but can further inform on the interactions and directionality of information transfer between different areas that form a brain network (Friston 2011). Effective connectivity methods, such as Granger Causality, are able to estimate the transfer of information from one brain region to another, thus allowing the assessment of causal relationships (Coben et al. 2014; Maximo et al. 2014).

One of the most robust findings in neuroimaging research of ASD is the atypical size of brain of ASD patients compared to TD individuals in the early phases of development. Prospective studies have documented lower total brain volumes in newborns that will be later diagnosed with ASD compared to TD controls (Hazlett et al. 2005; Sacco et al. 2015). Yet this abnormality has not been observed in toddlers with ASD, who instead show greater total brain volume, driven in particular by overgrowth in white matter, especially in frontal and temporal lobes (Courchesne et al. 2001; Sparks et al. 2002; Courchesne 2004). This trend of overgrowth seems not to continue later in the development, as smaller brain volumes, particularly in white matter, have been found in adolescents and adults with ASD compared to controls (Courchesne et al. 2001; Courchesne 2004). These results point to early, abnormally accelerated growth, resulting in greater brain volumes, during the first 2 years of life in the brains of individuals that will be later diagnosed with ASD, followed by an atypical trajectory leading to reduced brain volumes in ASD (Courchesne 2004; Courchesne et al. 2005). This early growth has been hypothesized to originate from neuroinflammation and a reduction in physiological synaptic pruning processes (Frith 2003; Herbert 2005). Importantly, such early abnormalities may prevent the formation of integrated networks between different regions of the brain, and result in the development of aberrant structural brain connectivity patterns in ASD (Frith 2003; Lewis and Elman 2008).

In line with brain volume studies and these early predictions, brain connectivity studies in ASD have documented widespread abnormalities in ASD, using both structural and functional approaches. However, several inconsistencies are present across studies with regard to which specific brain networks show dysconnectivity (over- or underconnectivity) within and between one another. Possible reasons for such inconsistencies are the use of different methodologies and modalities to characterize and statistically measure brain connectivity, as well as the use of small samples with wide age ranges. In addition, few longitudinal studies have been conducted, and several studies, to date, have failed to adopt a developmental perspective, which would likely aid in the identification of atypical age-related trajectories of connectivity in individuals with ASD compared to TD individuals (Uddin et al. 2013a). The present chapter will highlight the importance of brain connectivity in ASD, review the existing evidence of atypical brain connectivity patterns in individuals with ASD across development, explore the different research methods to characterize brain connections and networks, and discuss the clinical implication of studying brain connectivity abnormalities in ASD.

13.2 Review of findings in brain connectivity and autism

Brain connectivity and the formation of brain networks are key characteristics of the human brain and essential in order to undertake complex behaviors and higher-order cognitive functions, including language acquisition, executive control, and theory of mind operations (Catani 2006). Several of these high-level cognitive functions are impaired in ASD and thought to underlie the clinical presentation of the disorder, characterized by marked difficulties in the development of language skills, social communication and interaction, repetitive behaviors, and restricted interests (APA 2013). A lack of integrated brain networks, as well as inefficient communication between brain areas, have been proposed as core features in the etiopathogenesis of ASD in the cortical underconnectivity theory (Just et al. 2004, 2012). Yet, disrupted connectivity in ASD has also been associated with patterns of atypical overconnectivity, especially within local perceptual regions and short-range connections (Uddin et al. 2013a). Under- and overconnectivity findings, rather than being conflicting with each other, may be interpreted in light of a unified hypothesis of brain connectivity of ASD, which proposes the presence of long-range underconnectivity between different brain regions/networks, as well as short-range overconnectivity within brain regions/networks (Belmonte et al. 2004; Courchesne and Pierce 2005; Wass 2011). In this section, we will review the findings of structural, functional, and effective connectivity studies in ASD samples.

13.2.1 Structural connectivity studies

Over the last two decades, several structural connectivity studies, using various DTI-based analytic approaches, have identified several differences in anatomical connectivity in individuals with ASD compared to age-matched TD controls, especially in white matter tracts (Aoki et al. 2013; Hoppenbrouwers et al. 2014; Ameis and Catani 2015). DTI studies measure the integrity and organization of white matter fiber microstructure with a few indices, such as fractional anisotropy (quantifying the degree of coherence in directionality of water diffusion along white matter fibers), mean diffusivity (reflecting mean water diffusion within a voxel), and radial and axial diffusivity (measuring the movement of water molecules running, respectively, perpendicular or parallel to the principal axon of diffusion) (Basser and Pierpaoli 1996; Catani 2006). Lower functional anisotropy and greater mean, radial, and axial diffusivity indicate underconnectivity. Additionally, recent advanced structural connectivity techniques have enabled investigations of gray matter connectivity in ASD (Ecker et al. 2013; Balardin et al. 2015).

Reduced structural connectivity broadly affecting white matter tracts across frontal, temporal, and parietal cortical areas has been reported in studies investigating whole-brain white matter connectivity with voxel-based DTI techniques in ASD in childhood, adolescence, and adulthood, although the majority of studies used small samples. Studies with larger samples found lower fractional anisotropy (Keller et al. 2007; Kumar et al. 2010; Shukla et al. 2010; Gibbard et al. 2013) and greater mean and radial diffusivity (Ameis et al. 2011) in widespread white-matter tracts in ASD as compared to controls. Other studies, however, also found a mixed pattern of lower and higher fractional anisotropy in different white matter tracts in ASD (Cheng et al. 2010; Ellmore et al. 2013), and one study with a relatively large sample size found greater fractional anisotropy in inferior fronto-occipital fasciculus and optic radiation in adolescents with ASD (Bode et al. 2011).

Investigations using a region of interest (ROI) approach reveal a similar picture of broad aberrant structural connectivity in ASD. A meta-analysis of ROI DTI studies of the most investigated white matter tracts has found strong evidence of lower structural connectivity of white matter integrity in corpus callosum, left uncinate fasciculus, and left superior longitudinal fasciculus (including the arcuate fasciculus) in children, adolescents, and adults with ASD (Aoki et al. 2013) in at least three studies. Other studies with reasonably large samples also reported decreased fractional anisotropy in superior temporal gyrus and temporal stem (Lee et al. 2007), internal capsule, middle cerebellar peduncle (Shukla et al. 2010), and short-range frontal, parietal, and temporal tracts (Sundaram et al. 2008; Shukla et al. 2011). More recently, studies using DTI-based tractography (another ROI method) have provided further information on the macrostructural white matter properties by three-dimensionally reconstructing different white matter fibers (Catani 2006). These studies have reported decreased connectivity in several tracts, including corpus callosum, uncinate and arcuate fasciculi, cingulum, parieto-occipital tracts, forceps minor, and short-range cerebellar fibers in children, adolescents, and adults with ASD (Catani et al. 2008; Pugliese et al. 2009; Ameis et al. 2013; Chang et al. 2014; Hanaie et al. 2014; Bos et al. 2015).

In contrast with the underconnectivity shown in most DTI studies of children, adolescents, and adults with ASD, a few structural connectivity studies of infants and toddlers later diagnosed with ASD have reported higher fractional anisotropy within commissural (e.g., corpus callosum), association (e.g., uncinate fasciculus) and projection (e.g., internal capsule) fibers (Ben Bashat et al. 2007; Weinstein et al. 2011; Billeci et al. 2012; Wolff et al. 2012; Solso et al. 2016). The inconsistencies of findings across the development may be explained by initial evidence from a longitudinal study investigating the early developmental trajectories of white matter tract organization in infants at high risk for ASD (Wolff et al. 2012). This study observed transient short-range overconnectivity in most of the white matter tracts investigated throughout the brain, such that infants later diagnosed with ASD showed overconnectivity at 6 months, but underconnectivity at 24 months, compared to children who did not receive a diagnosis. This suggests a developmental trajectory of white matter overconnectivity followed by a shift toward underconnectivity around 2 years of age (Conti et al. 2015), as also suggested by studies of children from age 3 (Lee et al. 2007; Sundaram et al. 2008; Shukla et al. 2010; Walker et al. 2012). In another study, higher fractional anisotropy and volume of frontal tracts have been found at the youngest ages in a sample of young children with ASD aged 1–3 years compared to controls, and predicted greater symptom severity at age 3. Notably, an opposite trend of reduced fractional anisotropy and brain volume emerged in older participants with ASD, and also correlated with greater symptom severity (Solso et al. 2016). This indicates that early overgrowth and overconnectivity, as well as later volume reduction and underconnectivity, are associated with ASD symptoms, and may support an association between abnormal brain growth and connectivity in the etiopathogenesis of ASD (Frith 2003; Courchesne et al. 2005).

Taken together, the majority of structural connectivity studies of short- and long-range white matter fibers show widespread underconnectivity in white matter tracts in children, adolescents, and adults with ASD, while overconnectivity may characterize earlier development only. In contrast with the short-range overconnectivity and long-range underconnectivity model (Belmonte et al. 2004; Courchesne and Pierce 2005; Wass 2011), structural over- and underconnectivity may be present in both short- and long-range tracts at different developmental stages. One of the most investigated tracts that consistently show atypical connectivity in ASD is the corpus callosum (Shukla et al. 2010; Ameis et al. 2011; Aoki et al. 2013), the most prominent white matter commissural tract in the cortex, with a key role in integrating brain activity in the left and right hemispheres. Alterations in the uncinate and arcuate fasciculi are also particularly relevant for ASD as they connect fronto-temporal areas involved in socioemotional functioning and language, respectively (Pugliese et al. 2009; Fletcher et al. 2010; Aoki et al. 2013), and their integrity correlates with the level of ASD symptoms (Kumar et al. 2010; Cheon et al. 2011; Billeci et al. 2012).

13.2.2 Functional and effective connectivity studies

In recent years, there has been a surge in interest in better understanding the functional and effective relationships between the numerous complex networks of the brain. These relationships are typically described by temporal correlations of activity between brain regions during active processes or resting, providing insight into how spatially distant brain regions, which may or may not be structurally connected, are functionally segregated or integrated with each other (Friston 2011).

Neuroimaging methods such as fMRI, EEG, and MEG are typically utilized to measure these relationships, due to their respective spatial and temporal resolutions, which are necessary when evaluating the dense and dynamic networks of the brain. Such methods are applied to investigate the functional relationships between networks both during resting state and task performance. They may also be employed to describe how specific regions influence one another during a given task when testing a causal hypothesis.

13.2.2.1 Resting-state studies A number of fMRI resting-state studies have focused on connectivity in the default mode network (DMN), a network typically related to resting state activity or inattentiveness (Buckner et al. 2008), involving the medial prefrontal cortex, posterior cingulate cortex/retrosplenial cortex, inferior parietal lobule, lateral temporal cortex, and hippocampal formation. The DMN is often a network of interest due to its activity during the resting state, along with its involvement in certain social and memory functions which are often impaired in ASD (Buckner et al. 2008). In studies observing connectivity within the DMN, there have been conflicting reports of hypoconnectivity in samples of adolescents and adults with ASD (Assaf et al. 2010; Weng et al. 2010; Rudie et al. 2012) as well as hyperconnectivity in samples of affected children (Lynch et al. 2013; Uddin et al. 2013a). Other studies have shown concurrent patterns of both hypo- and hyperconnectivity in different regions and paths. Monk et al. (2009) showed diminished connections between the posterior cingulate cortex (PCC) and superior frontal gyrus, and stronger connections between the PCC, right temporal lobe, and right parahippocampal gyrus in adults with ASD compared to controls. An fMRI study on high-functioning adolescents and adults with ASD reported widespread hypoconnectivity compared to age-matched controls, with significantly lower connectivity associated with the anterior and posterior cingulate cortex (Cherkassky et al. 2006). An additional fMRI study with a large sample of individuals with ASD ranging from childhood to adulthood found diminished long-range functional connectivity within the DMN between anterior and posterior components, as well as between DMN components and adjacent regions (Di Martino et al. 2014). This study also reported overt cortico-cortical and interhemispheric hypoconnectivity, with hyperconnectivity being observed in subcortical regions.

Investigation of social processing circuits has shown similar trends of dysconnectivity in ASD populations. A seed-based fMRI study in adolescents with ASD reported impaired connectivity between limbic areas and communication and visuospatial/motor-related regions using a whole-brain connectivity approach (Gotts et al. 2012). Similar findings were obtained in a seed-based connectivity study in adults, with reduced connectivity between the insula and amygdala, additional regions associated with social processing (von dem Hagen et al. 2012). Discriminable connectivity differences have also been seen in other brain regions, including somatosensory, visual, and subcortical regions (Chen et al. 2015; Yerys et al. 2015), with symptom-correlated findings of hyperconnectivity between subcortical and sensory cortices being observed (Cerliani et al. 2015).

Analysis via EEG and MEG methods has led to additional insight in functional connectivity differences, often through measurements of amplitude coherence or phase coherence between different regions. Measurements of coherence are associated with the degree to which neural oscillations measured in spatially remote regions are synchronized with each other, with high synchronization implying communication between these regions (Fries 2005). At rest, these oscillations are thought to reflect levels of arousal, vigilance, and activation (Klimesch 1999; Basar 2001). Locally elevated theta coherence measured via EEG has been observed in adults with ASD in left hemisphere frontal and temporal regions (Murias et al. 2007), along with reduced left-anterior/right-posterior theta connectivity being reported in a sample of children (Kikuchi et al. 2013). Alpha coherence has been shown to be reduced locally within frontal regions and globally in adults between frontal and other regions (Murias et al. 2007), as well as over temporal regions in an EEG study in children (Coben et al. 2008). In a more recent EEG study, Orekhova et al. (2014) explored phase-lagged connectivity in alpha band in infants (14 months) at high risk for ASD, and found alpha-range hyperconnectivity in frontal and central regions, which also correlated with the severity of repetitive behaviors at 3 years, as measured by the Autism Diagnostic Interview–Revised (ADI–R) Restricted and repetitive behaviors (RBB) scale. Of note, a relationship between neural connectivity in the alpha band and white matter tract development over age has also been suggested, providing a possible explanation for the progression of alpha band hyperconnectivity seen in children to the hypoconnectivity seen in adolescents and adults (Murias et al. 2007; Catarino et al. 2013; Orekhova et al. 2014). Evidence has also emerged on disruptions during resting state in the delta band, with increased short-range connectivity in lateral-frontal regions and decreased long-range fronto-occipital connections in adults (Barttfeld et al. 2011) and in the gamma band, often associated with attention and working memory, in children with ASD (Jensen et al. 2007; Kikuchi et al. 2013).

13.2.2.2 Task-based studies Task-based studies may give additional insight into network patterns that emerge due to the presence of stimulus- and task-related cognitive demands and goal-directed processes, with the need for the brain to facilitate information transfer and communication between different regions (Bullmore and Sporns 2013; Di et al. 2013). Investigations into task-based studies have led to observed decrements in intra- and inter-regional brain connectivity in ASD involving a number of cognitive processes. During a theory of mind task, where participants were asked to choose logical endings to a comic strip storyline, causal connectivity paths have been observed to be significantly reduced in adolescents with ASD in social brain areas, namely the fusiform face area (FFA) and middle temporal gyrus (Deshpande et al. 2013). Khan et al. (2013) similarly reported decreased connectivity associated with the FFA during a face-processing task conducted with MEG in adolescents. The FFA has also been characterized with deficient connections to the amygdala and superior temporal sulcus in high-functioning adults with ASD, with degree of social impairment correlated with reduced connectivity between the FFA and amygdala and, additionally, increased connectivity between the FFA and right inferior frontal cortex (Kleinhans et al. 2008). Deficits in visual areas have been noted during tasks involving visuo-motor performance (Villalobos et al. 2005) and visual processing (Carson et al. 2014). Underconnectivity with the frontal lobe has been reported during set-shifting (Doesburg et al. 2013) and working memory tasks (Koshino et al. 2005; Urbain et al. 2016), supporting the idea of a disconnected frontal lobe (Courchesne and Pierce 2005). An fMRI study using language comprehension tasks in adults has further shown similarly compromised connections associated with the frontal lobe, notably between frontal and parietal regions (Kana et al. 2006).

In contrast, some studies have reported hyperconnectivity during the performance of different cognitive tasks. An fMRI study in adults with ASD reported increased connectivity between frontal regions and superior frontal and anterior cingulate gyri during an imitation task (Shih et al. 2010). Long-range fronto-posterior connections in the left hemisphere were shown to be significantly stronger in ASD children during a visual encoding memory task using EEG (Chan et al. 2011). An fMRI study in children during motor execution described stronger connections between primary motor and primary visual cortices, with a more rightward trend of overconnectivity being observed in the precentral gyrus (Carper et al. 2015).

Overall, studies on functional connectivity in ASD have to date shown potentially contrasting findings, with mixed reports of hypo- and hyperconnectivity. Recently, there have been attempts to provide insight into these discrepancies. Nair et al. (2014) investigated this further, analyzing two groups of adolescents with ASD: one performing separate visual search (VS) and rapid serial visual presentation (RSVP) tasks, and the other a resting-state paradigm. Through the use of different methodological variables in their analyses, such as type of pipeline (coactivation vs. intrinsic), seed selection, field of view (ROI vs. whole brain), and type of data set, the authors were able to produce results of both hypo- and hyperconnectivity. Further explanations have been put forth to explain the inconsistencies seen across studies and modalities. One possibility is differing developmental stages of networks examined, which has been supported by an observed trend of hyperconnectivity in children with ASD which progresses into hypoconnectivity through adolescence and adulthood over a number of studies (see Uddin et al. 2013b for review).

This viewpoint is also supported by recent studies which have replicated analyses on multiple samples, showing overconnectivity on both global and local scales in children (Supekar et al. 2013) with connectivity diminishing as age increases, relative to neurotypical networks (Nomi and Uddin 2015). In addition to the methodological variables proposed by Nair et al. described previously, others have proposed variables such as the use of task-regression as a proxy for resting state, the inclusion or high- or low-functioning individuals (Tyszka et al. 2014), and diagnostic subtype (Di Martino et al. 2014) as possible reasons for discrepancies across studies. Due to the complexity of the underlying disrupted networks as well as the heterogeneity of the disorder, we highlight the importance of carefully scrutinizing connectivity findings before making inferences across subject groups. Many of these studies, for example, have used coherence as an EEG/MEG metric across pairs of locations. This approach has been shown to be flawed in terms of the reality of effective connectivity measurements (Blinowska 2011; Coben et al. 2014).

13.3 How to characterize brain networks

Brain networks can be delineated from functional or structural brain data using the mathematical tools of graph theory, a field first pioneered by Leonhard Euler in the eighteenth century to describe the connectivity of city districts in Königsberg, Prussia (Sporns 2011). Graph theory considers abstract entities (nodes) by modeling the relationships (edges) between them as a network (graph). For example, nodes may be constructed from data channels in sensor space or source space in the case of EEG/MEG data, or from voxels in the case of fMRI. Edges are calculated as a single number quantifying the anatomical relationship (structural connectivity), statistical dependency (functional connectivity), or directed information transfer (effective connectivity) between two nodes. Edges are contained in a connectivity matrix $\mathbf{A}$ (also known as an adjacency matrix) describing all pairwise relationships between nodes in a graph. Where the relationship between any two nodes is not symmetrical, that is, $\mathbf{A}_{i,j} \neq \mathbf{A}_{j,i}$, a graph may be described as directed, as is the case with effective connectivity. For undirected graphs where $\mathbf{A}_{i,j} = \mathbf{A}_{j,i}$, connectivity between node i and node j is equal in both directions. Other special terms for graphs refer to the range of values edges may assume. For a weighted graph, an edge may assume the value of any real number, though edges are often normalized such that $\mathbf{A}_{i,j} \in [-1,1]$. By contrast, for an unweighted graph, edges assume Boolean values, that is, $\mathbf{A}_{i,j} \in \{0,1\}$. In practice, unweighted graphs are usually constructed by applying a thresholding scheme to edges in a weighted graph. This step creates a sparse matrix from $\mathbf{A}$ and simplifies the model network by allowing one to only examine strong or interesting relationships. Many measures described below, such as path length and clustering coefficient, can often be computed only for unweighted graphs.

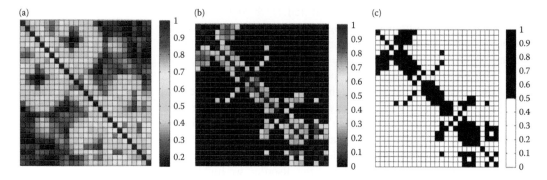

Figure 13.1 Visualization of connectivity matrix created from magnitude squared coherence between EEG channels. A connectivity matrix can be visualized using hot colors for strong edges and cool colors for weak edges. Below is an example connectivity matrix produced using coherence between EEG channels. (a) The connectivity matrix is created from a weighted graph. The main diagonal, that is, the line of identity, is saturated owing to the fact that $A_{i,i} = 1$. Note that the matrix is symmetrical about the line of identity, that is, $A_{i \cdot j} = A_{j,i}$. (b) The weighted graph has been pruned such that all edge weights with a z-score < +1 are set to 0, with only strong edges being kept. (c) An unweighted graph has been constructed by binarizing the values from (b), such that any nonzero value after pruning is assumed a value of 1. Such thresholding schemes are common for creating unweighted graphs.

Considering the high dimensionality of structural or functional brain data owing to a large number of sensors, a typical connectivity matrix might include thousands of edges. By analyzing all edges with standard statistical approaches, one risks the issue of multiple comparisons, as well as difficulty in understanding the meaning of the multiple results produced. How, then, does one quantify and analyze the brain network without testing a prohibitively large number of hypotheses? First, the connectivity matrix **A** can be visualized as seen in Figure 13.1 for qualitative inspection, allowing one to glean useful information for forming hypotheses. Second, a number of holistic measures can be used to describe the style of connectivity observed in the network using a single number. Path length is a measure of network efficiency that gives the average number of edges between any two nodes of a graph. The global clustering coefficient reflects the tendency of the graph to form "cliques" or modules. It is the arithmetic mean of each node's local clustering coefficient, a measure of "cliquishness," which is the probability that a node's neighbors are directly connected to each other. Networks with low path length and high clustering coefficient are efficient because they allow for information to spread between any two arbitrary nodes in a minimal number of steps. This is known as a small-world network, the preferred architecture of many networks in nature. Small-world networks commonly feature densely interconnected clusters with few connections to other clusters, a condition known as modularity. Hub nodes with many neighbors hold together such networks by serving as figurative way stations.

Having chosen a set of observations—for example, time series from electrodes, source localized signals, or MRI voxels—to serve as nodes, one next chooses a method for delineating edges. In structural connectivity analysis, edges reflect anatomical white matter fibers, typically estimated with fractional anisotropy in the context of diffusion MRI or diffusion tensor imaging (DTI). In functional connectivity analysis, edges reflect statistical dependencies captured by a number of possible techniques, including correlation, coherence, phase-locking statistic (PLS) (Lachaux et al. 1999), mutual information (Tononi et al. 1998), and synchronization likelihood (Stam and Van Dijk 2002). Coherence, the most commonly applied technique for EEG and MEG recordings, is a linear measure of synchronization between two stationary signals, where a stationary signal is one whose statistical properties are fixed with time. Put simply, coherence describes the degree of similarity between two brain signals recorded from different scalp or cortical locations. Specifically, magnitude squared coherence quantifies this relationship as a function of frequency for two broadband signals. It is given by

$$C_{xy}(f) = \frac{|G_{xy}(f)|^2}{G_{xx}(f)G_{yy}(f)}$$

where $G_{xy}(f)$ is the cross-spectral density of signal x and signal y, $G_{xx}(f)$ and $G_{yy}(f)$ are spectral densities of signal x and signal y, respectively, and $C_{xy}(f) \in [0,1]$. Note the similarity between this definition and that of the Pearson correlation coefficient

$$r_{xy} = \frac{\sigma_{xy}}{\sqrt{\sigma_{xx}\sigma_{yy}}}$$

where σ_{xy} is the covariance of signal x and signal y, and σ_{xx} and σ_{yy} are the variances of signal x and signal y, respectively, and $r_{xy} \in [-1,1]$. In theory, neuronal ensembles should oscillate coherently for temporal coordination of information transfer (Fries 2005; Buzsaki 2006), providing an attractive theoretical foundation for coherence as a brain connectivity measure. However, coherence is vulnerable to false-positive connectivity created by volume conduction, the tendency for electrical signals to be spatially smeared. Because volume conduction is essentially instantaneous, this limitation can be overcome using cross-correlation, that is, computing the correlation as a function of a time lag. In fact, $G_{xy}(f)$ in the coherence formula above is obtained using the Fourier transform of the cross correlation between signal x and signal y. For EEG signals, a time lag can be chosen to match time delays created by physiologically plausible synaptic conduction velocities. Alternatively, current source density (CSD) techniques can be applied to scalp EEG recordings to effectively create a high-pass spatial filter that minimizes volume conduction artifact.

While cross-correlation and coherence are arguably the simplest measures of functional connectivity, more sophisticated techniques—which capture nonlinear dependencies—include mutual information (Tononi et al. 1998), transfer entropy (Schreiber 2000), Granger causality

(Granger 1969), and synchronization likelihood (Stam and Van Dijk 2002). Although it is technically possible to use principal component analysis (PCA) for identification of component sources to serve as network nodes, PCA is not recommended for this purpose, as it will, by definition, create a network with minimal linear correlation between nodes. Instead, PCA can be used more appropriately to identify features in connectivity matrices for classifying subjects. For example, Duffy and Als used patterns of coherence identified with PCA from CSD estimates of resting-state EEG recordings as features to classify children with and without ASD (Duffy and Als 2012). Using 40 features identified with PCA, the study classified three age-specific subgroups of children (2 to 4 year olds, $n = 301$; 4 to 6 year olds, $n = 137$; 6- to 12-year olds, $n = 546$) with >90% accuracy.

13.4 Connectivity explanation

As we discussed earlier in this chapter, two brain regions or, more generally, two nodes of any network can be connected with each other by having either (1) a structural (physical) relationship; (2) a functional relationship, whereby their functions are similar; and (3) a causal or effective relationship, in that the activity of one node is the reason/cause for the activity of other node. We can illustrate the difference between functional and effective connectivity with an example.

Suppose there is a surveillance camera in operation in an airport. Two spies ("A" and "B") are trying to share information by waving their hands at each other with certain secret patterns from two opposite sides of the Duty Free area. Shortly after, another spy "C" starts waving his hand to signal his/her location. This activity looks suspicious to a security officer observing passengers from CCTV screens in the airport control room, and he wants to understand whether the three passengers have some form of connection with one another. In terms of functional connectivity analysis, if the three spies wave their hands with a similar pattern (e.g., in the same speed or direction) this suggests they may be communicating with each other. In our example, if A and B show the same hand waving patterns, but C shows a different one, the officer may conclude that "A" and "B" are most likely to have some relationship, while "C" does not have any connection with them. Now, suppose that the officer needs to know whether A is initiating the hand waving to B. In this case, the officer should look at the temporal precedence of the hand waving of A and B to examine (a) how similar the activity of A is compared to B, and (b) which activity has temporal (time) precedence to the other, that is, who waves first. Also, the officer may understand that hand waving of A can also initiate C's, even though his/her hand waving pattern is different. These two relationships between A and B and between A and C may be result of the effective or causal connectivity between these three passengers.

In the following section, causality analysis between nodes of a brain network has been discussed based on Coben and Mohammad-Rezazadeh (2015) and Mohammad-Rezazadeh et al. (2016).

Granger causality (GC) is a linear regression method and the most popular form of causality analyses. It was first introduced by Norbert Wiener (the father of cybernetics) in 1956 and later formalized by Clive W. J. Granger and can be simply defined as follows: at frequency f_0, if past values of one process X_2 help to predict future values of another process X_1 beyond what can be inferred from past values of recording X_1 alone, then (according to GC), X_2 has a Granger causal effect on X_1. While not true causality, GC is useful for inferring directionality of neural information transfer.

Some important prerequisites are needed for obtaining accurate GC estimation such as (1) linear interaction between network nodes. Thus, GC has been mostly applied using a multivariate autoregressive (MVAR) model by incorporating methods such as direct transfer function (DTF), partial directed coherence (PDC), and directed partial coherence (DPC). These approaches may cause misleading results when applied on network data that has nonlinear dependencies between its nodes' activities. In this case, either using the nonlinear GC method or implementing blind source separation (BSS) methods data (such as independent component analysis [ICA]) before applying GC on may help to extract maximally statistically independent sources; (2) relatively low noise level in data; and (3) low cross-talk between the measurements of network entities. In neuroimaging data processing, this issue happens because of the scalp volume conductance, which is a phenomenon whereby electrical signals are spread out widely as they travel through brain tissue and spatially smeared by the skull, like a narrow point of light viewed through frosted glass. As a result of volume conduction, spatial relationships measured from the scalp may not represent true neural connectivity but rather artifacts of volume conduction. Spatial filters such as current source density (CSD)—the second spatial derivative (Laplacian transformation) of sensor-space recordings—have been introduced by researchers to deal with the volume conductance issue. Alternatively, by using an inverse model approach such as standardized low-resolution brain electromagnetic tomography (sLORETA), beamforming, and independent components analysis for dipole localization, spatial locations of "cortical activity" sources can be estimated and considered as the nodes of the network.

13.5 Measuring functional or effective connectivity with graph theory methods

EEG recordings are often afflicted by numerous sources of noise, both physiological and external, which can negatively impact the ability to detect or analyze the true brain activity that may be embedded in this noise. Therefore, a number of cleaning processes must be applied to EEG recordings in order to remove any "nonbrain"-related EEG data. These processes can include (1) filtering, which may be used to remove near-DC (0 Hz) or nonbrain-related high-frequency activity; (2) artifact rejection, where large "nonneural" artifacts can be rejected from the data using methods such as independent component analysis (ICA). Once EEG data is cleaned and processed, analytical brain connectivity techniques, such as coherence or Granger causality described previously, may be applied to the data in order to better understand the brain activity occurring (Rubinov and Sporns 2010). Here, we describe the process of using such analysis techniques along with graph theory to analyze EEG data, as well as introduce the Biomarker and Neural Connectivity Toolbox (BioNeCT, available at https://sites.google.com/site/bionectweb), an in-house MATLAB® Toolbox created to perform such analyses.

Through analysis, as described in the previous sections, on an EEG data set, electrode relationships between one another are obtained. These relationships, or edges, are mapped to an $N \times N$ adjacency (or connectivity) matrix (Figure 13.2), where N is the number of electrodes

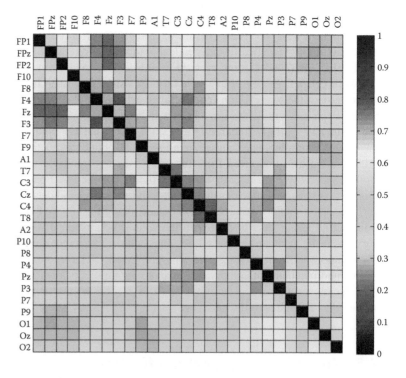

Figure 13.2 An example of an undirected and weighted connectivity matrix of coherence values ranging between 0 and 1 obtained from 27-channel EEG data in the theta band during the stimulus of a high-load working memory task.

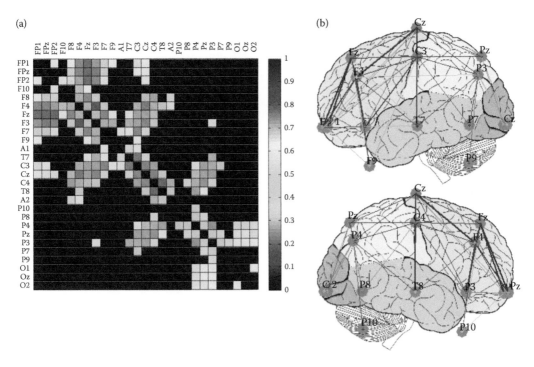

Figure 13.3 (a) Thresholded connectivity matrix from Figure 13.1, where connections of strength <0.6 are set to zero. (b) Connectivity from (a) mapped to lateral views of left (top) and right (bottom) hemispheres.

or channels, and value in matrix index (I, J) is the relationship calculated between any channel I and channel J. The matrix values assumed depend both on whether relationship parameters such as weight and directionality are being considered. Connectivity matrices may firstly be either binary or weighted, where binary connections are given values of 0 or 1, and weighted connections taking non-integer values, with larger values indicating a stronger relationship. Matrices may also display directionality (i.e., in causality relationships), where values can be either positive or negative, while maintaining one of the weight relationships described prior.

While complete connectivity matrices may give insight into certain parameters of the brain network as a whole, it is often necessary to threshold the matrix to remove either spurious or uninteresting connections. Thresholding is typically applied such that connections with a strength below a certain threshold value are set to be zero, allowing for analysis of only the strongest components of the network, as shown in Figure 13.3. Post-thresholding, network analysis techniques such as graph theory can be applied to detect underlying patterns in the network.

It is often of further interest to analyze how brain networks differ between different phenotypes (e.g., children with ASD and those

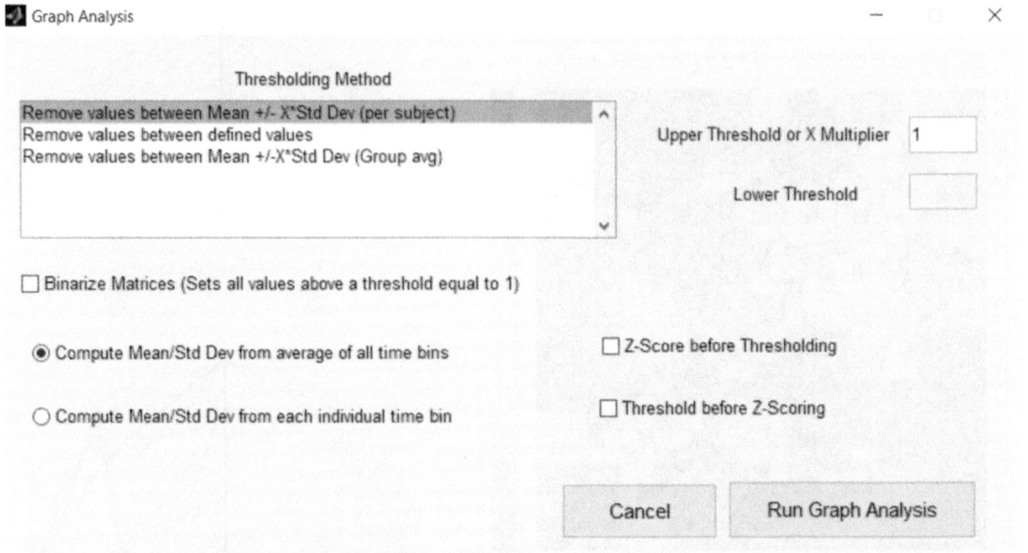

Figure 13.4 Screenshot from graph metric extraction stage of BioNeCT analysis pipeline. Depending on connections of interest, thresholding methods may be different and are often arbitrary, and can produce unique resulting networks.

typically developing) or psychological conditions, as well as the degree to which these brain networks are dissimilar. Using graph theory metrics, as mentioned above, is one way of quantitatively describing individual networks so that comparisons between different groups can be made (Figure 13.4).

These metrics can also be placed into machine-learning classifiers (such as a support vector machine) to estimate how differentiable networks of given phenotypes are, given a set of metrics. However, when a large number of metrics or features are available to use for classification, including features that do not differ greatly between compared groups, this may render the classifier ineffective due to excessive information. Feature selection and reduction methods are often used to accommodate this issue prior to the classification stage, so that group classification is performed using only discriminable features (Figure 13.5).

Following feature selection with one of the methods above, the resulting set of features are then fed into a classifier, to determine how effective these features are in discriminating between different phenotype groups (Figure 13.6). While feature/dimensionality reduction techniques such as principal component analysis (PCA) are possible methods for reducing the number of features fed to a classifier, such methods create features that are difficult to interpret.

Alternatively, performing different statistical analyses on data sets (such as graph metrics) may be of interest. BioNeCT provides within-toolbox

(a)

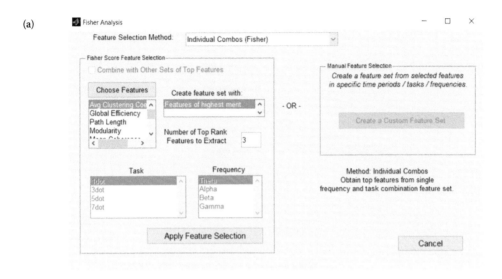

(b)

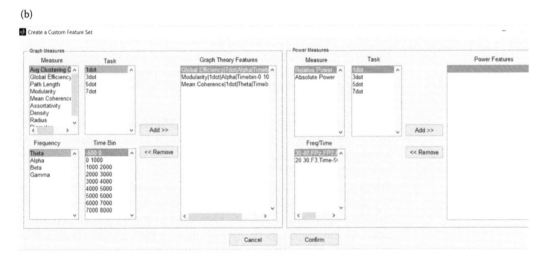

Figure 13.5 Screenshots from feature selection stage of BioNeCT analysis pipeline. (a) Selection of graph theory features from which to extract a specified number of most-discriminable (between-group) features. (b) Custom selection of graph theory features calculated from data set.

detection of significant differences between phenotypes, as well as the capability to export all calculated metrics for external analyses.

13.6 Measuring effective connectivity with Granger causality

We have previously presented and reviewed how Granger causality may be used and applied to measuring connectivity in both autism and

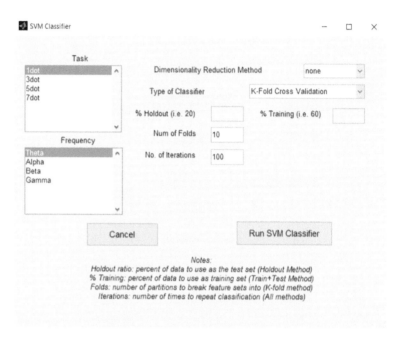

Figure 13.6 Screenshot from classifier stage of BioNeCT analysis pipeline. Options include dimensionality reduction, classifier type, and classifier parameters which may vary depending on size of the data set.

epilepsy (Coben et al. 2014; Coben and Mohammad-Rezazadeh 2015; Mohammad-Rezazadeh et al. 2016). Granger causality analysis (GCA) is a method for investigating whether one time series can correctly forecast another (Bressler and Seth 2011). Granger causality (GC) is a data-driven approach based on linear regressive models and requires only a few basic assumptions about the original data statistics. Recently in neuroscience applications, GC has been used to explore causal dependencies between brain regions by investigating directed information flow or causality in the brain. It uses the error prediction of autoregressive (AR) or multivariant autoregressive (MAR) models to estimate if a brain process is a Granger cause of another brain process. Effective connectivity, as defined as a measurement of the interdependence of brain signals that assesses its interactions and directionality of information transfer, is explicitly measured in Granger causality.

13.6.1 Definition

Suppose two stochastic processes $X_1(t)$ and $X_2(t)$ and future values of $X_1(t)$ are going to be predicted by using two different data sets: using only the past values of $X_1(t)$ and by incorporation of past values of $X_1(t)$ and $X_2(t)$. If incorporating the past knowledge of $X_2(t)$ permits more accurate prediction of X_1, then X_2 could be called a causal to X_1 (Cadotte et al. 2008).

13.6.2 Mathematical form of GC

Suppose X_1 and X_2 can be represented by single variable AR models:

$$X_1(t) = \sum_{j=1}^{m} a_j X_1(t-j) + \varepsilon_{11}(t)$$

$$X_2(t) = \sum_{j=1}^{m} b_j X_2(t-j) + \varepsilon_{22}(t)$$

A joint predictor of $X_1(t)$ can be defined as:

$$X_1^*(t) = \sum_{j=1}^{m} a_j^* X_1(t-j) + \sum_{j=1}^{m} b_j^* X_2(t-j) + \varepsilon_{12}(t)$$

which is a part of the multivariate model of the "process" that generates X_1 and X_2. Here, if the variance of prediction error $\delta_{12}^2(\varepsilon_{12})$ is less than the variance of $\delta_{12}^2(\varepsilon_{11})$ then it is an indication of a causal interaction from $X_2(t)$ to $X_1(t)$. The magnitude of causality from X_2 to X_1 is defined as

$$F_{X_2 \to X_1} = \ln\left(\frac{\delta_{12}^2}{\delta_1^2}\right)$$

thus if $\delta_1^2 = \delta_{12}^2$ then the magnitude of causality from X_2 to X_1 is 0. In a similar way, $F_{X_1 \to X_2}$ the causality from X_1 to X_2 also can be defined as well. The asymmetry in $F_{X_1 \to X_2}$ and $F_{X_2 \to X_1}$ indicates the directionality of causality between X_1 and X_2 (Vakorin et al. 2013):

$$\Delta F = F_{X_2 \to X_1} - F_{X_1 \to X_2}$$

If ΔF is positive then the net direction of causality (coupling) is from X_2 to X_1, and vice versa.

13.6.3 Conditional Granger causality

Now suppose a system with more than two variable time series. One question is whether in this system a causal influence between any pair of time series is directed or mediated by others (Dhamala et al. 2008). For example, if X_1 has causal influence on X_2 and X_2 has causal influence on X_3 then X_1 has indirect causal influence on X_3. Direct and indirect causation between two time series or in general two variables of a system can be defined by conditional GC

$$F_{X_1 \to X_3 | X_2} = \ln \frac{\delta_{1,3}^2}{\delta_{1,2,3}^2}$$

where $\delta_{1,2,3}^2$ is the variance of the error of predicting X_1 using the past values of X_1, X_2, and X_3.

13.6.4 Granger causality limitations

Granger causality needs three main prerequisites to be applied on brain data: (1) linear interaction model between network entities. Thus, GC has been mostly applied using a multivariate autoregressive (MVAR) model by incorporating methods such as direct transfer function (DTF), PDC, and directed partial coherence (DPC). These approaches may cause misleading results when applied in signals that have nonlinear dependencies such as EEG; thus applying blind source separation (BSS) methods like independent component analysis (ICA) can be helpful to have maximally independent data sources before applying GC method on the data (Liu and Aviyente 2012); (2) relatively low noise level in data. Again, data cleaning from bad components using methods such as ICA can be beneficial to obtain cleaner data; and (3) low cross-talk between the measurements of network entities. To tackle this issue, which arises mostly because of the scalp volume conductance, GC analyses can be performed by applying GC on ICA brain sources or current source density signals (also known as spatial Laplacians) instead of original brain voltages from scalp channels (Vicente et al. 2011; Coben et al. 2014).

It should also be noted that the accuracy of any GC model prediction may be positively influenced by higher sampling rates (Kayser et al. 2009), re-referencing to average or Laplacian methods (Nunez et al. 1997), using noncausal filters with zero phase lag (Mullen et al. 2012), accurate model ordering, and model stationarity (see Coben and Mohammad-Rezazadeh 2015).

13.7 Imaging GC connectivity in cases with autism spectrum disorder

We now present data from two cases on the autism spectrum illustrating imaging of their brain connectivity processes. In each case, EEG data were collected in the following manner. A stretchable electrode cap embedded with 19 sensors attached to the scalp was used to collect data, with frontal reference, prefrontal ground, and linked ears. Each recording lasted 10 minutes per condition (eyes closed or open). This included recording and digitizing EEG readings based on the International 10/20 System of electrode placement utilizing the Deymed Diagnostic (2004) TruScan 32 Acquisition EEG System. This system included 32 channels with sampling at 256 cycles per second and filtering between 0.1 and 40 Hz. All recordings were done with impedance <5 kΩ. The common mode rejection ratio for this system is 102 dB and the isolation mode rejection ratio is 140 dB. The methods of EEG analysis are reviewed in detail in our previous work (Coben et al. 2014; Coben and Mohammad-Rezazadeh 2015). Essentially, we used EEGLAB v13 (Delorme et al. 2011) and MVGC, an in-house MATLAB Toolbox for processing of Granger causality data. A key aspect of this approach is that it focuses on estimating and visualizing multivariate effective connectivity in the source domain rather than between scalp electrode signals. This should allow us to achieve finer spatial localization of the network components while minimizing the challenging signal processing confounds produced by broad volume conduction from "neural" sources to the scalp electrodes. From our EEG data, we have virtually epoched this stream into 1-s segments. Independent Component Analysis was then used to extract unique, independent components from the data. To fit multiple component dipoles and determine their locations, DIPFIT toolbox was then applied. Then by investigating the dipole locations and the components topographical maps, only good "neural" components that are related to neural process in the brain have been included for further processing. Following these procedures takes the EEG data from sensory to source space via independent component analysis and dipole localization. This diminishes the issue of volume conduction (see Astolfi et al. 2007; Acar and Makeig 2013). Once dipole localization has been performed, these data are subjected to MVAR and Granger causality (GC) analysis. Within a reasonable range of values, changes in model order may show little effect on the spectral density (and by extension coherence) (e.g., see Florian and Pfurtscheller 1995). Our model order has been based on Akaike information criterion (AIC) and Bayesian information criterion (BIC) criteria to maximize model effects. Statistically, the critical issue for GC is the ratio between the number of independent observations (i.e., samples) and the model complexity (i.e., number of parameters). If the number of observations is large relative to the number of parameters, then the model order selection criteria are still valid. If the number of observations is small, then we might run into problems with AIC and other asymptotic estimators, but there are corrections for that (corrected Akaike information criterion). In our data set (case epoching), we have plenty of data available and the ratio of observations (total data samples within a time window [x trials]) to parameters is >40 suggesting that we have a valid model using AIC (Burnham 2004).

13.7.1 Results

13.7.1.1 Case 1 Data from this 5-year-old boy diagnosed with Autism was processed as described above. He presented, being brought by his mother, with delays in language development, self-regulation, social awareness and skills, and poor attention and motor coordination. He had already been seen for multiple interventions including physical and occupational therapies and ABA intervention. Following the steps listed above including baseline correction, filtering of the data from 1 to 50 Hz, re-referencing to an average reference, and de-artifacting based on blind source separation, and reviewing of independent components, the data was cleaned. The result was a reduction from 19 to 8 brain-related components that are viewed below in Figure 13.7 with their associated dipole localizations. These source localizations show key brain activity over

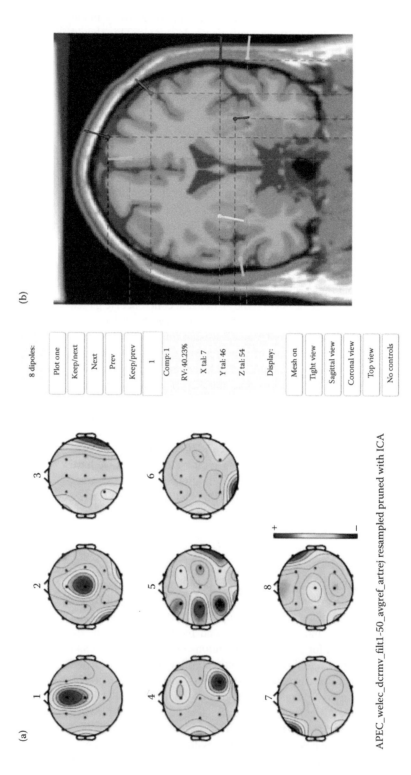

APEC_welec_dcrmv_filt1-50_avgref_artrej resampled pruned with ICA

Figure 13.7 ICA findings from Case 1 with Autism showing the remaining (a) independent components and their surface activations and (b) their dipole source localizations (coronal view).

bilateral hemispheres and frontal regions as well. These included the (1) right superior frontal gyrus, Brodmann 8; (2) right superior frontal gyrus, Brodmann 6; (3) right superior temporal gyrus, Brodmann 22; (4) right inferior parietal lobule, Brodmann 40; (5) right middle temporal gyrus, Brodmann 21; (6) left inferior frontal gyrus, Brodmann 10, and (7) right superior frontal gyrus, Brodmann 10. One of the components was removed as its dipole lay outside of significant brain space.

These component dipoles were then entered in as nodes for further Granger causality analysis processed by the MVGC toolbox. These data were processed with a designated frequency range of 6–11 Hz. due to spectral elevations and findings of concern. The findings may be viewed in Figure 13.8 showing some mild right superior frontal gyrus hyperconnectivity with other bilateral frontal localizations and dense areas of hypoconnectivity across and between parietal, temporal, and frontal regions of his brain. While the outflow from parietal and temporal nodes approaches 0.3 and the superior frontal outflow is closer to 0.6, the connectivity value across these regions is less than 0.1. These would suggest an effective connectivity system that is functioning at very low levels.

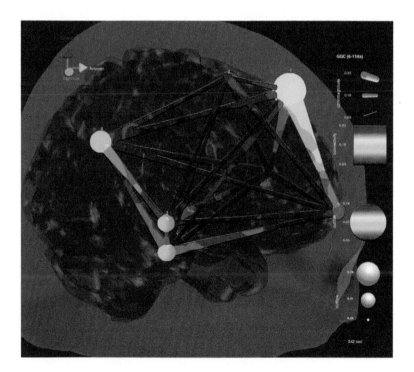

Figure 13.8 Findings of Granger causality connectivity on Case 1 with Autism. Nodes are indicated by ROI balls with greater size and brighter color indicating greater outflow. Connectivity is indicated by the size and brightness of the lines between the nodes.

13.7.1.2 Case 2   This boy was 14 years old at the time of his presentation. He presented, accompanied by his mother, with a lengthy history of social challenges and trouble regulating his emotions. He had been diagnosed with Asperger's syndrome 5 years prior, but has no cognitive or academic deficiencies. He was not taking any medication and was rated by his mother as being socially indifferent, not having any friends, and wanting to be by himself. His EEG data were processed in a similar manner as was described above. Nineteen original components were reduced to six after the de-artifacting procedure with a spectral analysis showing enhanced frontal to right posterior activity between 8 and 16 Hz (Figure 13.9).

The remaining six independent components and their dipole source localizations are shown in Figure 13.10. The majority of these are over right hemisphere and frontal regions as would be expected for such a case. These loci included (1) right middle occipital gyrus, Brodmann 18; (2) right middle temporal gyrus; (3) right middle frontal gyrus, Brodmann 6; (4) right superior frontal gyrus, Brodmann 8; (5) left inferior frontal gyrus, Brodmann 10; and (6) left superior temporal gyrus.

All six of these dipoles were judged to be in brain space and were entered as nodes for further GCC analysis in MVGC (Figure 13.11). These data were processed for a frequency from 8 to 16 Hz as discussed above. Again, there are regions with higher and lower degrees of connectivity. There is an outflow approaching 0.5 coming from the right middle temporal and frontal nodes. The connectivity between these locations approaches 0.2, while the connectivity from right occipital association

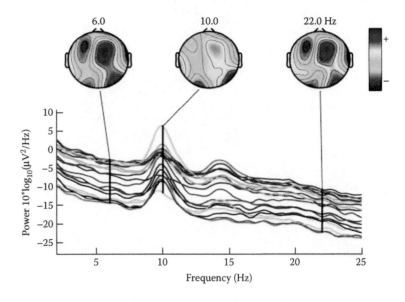

Figure 13.9 Post-artifacted spectral analysis for Case 2 with Asperger's syndrome.

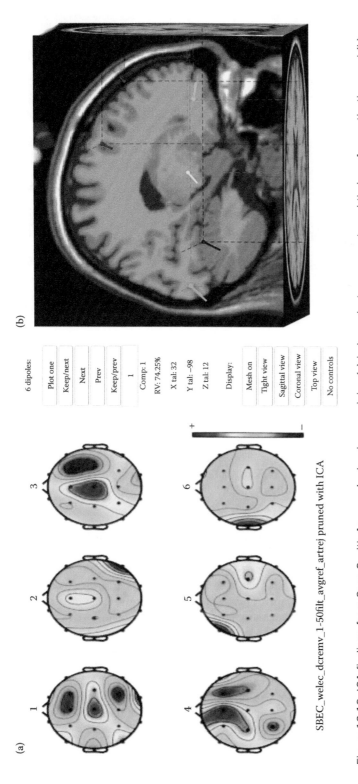

SBEC_welec_dcremv_1-50filt_avgref_artrej pruned with ICA

Figure 13.10 ICA findings from Case 2 with Asperger's showing remaining (a) independent components and their surface activations and (b) their dipole source localizations (sagittal view).

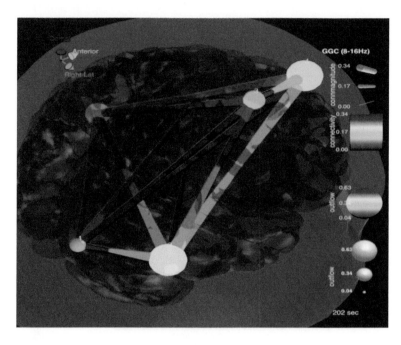

Figure 13.11 Findings of Granger causality connectivity on Case 2 with Asperger's. Nodes are indicated by ROI balls with greater size and brighter color indicating greater outflow. Connectivity is indicated by the size and brightness of the lines between the nodes.

cortex to frontal regions is severely low approaching 0. The same would appear to be true of cross-hemispheric communication over to the left middle temporal gyrus. This suggests a system with moderate levels of activity in some regions, but despite this a paucity of connectivity between other locations presumably needed for intact social and emotional regulation.

13.7.1.3 Discussion While these findings are fascinating, their true implications require further study. It is noteworthy in both of these cases that these representations of effective connectivity do not at all match findings of their respective measures of functional connectivity (pairwise coherence maps). This is not surprising given the evidence that pairwise estimates are incorrect estimates of true connectivity and that a complete set of signals processed with multivariate autoregressive techniques are needed to match the network activity (Kus et al. 2004). It is also quite interesting to consider that in our previous work (Coben et al. 2014) we showed an exemplar of how GCC estimates of effective connectivity very closed resembled findings of structural connectivity from MRI-DTI of the same individual. The regions of dysfunction shown in these connectivity analyses also tend to match those of autistic individuals reviewed above and the particular symptom expression in each case presented. These forms of face validity are certainly encouraging.

13.8 Clinical applications

We have shown how complex analytic techniques can be applied to the human EEG to measure brain connectivity. Ideally, this information would be of clinical or predictive value. For example, can we use such an approach to diagnose or classify individuals? Or, maybe more importantly, is this information useful in designing treatments that can improve the lives of persons on the autism spectrum? It seems apparent that the types of intervention that this might be most useful for are those that involve neuromodulation or attempts to directly and therapeutically alter brain activity (Coben and Evans 2010). Neuromodulation approaches typically include modern techniques of repetitive Transcranial Magnetic Stimulation (rTMS; see Sokhadze et al. 2012; Enticott et al. 2014), Transcranial Direct Current Stimulation (Tortella et al. 2015), and fMRI or EEG biofeedback (Neurofeedback) (Coben et al. 2010; Sulzer et al. 2013). Of these, rTMS and Neurofeedback have been researched as it relates to assisting those on the spectrum. To our knowledge there have not been significant applications of fMRI neurofeedback or TDCS applied to autism. The initial work that has been done with rTMS has been encouraging (Sokhadze et al. 2009, 2012). Neurofeedback (EEG) has been applied and studied related to the hope of reducing autism symptoms for almost 14 years now (Jarusiewicz 2002) with encouraging findings. Neurofeedback is also an attractive modality from the perspective of brain connectivity as it can be used to directly train to reduce or enhance brain connectivity as reflected by coherence measures.

Coben (2013) has recently reviewed the literature related to how neurofeedback has been empirically applied to the challenge of autism symptoms. Neurofeedback uses EEG and advanced computer technology to train individuals to improve poorly regulated brain activity. During a neurofeedback session, EEG electrodes are placed on the scalp and earlobes to measure brain activity. An individual then receives feedback in a game-like format in both auditory and visual modalities. Based on this feedback, they are encouraged and motivated to therapeutically change the amplitude or synchronization of brain activity. It was documented more than 40 years ago that individuals could use such feedback framed in a learning paradigm to lessen troubling symptoms (Sherlin et al. 2011). Several research groups have now demonstrated that this form of intervention can be used to lessen the symptoms associated with autism disorders (see e.g., Pineda et al. 2008; Kouijzer et al. 2009; Coben et al. 2014). Coben (2013) has classified neurofeedback as an intervention that may be possibly efficacious for autism and compared favorably to many others. There is also mounting evidence that the effects of this treatment may be long lasting (Coben et al. 2010).

In an interesting study, Coben and Myers (2010) showed that neurofeedback based on training coherence metrics was two to three times more effective than a model involved in training EEG amplitude alone.

273

With advancements in technology over the past several years, it has now become possible to train coherence with more sensors and greater complexity leading to even greater efficacy and time efficiency. Within this model, the decision of what brain networks to train and in what way becomes critical. The analysis of brain networks that we have discussed in this chapter may have predictive or proscriptive value in their ability to pinpoint brain networks to be trained and enhance the overall efficacy of this approach. The following case exemplar is shown to illustrate this approach.

13.8.1 Treatment case

This 20-year-old man was seen for an initial assessment, received 12 sessions of four channel multivariate coherence training, and was then seen for a follow-up assessment to attempt to measure any changes in brain connectivity. He has lived with a diagnosis of autism for most of his life having received many different forms of treatment including medication, ABA, special diets and other more traditional therapies as well. At the time of his presentation for the initial assessment, he was struggling with severe OCD behaviors (despite taking high dosages of Zoloft), anxiety and social alienation. Based on an analysis of his eyes open resting EEG following all the same procedures outline above, seven independent components and dipole localizations were identified (Figure 13.12). These were source localized to the (1) right inferior frontal gyrus, Brodmann 9; (2) right middle frontal gyrus, Brodmann 47; (3) right occipital lobe, cuneus; (4) left superior parietal lobule, Brodmann 7; (5) right middle temporal gyrus; (6) right middle occipital gyrus, Brodmann 19; and (7) right superior frontal gyrus, Brodmann 6. Three of these seven locations are in the frontal regions, the regions most closely related to OCD behaviors.

These dipoles were used as nodes in MVGC for GCC analysis with a frequency from 5 to 12 Hz. Images taken at different time sequences show evolving patterns of connectivity in Figure 13.13. Earlier in the recording, there is a generalized pattern of under connectivity greatest between right inferior pathways from the right occipital temporal to frontal regions. This connectivity never rises, at that time, above 0.07 with many paths close to 0. Later in the recording there is a dramatic increase in outflow to almost 0.4 and in connectivity to almost 0.2, all coming from anterior frontal locations. While this may not reach a level that we would refer to as hyperconnectivity, it is a dramatic shift in the system. Interestingly, Fitzgerald et al. (2011) have shown a mixed pattern of hypo- and hyperconnectivity in obsessive-compulsive disorder with hyperconnectivity being present in emotional pathways.

Based on these findings it was decided that he would participate in neurofeedback training with a focus on enhancing connectivity or coherence over right inferior pathways from anterior regions to posterior sites.

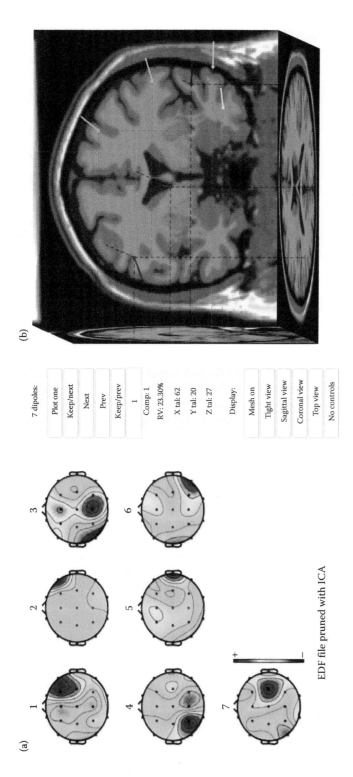

Figure 13.12 ICA findings from Treatment Case with Autism showing remaining (a) independent components and their surface activations and (b) their dipole source localizations (coronal view).

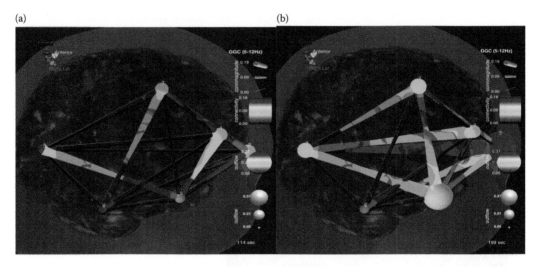

Figure 13.13 Findings of Granger causality connectivity on Treatment Case with Autism. Nodes are indicated by ROI balls with greater size and brighter color indicating greater outflow. Connectivity is indicated by the size and brightness of the lines between the nodes. On the left side of the figure (a) shows GCC findings at 114 seconds into the recording and on the right side (b) shows findings later at 199 seconds.

This was performed with the EEGer neurofeedback software suite (EEG Software, 2013) using a four channel multivariate coherence training module in which the coherences at all four sites are simultaneously averaged to provide multichannel estimates of connectivity. This training was performed over 10/20 EEG placement sites, inclusive of O2, T6, T4, and F8. Following 12 sessions, another EEG was gathered and analyzed to determine if there were any changes. Finally, Figure 13.14 shows the pre- and post-training GCC analyses for comparison.

These findings are interesting in that they no longer show significant nodes along the right inferior path or up to inferior or anterior frontal regions. The superior paths that are shown from posterior to anterior localizations show enhanced outflow from 0.07 to approximately 0.2 and enhanced connectivity from 0–0.07 to close to 0.15. These would appear to represent fairly sizeable changes in brain activity and connectivity measurable in this fashion. These were associated with reports of dramatically reduced OCD behaviors and enhanced emotional regulation and social interest.

13.9 Future directions

We have presented information on brain connectivity imaging applied to persons with ASD as a means to help understand and assess these features. These techniques may be helpful in further understanding these processes for both research and clinical purposes. Significantly more

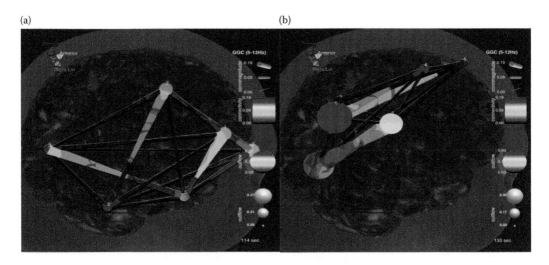

(a)   (b)

Figure 13.14 Findings of Granger causality connectivity on Treatment Case with Autism. Nodes are indicated by ROI balls with greater size and brighter color indicating greater outflow. Connectivity is indicated by the size and brightness of the lines between the nodes. On the left side, shows (a) the pretreatment findings and on the right (b) post-treatment.

research is needed into these approaches to understand their meaning and value. Research that looks at how these effective connectivity measures related to structural connectivity is desired. The limitations of these approaches must also be outlined and placed in the larger context of brain imaging in autism. Last, further work determining how such findings can be used to enhance the lives of those with autism spectrum disorder should be of the utmost priority.

References

Acar, Z. A. and S. Makeig. 2013. Effects of forward model errors on EEG source localization. *Brain Topogr.* 26:378–96.

Ameis, S. H. and M. Catani. 2015. Altered white matter connectivity as a neural substrate for social impairment in autism spectrum disorder. *Cortex* 62:158–81.

Ameis, S. H., J. Fan, C. Rockel, L. Soorya, A. T. Wang, and E. Anagnostou. 2013. Altered cingulum bundle microstructure in autism spectrum disorder. *Acta Neuropsychiatr.* 25:275–82.

Ameis, S. H., J. Fan, C. Rockel et al. 2011. Impaired structural connectivity of socioemotional circuits in autism spectrum disorders: A diffusion tensor imaging study. *PLoS One* 6:e28044.

Amiet, C., I. Gourfinkel-An, A. Bouzamondo et al. 2008. Epilepsy in autism is associated with intellectual disability and gender: Evidence from a meta-analysis. *Biol. Psychiatry* 64:577–82.

Aoki, Y., O. Abe, Y. Nippashi, and H. Yamasue. 2013. Comparison of white matter integrity between autism spectrum disorder subjects and typically developing individuals: A meta-analysis of diffusion tensor imaging tractography studies. *Mol. Autism* 4(1):25.

APA. 2013. *Diagnostic and Statistical Manual of Mental Disorders*, 5th ed. Arlington: American Psychiatric Publishing.

Assaf, M., K. Jagannathan, V. D. Calhoun et al. 2010. Abnormal functional connectivity of default mode sub-networks in autism spectrum disorder patients. *Neuroimage* 53:247–56.

Astolfi, L., F. Cincotti, D. Mattia et al. 2007. Comparison of different cortical connectivity estimators for high-resolution EEG recordings. *Hum. Brain Mapp.* 28:143–57.

Balardin, J. B., W. E. Comfort, E. Daly et al. 2015. Decreased centrality of cortical volume covariance networks in autism spectrum disorders. *J. Psychiatr. Res.* 69:142–9.

Barttfeld, P., B. Wicker, S. Cukier, S. Navarta, S. Lew, and M. Sigman. 2011. A big-world network in ASD: Dynamical connectivity analysis reflects a deficit in long-range connections and an excess of short-range connections. *Neuropsychologia* 49:254–63.

Başar, E., C. Başar-Eroglu, S. Karakaş, and M. Schürmann. 2001. Gamma, alpha, delta, and theta oscillations govern cognitive processes. *Int. J. Psychophysiol.* 39:241–8.

Basser, P. J. and C. Pierpaoli. 1996. Microstructural and physiological features of tissues elucidated by quantitative-diffusion-tensor MRI. *J. Magn. Reson. B.* 111:209–19.

Belmonte, M. K., G. Allen, A. Beckel-Mitchener, L. M. Boulanger, R. A. Carper, and S. J. Webb. 2004. Autism and abnormal development of brain connectivity. *J. Neurosci.* 24:9228–31.

Ben Bashat, D., V. Kronfeld-Duenias, D. A. Zachor, P. M. Ekstein, T. Hendler, R. Tarrasch et al. 2007. Accelerated maturation of white matter in young children with autism: A high b value DWI study. *Neuroimage* 37:40–7.

Billeci, L., S. Calderoni, M. Tosetti, M. Catani, and F. Muratori. 2012. White matter connectivity in children with autism spectrum disorders: A tract-based spatial statistics study. *BMC Neurol.* 12:148.

Blinowska, K. J. 2011. Review of the methods of determination of directed connectivity from multichannel data. *Med. Biol. Eng. Comput.* 49:521–9.

Bode, M. K., M. L. Mattila, V. Kiviniemi et al. 2011. White matter in autism spectrum disorders—Evidence of impaired fiber formation. *Acta. Radiol.* 52:1169–74.

Bos, D. J., J. Merchan-Naranjo, K. Martinez et al. 2015. Reduced gyrification is related to reduced interhemispheric connectivity in autism spectrum disorders. *J. Am. Acad. Child. Adolesc. Psychiatry* 54:668–76.

Bourgeron, T. 2015. From the genetic architecture to synaptic plasticity in autism spectrum disorder. *Nat. Rev. Neurosci.* 16:551–63.

Bressler, S. L. and A. K. Seth. 2011. Wiener–Granger causality: A well established methodology. *Neuroimage* 58:323–9.

Buckner, R. L., J. R. Andrews-Hanna, and D. L. Schacter. 2008. The brain's default network: Anatomy, function, and relevance to disease. *Ann. N. Y. Acad. Sci.* 1124:1–38.

Bullmore, E. and O. Sporns. 2013. The economy of brain network organization. *Nat. Rev. Neurosci.* 13:336–49.

Burnham, K. P. and D. R. Anderson. 2004. Multimodel inference understanding AIC and BIC in model selection. *Sociol. Methods Res.* 33:261–304.

Buzsaki, G. 2006. *Rhythms of the Brain.* New York: Oxford University Press.

Cadotte, A. J., T. B. DeMarse, P. He, and M. Ding. 2008. Causal measures of structure and plasticity in simulated and living neural networks. *PloS One* 3:e3355.

Carper, R. A., S. Solders, J. M. Treiber, I. Fishman, and R. A. Muller. 2015. Corticospinal tract anatomy and functional connectivity of primary motor cortex in autism. *J. Am. Acad. Child. Adolesc. Psychiatry* 54:859–67.

Carson, A. M., N. M. Salowitz, R. A. Scheidt, B. K. Dolan, and A. V. Van Hecke. 2014. Electroencephalogram coherence in children with and without autism spectrum disorders: Decreased interhemispheric connectivity in autism. *Autism Res.* 7:334–43.

Catani, M. 2006. Diffusion tensor magnetic resonance imaging tractography in cognitive disorders. *Curr. Opin. Neurol.* 19:599–606.

Catani, M., D. K. Jones, E. Daly et al. 2008. Altered cerebellar feedback projections in Asperger syndrome. *Neuroimage* 41:1184–91.

Catarino, A., A. Andrade, O. Churches, A. P. Wagner, S. Baron-Cohen, and H. Ring. 2013. Task-related functional connectivity in autism spectrum conditions: An EEG study using wavelet transform coherence. *Mol. Autism* 4:1.

Cerliani, L., M. Mennes, R. M. Thomas, A. Di Martino, M. Thioux, and C. Keysers. 2015. Increased functional connectivity between subcortical and cortical resting-state networks in autism spectrum disorder. *JAMA Psychiatry* 72:767–77.

Chan, A. S., Y. M. Han, S. L. Sze et al. 2011. Disordered connectivity associated with memory deficits in children with autism spectrum disorders. *Res. Autism Spectrum Disord.* 5:237–45.

Chang, Y. S., J. P. Owen, S. S. Desai et al. 2014. Autism and sensory processing disorders: Shared white matter disruption in sensory pathways but divergent connectivity in social-emotional pathways. *PLoS One* 9:e103038.

Chen, C. P., C. L. Keown, A. Jahedi et al. 2015. Diagnostic classification of intrinsic functional connectivity highlights somatosensory, default mode, and visual regions in autism. *Neuroimage. Clin.* 8:238–45.

Cheng, Y., K. H. Chou, I. Y. Chen, Y. T. Fan, J. Decety, and C. P. Lin. 2010. Atypical development of white matter microstructure in adolescents with autism spectrum disorders. *Neuroimage* 50:873–82.

Cheon, K. A., Y. S. Kim, S. H. Oh et al. 2011. Involvement of the anterior thalamic radiation in boys with high functioning autism spectrum disorders: A Diffusion Tensor Imaging study. *Brain Res.* 1417:77–86.

Cherkassky, V. L., R. K. Kana, T. A. Keller, and M. A. Just. 2006. Functional connectivity in a baseline resting-state network in autism. *Neuroreport* 17:1687–90.

Coben, R. 2013. Neurofeedback for autistic disorders: Emerging empirical evidence. In *Imaging the Brain in Autism*, eds. M. F. Casanova, A. S. El-Baz, and J. Suri, 107–34. New York: Springer.

Coben, R., M. Arns, and M. E. Kouijzer. 2010. Enduring effects of neurofeedback in children. In *Neurofeedback and Neuromodulation Techniques and Applications*, eds. R. Coben and J. R. Evans, 403–22. London: Academic Press.

Coben, R., A. R. Clarke, W. Hudspeth, and R. J. Barry. 2008. EEG power and coherence in autistic spectrum disorder. *Clin. Neurophysiol.* 119:1002–9.

Coben, R. and J. R. Evans, eds. 2010. *Neurofeedback and Neuromodulation Techniques and Applications*. London: Academic Press.

Coben, R. and I. Mohammad-Rezazadeh. 2015. Neural connectivity in epilepsy as measured by Granger causality. *Front. Hum. Neurosci.* 9:194.

Coben, R., I. Mohammad-Rezazadeh, and R. L. Cannon. 2014. Using quantitative and analytic EEG methods in the understanding of connectivity in autism spectrum disorders: A theory of mixed over- and under-connectivity. *Front. Hum. Neurosci.* 8:45.

Coben, R. and T. E. Myers. 2010. The relative efficacy of connectivity guided and symptom based EEG biofeedback for autistic disorders. *Appl. Psychophysiol. Biofeedback* 35:13–23.

Coben, R., M. Linden, and T. E. Myers. 2010. Neurofeedback for autistic spectrum disorder: A review of the literature. *Appl. Psychophysiol. Biofeedback.* 35:83–105.

Coben, R., L. Sherlin, W. J. Hudspeth, K. McKeon, and R. Ricca. 2014. Connectivity-guided EEG biofeedback for autism spectrum disorder: Evidence of neurophysiological changes. *Neuro. Regul.* 1:109.

Conti, E., S. Calderoni, V. Marchi, F. Muratori, G. Cioni, and A. Guzzetta. 2015. The first 1000 days of the autistic brain: A systematic review of diffusion imaging studies. *Front. Hum. Neurosci.* 9:159.

Courchesne, E. 2004. Brain development in autism: Early overgrowth followed by premature arrest of growth. *Ment. Retard. Dev. Disabil. Res. Rev.* 10:106–11.

Courchesne, E., C. M. Karns, H. R. Davis et al. 2001. Unusual brain growth patterns in early life in patients with autistic disorder: An MRI study. *Neurology* 57:245–54.

Courchesne, E., P. R. Mouton, M. E. Calhoun et al. 2011. Neuron number and size in prefrontal cortex of children with autism. *JAMA* 306:2001–10.

Courchesne, E. and K. Pierce. 2005. Why the frontal cortex in autism might be talking only to itself: Local over-connectivity but long-distance disconnection. *Curr. Opin. Neurobiol.* 15:225–30.

Courchesne, E., E. Redcay, J. T. Morgan, and D. P. Kennedy. 2005. Autism at the beginning: Microstructural and growth abnormalities underlying the cognitive and behavioral phenotype of autism. *Dev. Psychopathol.* 17:577–97.

Delorme, A., T. Mullen, C. Kothe, Z. A. Acar, N. Bigdely-Shamlo, A. Vankov, and S. Makeig. 2011. EEGLAB, SIFT, NFT, BCILAB, and ERICA: New tools for advanced EEG processing. *Comput. Intell. Neurosci.* 2011:10.

Deshpande, G., L. E. Libero, K. R. Sreenivasan, H. D. Deshpande, and R. K. Kana. 2013. Identification of neural connectivity signatures of autism using machine learning. *Front. Hum. Neurosci.* 7:670.

D'Gama, A. M., S. Pochareddy, M. Li et al. 2015. Targeted DNA sequencing from autism spectrum disorder brains implicates multiple genetic mechanisms. *Neuron* 88:910–17.

Dhamala, M., G. Rangarajan, and M. Ding. 2008. Analyzing information flow in brain networks with nonparametric Granger causality. *NeuroImage* 41:354–62.

Di, X., S. Gohel, E. H. Kim, and B. B. Biswal. 2013. Task vs. rest—Different network configurations between the coactivation and the resting-state brain networks. *Front. Human Neurosci.* 7:493.

Di Martino, A., K. Ross, L. Q. Uddin, A. B. Sklar, F. X. Castellanos, and M. P. Milham. 2009. Functional brain correlates of social and nonsocial processes in autism spectrum disorders: An activation likelihood estimation meta-analysis. *Biol. Psychiatry* 65:63–74.

Di Martino, A., C. G. Yan, Q. Li et al. 2014. The autism brain imaging data exchange: Towards a large-scale evaluation of the intrinsic brain architecture in autism. *Mol. Psychiatry* 19:659–67.

Doesburg, S. M., J. Vidal, and M. J. Taylor. 2013. Reduced theta connectivity during set-shifting in children with autism. *Front. Hum. Neurosci.* 7:785.

Duffy, F.H. and H. Als. 2012. A stable pattern of EEG spectral coherence distinguishes children with autism from neuro-typical controls-a large case control study. *BMC Med.* 10:64.

Ecker, C., L. Ronan, Y. Feng et al. 2013. Intrinsic gray-matter connectivity of the brain in adults with autism spectrum disorder. *Proc. Natl. Acad. Sci. USA* 110:13222–7.

EEG Software. 2013. *EEGer4 Neurofeedback Software: Technical Manual*, ver. 4.3.0. Granada Hills: EEG Education and Research.

Ellmore, T. M., H. Li, Z. Xue, S. T. Wong, and R. E. Frye. 2013. Tract-based spatial statistics reveal altered relationship between non-verbal reasoning abilities and white matter integrity in autism spectrum disorder. *J. Int. Neuropsychol. Soc.* 19:723–8.

Enticott, P. G., B. M. Fitzgibbon, H. A. Kennedy et al. 2014. A double-blind, randomized trial of deep repetitive transcranial magnetic stimulation (rTMS) for autism spectrum disorder. *Brain Stimul.* 7:206–11.

Fitzgerald, K. D., R. C. Welsh, E. R. Stern, M. Angstadt, G. L. Hanna, J. L. Abelson, and S. F. Taylor. 2011. Developmental alterations of frontal-striatal-thalamic connectivity in obsessive-compulsive disorder. *J. Am. Acad. Child. Adolesc. Psychiatry* 50:938–48.

Fletcher, P. T., R. T. Whitaker, R. Tao et al. 2010. Microstructural connectivity of the arcuate fasciculus in adolescents with high-functioning autism. *Neuroimage* 51:1117–25.

Florian, G. and G. Pfurtscheller. 1995. Dynamic spectral analysis of event-related EEG data. *Electroencephalogr. Clin. Neurophysiol.* 95:393–6. doi: 10.1016/0013-4694(95)00198-8.

Fries, P. 2005. A mechanism for cognitive dynamics: Neuronal communication through neuronal coherence. *Trends. Cogn. Sci.* 9:474–80.

Friston, K. J. 2011. Functional and effective connectivity: A review. *Brain Connect.* 1:13–36.

Frith, C. 2003. What do imaging studies tell us about the neural basis of autism? *Novartis. Found. Symp.* 251:149–66; discussion 166–76, 281–97.

Gibbard, C. R., J. Ren, K. K. Seunarine, J. D. Clayden, D. H. Skuse, and C. A. Clark. 2013. White matter microstructure correlates with autism trait severity in a combined clinical-control sample of high-functioning adults. *Neuroimage Clin.* 3:106–14.

Gotts, S. J., W. K. Simmons, L. A. Milbury, G. L. Wallace, R. W. Cox, and A. Martin. 2012. Fractionation of social brain circuits in autism spectrum disorders. *Brain* 135:2711–25.

Granger, C. W. 1969. Investigating causal relations by econometric models and cross-spectral methods. *Econometrica* 37:424–38.

Hanaie, R., I. Mohri, K. Kagitani-Shimono et al. 2014. Abnormal corpus callosum connectivity, socio-communicative deficits, and motor deficits in children with autism spectrum disorder: A diffusion tensor imaging study. *J. Autism Dev. Disord.* 44:2209–20.

Hazlett, H. C., M. Poe, G. Gerig et al. 2005. Magnetic resonance imaging and head circumference study of brain size in autism: Birth through age 2 years. *Arch. Gen. Psychiatry* 62:1366–76.

Herbert, M. R. 2005. Large brains in autism: The challenge of pervasive abnormality. *Neuroscientist* 11:417–40.

Hernandez, L. M., J. D. Rudie, S. A. Green, S. Bookheimer, and M. Dapretto. 2015. Neural signatures of autism spectrum disorders: Insights into brain network dynamics. *Neuropsychopharmacology* 40:171–89.

Hoppenbrouwers, M., M. Vandermosten, and B. Boets. 2014. Autism as a disconnection syndrome: A qualitative and quantitative review of diffusion tensor imaging studies. *Res. Autism Spectrum Disord.* 8:387–412.

Jarusiewicz, B. 2002. Efficacy of neurofeedback for children in the autistic spectrum: A pilot study. *J. Neurother.* 6:39–49.

Jensen, O., J. Kaiser, and J. P. Lachaux. 2007. Human gamma-frequency oscillations associated with attention and memory. *Trends Neurosci.* 30:317–24.

Jeste, S. S. 2011. The neurology of autism spectrum disorders. *Curr. Opin. Neurol.* 24:132–9.

Just, M. A., V. L. Cherkassky, T. A. Keller, and N. J. Minshew. 2004. Cortical activation and synchronization during sentence comprehension in high-functioning autism: Evidence of underconnectivity. *Brain* 127:1811–21.

Just, M. A., T. A. Keller, V. L. Malave, R. K. Kana, and S. Varma. 2012. Autism as a neural systems disorder: A theory of frontal-posterior underconnectivity. *Neurosci. Biobehav. Rev.* 36:1292–313.

Kana, R. K., T. A. Keller, V. L. Cherkassky, N. J. Minshew, and M. A. Just. 2006. Sentence comprehension in autism: Thinking in pictures with decreased functional connectivity. *Brain* 129:2484–93.

Kapur, S., A. G. Phillips, and T. R. Insel. 2012. Why has it taken so long for biological psychiatry to develop clinical tests and what to do about it? *Mol. Psychiatry* 17:1174–9.

Kayser, A. S., F. T. Sun, and M. D'Esposito. 2009. A comparison of Granger causality and coherency in fMRI-based analysis of the motor system. *Hum. Brain Mapp.* 30:3475–94.

Keller, T. A., R. K. Kana, and M. A. Just. 2007. A developmental study of the structural integrity of white matter in autism. *Neuroreport* 18:23–7.

Khan, S., A. Gramfort, N. R. Shetty et al. 2013. Local and long-range functional connectivity is reduced in concert in autism spectrum disorders. *Proc. Natl. Acad. Sci. USA* 110:3107–12.

Kikuchi, M., K. Shitamichi, Y. Yoshimura et al. 2013. Altered brain connectivity in 3-to 7-year-old children with autism spectrum disorder. *Neuroimage. Clin.* 2:394–401.

Kleinhans, N. M., T. Richards, L. Sterling, K. C. Stegbauer, R. Mahurin, L. C. Johnson, J. Greenson, G. Dawson, and E. Aylward. 2008. Abnormal functional connectivity in autism spectrum disorders during face processing. *Brain* 131:1000–12.

Klimesch, W. 1999. EEG alpha and theta oscillations reflect cognitive and memory performance: A review and analysis. *Brain Res. Rev.* 29:169–95.

Koshino, H., P. A. Carpenter, N. J. Minshew, V. L. Cherkassky, T. A. Keller, and M. A. Just. 2005. Functional connectivity in an fMRI working memory task in high-functioning autism. *Neuroimage* 24:810–21.

Kouijzer, M. E., J. M. de Moor, B. J. Gerrits, M. Congedo, and H. T. van Schie. 2009. Neurofeedback improves executive functioning in children with autism spectrum disorders. *Res. Autism Spectrum Disord.* 3:145–62.

Kumar, A., S. K. Sundaram, L. Sivaswamy et al. 2010. Alterations in frontal lobe tracts and corpus callosum in young children with autism spectrum disorder. *Cereb. Cortex.* 20:2103–13.

Kuś, R., M. Kamiński, and K. J. Blinowska. 2004. Determination of EEG activity propagation: Pair-wise versus multichannel estimate. *IEEE Trans. Biomed. Eng.* 51:1501–10.

Lachaux, J. P., E. Rodriguez, J. Martinerie, and F. J. Varela. 1999. Measuring phase synchrony in brain signals. *Hum. Brain Mapp.* 8:194–208.

Lee, J. E., E. D. Bigler, A. L. Alexander et al. 2007. Diffusion tensor imaging of white matter in the superior temporal gyrus and temporal stem in autism. *Neurosci. Lett.* 424:127–32.

Lefebvre, A., A. Beggiato, T. Bourgeron, and R. Toro. 2015. Neuroanatomical diversity of corpus callosum and brain volume in autism: Meta-analysis, analysis of the Autism Brain Imaging Data Exchange Project, and simulation. *Biol. Psychiatry* 78:126–34.

Lewis, J. D. and J. L. Elman. 2008. Growth-related neural reorganization and the autism phenotype: A test of the hypothesis that altered brain growth leads to altered connectivity. *Dev. Sci.* 11:135–55.

Liu, Y. and S. Aviyente. 2012. Quantification of effective connectivity in the brain using a measure of directed information. *Comput. Math. Methods. Med.* 2012:635103.

Loo, S. K., A. Lenartowicz, and S. Makeig. 2015. Research review: Use of EEG biomarkers in child psychiatry research—Current state and future directions. *J. Child. Psychol. Psychiatry.* in press. doi: 10.1111/jcpp.12435. PMID: 26099166.

Lynch, C. J., L. Q. Uddin, K. Supekar, A. Khouzam, J. Phillips, and V. Menon. 2013. Default mode network in childhood autism: Posteromedial cortex heterogeneity and relationship with social deficits. *Biol. Psychiatry* 74:212–9.

Maximo, J. O., E. J. Cadena, and R. K. Kana. 2014. The implications of brain connectivity in the neuropsychology of autism. *Neuropsychol. Rev.* 24:16–31.

Mohammad-Rezazadeh, I., J. Frohlich, S. K. Loo, and S. S. Jeste. 2016. Brain connectivity in autism spectrum disorder. *Curr. Opin. Neurol.* 29:137–47.

Monk, C. S., S. J. Peltier, J. L. Wiggins et al. 2009. Abnormalities of intrinsic functional connectivity in autism spectrum disorders. *Neuroimage* 47:764–72.

Mullen, T., G. Worrell, and S. Makeig. 2012. Multivariate principal oscillation pattern analysis of ICA sources during seizure. *Int. Conf. IEEE Eng. Med. Biol. Soc.* 34:2921–4.

Murias, M., S. J. Webb, J. Greenson, and G. Dawson. 2007. Resting state cortical connectivity reflected in EEG coherence in individuals with autism. *Biol. Psychiatry* 62:270–3.

Nair, A., C. L. Keown, M. Datko, P. Shih, B. Keehn, and R. A. Muller. 2014. Impact of methodological variables on functional connectivity findings in autism spectrum disorders. *Hum. Brain Mapp.* 35:4035–48.

Nomi, J. S. and L. Q. Uddin. 2015. Developmental changes in large-scale network connectivity in autism. *Neuroimage Clin.* 7:732–41.

Nunez, P. L., R. Srinivasan, A. F. Westdorp, R. S. Wijesinghe, D. M. Tucker, R. B. Silberstein, and P. J. Cadusch. 1997. EEG coherency: I: Statistics, reference electrode, volume conduction, Laplacians, cortical imaging, and interpretation at multiple scales. *Electroencephalogr. Clin. Neurophysiol.* 103:499–515.

Orekhova, E. V., M. Elsabbagh, E. J. Jones, G. Dawson, T. Charman, and M. H. Johnson. 2014. EEG hyper-connectivity in high-risk infants is associated with later autism. *J. Neurodev. Disord.* 6:40.

Pineda, J. A., D. Brang, E. Hecht et al. 2008. Positive behavioral and electrophysiological changes following neurofeedback training in children with autism. *Re. Autism Spectrum Disord.* 2:557–81.

Pugliese, L., M. Catani, S. Ameis et al. 2009. The anatomy of extended limbic pathways in Asperger syndrome: A preliminary diffusion tensor imaging tractography study. *NeuroImage* 47:427–34.

Rubinov, M. and O. Sporns. 2010. Complex network measures of brain connectivity: Uses and interpretations. *NeuroImage* 52:1059–69.

Rudie, J. D., J. A. Brown, D. Beck-Pancer et al. 2012. Altered functional and structural brain network organization in autism. *Neuroimage Clin.* 2:79–94.

Sacco, R., S. Gabriele, and A. M. Persico. 2015. Head circumference and brain size in autism spectrum disorder: A systematic review and meta-analysis. *Psychiatry Res.* 234:239–51.

Sanders, S. J. 2015. First glimpses of the neurobiology of autism spectrum disorder. *Curr. Opin. Genet. Dev.* 33:80–92.

Schreiber, T. 2000. Measuring information transfer. *Phys. Rev. Lett.* 85:461.

Sherlin, L. H., M. Arns, J. Lubar, H. Heinrich, C. Kerson, U. Strehl, and M. B. Sterman. 2011. Neurofeedback and basic learning theory: Implications for research and practice. *J. Neurother.* 15:292–304.

Shih, P., M. Shen, B. Ottl, B. Keehn, M. S. Gaffrey, and R. A. Müller. 2010. Atypical network connectivity for imitation in autism spectrum disorder. *Neuropsychologia* 48:2931–9.

Shukla, D. K., B. Keehn, A. J. Lincoln, and R. A. Müller. 2010. White matter compromise of callosal and subcortical fiber tracts in children with autism spectrum disorder: A diffusion tensor imaging study. *J. Am. Acad. Child. Adolesc. Psychiatry* 49:1269–78.e2.

Shukla, D. K., B. Keehn, D. M. Smylie, and R. A. Müller. 2011. Microstructural abnormalities of short-distance white matter tracts in autism spectrum disorder. *Neuropsychologia* 49:1378–82.

Sokhadze, E. M., J. M. Baruth, L. Sears, G. E. Sokhadze, A. S. El-Baz, and M. F. Casanova. 2012. Prefrontal neuromodulation using rTMS improves error monitoring and correction function in autism. *Appl. Psychophysiol. Biofeedback* 37:91–102.

Sokhadze, E. M., A. El-Baz, J. Baruth, G. Mathai, L. Sears, and M. F. Casanova. 2009. Effects of low frequency repetitive transcranial magnetic stimulation (rTMS) on gamma frequency oscillations and event-related potentials during processing of illusory figures in autism. *J. Autism Dev. Disord.* 39:619–34.

Solso, S., R. Xu, J. Proudfoot et al. 2016. Diffusion tensor imaging provides evidence of possible axonal overconnectivity in frontal lobes in autism spectrum disorder toddlers. *Biol. Psychiatry* 79:676–84.

Sparks, B. F., S. D. Friedman, D. W. Shaw et al. 2002. Brain structural abnormalities in young children with autism spectrum disorder. *Neurology* 59:184–92.

Sporns, O. 2011. *Networks of the Brain*. Cambridge: MIT Press.

Sporns, O. 2014. Contributions and challenges for network models in cognitive neuroscience. *Nat. Neurosci.* 17:652–60.

Sulzer, J., S. Haller, F. Scharnowski et al. 2013. Real-time fMRI neurofeedback: Progress and challenges. *Neuroimage* 76:386–99.

Sundaram, S. K., A. Kumar, M. I. Makki, M. E. Behen, H. T. Chugani, and D. C. Chugani. 2008. Diffusion tensor imaging of frontal lobe in autism spectrum disorder. *Cereb. Cortex* 18:2659–65.

Supekar, K., L. Q. Uddin, A. Khouzam et al. 2013. Brain hyperconnectivity in children with autism and its links to social deficits. *Cell. Rep.* 5:738–47.

Stam, C. and B. Van Dijk. 2002. Synchronization likelihood: An unbiased measure of generalized synchronization in multivariate data sets. *Physica D. Nonlin. Phenom.* 163:236–51.

Tick, B., P. Bolton, F. Happe, M. Rutter, and F. Rijsdijk. 2016. Heritability of autism spectrum disorders: A meta-analysis of twin studies. *J. Child. Psychol. Psychiatry* 57(5):585–95. doi: 10.1111/jcpp.12499.

Tononi, G., G. M. Edelman, and O. Sporns. 1998. Complexity and coherency: Integrating information in the brain. *Trends Cogn. Sci.* 2:474–84.

Tortella, G., R. Casati, L. V. Aparicio et al. 2015. Transcranial direct current stimulation in psychiatric disorders. *World. J. Psychiatry* 5:88–102.

Tyszka, J. M., D. P. Kennedy, L. K. Paul, and R. Adolphs. 2014. Largely typical patterns of resting-state functional connectivity in high-functioning adults with autism. *Cereb. Cortex* 24:1894–905.

Uddin, L. Q., K. Supekar, C. J. Lynch, A. Khouzam, J. Phillips, C. Feinstein, S. Ryali, and V. Menon. 2013a. Salience network-based classification and prediction of symptom severity in children with autism. *JAMA Psychiatry* 70:869–79.

Uddin, L. Q., K. Supekar, and V. Menon. 2013b. Reconceptualizing functional brain connectivity in autism from a developmental perspective. *Front. Hum. Neurosci.* 7:458.

Urbain, C., V. M. Vogan, A. X. Ye, E. W. Pang, S. M. Doesburg, and M. J. Taylor. 2016. Desynchronization of fronto-temporal networks during working memory processing in autism. *Hum. Brain Mapp.* 37:153–64.

Vakorin, V. A., B. Mišić, O. Krakovska, G. Bezgin, and A. R. McIntosh. 2013. Confounding effects of phase delays on causality estimation. *PLoS One* 8:e53588.

Vicente, R., M. Wibral, M. Lindner, and G. Pipa. 2011. Transfer entropy—A model-free measure of effective connectivity for the neurosciences. *J. Comput. Neurosci.* 30:45–67.

Villalobos, M. E., A. Mizuno, B. C. Dahl, N. Kemmotsu, and R. A. Müller. 2005. Reduced functional connectivity between V1 and inferior frontal cortex associated with visuomotor performance in autism. *Neuroimage* 25:916–25.

Viscidi, E. W., E. W. Triche, M. F. Pescosolido et al. 2013. Clinical characteristics of children with autism spectrum disorder and co-occurring epilepsy. *PLoS One* 8:e67797.

von dem Hagen, E. A., R. S. Stoyanova, S. Baron-Cohen, and A. J. Calder. 2012. Reduced functional connectivity within and between "social" resting state networks in autism spectrum conditions. *Soc. Cogn. Affect. Neurosci.* 8:694–701.

Walker, L., M. Gozzi, R. Lenroot et al. 2012. Diffusion tensor imaging in young children with autism: Biological effects and potential confounds. *Biol. Psychiatry* 72:1043–51.

Warrier, V., V. Chee, P. Smith, B. Chakrabarti, and S. Baron-Cohen. 2015. A comprehensive meta-analysis of common genetic variants in autism spectrum conditions. *Mol. Autism* 6:49.

Wass, S. 2011. Distortions and disconnections: Disrupted brain connectivity in autism. *Brain. Cogn.* 75:18–28.

Weinstein, M., L. Ben-Sira, Y. Levy et al. 2011. Abnormal white matter integrity in young children with autism. *Hum. Brain. Mapp.* 32:534–43.

Weng, S. J., J. L. Wiggins, S. J. Peltier et al. 2010. Alterations of resting state functional connectivity in the default network in adolescents with autism spectrum disorders. *Brain Res.* 1313:202–14.

Willsey, A. J. and M. W. State. 2015. Autism spectrum disorders: From genes to neurobiology. *Curr. Opin. Neurobiol.* 30:92–9.

Wolff, J. J., H. Gu, G. Gerig et al. 2012. Differences in white matter fiber tract development present from 6 to 24 months in infants with autism. *Am. J. Psychiatry* 169:589–600.

Yerys, B. E., E. M. Gordon, D. N. Abrams et al. 2015. Default mode network segregation and social deficits in autism spectrum disorder: Evidence from nonmedicated children. *Neuroimage Clin.* 9:223–32.

Zikopoulos, B. and H. Barbas. 2010. Changes in prefrontal axons may disrupt the network in autism. *J. Neurosci.* 30:14595–609.

Chapter 14 Brain network organization in ASD
Evidence from functional and diffusion weighted MRI

Ralph-Axel Müller and
Ruth A. Carper

Contents

Abstract 288
14.1 Introduction 288
14.2 Functional connectivity 289
    14.2.1 Why do findings diverge? 290
    14.2.2 Challenge no. 1: "Resting" state 294
    14.2.3 Challenge no. 2: Dynamic connectivity 295
14.3 Anatomical connectivity 297
    14.3.1 Findings in children, adolescents, and adults 298
    14.3.2 Findings in infants and toddlers 299
    14.3.3 Challenge no. 1: Understanding microstructural
            underpinnings 299
    14.3.4 Challenge no. 2: Complex fiber orientations 300
    14.3.5 Challenge no. 3: Motion 301
14.4 Perspectives 302
    14.4.1 A developmental model of neurofunctional
            organization in ASD 302
    14.4.2 From genes to treatment: Can neuroimaging
            bridge the gap? 304
Acknowledgments 307
References 307

Abstract

Beyond the general consensus of ASD being a brain-based disorder, there is increasing evidence of anomalies in network organization and connectivity. However, the abundance of findings is coupled with low replication rates. In this chapter, we review some main findings from functional and anatomical connectivity research in ASD. Major methodological challenges in functional connectivity and diffusion weighted MRI and potential solutions are discussed. A developmental model of dual network impairment is presented that reconciles some apparent inconsistencies in findings, followed by a discussion of conceptual challenges and the importance of data-driven approaches.

14.1 Introduction

Although the insight that autistic symptomatology reflects neurological disturbances, rather than bad parenting (Bettelheim 1967), is decades old, to the present day neither *in vivo* imaging techniques nor postmortem cellular analyses permit a diagnostic decision based on brain markers alone. Simply put, we still cannot look at a brain scan and point to a specific anomaly or pattern of anomalies to determine: "This child has autism." Paradoxically, as much as we are convinced that autism is in the brain, it appears to be nowhere (in particular) in the brain. At the same time, exacerbating the paradox (as we will discuss further down) autism appears to be everywhere in the brain.

Many proposals have been put forward. Some of them have been comparatively simple in neuroanatomical terms, focusing on a single brain structure, such as the amygdala (Baron-Cohen et al. 2000) or the cerebellum (Courchesne et al. 1988). However, as we shall see, such proposals are incompatible with the extensive evidence implicating numerous other brain loci and systems. Following a general shift of focus in the cognitive and clinical neurosciences, the modern view of autism spectrum disorders (ASD) refers to atypical brain organization at the level of distributed networks and interconnectivity (Menon 2011). Even within this contemporary paradigm, some relatively simple hypotheses have been proposed, such as a specific underconnectivity between frontal and parietal lobes (Just et al. 2012) or a dichotomy of increased local but reduced long-distance connectivity (Belmonte et al. 2004; Courchesne and Pierce 2005). While such proposals may be useful in the Popperian sense (Popper 1965) that only falsifiable hypotheses promote scientific advance, they can easily mislead the large lay community (in particular, the parents of children with ASD) to believe that we have firm knowledge when in truth the evidence is inconclusive at best.

In this chapter, we first provide an overview of the available literature on functional and anatomical connectivity in ASD, with focus on MRI techniques. Many of the uncountable findings lack replication, and our review will therefore not even attempt completeness. Instead, we will aim to outline patterns in the multitude of findings, before turning to issues and caveats, as well as broader perspectives.

14.2 Functional connectivity

Functional connectivity was originally defined as "temporal correlations between spatially remote neurophysiological events" (Friston et al. 1993), but a more recent and broader definition refers to any "statistical dependence between remote neural processes" (Honey et al. 2007). The dominant technique has been functional connectivity MRI (fcMRI), although a few early studies used positron emission tomography (PET; Horwitz et al. 1988; Castelli et al. 2002). However, the temporal resolution of PET is effectively nonexistent, whereas it is typically in the range of 2–3 sec in functional MRI. The serendipitous observations triggered by the pioneering work in Biswal et al. (1995) showed that low-frequency fluctuations in the blood oxygen level dependent (BOLD) signal, which can be detected even at the modest temporal resolution of fMRI, are highly informative of brain network organization. Correlations in very low-frequency domains (c. $0.1 > f > 0.01$ Hz; Cordes et al. 2001) probably reflect network-specific fluctuations in local field potentials, that is, the local summation of neuronal electrical activity (Leopold et al. 2003; Schölvinck et al. 2010). Outside the ASD literature, the dominant fcMRI approach, commonly called intrinsic fcMRI (Van Dijk et al. 2010), has focused on such spontaneous, low-frequency BOLD fluctuations in resting state fMRI data. This approach has been successfully implemented in the study of numerous networks, such as motor (Jiang et al. 2004; Kim et al. 2010), visual (Lowe et al. 1998; Cordes et al. 2000; Nir et al. 2006), auditory (Saur et al. 2010), language (Hampson et al. 2002), reading (Koyama et al. 2011), working memory (Lowe et al. 2000), task control (Dosenbach et al. 2007; Seeley et al. 2007), default mode (Greicius et al. 2003; Wang et al. 2012), and attention (Fox et al. 2006) systems.

In the very first fcMRI study of ASD, Just and colleagues (2004) showed that BOLD signal correlations associated with sentence comprehension were reduced between a number of region pairs in adults with ASD and proposed an "underconnectivity theory" of autism. Consistent with this, the evidence of reduced functional connectivity in ASD has been reported in many studies that tested finger movement (Mostofsky et al. 2009), visuomotor coordination (Villalobos et al. 2005), face processing (Kleinhans et al. 2008), sentence comprehension (Kana et al. 2006), response inhibition (Kana et al. 2007; Lee et al. 2009; Agam et al. 2010), verbal working memory (Koshino et al. 2005), problem solving (Just et al. 2007), attention orienting (Fitzgerald et al. 2014), cognitive control (Solomon et al. 2009), self-representation (Lombardo et al. 2010; Mizuno et al. 2011), and theory of mind tasks (Mason et al. 2008; Kana et al. 2009, 2012). The apparent convergence of these findings led to the tentative conclusion of a "first firm finding" in ASD (Hughes 2007).

A closer look at the long list of studies cited above, however, shows a methodological complication that greatly impacts the interpretation of the findings. In all of the above studies, BOLD signal changes were prompted by domain-specific tasks. As described above, this differs from the intrinsic functional connectivity (iFC) approach. While the iFC paradigm has generally dominated the functional connectivity literature of the past two decades (Biswal et al. 1995; Fox and Raichle 2007; Van Dijk et al. 2010; Buckner et al. 2013; Power et al. 2014b), this has not been the case in ASD connectivity research. More recently, however, the early predominance of task-related "co-activation" fcMRI studies of ASD has been superseded by a growing number of iFC studies. Results from these have been much more complex. A number of studies that statistically regressed out task-related effects in order to isolate intrinsic low-frequency fluctuations reported extensive overconnectivity effects in ASD (Mizuno et al. 2006; Noonan et al. 2009; Shih et al. 2010, 2011; Shen et al. 2012; Keehn et al. 2013a). This suggests that removal of task-related or stimulus-driven effects shifts the distribution of findings from under- to overconnectivity, consistent with a meta-analysis (Müller et al. 2011) and two empirical comparative method studies (Jones et al. 2010; Nair et al. 2014). However, this approach of isolating intrinsic BOLD fluctuations from data acquired during task performance—though legitimate in principle (Fair et al. 2007)—has been implemented in ASD primarily only by a single group (our own)—warranting caution. A much larger number of studies have instead implemented a resting state fcMRI approach. Findings from this literature are by no means conclusive, ranging from predominant underconnectivity (Anderson et al. 2011a; Gotts et al. 2012; von dem Hagen et al. 2012; Abrams et al. 2013; Di Martino et al. 2014) to mixed findings (Monk et al. 2009; Keown et al. 2013; Lynch et al. 2013; Washington et al. 2013; Fishman et al. 2014, 2015; Abbott et al. 2015; Doyle-Thomas et al. 2015; Nair et al. 2015) and even to predominant overconnectivity (Di Martino et al. 2011; Delmonte et al. 2013; Supekar et al. 2013; Carper et al. 2015; Cerliani et al. 2015; Chien et al. 2015; Khan et al. 2015a). While they suggest that a generalized underconnectivity account of ASD is too simple, the question remains what may explain the divergent findings. Aside from effects of task, which, as described above, demonstrably tend to boost "underconnectivity" effects in ASD (unless the task taps into an "island of strength," Keehn et al. 2013a), there must be other factors, which we will now discuss.

14.2.1 Why do findings diverge?

The fcMRI technique had been implemented in ASD for many years before the field grew aware of issues related to head motion. While, in conventional activation fMRI, head motion of 2–3 mm (quite common in children or clinical populations) may be acceptable, several groups

Default mode network   Salience network

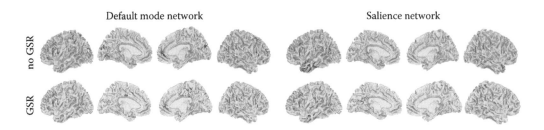

Figure 14.1 Whole brain intrinsic functional connectivity for representative seeds of default mode network (DMN: medial posterior cingulate cortex) and salience network (SN: right anterior insula). While, for analyses without global signal regression (GSR; top row), a distinctive pattern of predominant overconnectivity for DMN, but predominant underconnectivity for SN is observed, this pattern is lost with application of GSR. Since findings are from the identical resting fMRI data set, network-specific findings cannot be accounted for by differences in motion or other noise and therefore likely reflect true activity differences, which are obscured by GSR. (Adapted from Abbott, A. E. et al. 2015. *Cereb. Cortex.* DOI: 10.1093/cercor/bhv191.)

(Power et al. 2011; Van Dijk et al. 2012; Satterthwaite et al. 2013) demonstrated that even micromotion in the submillimeter range had a dramatic effect on fcMRI findings because motion-related signal changes may co-occur in many voxels across the brain, resulting in mostly inflated signal correlations (Power et al. 2015).

The ASD community was not prepared for this. By late 2010, only 4 out of 32 published fcMRI studies had presented statistical tests of potential group differences in motion (Müller et al. 2011). The conclusion that underconnectivity in early studies may have been an artifact of group differences in motion was obvious (Deen and Pelphrey 2012), but this account is clearly too simple. First, greater head motion in ASD groups would be overall more likely to inflate (not deflate) signal correlations (Power et al. 2014a), resulting in pseudo-overconnectivity. Second, some more recent iFC studies that carefully removed motion effects and matched groups for motion still had predominant underconnectivity findings (Nair et al. 2013; Starck et al. 2013; Di Martino et al. 2014). While scrupulous treatment of head motion is surely crucial in fcMRI (Power et al. 2015), it will not fully resolve apparent inconsistencies in the ASD literature.

Another proposal in this regard relates to global signal regression (GSR), that is, the use of mean brain signal fluctuations across time points as a nuisance regressor. An initial study (Jones et al. 2010) suggested that overconnectivity effects were an artifact of GSR. While clearly a powerful tool for noise reduction (Power et al. 2014a), GSR may distort group differences (Saad et al. 2012; Gotts et al. 2013), possibly because global signal fluctuations, in part, reflect true neuronal activity changes (Schölvinck et al. 2010). An example is provided in Figure 14.1. However, many studies have reported overconnectivity findings in the absence of GSR (Shih et al. 2011; Keehn et al. 2013a; Redcay et al. 2013; Supekar et al. 2013; Fishman et al. 2014), contrary to the hypothesis by Jones and colleagues.

Yet another account of fcMRI inconsistencies concerns developmental stage. Uddin et al. (2013) hypothesized that overconnectivity in younger children with ASD may be followed by underconnectivity in adolescents and adults. The proposal rightly points to the importance of maturational schedules, which probably differ between typically developing (TD) children and those with ASD. It also presents an interesting analogy to well-established anomalies in anatomical growth, with early overgrowth in ASD between 2 and 4 years (Schumann et al. 2010; Hazlett et al. 2011; Shen et al. 2013), and preliminary findings from DTI studies that may suggest accelerated white matter development in the first few years in ASD (Weinstein et al. 2011; Wolff et al. 2012a; Solso et al. 2015). Using near-infrared spectroscopy, Keehn et al. (2013b) also reported increased functional connectivity in 3-month-old infants with high-risk of ASD (compared to low-risk infants) and a "cross-over" to underconnectivity in these infants by age 12 months. All these latter findings highlight the need to interpret findings with respect to maturational changes. However, they are not readily consistent with the timeline proposed by Uddin et al. (2013) because they suggest "cross-over" from early overgrowth and overconnectivity to later flattened growth and underconnectivity in infancy or during the toddler years. In addition, some empirical evidence from fcMRI appears to directly contradict the hypothesis: For example, Dinstein et al. (2011) report interhemispheric underconnectivity in 12- to 46-month-old toddlers with ASD. Some studies including adolescents and adults have reported overconnectivity in ASD (Monk et al. 2009; Shen et al. 2012; Fishman et al. 2014, 2015; Abbott et al. 2015; Cerliani et al. 2015; Khan et al. 2015a). Di Martino et al. (2014), in the largest available iFC study incorporating 360 ASD participants (7–56 year old), found that differences from TD controls were mostly stable across different ages. Surveying the entire ASD fcMRI literature, a preponderance of underconnectivity findings in adults can indeed be found. However, this is partly due to the fact that one highly productive group, which applied coactivation methods testing for task-related BOLD correlations, happened to study adolescents and adults (Just et al. 2004, 2007; Koshino et al. 2005, 2008; Kana et al. 2006, 2007, 2009; Mason et al. 2008; Damarla et al. 2010; Mizuno et al. 2011). The appearance of a "developmental" pattern in the literature may therefore be, in part, methodological in nature.

Findings from Nair et al. (2014) suggest that methodological factors (other than GSR) have dramatic impact on group differences detected between ASD and TD samples. This study comparatively analyzed three data sets along competing pipelines. The most striking finding was that, for each data set, effects ranged from robust underconnectivity to robust overconnectivity in ASD, depending on methodological choices. Significant variables were type of analysis (coactivation vs. intrinsic fcMRI, as described above) and field of view (regions of interest vs. whole brain). Coactivation analyses limited to regions of interest tended to detect underconnectivity, whereas intrinsic fcMRI analyses testing for effects across the whole brain yielded mostly overconnectivity (Figure 14.2 for an example). Three

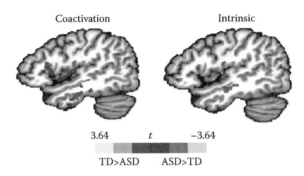

Coactivation   Intrinsic

3.64   t   −3.64

TD>ASD   ASD>TD

Figure 14.2 Significant BOLD correlations for a seed in left fusiform gyrus. Data are taken from a study by Keehn, B. et al. 2013a. *Hum. Brain Mapp.*, 34:2524–37, which also provided seed location based on activation peak for a visual search task. While task-driven correlations are greater in the TD group, suggesting greater functional connectivity, the opposite is found in an intrinsic functional connectivity analysis (with low bandpass filtering and after regressing out effects of task paradigm). (Adapted from Nair, A. et al. 2014. *Hum. Brain Mapp.*, 35:4035–48.)

drastic conclusions could be drawn. (1) *You find what you'd like to find*: Investigators predetermine through methodological choices the probability of detecting under- or overconnectivity in ASD. (2) *If you don't look, you won't find*: Studies limited to regions of expected effects may miss the bigger picture of overconnectivity elsewhere in the brain. (3) *fcMRI doesn't really work*: The fcMRI approach produces such unstable results that it may be unsuitable for investigating abnormalities of the autistic brain.

However, such conclusions would be overly pessimistic and unwarranted. While lack of replication is a serious problem in ASD (as discussed below), the same problem applies to ASD studies using other techniques and approaches (Fletcher and Grafton 2013; Yerys and Herrington 2014). Given evidence of the general reliability of fcMRI (Shehzad et al. 2009; Van Dijk et al. 2010; Birn et al. 2013; Buckner et al. 2013), it is more likely that inconsistencies actually reflect the sensitivity of the technique to subtle variability in study cohorts or methods. Such sensitivity can be a strength, if critical variables are controlled. The methodological literature has made some first steps toward such control, as described above, but deeper issues remain, as will be discussed below. Differential results from coactivation and intrinsic fcMRI approaches should not be contrasted as "right" or "wrong." The challenge is to understand why task-induced BOLD correlations may tell an often completely different story from intrinsic low frequency fluctuations observed during the "resting" state.

The advantages of coactivation (task-induced) fcMRI are relatively good control over cognitive state and its changes (which may be largely determined by response to the known sequence of task trials) and specificity of the functional domain under study (with a task designed to tap into a domain of interest, e.g., face processing). However, skeptics may point

293

out that stimulus-induced BOLD changes can be correlated between two regions even if these are not connected to each other, simply because they receive concurrent input from a third region (Jones et al. 2010). In addition, coactivation fcMRI primarily reflects online processing, rather than underlying functional architecture. This latter issue points to the potential main strength of intrinsic fcMRI, which may provide insight into the nature of network organization because of its sensitivity to activity- and experience-driven Hebbian mechanisms of plasticity (Lewis et al. 2009; Luo et al. 2012; Schultz et al. 2012; Jolles et al. 2013; Vidyasagar et al. 2014). While task-induced FC measures may thus be limited to a relatively "shallow" and transient measure of online cooperation between brain regions, iFC may provide "deeper" insight into the brain's functional architecture and its plasticity. However, the focus on spontaneous BOLD fluctuations comes at a cost, related to the condition under which data are acquired.

14.2.2 Challenge no. 1: "Resting" state

The study of iFC is often equated with the use of data acquired in a "resting" state. However, when instructing participants to relax, think of nothing in particular, and keep their eyes closed (without falling asleep) or open and fixated on a cross on a screen, one actually gives them a task (to abide by the instructions, while at the same time keeping very still, not falling asleep, etc.). There is awareness of the problem in the field (Buckner et al. 2013), but there are only partial solutions (e.g., video-recording participants to monitor awake state). This is so because the resting state fundamentally discards principles of experimental cognitive psychology that have dominated functional neuroimaging for decades (e.g., Petersen et al. 1989). These principles demand the tightest possible control of cognitive state during an experiment. In other words, an experiment needs to be designed in a way to transparently drive the brain to perform certain well-defined operations, usually in a subtraction design, in which task conditions differ by only a single-added cognitive component (Price and Friston 1997). None of these iron rules apply to the resting state. Instead, resting-state fcMRI emerged from a haphazard observation that error residuals in conventional fMRI data analyses, usually considered noise, actually had surprising spatial specificity (Biswal et al. 1995; Hyde and Biswal 1999). The exponential growth of iFC in the past 20 years was not founded on incremental hypothesis-driven advances, but on a serendipitous discovery. There was never a plan, but the technique proved to be miraculously powerful. Given its success in the study of the healthy adult brain, it was soon applied to clinical populations, including ASD. Ten years after the first resting state fcMRI study of ASD (Cherkassky et al. 2006), the field now has to go back and do the groundwork because a crucial question remains unanswered: Although resting-state iFC works so well in the healthy adult brain, could it work differently in a disorder such as ASD, which is known for its atypical response to environmental setting and stimulation?

The question has many facets. Some belong to basic science. The iFC methods field is still working to uncover the basic neurophysiological mechanisms at the root of synchronized low-frequency BOLD fluctuations (Schölvinck et al. 2010; Schmithorst et al. 2014). Even if these were completely understood, we could not assume that they work exactly the same way in the autistic brain. Functional MRI has been used in ASD for almost 20 years (Baron-Cohen et al. 1999; Ring et al. 1999). However, to the present day, little research has been done to test whether neurovascular mechanisms generating the BOLD effect may be different in ASD. Given changes in these mechanisms during typical development (Schmithorst et al. 2014) and the frequent observation that children with ASD appear neurofunctionally immature (Shih et al. 2011; Nair et al. 2013; Fishman et al. 2014; Ben-Ari 2015), an atypical BOLD effect in ASD is not at all unlikely. A recent study using arterial spin labeling, an MRI technique for quantitative measurements of regional perfusion, tantalizingly reported that robust correlations between local perfusion and local iFC detected in TD children were absent in children with ASD, suggesting an atypical relation between baseline blood flow and BOLD correlations (Jann et al. 2015).

Other facets of the question are more practical. For example, does the uncomfortable, constricted, and noisy environment inside the MRI bore affect people with ASD differently from neurotypical people? Eilam-Stock and colleagues (2014) recently reported reduced skin-conductance responses (SCRs) during resting-state fMRI in adults with ASD. Furthermore, SCRs were correlated with FC of visual and medial temporal regions in people with ASD, whereas in neurotypical adults, they correlated with regions of default mode and salience networks (including posterior cingulate gyrus and anterior insula). This suggests that autonomic states and links between these states and observed FC patterns may be atypical in ASD. A related question is whether participants with ASD may experience more (or less) anxiety or stress than control counterparts during scanning. Any such differences would be expected to affect the BOLD signal and its low-frequency fluctuations (Bijsterbosch et al. 2015; McMenamin and Pessoa 2015).

Yet another aspect of the question has to do with the low sampling rate in fMRI (typically around 2 sec) and the common, indeed almost ubiquitous, practice of analyzing data sets for activation or connectivity effects across the prolonged period of one (or even several) acquisition runs (i.e., ≥5 mins). However, the brain does not work statically, but constantly undergoes dynamic change.

14.2.3 Challenge no. 2: Dynamic connectivity

fcMRI studies of ASD have almost exclusively reported BOLD correlations (or some other measure of signal synchronization) for time series of five or more minute duration. In the methods literature at large, the limitation of this static fcMRI approach has been recognized (Hutchison et al. 2013). An alternative dynamic fcMRI approach uses a sliding window technique that detects BOLD correlations for each time window (e.g., 40 sec), successively shifted forward. This yields a higher-order time series of correlations that reflects dynamic changes (Chang and Glover 2010). Using this approach in healthy adults, FC within the default mode network (DMN) was found to be variable across time (Chang and Glover 2010; Handwerker et al. 2012), possibly reflecting mind-wandering (Christoff et al. 2009). Allen et al. (2014) expanded these findings identifying large "zones of instability" (changes across time), not only in the DMN, but also in lateral parietal, extrastriate, and prefrontal regions bilaterally, which they attribute to changes in vigilance (cf. Stamatakis et al. 2010). Given these spatially extensive findings, it is possible that most static fcMRI findings in ASD may have been affected by undetected differences in temporal variability. An obvious example concerns FC between posterior cingulate/precuneus and medial prefrontal nodes of the DMN, which is extremely robust in the TD brain, but has been found reduced in ASD (Monk et al. 2009; Assaf et al. 2010; Murdaugh et al. 2012; von dem Hagen et al. 2012; Starck et al. 2013; Washington et al. 2013; Abbott et al. 2015; Doyle-Thomas et al. 2015). This represents one of the most replicated fcMRI findings in ASD; yet does such a finding from static fcMRI truly imply "underconnectivity"? Since it reflects reduced correlation across a long time series, an alternative explanation of greater variability across time could equally apply. This latter account would not imply any architectural impairment of the DMN in ASD, but could be related to more frequent changes in default mode-related cognitive states (e.g., in mind wandering) in people with ASD (Falahpour et al. 2016).

Dynamic fcMRI will surely play a role in the exploration of iFC changes across time, which promises to enrich our understanding of network abnormalities in ASD. However, given limits in temporal sampling rate and sluggishness of the BOLD response, even advanced multiband fMRI protocols cannot rival the temporal resolution of electrophysiological techniques. A review of the EEG and magnetoencephalography (MEG) literature on connectivity in ASD is beyond the scope of this chapter. We will therefore solely mention a few studies that serve as examples of how MEG data can enrich our understanding of functional connectivity in ASD, in at least four respects. First, MEG can identify not only regions in a functional circuit that may activate at atypical levels (detectable also in fMRI), but also those activating at normal levels but with atypical latency (beyond the temporal resolution of fMRI). For example, Pang et al. (2016) showed atypical activation in left cuneus during production of meaningless syllables in children with ASD, accompanied by normal-level activation in right inferior frontal gyrus that occurred at atypically short latency. Second, MEG permits the investigation of signal coherence or synchronization in high-frequency domains that are thought to be crucial for online cognitive processing, in particular the γ range (>30 Hz) (Canolty et al. 2007). The finding of reduced γ power in response to simple auditory clicks in children and adolescents with

ASD may, therefore, indicate reduced binding between crucial perceptual brain regions (Wilson et al. 2007). Another recent finding was reduced fronto-temporal synchronization in the α band during a working memory task in children with ASD (Urbain et al. 2015). Third, MEG detects signals in several high-frequency bands and patterns of anomaly in ASD may differ across these. For example, Kitzbichler and colleagues (2014) found widespread higher global efficiency (increased connectivity) in α (8–12 Hz) and γ (30–70 Hz) bands, but reduced efficiency for β (13–30 Hz) and δ bands (1–2 Hz) in frontal and occipital lobes in participants with ASD during rest. Fourth, divergent patterns in different frequency bands may elucidate organizational principles to which fcMRI is largely blind. For example, Khan et al. (2015b) reported differential effects in γ and mu-β bands, possibly suggesting increased feedforward, but reduced feedback connectivity in the somatosensory system in ASD. Based on these examples from the as yet small MEG literature, major contributions to an improved understanding of network dynamics and its abnormalities in ASD can be expected.

14.3 Anatomical connectivity

As mentioned previously, intrinsic fcMRI examines correlated activity between distal regions as a method of assessing stable networks that have evolved as a result of Hebbian processes. Of course, this correlated activity requires some form of underlying structural connectivity, that is, physical (axonal) connections. Such connections need not be direct, however, which is an important caveat to the interpretation of intrinsic fcMRI studies. Simultaneous input from a third region, or multiple regions, could also drive correlated (or inversely correlated) activity. Diffusion weighted MRI (dMRI) is one method allowing *in vivo* examination of the white matter connections underlying functional networks. This may also help to disambiguate typical functional networks from those that reflect compensatory networks (i.e., those that show typical correlated activity via atypical physical connections).

Diffusion MRI works by measuring the Brownian motion of water molecules within tissue at the subvoxel level (Le Bihan et al. 1986). This random motion is impeded when it encounters structures such as cellular membranes, intracellular filaments, or proteins. When such structures are highly organized, for example when a bundle of axons run parallel to each other, diffusion will be hindered perpendicular to the axons, but comparatively free parallel to the bundle. By applying a series of differentially oriented field gradients during data acquisition, dMRI samples the diffusion at multiple directions (from 6 in early dMRI sequences, to ≥60 in more recent high angular resolution diffusion imaging [HARDI], to 270 within the Human Connectome Project [Sotiropoulos et al. 2013]). Microstructural changes such as differences in myelination, organization, or axon caliber are reflected in changes of the quantities derived from dMRI (Beaulieu 2002, and see below for limitations in interpretation). The most commonly reported diffusion measures are derived from the mathematical tensor and referred to as diffusion tensor imaging (DTI). While axial diffusivity (AD) reflects the direction of greatest diffusion within a voxel and the magnitude of that diffusion, radial diffusivity (RD) quantifies diffusion in the orthogonal plane, and mean diffusivity (MD) measures the overall diffusion, regardless of direction. The most commonly reported tensor measure, fractional anisotropy (FA), varies between 0 and 1 and provides an index of the degree to which water preferentially diffuses in the axial rather than the radial direction. Eigen-vectors are also derived from the tensor to describe the predominant direction of diffusion (on average) within each voxel and are often interpreted as indicators of the primary axon orientation. Below we review the current DTI literature on ASD, discuss some of the challenges faced in this methodology, and briefly mention some of the ways these challenges are being addressed.

14.3.1 Findings in children, adolescents, and adults

The first dMRI study in ASD (Barnea-Goraly et al. 2004) reported reduced FA diffusely throughout white matter in adolescents with ASD compared to TD peers. Reduced FA, as well as increased MD, has been observed in most subsequent diffusion studies of school-age children, adolescents, and adults, including studies using region or tract of interest approaches (Sundaram et al. 2008; Sahyoun et al. 2010b), voxel-based morphology (VBM, Keller et al. 2007; Barnea-Goraly et al. 2010), and Tract-Based Spatial Statistics (TBSS, a VBM approach adapted specifically for use in cerebral white matter; Jou et al. 2011; Shukla et al., 2011; see review in Travers et al. 2012). However, the localization of reported differences has varied across studies, with significant effects reported in uncinate (Cheon et al. 2011; Poustka et al. 2012; Jou et al. 2015), superior and inferior longitudinal fasciculi (Shukla et al. 2010; Jou et al. 2011; Poustka et al. 2012), corpus callosum (Alexander et al. 2007; Keller et al. 2007; Shukla et al. 2010), cerebellum (Cheung et al. 2009), and projection tracts (Keller et al. 2007; Nair et al. 2015). A meta-analysis of ROI-based studies including data from several hundred participants (Aoki et al. 2013) found significantly reduced FA or increased MD in corpus callosum, uncinate, and superior longitudinal fasciculus either unilaterally or bilaterally, but not cingulum, inferior longitudinal, or inferior fronto-occipital fasciculus. However, not all tracts were equally represented in the literature and only association tracts were considered in the report. Spatial specificity of the meta-analysis was therefore limited, and age effects were not considered. A handful of studies have reported more mixed effects, including increased FA or decreased MD in some white matter tracts, but even these varied spatially (Cheung et al. 2009; Sahyoun et al. 2010a; Sivaswamy et al. 2010). This variability may be due, in part, to methodological limitations such as intersubject alignment, motion artifacts and biases, and complex fiber crossings (discussed below).

14.3.2 Findings in infants and toddlers

Diffusion studies in infants and toddlers with ASD are still limited, but indicate increased FA compared to TD children during the earliest years (Ben Bashat et al. 2007; Weinstein et al. 2011). These findings appear to mirror the atypical developmental trajectory seen in volumetric studies of early ASD, with accelerated development in the first years of life, but atypically slow growth following (Carper and Courchesne 2000, 2005; Courchesne et al. 2001; Hazlett et al. 2011, 2012; Schumann and Nordahl 2011; Zielinski et al. 2014). In toddlers around 3 years of age, Weinstein et al. (2011) found significantly greater FA in corpus callosum, left superior longitudinal fasciculus, and cingulum. Partially supportive findings come from a longitudinal examination of at-risk infants (younger siblings of children diagnosed with ASD) comparing those who met ASD criteria at 24 months to those who did not (Wolff et al. 2012b). FA tended to be higher for the ASD-positive group at the first (6 months) time point; however, developmental slopes for FA were steeper (increasing more rapidly) for the ASD-negative than the ASD-positive group in both projection and association tracts, resulting in a "cross-over" of effects during the second postnatal year. A similar difference in developmental trajectories for FA was found in several frontal tracts (but not posterior tracts) in a cohort-sequential study of 1 to 4 year olds (Solso et al. 2015) and in the corpus callosum in a cohort-sequential study of 3 to 41 year olds (Travers et al. 2015). This pattern of precocious development followed by a relative slowing emphasizes the necessity of considering cohort age in all studies of neurodevelopment in ASD. Differences present at one age may appear reversed at a different maturational stage or may simply disappear during the cross-over period or when a wide age range is included.

14.3.3 Challenge no. 1: Understanding microstructural underpinnings

The advent of dMRI was a boon for neuroimaging, providing previously inaccessible insight into the organization and condition of the network of axonal connections that make up white matter from *in vivo* studies across early development. Our ability to interpret quantitative dMRI findings in microstructural terms is still limited, however (see Beaulieu [2002, 2011] for review). We may wish to draw conclusions about the "strength" of anatomical connections, the number of axons in a fascicle, or the degree of axonal myelination, but dMRI only measures the diffusion of water molecules in tissue, and any interpretation regarding the neuroanatomical parameters of interest remains indirect. Water diffusion is hindered by various cellular and extracellular structures—such as cell membranes, filaments, or proteins—and it is this hindrance that is detected in dMRI. A single 1 mm^3 voxel may contain 3×10^5 axons of various diameters (e.g., in corpus callosum, Aboitiz et al. 1992), as well as oligodendrocytes (myelin) and other glial cells, whereas measured quantities (e.g., FA, MD, or RD) reflect average diffusion within a voxel, that is, diffusion within and between all of these cells types. In organized axonal bundles, FA and AD are high compared to gray matter. The proportion of myelin is one important contributor to this difference, but not the only one. Boundaries provided by axonal membranes are also key, as evidenced by animal studies comparing anisotropy in myelinated and unmyelinated nerves (Beaulieu and Allen 1994). Intra-axonal neurofibrils also make a distinct (though quantitatively smaller) contribution, and in animal models, selected loss of axonal neurofibrils can lead to an increase in AD without affecting RD (Kinoshita et al. 1999). Differences in axonal caliber or packing density can alter these dependent measures as well (Takahashi et al. 2002), as does the overall homogeneity of axonal organization within a given voxel (see below).

Any or all of these microstructural differences can lead to a change in the measureable characteristics of water diffusion. Because it is unknown in an *in vivo* sample, which of these subvoxel factors drives a change or group difference in the voxel average, vague terms like "white matter compromise" are frequently used in DTI studies. Unfortunately, such nonspecific descriptions seem to imply neuronal breakdown or poor myelination that simply cannot be concluded from the data available (Jbabdi and Johansen-Berg 2011; Jones et al. 2013). The most commonly reported DTI measures, FA and MD, seem to be most susceptible to this overinterpretation. AD and RD may be slightly less ambiguous and now appear more frequently in DTI reports, but still reflect within-voxel averages. Findings from conventional DTI have improved our understanding of network organization in ASD—but, at present, we cannot conclusively determine what exact microstructural differences the findings reflect. Recent development and implementation of multishell diffusion sequences, which rapidly sample at multiple b-values (gradient strengths), will help to improve this. These techniques allow quantification of different water compartments within a single voxel (Zhang et al. 2012; Sotiropoulos et al. 2013; White et al. 2013), with different models estimating intracellular and extracellular water fractions, orientation distribution functions of these compartments, or neurite density within a voxel.

14.3.4 Challenge no. 2: Complex fiber orientations

Another challenge of dMRI arises from the presence of multiple fiber orientations within sampled voxels. As with scalar measures (FA, AD, RD) estimates of diffusion direction within a voxel reflect the average of the axons contained, which may be in the hundreds of thousands. Axons may not all be in parallel, two or more bundles may cross within a voxel, or "kiss," fan-out, or bend, any of which can result in nearly identical diffusion measures from traditional tensor-based analytic approaches (Jbabdi and Johansen-Berg 2011; Jones et al. 2013). Tractography cannot, therefore, reliably trace true axonal pathways since generated streamlines (the computational approximations of axonal pathways) may fail to extend through areas of crossings or may go off-course and "jump" from one axonal bundle to another. For this reason, it is vital

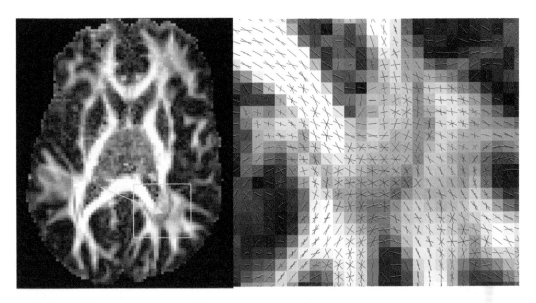

Figure 14.3 Whereas traditional DTI (A: FA image) struggles with areas of crossing fibers (arrow, low FA values), multishell diffusion acquisitions and analysis algorithms model multiple fiber directions within a single voxel (B primary fiber direction in blue, secondary and tertiary in red/fuchsia when present). Acquisition: 2 shells ($b = 1500, 3000$) with 46 diffusion directions each.

to compare dMRI-derived tracts (streamlines) to gold-standard axonal anatomy (e.g., axonal tracing through autoradiography) to verify anatomical validity. However, even this may be inadequate when studying clinical populations with potential deviations from normal anatomy.

Methodological advances in both acquisition and analysis of dMRI are improving our ability to resolve and interpret complex fiber crossings. Improvements in gradient hardware and sequence programming allow higher angular resolution. At the same time, a diversity of higher-order modeling approaches are moving beyond tensor-based calculations, particularly in conjunction with the multishell diffusion acquisitions mentioned above (Figure 14.3). Whereas tensor-based tractography usually models only one or at best two fiber directions within a voxel, newer algorithms assess the likelihood of complex fiber architectures and attempt to model them (Tournier et al. 2008, 2011; Jbabdi et al. 2012; Farquharson et al. 2013). This leads to estimation of more complex orientation distribution functions rather than eigenvectors, and is more successful at tracking through these regions.

14.3.5 Challenge no. 3: Motion

Similar to issues in fcMRI described above, diffusion results can also be adversely affected by head motion (Figure 14.4), which commonly occurs in the study of children and clinical populations. Limited artifacts can be filtered out by removing affected portions of the data, a

301

(a)   (b)   (c)

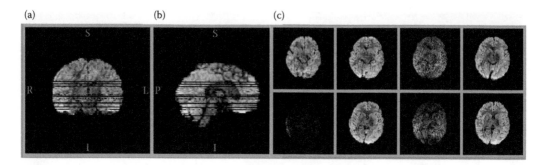

Figure 14.4 Example of motion-induced slice dropout seen in diffusion weighted imaging. Coronal (a) and sagittal (b) views with signal loss evident in several slices. Sequential axial slices from the same scan session shown in (c). Dropouts of this type may be seen in one or many diffusion sensitization directions examined in a single EPI examination and may bias the eigenvectors calculated from the tensor.

standard step in data processing, but subtle differences may remain and may bias quantitative findings. In a methodological study, Yendiki et al. (2013) reported that group-wise differences in small amounts of head motion could lead to spurious between-group findings (such as the commonly reported finding of reduced FA in ASD). Remarkably, this was also observed when a single TD group was split solely on the basis of head motion (i.e., the subsample with greater head motion appeared to have significantly higher RD, but lower FA and AD than the subsample with less motion). This is further supported by a study of healthy adults in which subject motion was found to bias DTI measures, particularly MD (Ling et al. 2012). These studies raise the possibility that inconsistencies in the ASD literature may be partly explained by insufficient motion matching between groups and some reported differences may be artifactual (Koldewyn et al. 2014). It remains to be determined whether larger sample sizes or other analytic approaches will be more sensitive to group differences and therefore more robust to motion.

14.4 Perspectives

Much of the previous sections on functional and anatomical connectivity in ASD have focused on methodological complexities resulting in nonreplications or inconsistencies in the data (Fletcher and Grafton 2013). In the remainder of this chapter, we will first outline a model that may accommodate many (though not all) connectivity findings described above, and will then sketch a roadmap of how neuroimaging findings may ultimately bridge the gap between basic science and treatment of ASD.

14.4.1 A developmental model of neurofunctional organization in ASD

Typical development is characterized by the interplay between constructive processes (e.g., synaptic strengthening, axonal myelination) and regressive events (e.g., synaptic pruning, axonal loss), which are governed by activity and experiential interaction with the environment (Quartz and Sejnowski 1997; Kandel et al. 2000). These principles determine changes in individual neurons and synapses, but also in larger functional networks, which become progressively more integrated (more strongly connected internally), and also more differentiated from other networks (through pruning of connections whose activity levels do not warrant inclusion within the increasingly specialized network). Much of the fcMRI literature suggests that both constructive and regressive processes are diminished in the functional development of the autistic brain, resulting in a dual impairment of reduced integration and differentiation (or segregation) of networks (Shih et al. 2011; Rudie et al. 2012; Fishman et al. 2015), which may be described as reduced "network sculpting" (Figure 14.5). In support, many (though not all) underconnectivity findings have been reported between regions that belong to one network or can be expected to coactivate, whereas overconnectivity findings have been frequently reported for regions outside the bounds of a neurotypical network (Nair et al. 2014; Doyle-Thomas et al. 2015). Both underconnectivity (e.g., Abrams et al. 2013) and overconnectivity (Fishman et al. 2014) have been found to be associated with symptom severity, suggesting that both aspects of the hypothesized dual impairment have clinical relevance.

Although the network sculpting model may grossly account for neurofunctional patterns detected in children and adults with ASD, it has limited depth of causality because it does not capture why constructive and regressive processes may be impaired in ASD. A link with

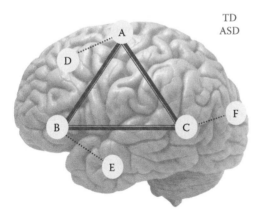

Figure 14.5 Diagrammatic illustration of the reduced network sculpting hypothesis. An exemplary network with three nodes (A–C) is shown. Interconnectivity between these nodes (network integration) is robust in the TD brain and reduced in the autistic brain. However, in ASD the brain maintains residual connectivity with extraneous regions (D–F) that do not participate in the network of the mature TD brain (but may have been connected to it at immature stages of development). This residual connectivity reflects impaired network differentiation (or segregation).

early disturbances of brain growth (Courchesne et al. 2001), possibly accompanied by precocious development of anatomical substrates of connectivity (Wolff et al. 2012a) at a time when experiential input cannot yet guide the formation of fine-tuned and fully functional networks, is conceivable, but confirmation will have to await long-term longitudinal studies following individuals with ASD from infancy into adolescence. Given the strong (though by far not absolute) heritability of ASD (Hallmayer et al. 2011), the ultimate causes surely involve genetic risk.

14.4.2 From genes to treatment: Can neuroimaging bridge the gap?

The number of genes that have been identified to convey some risk of ASD is in the hundreds and growing (Geschwind and State 2015). The task of developing mechanistic models linking these numerous genes with the emergence of idiopathic autism is thus highly complex. On the upside, many of the risk genes appear to converge functionally, as they affect synaptic formation and function (Toro et al. 2010; Lanz et al. 2013; Baudouin 2014; De Rubeis et al. 2014; Sahin and Sur 2015). A similar convergence argument can be made with respect to genetic causes of syndromic forms of ASD (fragile X, tuberous sclerosis, or Angelman syndrome; Ebrahimi-Fakhari and Sahin 2015). While this supports the importance of connectivity science in ASD, the convergence claim requires more than simple counting of the many risk genes that somehow relate to the synapse and circuit formation. The question is whether the number of genes affecting the synapse among all ASD risk genes is actually significantly higher than expected when compared to the proportion of genes with such function within the entire human genome.

Regardless of the answer to this question, genetics alone can at present not fully achieve either of two crucial goals in research on idiopathic ASD: (1) To provide diagnostic markers (sets of risk genes) that would predict ASD before a behavioral diagnosis is possible; (2) to differentiate subtypes of the disorder, which are presumed to exist (Happé et al. 2006). The problem, in simple terms, is that each susceptibility gene for idiopathic ASD, if affected in isolation, may carry only minimal risk. ASD may emerge when there is polygenic burden (multiple hit scenario), with a critical number of risk genes being affected (Brandler and Sebat 2015), possibly accompanied by environmental risks (Braunschweig et al. 2013; Kalkbrenner et al. 2015) and risks involving nonbrain bodily systems (such as gut microbiome; Hsiao et al. 2013).

Neuroimaging may play a pivotal role in linking genetic risk and phenotypic symptomatology. As explained in the previous section, imaging in children or adults cannot have the same "causal depth" as the study of genetic and epigenetic risk factors. This only partial causal depth, however, may be exactly what is needed to bridge the gap between the depth of the genetic approach and the causal shallowness of behavioral features.

Any neuroimaging feature reflects causal disturbances (prenatal or early postnatal) only indirectly because it is compounded by maturational, environmental, and therapeutic effects. Imaging features thus combine cause and outcome, although in ways that are probably so complex as to limit the success of hypothesis-driven research. An important alternative is, therefore, to resort to data-driven approaches that can extract complex patterns of interest from highly multivariate data sets.

Data-driven machine-learning approaches have been implemented in a number of ASD studies in the past few years. For example, Ecker and colleagues (2010) reported that distributed patterns of cortical thickness differences predicted diagnostic status (ASD vs. TD) with c. 85% accuracy in small samples of adults. Ingalhalikar et al. (2011) applied a similar approach to DTI data in a larger sample of children ($N = 75$), achieving approximately 80% diagnostic prediction accuracy, based on widely distributed white matter differences. However, common leave-one-out validation in these studies may overestimate predictive accuracy through overfitting to the idiosyncrasies of the data set at hand. Some recent machine-learning studies using iFC data have instead used external validation data sets (i.e., strict separation of data used for training and validation). One group first achieved approximately 70% prediction accuracy for a large iFC matrix (including >26 million ROI pairings) in a very small validation sample (Anderson et al. 2011b). They followed up with a study implementing the same approach in a much larger sample ($N = 964$) from the Autism Brain Imaging Data Exchange (ABIDE) (Di Martino et al. 2014), reporting an accuracy of only 60% (Nielsen et al. 2013). However, this disappointing result does not imply that iFC is inadequate for diagnostic prediction. The modest accuracy in the study by Nielsen et al. (2013) can be primarily attributed to two fundamental problems. The first concerns the use of multisite data, which boosts sample size, but introduces numerous factors of variability beyond those already present in single-site data sets. A second issue concerns the validation process. While use of an external validation data set is clearly preferable (as it prevents inflated accuracy through overfitting and may thus generate findings for the ASD population at large), it can result in overly conservative estimates of accuracy. If a prediction algorithm is trained on one data set, validation in a separate data set will likely be successful only if that data set is actually comparable, that is, tightly matched to the training set on all relevant demographic and clinical variables. Crucially, both sets would need to be matched on their composition with respect to ASD subtypes. Yet although such subtypes are generally expected (Happé et al. 2006; Geschwind and Levitt 2007), they remain unknown and cannot therefore be matched (cf. Chen et al. 2015). Ultimately, diagnostic prediction from imaging data may be an elusive goal because of a faulty premise: There can be no unique set of brain features for a disorder that is not unique, but is instead defined by a clinical umbrella term that is derived from behavioral observation and probably encompasses an unknown number of neurobiologically distinct disorders.

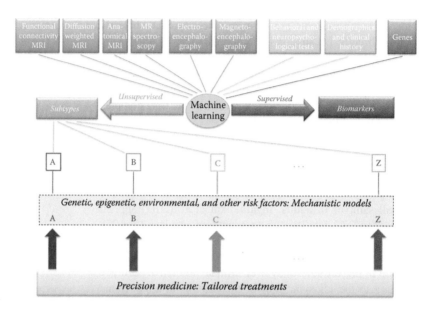

Figure 14.6 Rich data approach to diagnostic prediction (through supervised machine learning, on the right) and subtype identification (through unsupervised machine learning, on the left). Example input data types included in multivariate analyses are shown at the top. For each subtype A to Z detected in unsupervised clustering analyses, a mechanistic model linked to a specific set of causal factors (gray dotted rectangle) may be developed and treatments may be fine-tuned to each subtype and its etiological model.

Identifying subtypes that are defined by differential neurodevelopmental etiology is therefore of utmost importance. It will help resolve some methodological issues, such as the validation problem described above or the need for more homogeneous ASD samples to be compared to TD samples in hypothesis-driven imaging (or other) studies. A more important implication relates to the baffling complexity of genetic findings mentioned above. Some of this complexity is likely a reflection of the "umbrella status" of ASD and shallow diagnostic procedures ("shallow" in the same sense as above, because far removed from developmental causation). Why would anyone expect tractable genetic and epigenetic causation for a set of disorders that is only loosely held together by a wide range of outcome observations? On the other hand, for any biologically defined subtype, causation may be more tractably linked to risk genes and environmental factors. However, the field is facing a vicious circle: In order to optimally analyze data in the pursuit of subtypes, we would first need to know the subtypes. A way out may be the use of large (sample size) and rich data (large number of features for each participant) combining genetic, environmental, neuroimaging, and behavioral variables with multivariate pattern recognition tools (Figure 14.6).

However, as much of a scientific advance as all of the above would mean, the ultimate question remains: How does this help children with ASD and their parents? Knowledge of subtypes would open up the possibility of fully mechanistic developmental models of each type of disorder on the autism spectrum. Such efforts are already underway for ASD-related syndromes, such as Fragile-X, whose genetic causes are known (Fung and Reiss 2015). However, these syndromes account for only a small fraction of the population under the ASD umbrella. Large and rich imaging data in particular those capturing brain connectivity—in combination with genetic, epigenetic, and behavioral data—may eventually isolate subtypes of the disorder on the way to a full understanding of causation and the development of optimally tailored treatments.

Acknowledgments

Preparation of this chapter was in part supported by funding from the National Institutes of Health (R01 MH101173 and R01 MH103494).

References

Abbott, A. E., A. Nair, C. L. Keown, M. C. Datko, A. Jahedi, I. Fishman, and R.-A. Müller. 2015. Patterns of atypical functional connectivity and behavioral links in autism differ between default, salience, and executive networks. *Cerebral Cortex*. DOI: 10.1093/cercor/bhv191.

Aboitiz, F., A. B. Scheibel, R. S. Fisher, and E. Zaidel. 1992. Fiber composition of the human corpus callosum. *Brain Res*. 598:143–53.

Abrams, D. A., C. J. Lynch, K. M. Cheng, J. Phillips, K. Supekar, S. Ryali, L. Q. Uddin, and V. Menon. 2013. Underconnectivity between voice-selective cortex and reward circuitry in children with autism. *Proc. Natl. Acad. Sci. USA* 110:12060–5.

Agam, Y., R. M. Joseph, J. J. Barton, and D. S. Manoach. 2010. Reduced cognitive control of response inhibition by the anterior cingulate cortex in autism spectrum disorders. *NeuroImage* 52:336–47.

Alexander, A. L., J. E. Lee, M. Lazar et al. 2007. Diffusion tensor imaging of the corpus callosum in Autism. *NeuroImage* 34:61–73.

Allen, E. A., E. Damaraju, S. M. Plis, E. B. Erhardt, T. Eichele, and V. D. Calhoun. 2014. Tracking whole-brain connectivity dynamics in the resting state. *Cereb. Cortex*. 24:663–76.

Anderson, J. S., T. J. Druzgal, A. Froehlich et al. 2011a. Decreased interhemispheric functional connectivity in autism. *Cereb. Cortex*. 21:1134–46.

Anderson, J. S., J. A. Nielsen, A. L. Froehlich et al. 2011b. Functional connectivity magnetic resonance imaging classification of autism. *Brain* 134:3742–54.

Aoki, Y., O. Abe, Y. Nippashi, and H. Yamasue. 2013. Comparison of white matter integrity between autism spectrum disorder subjects and typically developing individuals: A meta-analysis of diffusion tensor imaging tractography studies. *Molecular Autism*, 4(25):1–17. DOI: 10.1186/2040-2392-4-25.

Assaf, M., K. Jagannathan, V. D. Calhoun, L. Miller, M. C. Stevens, R. Sahl, J. G. O'Boyle, R. T. Schultz, and G. D. Pearlson. 2010. Abnormal functional connectivity of default mode sub-networks in autism spectrum disorder patients. *NeuroImage* 53:247–56.

Barnea-Goraly, N., H. Kwon, V. Menon, S. Eliez, L. Lotspeich, and A. L. Reiss. 2004. White matter structure in autism: Preliminary evidence from diffusion tensor imaging. *Biol. Psychiatry* 55:323–6.

307

Barnea-Goraly, N., L. J. Lotspeich, and A. L. Reiss. 2010. Similar white matter aberrations in children with autism and their unaffected siblings: A diffusion tensor imaging study using tract-based spatial statistics. *Arch. Gen. Psychiatry* 67:1052–60.

Baron-Cohen, S., H. A. Ring, E. T. Bullmore, S. Wheelwright, C. Ashwin, and S. C. Williams. 2000. The amygdala theory of autism. *Neurosci. Biobehav. Rev.* 24:355–64.

Baron-Cohen, S., H. A. Ring, S. Wheelwright, E. T. Bullmore, M. J. Brammer, A. Simmons, and S. C. Williams. 1999. Social intelligence in the normal and autistic brain: An fMRI study. *Eur. J. Neurosci.* 11:1891–8.

Baudouin, S. J. 2014. Heterogeneity and convergence: The synaptic pathophysiology of autism. *Eur. J. Neurosci.* 39:1107–13.

Beaulieu, C. 2002. The basis of anisotropic water diffusion in the nervous system—A technical review. *NMR Biomed.* 15:435–55.

Beaulieu, C. 2011. What makes diffusion anisotropic in the nervous system? In *Diffusion MRI: Theory, Methods, and Applications*, ed. D. K. Jones, 92–109. New York: Oxford University Press.

Beaulieu, C. and P. S. Allen. 1994. Determinants of anisotropic water diffusion in nerves. *Magn. Reson. Med.* 31:394–400.

Belmonte, M. K., G. Allen, A. Beckel-Mitchener, L. M. Boulanger, R. A. Carper, and S. J. Webb. 2004. Autism and abnormal development of brain connectivity. *J. Neurosci.* 24:9228–31.

Ben Bashat, D., V. Kronfeld-Duenias, D. A. Zachor, P. M. Ekstein, T. Hendler, R. Tarrasch, A. Even, Y. Levy, and L. Ben Sira. 2007. Accelerated maturation of white matter in young children with autism: A high b value DWI study. *NeuroImage* 37:40–7.

Ben-Ari, Y. 2015. Is birth a critical period in the pathogenesis of autism spectrum disorders? *Nat. Rev. Neurosci.* 16:498–505.

Bettelheim, B. 1967. *The Empty Fortress: Infantile Autism and the Birth of the Self.* New York: Free Press.

Bijsterbosch, J., S. Smith, and S. J. Bishop. 2015. Functional connectivity under anticipation of shock: Correlates of trait anxious affect versus induced anxiety. *J. Cogn. Neurosci.* 27:1840–53.

Birn, R. M., E. K. Molloy, R. Patriat, T. Parker, T. B. Meier, G. R. Kirk, V. A. Nair, M. E. Meyerand, and V. Prabhakaran. 2013. The effect of scan length on the reliability of resting-state fMRI connectivity estimates. *NeuroImage* 83:550–8.

Biswal, B., F. Z. Yetkin, V. M. Haughton, and J. S. Hyde. 1995. Functional connectivity in the motor cortex of resting human brain using echo-planar MRI. *Magn. Reson. Med.* 34:537–41.

Brandler, W. M. and J. Sebat. 2015. From *de novo* mutations to personalized therapeutic interventions in autism. *Annu. Rev. Med.* 66:487–507.

Braunschweig, D., P. Krakowiak, P. Duncanson, R. Boyce, R. L. Hansen, P. Ashwood, I. Hertz-Picciotto, I. N. Pessah, and J. Van de Water. 2013. Autism-specific maternal autoantibodies recognize critical proteins in developing brain. *Transl. Psychiatry* 3:e277.

Buckner, R. L., F. M. Krienen, and B. T. Yeo. 2013. Opportunities and limitations of intrinsic functional connectivity MRI. *Nat. Neurosci.* 16:832–7.

Canolty, R. T., M. Soltani, S. S. Dalal, E. Edwards, N. F. Dronkers, S. S. Nagarajan, H. E. Kirsch, N. M. Barbaro, and R. T. Knight. 2007. Spatiotemporal dynamics of word processing in the human brain. *Front. Neurosci.* 1:185–96.

Carper, R. A. and E. Courchesne. 2000. Inverse correlation between frontal lobe and cerebellum sizes in children with autism. *Brain* 123 (Pt 4):836–44.

Carper, R. A. and E. Courchesne. 2005. Localized enlargement of the frontal cortex in early autism. *Biol. Psychiatry* 57:126–33.

Carper, R. A., S. Solders, J. M. Treiber, I. Fishman, and R. A. Muller. 2015. Corticospinal tract anatomy and functional connectivity of primary motor cortex in autism. *J. Am. Acad. Child Adolesc. Psychiatry* 54:859–67.

Castelli, F., C. Frith, F. Happe, and U. Frith. 2002. Autism, Asperger syndrome and brain mechanisms for the attribution of mental states to animated shapes. *Brain* 125:1839–49.

Cerliani, L., M. Mennes, R. M. Thomas, A. Di Martino, M. Thioux, and C. Keysers. 2015. Increased functional connectivity between subcortical and cortical resting-state networks in autism spectrum disorder. *JAMA Psychiatry* 72(8):767–77.

Chang, C. and G. H. Glover. 2010. Time-frequency dynamics of resting-state brain connectivity measured with fMRI. *NeuroImage*, 50:81–98.

Chen, C. P., C. L. Keown, A. Jahedi, A. Nair, M. E. Pflieger, B. A. Bailey, and R.-A. Müller. 2015. Diagnostic classification of intrinsic functional connectivity highlights somatosensory, default mode, and visual regions in autism. *NeuroImage: Clinical* 8:238–45.

Cheon, K. A., Y. S. Kim, S. H. Oh et al. 2011. Involvement of the anterior thalamic radiation in boys with high functioning autism spectrum disorders: A diffusion tensor imaging study. *Brain Res.* 1417:77–86.

Cherkassky, V. L., R. K. Kana, T. A. Keller, and M. A. Just. 2006. Functional connectivity in a baseline resting-state network in autism. *NeuroReport* 17:1687–90.

Cheung, C., S. E. Chua, V. Cheung, P. L. Khong, K. S. Tai, T. K. W. Wong, T. P. Ho, and G. M. McAlonan. 2009. White matter fractional anisotrophy differences and correlates of diagnostic symptoms in autism. *J. Child Psychol. Psychiatry Allied Disciplines* 50:1102–12.

Chien, H. Y., H. Y. Lin, M. C. Lai, S. S. Gau, and W. Y. Tseng. 2015. Hyperconnectivity of the right posterior temporo-parietal junction predicts social difficulties in boys with autism spectrum disorder. *Autism Res* 8(4):427–41.

Christoff, K., A. M. Gordon, J. Smallwood, R. Smith, and J. W. Schooler. 2009. Experience sampling during fMRI reveals default network and executive system contributions to mind wandering. *Proc. Natl. Acad. Sci. USA* 106:8719–24.

Cordes, D., V. M. Haughton, K. Arfanakis, J. D. Carew, P. A. Turski, C. H. Moritz, M. A. Quigley, and M. E. Meyerand. 2001. Frequencies contributing to functional connectivity in the cerebral cortex in "resting-state" data. *AJNR Am. J. Neuroradiol.* 22:1326–33.

Cordes, D., V. M. Haughton, K. Arfanakis, G. J. Wendt, P. A. Turski, C. H. Moritz, M. A. Quigley, and M. E. Meyerand. 2000. Mapping functionally related regions of brain with functional connectivity MR imaging. *AJNR Am. J. Neuroradiol.* 21:1636–44.

Courchesne, E., C. M. Karns, H. R. Davis et al. 2001. Unusual brain growth patterns in early life in patients with autistic disorder: An MRI study. *Neurology* 57:245–54.

Courchesne, E. and K. Pierce. 2005. Why the frontal cortex in autism might be talking only to itself: Local over-connectivity but long-distance disconnection. *Curr. Opin. Neurobiol.* 15:225–30.

Courchesne, E., R. Yeung-Courchesne, G. A. Press, J. R. Hesselink, and T. L. Jernigan. 1988. Hypoplasia of cerebellar vermal lobules VI and VII in autism. *New Engl. J. Med.* 318:1349–54.

Damarla, S. R., T. A. Keller, R. K. Kana, V. L. Cherkassky, D. L. Williams, N. J. Minshew, and M. A. Just. 2010. Cortical underconnectivity coupled with preserved visuospatial cognition in autism: Evidence from an fMRI study of an embedded figures task. *Autism Res.* 3:273–9.

De Rubeis, S., X. He, A. P. Goldberg et al. 2014. Synaptic, transcriptional and chromatin genes disrupted in autism. *Nature* 515:209–15.

309

Deen, B. and K. Pelphrey. 2012. Perspective: Brain scans need a rethink. *Nature* 491:S20.

Delmonte, S., L. Gallagher, E. O'Hanlon, J. McGrath, and J. H. Balsters. 2013. Functional and structural connectivity of frontostriatal circuitry in autism spectrum disorder. *Front. Hum. Neurosci.* 7:430.

Di Martino, A., C. Kelly, R. Grzadzinski, X. N. Zuo, M. Mennes, M. A. Mairena, C. Lord, F. X. Castellanos, and M. P. Milham. 2011. Aberrant striatal functional connectivity in children with autism. *Biol. Psychiatry* 69:847–56.

Di Martino, A., C. G. Yan, Q. Li et al. 2014. The autism brain imaging data exchange: Towards a large-scale evaluation of the intrinsic brain architecture in autism. *Mol. Psychiatry* 19:659–67.

Dinstein, I., K. Pierce, L. Eyler, S. Solso, R. Malach, M. Behrmann, and E. Courchesne. 2011. Disrupted neural synchronization in toddlers with autism. *Neuron* 70:1218–25.

Dosenbach, N. U., D. A. Fair, F. M. Miezin et al. 2007. Distinct brain networks for adaptive and stable task control in humans. *Proc. Natl. Acad. Sci. USA* 104:11073–8.

Doyle-Thomas, K. A., W. Lee, N. E. Foster et al. 2015. Atypical functional brain connectivity during rest in autism spectrum disorders. *Ann. Neurol.* 77:866–76.

Ebrahimi-Fakhari, D. and M. Sahin. 2015. Autism and the synapse: Emerging mechanisms and mechanism-based therapies. *Curr. Opin. Neurol.* 28:91–102.

Ecker, C., A. Marquand, J. Mourao-Miranda et al. 2010. Describing the brain in autism in five dimensions—Magnetic resonance imaging-assisted diagnosis of autism spectrum disorder using a multiparameter classification approach. *J. Neurosci.* 30:10612–23.

Eilam-Stock, T., P. Xu, M. Cao et al. 2014. Abnormal autonomic and associated brain activities during rest in autism spectrum disorder. *Brain* 137:153–71.

Fair, D. A., B. L. Schlaggar, A. L. Cohen, F. M. Miezin, N. U. Dosenbach, K. K. Wenger, M. D. Fox, A. Z. Snyder, M. E. Raichle, and S. E. Petersen. 2007. A method for using blocked and event-related fMRI data to study "resting state" functional connectivity. *NeuroImage* 35:396–405.

Falahpour, M., Thompson, W.K., Abbott, A.E., Jahedi, A., Mulvey, M.E., Datko, M., Liu, T.T., and Müller, R-A. 2016. Underconnected, But Not Broken? Dynamic Functional Connectivity MRI Shows Underconnectivity in Autism Is Linked to Increased Intra-Individual Variability Across Time. *Brain Connectivity* 6:403–14.

Farquharson, S., J.-D. Tournier, F. Calamante, G. Fabinyi, M. Schneider-Kolsky, G. D. Jackson, and A. Connelly. 2013. White matter fiber tractography: Why we need to move beyond DTI. *J. Neurosurg.* 118:1367–77.

Fishman, I., M. Datko, Y. Cabrera, R. A. Carper, and R. A. Müller. 2015. Reduced integration and differentiation of the imitation network in autism: A combined fcMRI and DWI study. *Ann. Neurol.* 78:958–69.

Fishman, I., C. L. Keown, A. J. Lincoln, J. A. Pineda, and R.-A. Müller. 2014. Atypical cross talk between mentalizing and mirror neuron networks in autism spectrum disorder. *JAMA Psychiatry* 71(7):751–60.

Fitzgerald, J., K. Johnson, E. Kehoe, A. L. Bokde, H. Garavan, L. Gallagher, and J. McGrath. 2014. Disrupted functional connectivity in dorsal and ventral attention networks during attention orienting in autism spectrum disorders. *Autism Res.* 8(2):136–52.

Fletcher, P. C. and S. T. Grafton. 2013. Repeat after me: Replication in clinical neuroimaging is critical. *NeuroImage Clin.* 2:247–8.

Fox, M. D., M. Corbetta, A. Z. Snyder, J. L. Vincent, and M. E. Raichle. 2006. Spontaneous neuronal activity distinguishes human dorsal and ventral attention systems. *Proc. Natl. Acad Sci. USA* 103:10046–51.

Fox, M. D. and M. E. Raichle. 2007. Spontaneous fluctuations in brain activity observed with functional magnetic resonance imaging. *Nat. Rev. Neurosci.* 8:700–11.

Friston, K. J., C. D. Frith, and R. S. J. Frackowiak. 1993. Time-dependent changes in effective connectivity measured with PET. *Hum. Brain Mapp.* 1:69–79.

Fung, L. K. and A. L. Reiss. 2015. Moving toward integrative, multidimensional research in modern psychiatry: Lessons learned from fragile X syndrome. *Biol. Psychiatry* 80(2):100–11.

Geschwind, D. H. and P. Levitt. 2007. Autism spectrum disorders: Developmental disconnection syndromes. *Curr. Opin. Neurobiol.* 17:103–11.

Geschwind, D. H. and M. W. State. 2015. Gene hunting in autism spectrum disorder: On the path to precision medicine. *Lancet Neurol* 14(11):1109–20.

Gotts, S. J., Z. S. Saad, H. J. Jo, G. L. Wallace, R. W. Cox, and A. Martin. 2013. The perils of global signal regression for group comparisons: A case study of autism spectrum disorders. *Front Hum. Neurosci.* 7:356.

Gotts, S. J., W. K. Simmons, L. A. Milbury, G. L. Wallace, R. W. Cox, and A. Martin. 2012. Fractionation of social brain circuits in autism spectrum disorders. *Brain* 135:2711–25.

Greicius, M. D., B. Krasnow, A. L. Reiss, and V. Menon. 2003. Functional connectivity in the resting brain: A network analysis of the default mode hypothesis. *Proc. Natl. Acad Sci. USA* 100:253–8.

Hallmayer, J., S. Cleveland, A. Torres et al. 2011. Genetic heritability and shared environmental factors among twin pairs with autism. *Arch. Gen. Psychiatry* 68:1095–102.

Hampson, M., B. S. Peterson, P. Skudlarski, J. C. Gatenby, and J. C. Gore. 2002. Detection of functional connectivity using temporal correlations in MR images. *Hum. Brain Mapp.* 15:247–62.

Handwerker, D. A., V. Roopchansingh, J. Gonzalez-Castillo, and P. A. Bandettini. 2012. Periodic changes in fMRI connectivity. *NeuroImage* 63:1712–9.

Happé, F., A. Ronald, and R. Plomin. 2006. Time to give up on a single explanation for autism. *Nat. Neurosci.* 9:1218–20.

Hazlett, H. C., M. D. Poe, G. Gerig, M. Styner, C. Chappell, R. G. Smith, C. Vachet, and J. Piven. 2011. Early brain overgrowth in autism associated with an increase in cortical surface area before age 2 years. *Arch. Gen. Psychiatry* 68:467–76.

Hazlett, H. C., M. D. Poe, A. A. Lightbody, M. Styner, J. R. MacFall, A. L. Reiss, and J. Piven. 2012. Trajectories of early brain volume development in fragile X syndrome and autism. *J. Am. Acad Child Adolesc Psychiatry* 51:921–33.

Honey, C. J., R. Kotter, M. Breakspear, and O. Sporns. 2007. Network structure of cerebral cortex shapes functional connectivity on multiple time scales. *Proc. Natl. Acad. Sci. USA* 104:10240–5.

Horwitz, B., J. M. Rumsey, C. L. Grady, and S. I. Rapoport. 1988. The cerebral metabolic landscape in autism: Intercorrelations of regional glucose utilization. *Arch. Neurol.* 45:749–55.

Hsiao, E. Y., S. W. McBride, S. Hsien et al. 2013. Microbiota modulate behavioral and physiological abnormalities associated with neurodevelopmental disorders. *Cell* 155:1451–63.

Hughes, J. R. 2007. Autism: The first firm finding = underconnectivity? *Epilepsy Behav.* 11:20–4.

Hutchison, R. M., T. Womelsdorf, E. A. Allen et al. 2013. Dynamic functional connectivity: Promise, issues, and interpretations. *NeuroImage* 80:360–78.

Hyde, J. S. and B. B. Biswal. 1999. Functionally related correlation in the noise. In *Functional MRI*, eds. C. T. W. Moonen and P. A. Bandettini, 263–75. New York: Springer.

Ingalhalikar, M., D. Parker, L. Bloy, T. P. Roberts, and R. Verma. 2011. Diffusion based abnormality markers of pathology: Toward learned diagnostic prediction of ASD. *NeuroImage* 57:918–27.

Jann, K., L. M. Hernandez, D. Beck-Pancer, R. McCarron, R. X. Smith, M. Dapretto, and D. J. Wang. 2015. Altered resting perfusion and functional connectivity of default mode network in youth with autism spectrum disorder. *Brain Behav.* 5:e00358.

Jbabdi, S. and H. Johansen-Berg. 2011. Tractography: Where do we go from here? *Brain Connectivity* 1:169–83.

Jbabdi, S., S. N. Sotiropoulos, A. M. Savio, M. Graña, and T. E. J. Behrens. 2012. Model-based analysis of multishell diffusion MR data for tractography: How to get over fitting problems. *Magn. Reson. Med.* 68:1846–55.

Jiang, T., Y. He, Y. Zang, and X. Weng. 2004. Modulation of functional connectivity during the resting state and the motor task. *Hum. Brain Mapp.* 22:63–71.

Jolles, D. D., M. A. van Buchem, E. A. Crone, and S. A. Rombouts. 2013. Functional brain connectivity at rest changes after working memory training. *Hum. Brain Mapp.* 34:396–406.

Jones, D. K., T. R. Knösche, and R. Turner. 2013. White matter integrity, fiber count, and other fallacies: The do's and don'ts of diffusion MRI. *NeuroImage* 73:239–254.

Jones, T. B., P. A. Bandettini, L. Kenworthy, L. K. Case, S. C. Milleville, A. Martin, and R. M. Birn. 2010. Sources of group differences in functional connectivity: An investigation applied to autism spectrum disorder. *NeuroImage* 49:401–14.

Jou, R. J., N. Mateljevic, M. D. Kaiser, D. R. Sugrue, F. R. Volkmar, and K. A. Pelphrey. 2011. Structural neural phenotype of autism: Preliminary evidence from a diffusion tensor imaging study using tract-based spatial statistics. *AJNR Am. J. Neuroradiol.* 32:1607–13.

Jou, R. J., H. E. Reed, M. D. Kaiser, A. C. Voos, F. R. Volkmar, and K. A. Pelphrey. 2015. White matter abnormalities in autism and unaffected siblings. *J Neuropsychiatry Clin Neurosci*: appineuropsych15050109.

Just, M. A., V. L. Cherkassky, T. A. Keller, R. K. Kana, and N. J. Minshew. 2007. Functional and anatomical cortical underconnectivity in autism: Evidence from an FMRI study of an executive function task and corpus callosum morphometry. *Cereb. Cortex* 17:951–61.

Just, M. A., V. L. Cherkassky, T. A. Keller, and N. J. Minshew. 2004. Cortical activation and synchronization during sentence comprehension in high-functioning autism: Evidence of underconnectivity. *Brain* 127:1811–21.

Just, M. A., T. A. Keller, V. L. Malave, R. K. Kana, and S. Varma. 2012. Autism as a neural systems disorder: A theory of frontal-posterior underconnectivity. *Neurosci. Biobehav. Rev.* 36:1292–313.

Kalkbrenner, A. E., G. C. Windham, M. L. Serre, Y. Akita, X. Wang, K. Hoffman, B. P. Thayer, and J. L. Daniels. 2015. Particulate matter exposure, prenatal and postnatal windows of susceptibility, and autism spectrum disorders. *Epidemiology* 26:30–42.

Kana, R. K., T. A. Keller, V. L. Cherkassky, N. J. Minshew, and M. A. Just. 2009. Atypical frontal-posterior synchronization of Theory of Mind regions in autism during mental state attribution. *Soc. Neurosci.* 4:135–52.

Kana, R. K., T. A. Keller, V. L. Cherkassky, N. J. Minshew, and M. A. Just. 2006. Sentence comprehension in autism: Thinking in pictures with decreased functional connectivity. *Brain* 129:2484–93.

Kana, R. K., T. A. Keller, N. J. Minshew, and M. A. Just. 2007. Inhibitory control in high-functioning autism: Decreased activation and underconnectivity in inhibition networks. *Biol. Psychiatry* 62:198–206.

Kana, R. K., L. E. Libero, C. P. Hu, H. D. Deshpande, and J. S. Colburn. 2012. Functional brain networks and white matter underlying theory-of-mind in autism. *Soc. Cogn. Affect. Neurosci* 9(1):98–105.

Kandel, E. R., T. M. Jessell, and J. R. Sanes. 2000. Sensory experience and the fine tuning of synaptic connections. In *Principles of Neural Science*, eds. E. R. Kandel, J. H. Schwartz, and T. M. Jessell, 1115–30. New York: Elsevier.

Keehn, B., P. Shih, L. Brenner, J. Townsend, and R.-A. Müller. 2013a. Functional connectivity for an "island of sparing" in autism spectrum disorder: An fMRI study of visual search. *Hum. Brain Mapp.* 34:2524–37.

Keehn, B., J. B. Wagner, H. Tager-Flusberg, and C. A. Nelson. 2013b. Functional connectivity in the first year of life in infants at-risk for autism: A preliminary near-infrared spectroscopy study. *Front. Hum. Neurosci.* 7:444.

Keller, T. A., R. K. Kana, and M. A. Just. 2007. A developmental study of the structural integrity of white matter in autism. *NeuroReport* 18:23–7.

Keown, C. L., P. Shih, A. Nair, N. Peterson, and R.-A. Müller. 2013. Local functional overconnectivity in posterior brain regions is associated with symptom severity in autism spectrum disorders. *Cell Reports* 5:567–72.

Khan, A. J., A. Nair, C. L. Keown, M. C. Datko, A. J. Lincoln, and R. A. Müller. 2015a. Cerebro-cerebellar resting-state functional connectivity in children and adolescents with autism spectrum disorder. *Biol. Psychiatry* 78:625–34.

Khan, S., A. Gramfort, N. R. Shetty et al. 2013. Local and long-range functional connectivity is reduced in concert in autism spectrum disorders. *Proc. Natl. Acad. USA* 110:3107–12.

Khan, S., K. Michmizos, M. Tommerdahl, S. Ganesan, M. G. Kitzbichler, M. Zetino, K. L. Garel, M. R. Herbert, M. S. Hamalainen, and T. Kenet. 2015b. Somatosensory cortex functional connectivity abnormalities in autism show opposite trends, depending on direction and spatial scale. *Brain* 138(Pt 5): 1394–409.

Kim, J. H., J. M. Lee, H. J. Jo et al. 2010. Defining functional SMA and pre-SMA subregions in human MFC using resting state fMRI: Functional connectivity-based parcellation method. *NeuroImage* 49:2375–86.

Kinoshita, Y., A. Ohnishi, K. Kohshi, and A. Yokota. 1999. Apparent diffusion coefficient on rat brain and nerves intoxicated with methylmercury. *Environ. Res.* 80:348–54.

Kitzbichler, M. G., S. Khan, S. Ganesan, M. G. Vangel, M. R. Herbert, M. S. Hamalainen, and T. Kenet. 2014. Altered development and multifaceted band-specific abnormalities of resting state networks in autism. *Biol. Psychiatry* 77(9):794–804.

Kleinhans, N. M., T. Richards, L. Sterling, K. C. Stegbauer, R. Mahurin, L. C. Johnson, J. Greenson, G. Dawson, and E. Aylward. 2008. Abnormal functional connectivity in autism spectrum disorders during face processing. *Brain* 131:1000–12.

Koldewyn, K., A. Yendiki, S. Weigelt, H. Gweon, J. Julian, H. Richardson, C. Malloy, R. Saxe, B. Fischl, and N. Kanwisher. 2014. Differences in the right inferior longitudinal fasciculus but no general disruption of white matter tracts in children with autism spectrum disorder. *Proc. Natl. Acad. Sci. USA* 111:1981–6.

Koshino, H., P. A. Carpenter, N. J. Minshew, V. L. Cherkassky, T. A. Keller, and M. A. Just. 2005. Functional connectivity in an fMRI working memory task in high-functioning autism. *NeuroImage* 24:810–21.

Koshino, H., R. K. Kana, T. A. Keller, V. L. Cherkassky, N. J. Minshew, and M. A. Just. 2008. fMRI investigation of working memory for faces in autism: Visual coding and underconnectivity with frontal areas. *Cereb. Cortex* 18:289–300.

Koyama, M. S., A. Di Martino, X. N. Zuo, C. Kelly, M. Mennes, D. R. Jutagir, F. X. Castellanos, and M. P. Milham. 2011. Resting-state functional connectivity indexes reading competence in children and adults. *J. Neurosci.* 31:8617–24.

Lanz, T. A., E. Guilmette, M. M. Gosink, J. E. Fischer, L. W. Fitzgerald, D. T. Stephenson, and M. T. Pletcher. 2013. Transcriptomic analysis of genetically defined autism candidate genes reveals common mechanisms of action. *Mol. Autism* 4:45.

Le Bihan, D., E. Breton, D. Lallemand, and P. Grenier. 1986. MR imaging of intra-voxel incoherent motions: Application to diffusion and perfusion in neurologic disorders. *Radiology* 161:401–7.

Lee, P. S., B. E. Yerys, A. Della Rosa, J. Foss-Feig, K. A. Barnes, J. D. James, J. VanMeter, C. J. Vaidya, W. D. Gaillard, and L. E. Kenworthy. 2009. Functional connectivity of the inferior frontal cortex changes with age in children with autism spectrum disorders: A fcMRI study of response inhibition. *Cereb. Cortex* 19:1787–94.

Leopold, D. A., Y. Murayama, and N. K. Logothetis. 2003. Very slow activity fluctuations in monkey visual cortex: Implications for functional brain imaging. *Cereb. Cortex* 13:422–33.

Lewis, C. M., A. Baldassarre, G. Committeri, G. L. Romani, and M. Corbetta. 2009. Learning sculpts the spontaneous activity of the resting human brain. *Proc. Natl. Acad. Sci. USA* 106:17558–63.

Ling, J., F. Merideth, A. Caprihan, A. Pena, T. Teshiba, and A. R. Mayer. 2012. Head injury or head motion? Assessment and quantification of motion artifacts in diffusion tensor imaging studies. *Hum. Brain Mapp.* 33:50–62.

Lombardo, M. V., B. Chakrabarti, E. T. Bullmore, S. A. Sadek, G. Pasco, S. J. Wheelwright, J. Suckling, and S. Baron-Cohen. 2010. Atypical neural self-representation in autism. *Brain* 133:611–24.

Lowe, M. J., M. Dzemidzic, J. T. Lurito, V. P. Mathews, and M. D. Phillips. 2000. Correlations in low-frequency BOLD fluctuations reflect cortico-cortical connections. *NeuroImage* 12:582–7.

Lowe, M. J., B. J. Mock, and J. A. Sorenson. 1998. Functional connectivity in single and multislice echoplanar imaging using resting-state fluctuations. *NeuroImage* 7:119–32.

Luo, C., Z. W. Guo, Y. X. Lai, W. Liao, Q. Liu, K. M. Kendrick, D. Z. Yao, and H. Li. 2012. Musical training induces functional plasticity in perceptual and motor networks: Insights from resting-state FMRI. *PLoS One* 7:e36568.

Lynch, C. J., L. Q. Uddin, K. Supekar, A. Khouzam, J. Phillips, and V. Menon. 2013. Default mode network in childhood autism: Posteromedial cortex heterogeneity and relationship with social deficits. *Biol. Psychiatry* 74(3):212–19.

Mason, R. A., D. L. Williams, R. K. Kana, N. Minshew, and M. A. Just. 2008. Theory of Mind disruption and recruitment of the right hemisphere during narrative comprehension in autism. *Neuropsychologia* 46:269–80.

Maximo, J. O., C. L. Keown, A. Nair, and R.-A. Müller. 2013. Approaches to local connectivity in autism using resting state functional connectivity MRI. *Front. Hum. Neurosci.* 7(605):1–13. DOI: 10.389/ fnhum.2013.00605.

McMenamin, B. W. and L. Pessoa. 2015. Discovering networks altered by potential threat ("anxiety") using quadratic discriminant analysis. *NeuroImage* 116:1–9.

Menon, V. 2011. Large-scale brain networks and psychopathology: A unifying triple network model. *Trends. Cogn. Sci.* 15:483–506.

Mizuno, A., Y. Liu, D. L. Williams, T. A. Keller, N. J. Minshew, and M. A. Just. 2011. The neural basis of deictic shifting in linguistic perspective-taking in high-functioning autism. *Brain* 134:2422–35.

Mizuno, A., M. E. Villalobos, M. M. Davies, B. C. Dahl, and R.-A. Müller. 2006. Partially enhanced thalamo-cortical functional connectivity in autism. *Brain Res.* 1104:160–74.

Monk, C. S., S. J. Peltier, J. L. Wiggins, S. J. Weng, M. Carrasco, S. Risi, and C. Lord. 2009. Abnormalities of intrinsic functional connectivity in autism spectrum disorders. *NeuroImage* 47:764–72.

Mostofsky, S. H., S. K. Powell, D. J. Simmonds, M. C. Goldberg, B. Caffo, and J. J. Pekar. 2009. Decreased connectivity and cerebellar activity in autism during motor task performance. *Brain* 132:2413–25.

Müller, R.-A., P. Shih, B. Keehn, J. R. Deyoe, K. M. Leyden, and D. K. Shukla. 2011. Underconnected, but how? A survey of functional connectivity MRI studies in autism spectrum disorders. *Cereb. Cortex* 21:2233–43.

Murdaugh, D. L., S. V. Shinkareva, H. R. Deshpande, J. Wang, M. R. Pennick, and R. K. Kana. 2012. Differential deactivation during mentalizing and classification of autism based on default mode network connectivity. *PLoS One* 7:e50064.

Nair, A., R. A. Carper, A. E. Abbott, C. P. Chen, S. Solders, S. Nakutin, M. C. Datko, I. Fishman, and R. A. Muller. 2015. Regional specificity of aberrant thalamo-cortical connectivity in autism. *Hum. Brain Mapp.* 36:4497–511.

Nair, A., C. L. Keown, M. Datko, P. Shih, B. Keehn, and R. A. Müller. 2014. Impact of methodological variables on functional connectivity findings in autism spectrum disorders. *Hum. Brain Mapp.* 35:4035–48.

Nair, A., J. M. Treiber, D. K. Shukla, P. Shih, and R.-A. Müller. 2013. Thalamocortical connectivity in autism spectrum disorder: A study of functional and anatomical connectivity. *Brain* 136:1942–55.

Nielsen, J. A., B. A. Zielinski, P. T. Fletcher, A. L. Alexander, N. Lange, E. D. Bigler, J. E. Lainhart, and J. S. Anderson. 2013. Multisite functional connectivity MRI classification of autism: ABIDE results. *Front Hum. Neurosci.* 7:599.

Nir, Y., U. Hasson, I. Levy, Y. Yeshurun, and R. Malach. 2006. Widespread functional connectivity and fMRI fluctuations in human visual cortex in the absence of visual stimulation. *NeuroImage* 30:1313–24.

Noonan, S. K., F. Haist, and R.-A. Müller. 2009. Aberrant functional connectivity in autism: Evidence from low-frequency BOLD signal fluctuations. *Brain Res.* 1262:48–63.

Pang, E. W., T. Valica, M. J. MacDonald, M. J. Taylor, J. Brian, J. P. Lerch, and E. Anagnostou. 2016. Abnormal brain dynamics underlie speech production in children with autism spectrum disorder. *Autism Res.* 9:249–61.

Petersen, S. E., P. T. Fox, M. I. Posner, M. Mintun, and M. E. Raichle. 1989. Positron emission tomographic studies of the processing of single words. *J. Cogn. Neurosci.* 1:153–70.

Popper, K. R. 1965. *Conjectures and Refutations: The Growth of Scientific Knowledge*. Neuw York: Routledge & Kegan Paul.

Poustka, L., C. Jennen-Steinmetz, R. Henze, K. Vomstein, J. Haffner, and B. Sieltjes. 2012. Fronto-temporal disconnectivity and symptom severity in children with autism spectrum disorder. *World J. Biol. Psychiatry* 13:269–80.

Power, J. D., A. L. Cohen, S. M. Nelson et al. 2011. Functional network organization of the human brain. *Neuron* 72:665–78.

Power, J. D., A. Mitra, T. O. Laumann, A. Z. Snyder, B. L. Schlaggar, and S. E. Petersen. 2014a. Methods to detect, characterize, and remove motion artifact in resting state fMRI. *NeuroImage* 84:320–41.

Power, J. D., B. L. Schlaggar, and S. E. Petersen. 2014b. Studying brain organization via spontaneous fMRI signal. *Neuron* 84:681–96.

Power, J. D., B. L. Schlaggar, and S. E. Petersen. 2015. Recent progress and outstanding issues in motion correction in resting state fMRI. *NeuroImage* 105C:536–51.

Price, C. J. and K. J. Friston. 1997. Cognitive conjunction: A new approach to brain activation experiments. *NeuroImage* 5:261–70.

Quartz, S. R. and T. J. Sejnowski. 1997. The neural basis of cognitive development: A constructivist manifesto. *Behav. Brain Sci.* 20:537–96.

Redcay, E., J. M. Moran, P. L. Mavros, H. Tager-Flusberg, J. D. Gabrieli, and S. Whitfield-Gabrieli. 2013. Intrinsic functional network organization in high-functioning adolescents with autism spectrum disorder. *Front. Hum. Neurosci.* 7:573.

Ring, H. A., S. Baron-Cohen, S. Wheelwright, S. C. Williams, M. Brammer, C. Andrew, and E. T. Bullmore. 1999. Cerebral correlates of preserved cognitive skills in autism: A functional MRI study of embedded figures task performance. *Brain* 122:1305–15.

Rudie, J. D., Z. Shehzad, L. M. Hernandez, N. L. Colich, S. Y. Bookheimer, M. Iacoboni, and M. Dapretto. 2012. Reduced functional integration and segregation of distributed neural systems underlying social and emotional information processing in autism spectrum disorders. *Cereb. Cortex* 22:1025–37.

Saad, Z. S., S. J. Gotts, K. Murphy, G. Chen, H. J. Jo, A. Martin, and R. W. Cox. 2012. Trouble at rest: How correlation patterns and group differences become distorted after global signal regression. *Brain Connect.* 2:25–32.

Sahin, M. and M. Sur. 2015. Genes, circuits, and precision therapies for autism and related neurodevelopmental disorders. *Science* 350(6263):926–35.

Sahyoun, C. P., J. W. Belliveau, and M. Mody. 2010a. White matter integrity and pictorial reasoning in high-functioning children with autism. *Brain Cogn.* 73:180–8.

Sahyoun, C. P., J. W. Belliveau, I. Soulières, S. Schwartz, and M. Mody. 2010b. Neuroimaging of the functional and structural networks underlying visuospatial vs. linguistic reasoning in high-functioning autism. *Neuropsychologia* 48:86–95.

Satterthwaite, T. D., M. A. Elliott, R. T. Gerraty et al. 2013. An improved framework for confound regression and filtering for control of motion artifact in the preprocessing of resting-state functional connectivity data. *NeuroImage* 64:240–56.

Saur, D., B. Schelter, S. Schnell et al. 2010. Combining functional and anatomical connectivity reveals brain networks for auditory language comprehension. *NeuroImage* 49:3187–97.

Schmithorst, V. J., J. Vannest, G. Lee, L. Hernandez-Garcia, E. Plante, A. Rajagopal, S. K. Holland, and C. A. C. The. 2014. Evidence that neurovascular coupling underlying the BOLD effect increases with age during childhood. *Hum. Brain Mapp* 36(1):1–15.

Schölvinck, M. L., A. Maier, F. Q. Ye, J. H. Duyn, and D. A. Leopold. 2010. Neural basis of global resting-state fMRI activity. *Proc Natl. Acad. Sci. USA* 107:10238–43.

Schultz, D. H., N. L. Balderston, and F. J. Helmstetter. 2012. Resting-state connectivity of the amygdala is altered following Pavlovian fear conditioning. *Front Hum. Neurosci.* 6:242.

Schumann, C. M., C. S. Bloss, C. C. Barnes et al. 2010. Longitudinal magnetic resonance imaging study of cortical development through early childhood in autism. *J. Neurosci.* 30:4419–27.

Schumann, C. M. and C. W. Nordahl. 2011. Bridging the gap between MRI and postmortem research in autism. *Brain Res.* 1380:175–86.

Seeley, W. W., V. Menon, A. F. Schatzberg, J. Keller, G. H. Glover, H. Kenna, A. L. Reiss, and M. D. Greicius. 2007. Dissociable intrinsic connectivity networks for salience processing and executive control. *J. Neurosci.* 27:2349–56.

Shehzad, Z., A. M. Kelly, P. T. Reiss et al. 2009. The resting brain: Unconstrained yet reliable. *Cereb. Cortex* 19:2209–29.

Shen, M. D., C. W. Nordahl, G. S. Young, S. L. Wootton-Gorges, A. Lee, S. E. Liston, K. R. Harrington, S. Ozonoff, and D. G. Amaral. 2013. Early brain enlargement and elevated extra-axial fluid in infants who develop autism spectrum disorder. *Brain* 136:2825–35.

Shen, M. D., P. Shih, B. Ottl, B. Keehn, K. M. Leyden, M. S. Gaffrey, and R. A. Muller. 2012. Atypical lexicosemantic function of extrastriate cortex in autism spectrum disorder: Evidence from functional and effective connectivity. *NeuroImage* 62:1780–91.

Shih, P., B. Keehn, J. K. Oram, K. M. Leyden, C. L. Keown, and R.-A. Müller. 2011. Functional differentiation of posterior superior temporal sulcus in autism: A functional connectivity magnetic resonance imaging study. *Biol. Psychiatry* 70:270–7.

Shih, P., M. Shen, B. Öttl, B. Keehn, M. S. Gaffrey, and R.-A. Müller. 2010. Atypical network connectivity for imitation in autism spectrum disorder. *Neuropsychologia* 48:2931–9.

Shukla, D. K., B. Keehn, and R.-A. Müller. 2010. Tract-specific analyses of diffusion tensor imaging show widespread white matter compromise in autism spectrum disorder. *J. Child Psychol. Psychiatry Allied Discipl.* 52:286–95.

Shukla, D. K., Keehn, B., Smylie, D. M., and Müller, R.-A. 2011. Microstructural abnormalities of short-distance white matter tracts in autism spectrum disorder. *Neuropsychologia* 49(5):1378–1382.

Sivaswamy, L., A. Kumar, D. Rajan, M. Behen, O. Muzik, D. Chugani, and H. Chugani. 2010. A diffusion tensor imaging study of the cerebellar pathways in children with autism spectrum disorder. *J. Child Neurol.* 25:1223–31.

Solomon, M., S. J. Ozonoff, S. Ursu, S. Ravizza, N. Cummings, S. Ly, and C. S. Carter. 2009. The neural substrates of cognitive control deficits in autism spectrum disorders. *Neuropsychologia* 47:2515–26.

Solso, S., R. Xu, J. Proudfoot et al. 2015. Diffusion tensor imaging provides evidence of possible axonal overconnectivity in frontal lobes in autism spectrum disorder toddlers. *Biol. Psychiatry.*

Sotiropoulos, S. N., S. Jbabdi, J. Xu et al. 2013. Advances in diffusion MRI acquisition and processing in the human connectome project. *NeuroImage* 80:125–43.

Stamatakis, E. A., R. M. Adapa, A. R. Absalom, and D. K. Menon. 2010. Changes in resting neural connectivity during propofol sedation. *PLoS One* 5:e14224.

Starck, T., J. Nikkinen, J. Rahko et al. 2013. Resting state fMRI reveals a default mode dissociation between retrosplenial and medial prefrontal subnetworks in ASD despite motion scrubbing. *Front Hum. Neurosci.* 7:802.

Sundaram, S. K., A. Kumar, M. I. Makki, M. E. Behen, H. T. Chugani, and D. C. Chugani. 2008. Diffusion tensor imaging of frontal lobe in autism spectrum disorder. *Cereb. Cortex* 18:2659–65.

Supekar, K., L. Q. Uddin, A. Khouzam, J. Phillips, W. D. Gaillard, L. E. Kenworthy, B. E. Yerys, C. J. Vaidya, and V. Menon. 2013. Brain hyperconnectivity in children with autism and its links to social deficits. *Cell Rep.* 5:738–47.

Takahashi, M., D. B. Hackney, G. Zhang, S. L. Wehrli, A. C. Wright, W. T. O'Brien, H. Uematsu, F. W. Wehrli, and M. E. Selzer. 2002. Magnetic resonance microimaging of intraaxonal water diffusion in live excised lamprey spinal cord. *Proc. Natl. Acad. Sci. USA* 99:16192–6.

Toro, R., M. Konyukh, R. Delorme, C. Leblond, P. Chaste, F. Fauchereau, M. Coleman, M. Leboyer, C. Gillberg, and T. Bourgeron. 2010. Key role for gene dosage and synaptic homeostasis in autism spectrum disorders. *Trends Genet.* 26:363–72.

Tournier, J.-D., S. Mori, and A. Leemans. 2011. Diffusion tensor imaging and beyond. *Magn. Reson. Med.* 65:1532–56.

Tournier, J.-D., C.-H. Yeh, F. Calamante, K.-H. Cho, A. Connelly, and C.-P. Lin. 2008. Resolving crossing fibres using constrained spherical deconvolution: Validation using diffusion-weighted imaging phantom data. *NeuroImage* 42:617–25.

Travers, B. G., N. Adluru, C. Ennis, D. P. M. Tromp, D. Destiche, S. Doran, E. D. Bigler, N. Lange, J. E. Lainhart, and A. L. Alexander. 2012. Diffusion tensor imaging in autism spectrum disorder: A review. *Autism Res.* 5:289–313.

Travers, B. G., P. M. Tromp do, N. Adluru et al. 2015. Atypical development of white matter microstructure of the corpus callosum in males with autism: A longitudinal investigation. *Mol. Autism* 6:15.

Uddin, L. Q., K. Supekar, and V. Menon. 2013. Reconceptualizing functional brain connectivity in autism from a developmental perspective. *Front. Hum. Neurosci.* 7:458.

Urbain, C., V. M. Vogan, A. X. Ye, E. W. Pang, S. M. Doesburg, and M. J. Taylor. 2015. Desynchronization of fronto-temporal networks during working memory processing in autism. *Hum. Brain Mapp* 37(1):153–164.

Van Dijk, K. R., T. Hedden, A. Venkataraman, K. C. Evans, S. W. Lazar, and R. L. Buckner. 2010. Intrinsic functional connectivity as a tool for human connectomics: Theory, properties, and optimization. *J. Neurophysiol* 103:297–321.

Van Dijk, K. R., M. R. Sabuncu, and R. L. Buckner. 2012. The influence of head motion on intrinsic functional connectivity MRI. *NeuroImage* 59:431–8.

Vidyasagar, R., S. E. Folger, and L. M. Parkes. 2014. Re-wiring the brain: Increased functional connectivity within primary somatosensory cortex following synchronous co-activation. *NeuroImage* 92:19–26.

Villalobos, M. E., A. Mizuno, B. C. Dahl, N. Kemmotsu, and R.-A. Müller. 2005. Reduced functional connectivity between V1 and inferior frontal cortex associated with visuomotor performance in autism. *NeuroImage* 25:916–25.

Von dem Hagen, E. A., R. S. Stoyanova, S. Baron-Cohen, and A. J. Calder. 2012. Reduced functional connectivity within and between "social" resting state networks in autism spectrum conditions. *Soc. Cogn. Affect Neurosci* 8(6):694–701.

Wang, Z., J. Liu, N. Zhong, Y. Qin, H. Zhou, and K. Li. 2012. Changes in the brain intrinsic organization in both on-task state and post-task resting state. *NeuroImage* 62:394–407.

Washington, S. D., E. M. Gordon, J. Brar et al. 2013. Dysmaturation of the default mode network in autism. *Hum. Brain Mapp* 35(4):1284–96.

Weinstein, M., L. Ben-Sira, Y. Levy, D. A. Zachor, E. Ben Itzhak, M. Artzi, R. Tarrasch, P. M. Eksteine, T. Hendler, and D. Ben Bashat. 2011. Abnormal white matter integrity in young children with autism. *Hum. Brain. Mapp* 32:534–43.

White, N. S., T. B. Leergaard, H. D'Arceuil, J. G. Bjaalie, and A. M. Dale. 2013. Probing tissue microstructure with restriction spectrum imaging: Histological and theoretical validation. *Hum. Brain Mapp.* 34:327–46.

Wilson, T. W., D. C. Rojas, M. L. Reite, P. D. Teale, and S. J. Rogers. 2007. Children and adolescents with autism exhibit reduced MEG steady-state gamma responses. *Biol. Psychiatry* 62:192–7.

Wolff, J. J., H. Gu, G. Gerig, et al. 2012a. Differences in white matter fiber tract development present from 6 to 24 months in infants with autism. *Am. J. Psychiatry* 169:589–600.

Wolff, J. J., H. Gu, G. Gerig et al. 2012b. Differences in white matter fiber tract development present from 6 to 24 months in infants with autism. *Am. J. Psychiatry* 169:589–600.

Yendiki, A., K. Koldewyn, S. Kakunoori, N. Kanwisher, and B. Fischl. 2013. Spurious group differences due to head motion in a diffusion MRI study. *NeuroImage* 88C:79–90.

Yerys, B. E. and J. D. Herrington. 2014. Multimodal imaging in autism: An early review of comprehensive neural circuit characterization. *Curr. Psychiatry Rep.* 16:496.

Zhang, H., T. Schneider, C. A. Wheeler-Kingshott, and D. C. Alexander. 2012. NODDI: Practical in vivo neurite orientation dispersion and density imaging of the human brain. *NeuroImage* 61:1000–16.

Zielinski, B. A., M. B. D. Prigge, J. A. Nielsen et al. 2014. Longitudinal changes in cortical thickness in autism and typical development. *Brain* 137:1799–812.

Chapter 15 Behavioral signal processing and autism

Learning from multimodal behavioral signals

Daniel Bone, Theodora Chaspari, and Shrikanth Narayanan

Contents

Abstract 320
15.1 Introduction 320
15.2 Audio signal processing (audio, speech, text, contextual
  events, interaction modeling) 322
  15.2.1 Audio acquisition 323
  15.2.2 Automatic speech recognition and synthesis 324
  15.2.3 Affective speech processing 325
  15.2.4 Speech prosody 326
  15.2.5 Modeling interaction with speech cues 329
  15.2.6 Speech: Future directions and open challenges 331
15.3 Visual signal processing (facial expressions, eye tracking,
  gestures) 331
  15.3.1 Facial processing 332
15.4 Physiological signal processing (heart rate and skin
  conductance) 333
  15.4.1 Signal fundamentals 334
  15.4.2 Collecting physiological signals 334
  15.4.3 Physiological signal-processing techniques 335
  15.4.4 Behavioral signal processing for physiological data . . . 336
15.5 Meta-data processing with machine learning 338
15.6 Conclusion 339
References 340

Abstract

Human communication is an intricate exchange of information occurring at different timescales through the coordination of several modalities; facial expressions, body language, and intonation coincide with spoken words for effective transferal of information. For children with autism spectrum disorder (ASD), the subtle coordination between modalities, which seems so natural to the experienced communicator, can be difficult to ascertain and master. In this chapter, we discuss the ways in which signal processing of behavioral data can aid in our understanding and treatment of autism and other behavioral disorders.

15.1 Introduction

Autism spectrum disorder is behaviorally defined, and thus is assessed through behavioral observation. While there is a push to create biological definitions of autism, success has been limited; this research domain still relies on detailed behavioral phenotyping, as does measuring the effectiveness of intervention. In particular, biological research indicates that simple syndromic conditions cannot account for the extreme heterogeneity observed in autism (i.e., it is suspected that they account for no more than 15% of ASD cases; Abrahams and Geschwind 2010); rather, many researchers believe that genetic variants will map to intermediate phenotypes, which collectively present as ASD. Consequently, dimensional behavioral descriptors are needed for enhanced phenotyping of ASD, both to support such biological efforts and to aid clinical practice; these include more specific representations of social-communication deficits and repetitive/restrictive behaviors (Lord and Jones 2012, cf. Figure 15.2B).

Behavioral assessment currently relies solely on trained clinicians. Humans are excellent signal processors, with the ability to make sense of complex scenes and attune to salient information; yet, human behavioral observation has its limits. Humans are subjective, are constrained by limited processing and multitasking capabilities, and are dependent on mood and noncontextual factors—all traits which computers can (arguably) overcome. Clinicians will always be critical to ASD diagnosis and treatment—they can adaptively interpret a subject's mood based on relevant contextual factors, drawing from an array of cultural and social experiences that are difficult to "teach" a computer. But, there is a role for computational technique in supporting and augmenting human perceptual and decision-making capabilities. In areas where humans disagree or physically cannot observe behavior, we can create signal-derived dimensional descriptors of behavior. These signal-derived measures can objectively answer, reliably and at large scale, the "what" and "how" of subjective behavioral constructs in ASD such as atypical prosody (Figure 15.1) and inappropriate use of eye contact.

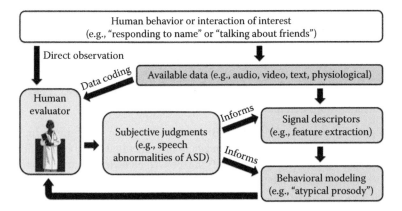

Figure 15.1 Human-in-the-loop approach to incorporating expert knowledge to develop novel behavioral measures. (Adapted from Narayanan, S. and P. G. Georgiou. 2013. *Proc. IEEE* 101:1203–33.)

In fact, informing human assessment and decision making is the primary goal of behavioral signal processing (BSP; Narayanan and Georgiou 2013): the technical and computational methods for measuring, analyzing, and modeling overt and covert human behavior. BSP aims to support clinicians in two key ways. The first is objective modeling of subjective behavioral constructs, through which we can automate annotation and learn about the human coding process. The second is through the creation of novel behavioral measures, which perform suprahuman processing of signal data. We will discuss applications in detail throughout this chapter.

Since human behavior is inherently multimodal, computational analysis of it should consider several behavioral signals. In particular, we will discuss BSP that uses audio (speech, language, nonverbal vocalization), video (bodily gestures, facial expression, proxemics), physiology (electrodermal activity [EDA] and electrocardiogram [ECG]), and meta-data (contextual elements of the interaction). Signal-processing practice is quite mature for these signals, making domain-specific applications viable. Furthermore, since it is often the coordination between multiple behavioral modalities that may appear awkward in individuals with ASD, machine-learning joint analysis and modeling techniques can be used to fuse the information in these behavioral signals.

Many notable examples exist for the first BSP outcome of re-creating human judgments beginning with low-lever behavioral signal cues. Consider our lab's work (SAIL, the Signal Analysis and Interpretation Lab at USC, sail.usc.edu/care/) on defining "atypical" prosody in autism (Bone et al. 2014a); prosody itself is an abstract concept, and determining the limits of "typicality" is a highly subjective decision that depends on context as well as the individual listener's physical attributes and domain knowledge (the sensor). We are working to define more objective parameters of atypical prosody from the acoustic waveform in order to overcome poor inter-rater agreement of this construct and to support personalized intervention. Another example is the quantitative measurement of bids for eye contact using point-of-view eyeglass cameras (Ye et al. 2015). Both of these targets have clear clinical applications. Concerning stereotypical behaviors relevant to autism, Goodwin (2008) presented experiments using pattern recognition with wearable accelerometers toward automated long-term monitoring.

Regarding the second goal of BSP, novel tools are emerging which extract information that is beyond human perceptual capabilities. For instance, researchers are quantifying covert behaviors that are only observable through advanced signal capture devices like wearable EDA and ECG. Goodwin et al. (2006) observed atypical arousal responses (i.e., heart rate) to stressful stimuli in ASD individuals; this work provided support for the potential utility of physiological stress monitoring as feedback for caregivers. More recently, we have investigated the dyadic synchrony in EDA signals of a child with autism and their interacting partner (Chaspari et al. 2014). Aside from covert signals, BSP methodology can be used to create knowledge-inspired tools that measure human-defined qualitative concepts. For example, Lee et al. (2014) presented a bottom-up definition of vocal entrainment entirely based on acoustic features. Entrainment is an aspect of positive interactions in which the participants match behavioral characteristics; in the case of vocal entrainment, they begin to speak like one another.

BSP can be seen as a specific approach of Computational behavioral science (CBS; http://www.cbs.gatech.edu), wherein the end-goal is a high-level behavioral construct (not an individual behavior), and that goal precludes all methodological decisions. More precisely, behavioral informatics, the high-level construct that is the output of BSP, is the priority; and the specific methods to get these outputs need not be generally applicable outside of the target domain, nor of scientific merit to the general engineering community.

In this chapter, we discuss the individual strengths of each sensing modality, the current state of the art, and detail applications in the domain of autism. Emphasis is given to work from our lab, the Signal Analysis and Interpretation Laboratory (SAIL) at University of Southern California.

15.2 Audio signal processing (audio, speech, text, contextual events, interaction modeling)

Speech signal-processing applications have evolved over the decades from simple tasks like detecting speech activity in controlled laboratory settings to the creation of tools that support autonomous interactions in diverse settings, like Apple's Siri; but there are many other facets to speech, a rich signal modulated by emotions and other paralinguistic intentions. Congruent with the complexities of spoken communication, a diversity of subdomains relevant to human–human and human–machine communication have emerged, such as automatic speech recognition (ASR), the process of converting an audio waveform into corresponding text; speech synthesis, the inverse process of converting text into machine speech; speaker diarization, determination of who spoke an utterance; automatic affect recognition and synthesis, the development of computational models of emotional speech; text analysis, methods of interpreting and learning linguistic tendencies from either spoken or written text; and speech prosody modeling, the study of "how" something is spoken, not "what" is spoken, through modeling of intonation, volume, and rhythm. In addition, audio event analysis can infer valuable context of human behavior; for example, we may automatically recognize from an audio signal if a child's parents are talking, if the location is outdoors or indoors, if a television is on, if someone is playing with toys, or if the child is in a crowded or a quiet environment.

In this section, we will discuss speech-processing methods and their relevance (including specific examples) to ASD research, including methods of audio acquisition, automatic speech recognition and synthesis, emotional speech modeling, quantification of "atypical" speech prosody, and the importance of a communicative partner's speech and language cues.

15.2.1 Audio acquisition

Behavior modeling of speech data begins with the initial step of acquiring ecologically valid data (Narayanan and Georgiou 2013). To ensure ecological validity, the audio collection system should be an invisible bystander, not distracting to the communicative partners. In the realm of children's research, this can be a challenging task, especially when compounded with the additional set of concerns that accompany ASD research.

A variety of recording options are available, each with benefits and drawbacks. Close-talking microphones may capture data with optimal signal-to-noise ratio (SNR), but they are generally obtrusive since they must be placed directly in front of the speaker. Lapel microphones can produce high SNR recordings, but are a tactile distraction for some subjects. Lightweight wearable microphones that fit into clothing may be a suitable solution for toddlers (e.g., LENA recording devices, Warren et al. 2010), although there is evidence that clothing can affect recordings (Bentler et al. 2010). One advantage of wearable microphones is that they can record an individual throughout their daily activities—this leads to a host of new, unsolved computational challenges regarding changing audio quality and context. Alternatively, there are far-field directional microphones that can capture audio from a longer distance and may be placed out of the child's line of sight (e.g., mounted on walls). Far-field audio may limit speech capture quality, reducing accuracy of certain speech features that rely on very accurate computation of vocal-fold opening and closing cycles (i.e., inverse filtering and voice quality features). We successfully employed far-field microphones to record Autism Diagnostic Observation Schedule (ADOS) interactions (Black et al. 2011); we will discuss studies that utilized this data later in this section.

15.2.2 Automatic speech recognition and synthesis

Automatic speech recognition (ASR) has matured to the point of general applicability in daily life as evidenced by Apple's Siri or Google Web-based speech recognition. Traditional methods of speech recognition involving hidden Markov models (HMMs) are being replaced by neural networks (i.e., deep neural networks, or DNNs) capable of learning complex, nonlinear acoustic properties of continuous speech. DNN-based speech processing is a big data application, because it relies on learning from immense amounts of data, such as that captured by Apple and Google software during product use. However, application to unique domains with small training data is still a challenge. For example, in the interview conversations that occur during the ADOS, children sporadically talk about pop culture, discuss friends and family, and quote movies. Moreover, recognition of children's speech will require novel computational techniques. Children's speech can be difficult to recognize due to speech impairments and disfluencies that reduce over time as the child's language and motor skills develop and their speech becomes more adult-like (Lee et al. 1999). This is an exceedingly difficult recognition task for a computer. Additionally, the related task of creating naturalistic speech from text is still an unsolved problem that relies on automatic recognition of appropriate intonation and affect in order to appear human-like.

What potential applications do speech recognition and synthesis have to autism? First, many manual speech-analytic techniques are dependent on an initial lexical transcription; automatic transcription through ASR would save significant time and money. Furthermore, ASR can facilitate fully automatic speech analysis systems, since many of the other methods that we will discuss depend on speech transcription or word-level segmentation of the audio. For example, a person's mood can be tracked throughout the day based on the language that they use. Second, speech synthesis is central to assistive speech-generating devices that allow a nonverbal or minimally verbal ASD child to have a voice; these devices have been shown effective in communicative interventions (Franco et al. 2009). In the future, it may benefit some children with autism to be able to "speak" with a voice that sounds like their own; this is a possibility with current speech-processing technology, but we are currently unaware of any comparable ASD applications.

15.2.3 Affective speech processing

Emotional speech research in engineering is a relatively young domain with a rich history. The initial motivation for engineers to investigate emotion was to create advanced human–machine systems that could interpret the state of the user and thus better communicate. Lee et al. (2001) developed classifiers to identify negative emotions (i.e., anger) in phone-recorded audio from call centers using only acoustic cues. This work was later expanded to include manually transcribed lexical and discourse features (Lee and Narayanan 2005). Numerous affective recognition methods have been considered, including global acoustic statistics of an utterance (e.g., pitch and loudness), HMMs (Schuller et al. 2003), and hierarchical classifiers (Lee et al. 2011). Affect recognition is highly dependent on the attributes of a given data collection; and thus to improve performance within a corpus typically means to decrease generalization to new data. To combat this issue, some robust cross-corpus applications are being developed. For instance, Bone et al. (2014b) developed a rule-based automatic system to rate vocal arousal (activation, excitement) from a speaker's voice, depicted in Figure 15.2.

Emotional production and perception deficits are commonly reported in ASD. Engineered emotional games for ASD children that incorporate multiple behavioral modalities are already appearing. Engineers began investigating emotion through multiple modalities over a decade ago; for example, Busso et al. (2004) jointly modeled speech and facial expressions during affective productions. This type of research has been translated into emotional human–machine systems. Mower et al. (2011) presented an Embodied Conversational Agent (ECA) that participates in

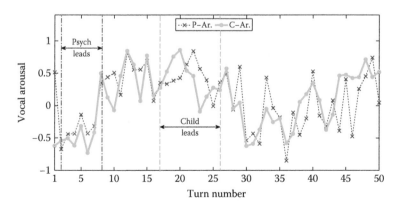

Figure 15.2 Sample of vocal arousal streams from child (C) and psychologist (P), with regions of psychologist leads and child leads indicated. *Note*: Turns occur asynchronously, and by convention turn N for the psychologist occurs before turn N for the child. (From Bone, D. et al. 2014c. *Proc. Interspeech* 15:218–22.)

a set of emotional games with a child with ASD. A researcher controlled the device in a Wizard of Oz format. Schuller et al. (2014) created an interactive emotional game system aimed at preventing social exclusion for adolescents with autism through the EU-funded ASC Inclusion project. The system uses state-of-the-art speech, gesture, and facial processing to interpret the emotions expressed by a user and provide feedback. Given the importance of emotion to ASD, the number of translational engineering systems is sure to grow.

15.2.4 Speech prosody

Speech prosody—the rhythm, stress, and intonation of speech that convey a speaker's meaning and affect—is critical to effective communication. Deficits in producing appropriate prosody can make listening an arduous task, and lead to perceptual errors that can reduce the quality of an interaction. Prosodic impairment is commonly reported in autism spectrum disorder; yet, since so little is well understood, it is regarded as an understudied and high-impact research area (McCann and Peppe 2003). Both perceptual and production deficits have been observed (Paul et al. 2005). Impairment in prosody may have links to social causes (Theory of Mind, ToM, Baron-Cohen et al. 1985) or motor causes—although there is growing counterevidence to motor theories (Shriberg et al. 2011). Still, it is certainly possible that the etiology of prosodic impairment in ASD is as complex and diverse as the behavioral presentation appears to be.

Remarkably, while "atypical" prosody is regularly reported in the ASD literature, it is often excluded from diagnostic instrument algorithms due to poor subjective reliability (Lord et al. 2000). The principal commonality between perceptual accounts of the autistic prosody is simply that a deficit is present, generally referred to as "atypical," "odd," or "awkward." The descriptions are often vague and even contrasting, indicating a characteristic out of the norm (above or below). For example, individuals with ASD have been reported in the same study as having either exaggerated or monotone pitch range (Baltaxe et al. 1984); and the Autism Diagnostic Observation Schedule (ADOS; Lord et al. 2000) seeks, among other perceptions, a speaking rate that is either too fast or too slow.

Scientific measures for atypical prosody are primarily rooted in human perception. Since "atypicality" is quite subjective and prosody is an abstract concept, this has led to a series of measures that are poorly specified and not comparable across studies; compounded with relatively small sample sizes (due to IRB restrictions, financial constraints, and time-intensive manual labeling), many contradictory findings have been presented (McCann and Peppe 2003). Perceptual studies often try to constrain the linguistic material through read sentences or paired-word tasks (Pronovost et al. 1966; Paul et al. 2005; Peppé et al. 2007);

the drawback is that the speech is unnatural, not spontaneous, and may not reflect those aspects of prosody that are most relevant to interaction. A broad perceptual rating tool (Shriberg et al. 1992, 2001) has been utilized to rate spontaneous utterances; but this process is very time-intensive and certain aspects of prosody still have low inter-rate reliability. Since the great heterogeneity of autistic symptoms extends to atypical prosody, a necessary next step to understand and possibly treat prosodic impairment is to obtain population prevalence estimates of various prosodic impairments; to our knowledge, no very large-scale studies (over 100 subjects per group) which test for highly specified prosodic abnormalities have been conducted. We propose that objective computational cues of prosody are a scalable alternative and counter to subjective disagreements between human raters. To date, there have been very few investigations that use objective computational cues of prosody (e.g., Diehl et al. 2009; Van Santen et al. 2010; Grossman et al. 2013). We believe speech signal processing has the potential to revolutionize the understanding of prosody, particularly its assessment and treatment in ASD.

In our initial work involving child–adult (psychologist) interactions as part of the ADOS Module 3 social interviews, we developed a set of acoustic–prosodic elements of conversational speech which were found to vary according to the child's level of severity (Bone et al. 2014a). Specifically, we computed 24 perceptually inspired prosodic cues, aggregated over a whole session, along the domains of intonation, volume, rate, and voice quality; the cues were motivated through the convergence of ASD perceptual literature and computational linguistics literature. In this sample, children with higher ASD severity judged by the ADOS also had more negative end-of-sentence pitch slopes and less typical voice quality (i.e., higher jitter and harmonics-to-noise ratio [HNR]). These findings demonstrated the feasibility of semiautomatic computational analysis of naturalistic speech. A limitation of this study is that there were no neurotypically developing (NTD) controls with which to define "normal" prosody characteristics. Instead, we were able to see the general trends in our data, which may correspond to general prevalence in the population. An illustration of the types of features that we extract is provided in Figure 15.3.

Although prosodic abnormalities are prevalent in ASD, not all individuals with ASD have them; as such, the typical design of dividing individuals into ASD and non-ASD groups has a noted drawback. One alternative approach we have taken is to ask raters to judge global aspects of prosody, which we then relate to objective acoustic–prosodic measures (Bone et al. 2015a). In this study, using crowdsourcing techniques, we asked naïve Amazon Mechanical Turk workers to judge general and specific notions of "awkward" prosody, motivated by the observation that peers of ASD individuals can detect something "odd" in their speech. As expected, we obtained higher agreement for the more

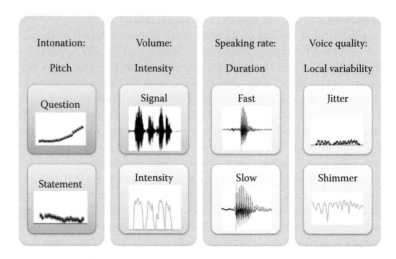

Figure 15.3 Types of prosodic features that were extracted in Bone et al. (2014a): intonation, turn-end final rise or fall; volume, high or low variability; speaking rate, too fast or too slow; and voice quality, atypically high jitter and shimmer.

general ratings. We found that more "awkward" prosody was judged as less expressive (more monotone) and was attributable to perceived awkward rate/rhythm, volume, and intonation. Regarding acoustic features, we reported that perceived expressivity could be quantified through intonation variability features (the more variable your intonation, the more expressive you sound), and that objective speaking rate and rhythm cues predict perceived awkwardness. A novel approach in this work was to compare perceived "awkward" prosody to expected production; specifically, we computed distance metrics (i.e., correlation and mean absolute difference) between expected and realized speaking rate across an utterance (Figure 15.4).

Computational researchers are also beginning to analyze text from spoken language, which not only indicates a speaker's skill or communicative intention, but also provides a window into their mental state. Assessing language use is a significant undertaking that practically might only be realized through automated quantitative methods. Heeman et al. (2010) counted the occurrence of different linguistic units in discourse segments taken from the ADOS, then compared between ASD and NTD groups. Children with ASD were observed to use the filler "um," acknowledgements, and the discourse marker and less often, while usage of the filler "uh" was similar between groups. The filler "um" is expected to signal a longer delay to the listener in order to maintain the floor during a moment of thought. Together with the other results, it is suspected that the ASD group had less back-and-forth conversation with their partner. Complementing these findings, we investigated language usage in our ADOS data, concluding that the conversation quality degrades for children with higher severity ASD (Bone et al. 2013). We found that children

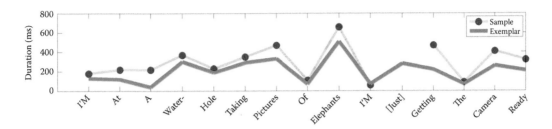

Figure 15.4 Word duration for a sample utterance versus an expected exemplar production. The word "just" was missing from the sample production, so we penalized the distance metric. (From Bone, D. et al. 2015a. *Proc. Interspeech* 16:1616–20.)

with greater ASD severity spoke less, spoke slower, responded later (i.e., longer latencies), and used personal pronouns, affective language, and fillers (e.g., "I mean," "you know") less often. With increasingly sophisticated techniques for language analysis being developed, the future is promising for textual analysis in ASD research using natural language processing.

15.2.5 Modeling interaction with speech cues

A novel view we have taken is to consider computationally the dynamic behavior of the interacting partner. Human interactional behavior does not happen in isolation, and so should not be viewed in isolation. For example, in clinical interactions, providers are not identical in the strategies they use, or even their ability to gain rapport with individual children. Still, we may find general trends in the behavior of the clinician in response to a child's actions, or lack thereof. Using recordings obtained during the administration of ADOS as a testbed, we have focused on computing the behavior of the clinician in these interactions and observing how it depends on the child's symptom severity (Bone et al. 2012, 2013, 2014a). This view is illustrated in Figure 15.5, wherein we can imagine that the clinician's behavior can inform the child's internal state, even when the child's behavior is not directly captured in signal data.

Overall, we find that the clinician, who acts as both evaluator and interlocutor, adjusts her behavior in predictable ways based on the child's social-communicative impairments (Bone et al. 2014a). Specifically, we observed that, when interacting with a child with higher ASD severity, the psychologist's speech prosody became more variable—possibly reflecting varying strategies for engagement and exaggerated affect. Furthermore, the psychologist was seen to adapt her behavior to that of the child in a surprising way; the more atypical the child's voice quality features (i.e., harmonics-to-noise ratio and jitter), the more atypical (higher) the psychologist's voice quality features (depicted for jitter in Figure 15.6). In addition to our conversation and language analysis of the child (Bone et al. 2013), we jointly modeled the psychologist's behavior. Aside from

329

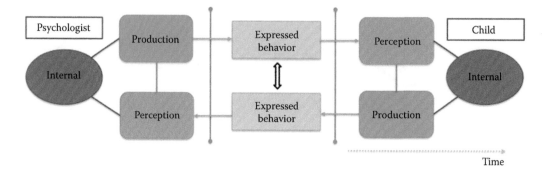

Figure 15.5 Visualization of dyadic interaction between a child and a psychologist: the internal states of the individuals (e.g., emotions, neurological conditions) are not observable, but expressed behaviors, which are linked through interaction, are observable.

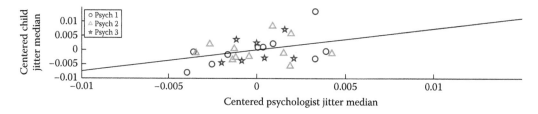

Figure 15.6 Coordination between paired child and psychologist jitter median, after controlling for individual psychologist jitter median.

the previously discussed prosodic elements, we found that the psychologist (when interacting with children with higher ASD severity) increased pausing, spoke more often, and used fewer assents and nonfluencies; all the while the child spoke less often, spoke slower, and responded later. Together, the conversational portrait becomes quite clear and indicates that the conversational quality degraded in those interactions.

Interestingly, we were able to better predict the child's symptom severity from the psychologist's acoustic–prosodic cues than from the child's own prosodic behavior (Bone et al. 2014a); this astounding finding highlights the importance of the psychologist's behavior in these interactions and even for translational applications. In addition, we used this classification framework to identify the most informative portions of the ADOS interaction (Bone et al. 2013).

Referring back to the vocal arousal measures of Figure 15.2 (Bone et al. 2014b), we used these time-continuous measures of affect to investigate child–psychologist synchrony (Bone et al. 2014c). We observed that children with higher ASD severity tended to lead the interaction (i.e., arousal dynamics) more, potentially because the children were not as responsive to the psychologist's affective cues. Thus, we were able to discover novel information about the interaction through the use of a signal-derived tool. Future BSP efforts should likely focus on creating more tools for discovery, or applying already available tools to ASD research. For instance, Lee et al. (2014) presented a measure of dyadic entrainment (synchrony) based on speech; the fully automatic, theory-based method correlated with positive and negative affect in couple's therapy interactions.

In the realm of ASD research, joint modeling of human–human interaction has previously focused on parent–child interaction. For example, Messinger et al. (2009) investigated synchrony of mother–infant facial expressions through windowed cross-correlation of smile intensity; a continuous index of smile intensity was formed based on automatically extracted smile strength and eye constriction (Duchenne smile). They reported that the individual streams were correlated over time for both infants and mothers, and "mutual repair and dissolution of affective synchrony" occurred based on temporal changes in dyadic smile activity. Franklin et al. (2014) compared infant vocalization patterns between interactive and noninteractive contexts. The researchers asserted that by 6 months of age infants have determined social value in their vocalizations, since they increased volubility during still face periods from their parents. Interaction-based research may support novel designs for ASD assessments and interventions, given the empirical support provided on the importance of clinician and caregiver actions.

15.2.6 Speech: Future directions and open challenges

Speech is an incredibly rich signal that not only communicates ostensible lexical information, but also is layered with mood, affect, and intention. Difficulties in processing audio remain, such as in robust ASR in noisy and novel domains, automatic speaker diarization or segmentation in real-world settings, and computational models of speech prosody. Each area has its own unique obstacles. Speech prosody, for example, can only be understood through appropriate modeling of context and through modeling the baseline of a speaker, which are both difficult to infer automatically. Also, speaker segmentation, even in commercially available devices, is often unreliable to use out-of-the-box. Still, since speech is so integral to human communication, quantitative behavioral signal-processing methods stand to teach us much about communication in general, and specifically those aspects that are impaired in ASD. Further research can aid in assessment as well as intervention, for which speech-based devices already exist.

15.3 Visual signal processing (facial expressions, eye tracking, gestures)

Facial expressions and gestures are informative behavioral units in social communication; understandably, production and perception deficits in these modalities are present in ASD. For example, individuals with ASD have been observed to perform worse in facial expression recognition tasks (Celani et al. 1999) and to have atypical brain responses to fearful versus neutral images (Dawson et al. 2004). This worthy research area is burgeoning with new computational applications that make use of visual sensors. Visual signal processing and pattern recognition include many domains that have relevance to ASD, such as facial and body recognition, motion, and tracking; action recognition; 3-D computer vision (e.g., Microsoft Kinect); medical image analysis; and egocentric (point-of-view) vision.

It is worth noting that standard video-based behavioral signal processing presently lacks the precision and reliability necessary to serve as a general-use tool for learning about complex human behavior. This visual signal processing can be sensitive to camera and subject position, occlusions, lighting changes, and recording quality; these confounding factors must be carefully controlled. Still, this is a promising research domain despite its challenges. Nevertheless, researchers are creating viable systems through the use of alternative visual sensors: wearable point-of-view cameras, facial motion capture, and Microsoft Kinect. Gesture processing is only beginning to be studied in ASD (e.g., Rehg et al. 2013), so our analysis will focus on facial processing.

15.3.1 Facial processing

In the study by Messinger et al. (2009), the researchers relied on automatic detection of smiles to create a scalable solution to the time-intensive task of annotation. The researchers used computer vision and machine learning on controlled lab-based video to create smile strength, eye constriction, and mouth-opening measurements.

More recently, Ye et al. (2015) developed a computer vision method for detecting bids for eye contact between toddlers and clinicians who were interacting as part of the Rapid ABC protocol. According to the authors, wearable point-of-view (POV) cameras are especially suited for detecting eye contact because they provide high-quality visual data with consistent frontal views of the face, high-resolution capture of the subject's eyes, and minimal occlusion. The method takes in an image sequences and output moments of eye contact. The proposed algorithm involves facial detection and head pose estimation, followed by temporal sequence modeling with condition random fields (CRFs). Training and evaluation were based on manual annotations of eye contact. While human raters were more reliable than the algorithm, the results support the plausible translation of this technique for clinical research and intervention evaluation; this is particularly impressive given the centrality of eye contact to ASD phenotypes.

Researchers at USC SAIL, collaborating with ASD clinical experts, are seeking to determine what evokes perceptions of awkwardness in the

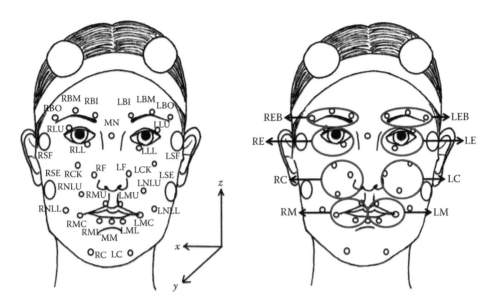

Figure 15.7 (a) Facial marker positions. (b) Divisions of markers into eight facial regions. (From Guha, T. et al. 2015. *IEEE Int. Conf. Acoustics, Speech Signal Process.* 40:803–7.)

facial expressions of children with ASD. Objective computational measures can provide higher precision measurements of minor facial movements, which, in turn, can lead to detailed tracking of facial dynamics that is comparable across subjects. Guha et al. (2015) analyzed the atypicality of emotional facial expressions of children with ASD in a mimicry task based on facial motion capture (MoCap; Figure 15.7). The authors employed methods from information theory, time-series modeling, and statistical analysis in their analysis; they reported that children with ASD exhibited lower complexity in facial dynamics, particularly in the eye region.

15.4 Physiological signal processing (heart rate and skin conductance)

Physiological signals can afford us new insights into behavior and complement the information provided from observable cues from audition and vision. Especially for individuals with autism, physiological signals can yield valuable feedback for social interactions, sensory reactivity, and emotional self-awareness (Picard 2009; Welch 2012). Our main focus in this section is the physiology related to the autonomous nervous system (ANS), which is captured through electrodermal activity (EDA) and electrocardiogram (ECG) signals. These signals have been widely studied in relation to ASD (Hirstein et al. 2001; Kushki et al. 2013). The ANS plays a regulatory role, helping the body maintain homeostasis

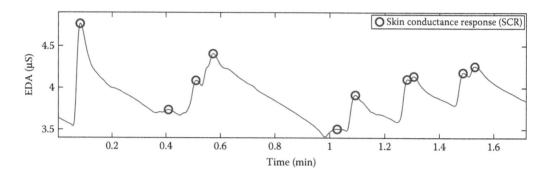

Figure 15.8 Example of electrodermal activity signal (EDA) with skin conductance responses (SCRs).

while adapting to internal and external demands. It consists of two inter-dependent branches: the sympathetic and the parasympathetic (Mendes 2009). Signals associated with the ANS may be recorded less obtrusively and over long periods of time compared to others, such as the electroen-cephalography (EEG) signal.

15.4.1 Signal fundamentals

EDA is one of the most frequently used psychophysiological signals. It is related to the sympathetic ANS activity that is responsible for the "fight-or-flight" responses and is measured through the changes in the levels of sweat on the skin. It has been related to memory, anxiety, attention, and other psychological constructs (Dawson et al. 2007; Boucsein 2012). EDA can be decomposed into a tonic and a phasic component. The for-mer depicts the signal's general trend and is called skin conductance level (SCL), while the latter reflects the short-term fluctuations superimposed onto the tonic part—referred to as skin conductance responses (SCRs; Figure 15.8). Traditional EDA measurements include the mean SCL and the frequency of SCR events computed over fixed time intervals.

ECG is the electrical signal produced by the activity of the heart and is relevant to various clinical factors and psychological processes (Berntson et al. 1997; Berntson and Cacioppo 2004). It comprises vari-ous facets—commonly referred as the P, Q, R, S, and T waves—that are created from the polarization and depolarization mechanisms of the heart. These points can serve to determine a variety of time-based ECG measures. Most commonly used are the interbeat interval (IBI; i.e., the time interval between two consecutive QRS complexes) and the heart-rate variability ([HRV]; depicting the variations in heart rate) measures.

15.4.2 Collecting physiological signals

Accurate and reliable data collection is a fundamental step toward infor-mative data analysis. Particularly for physiological signals, which tend to be noisy and affected by various external conditions (such as temperature, time of day, medication, etc.), it is important to be aware of the potentials and limitations of the various data capture configurations.

In-lab EDA measurements traditionally use silver–silver chloride electrodes placed on the thenar and hypothenar eminences of the palms or the solar surface of the medial or distal phalanges of the fingers (Dawson et al. 2007). Wet gel electrodes have also been widely used, since they can be disposable and more sensitive to skin conductance changes. On the other hand, this might lead to gel leakage and electrode detachment, especially during long-term recordings (Boucsein 2012). Recently, the focus has shifted to ambulatory EDA sensors that can record unobtrusively over long periods of time (Burns et al. 2010; Lee et al. 2010; Poh et al. 2010). These hold in terms of longitudinal monitoring of individuals outside the lab during their daily activities, but they also come with a wide set of challenges regarding electrode placement and data reliability (Van Dooren et al. 2012; Ranogajec and Geršak 2014).

ECG is recorded using electrodes positioned on the surface of the chest and the limb. Depending on the application of interest, several lead configurations have been proposed, the most well-known being the Einthoven triangle (Wasilewski and Lech 2012). Wireless devices have been also recently introduced for long-term unobtrusive ECG monitoring (Lucani et al. 2006; Lobodzinski and Laks 2012; Wang et al. 2015).

15.4.3 Physiological signal-processing techniques

Physiological signal processing typically includes detection of artifacts, denoising, and extraction of informative measures. EDA signals are usually affected by movement artifacts, drop-outs, and high-frequency noise (Dawson et al. 2007). Artifact detection in EDA has been performed using derivative-based and wavelet transform methods (Chellali and Hennig 2013; Jaimovich and Knapp 2015; Taylor et al. 2015). For the ECG signals, most common sources of noise include low-frequency, muscle, and electromagnetic interferences (Gacek 2012). Several ECG signal denoising techniques have been proposed that take advantage of wavelet transforms, fuzzy logic, or empirical mode decomposition (Kabir and Celia 2012; Joshi et al. 2013).

Previous studies have attempted fitting parameterized functions to explicitly quantify the shape of EDA (Lim et al. 1997), using inversion techniques to model the causal relation between the sudomotor activity and the resulting SCRs (Benedek and Kaernbach 2010; Bach et al. 2013), and designing parametric knowledge-driven dictionaries to find sparse approximations of EDA signals (Chaspari et al. 2015; Figure 15.9). A detailed review on EDA modeling methods can be found in Bach et al. (2011). Automatic SCR scoring is also possible with publicly available toolboxes, such as Ledalab (http://www.ledalab.de; Benedek and Kaernbach 2010) and SCRalyze (http://scralyze.sourceforge.net; Bach et al. 2013).

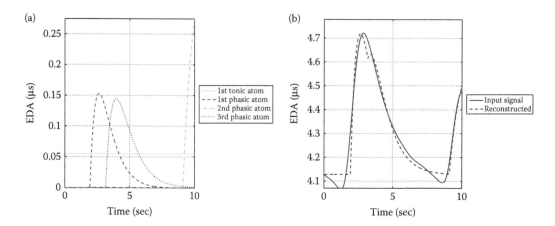

Figure 15.9 EDA representation scheme. (a) Input and reconstructed signal with solid blue and dashed red lines. (b) The dictionary atoms used to represent the EDA signal. The first tonic atom (solid cyan line) captures the *signal level*; the first and third phasic atoms (dashed magenta and dash-dotted green lines) capture the first SCR; and the second phasic atom (black dotted line) models the second SCR.

Automatic QRS detection has been performed using derivative (Pan and Tompkins 1985; Hamilton and Tompkins 1986), Hilbert-transform and phasor-transform (Martínez et al. 2000) based methods (Benitez et al. 2000). Recent studies have found that these algorithms are comparable in terms of performance, with the Hilbert-based one being slightly less accurate but more efficient for real-time applications (Arzeno et al. 2008). Another comparative study between the three approaches can be found in Álvarez et al. (2013). Various methods have also been proposed for HRV estimation, most commonly of which include time and spectral-based analysis. A complete review into QRS detection and HRV computation techniques can be found in Oweis and Tabbaa (2014). Publicly available ECG processing toolboxes include the BioSig (http://biosig.sourceforge.net), the PhysioToolkit (http://physionet.org/physiotools/; Goldberger et al. 2000), and the ECG-kit (http://marianux.github.io/ecg-kit/).

15.4.4 Behavioral signal processing for physiological data

Autism is often characterized through deficits in social interaction and communication. Monitoring the internal affect of individuals with ASD can provide better insight about observable behavior and the nature of their interactions (Picard 2009; Welch 2012). Several studies have proposed the use of physiological sensors for monitoring the affective state focused on providing objective feedback of arousal indices to therapists and caregivers and assisting ASD individuals toward better understanding and communicating their emotions.

Physiological signals are frequently related to stress and anxiety, which are of particular interest in the case of autism (Hirstein et al. 2001; Welch 2012). Various studies have discussed continuous monitoring of such affective cues in order to provide real-time feedback in therapy and intervention. Herman et al. (2012) discussed the effect of several activities from an occupational therapy session on a child's EDA state. Chaspari et al. (2014) modeled the occurrence of SCRs during therapy sessions in relation to regulatory behaviors from the child and the interacting psychologist, in an effort to assess therapeutic change and quantify effective child–therapist interaction (Figure 15.10). Hernandez et al. (2014) sought to automatically identify children's engagement levels from EDA-derived features with the aim to assess interactive synchrony and social coordination. Other studies have focused on sensing affect during human–computer and human–robot interactions in the context of ASD (Liu et al. 2008; Chaspari et al. 2013; Figure 15.11). Finally, Cermak et al. (2015) incorporated biosensors into an adaptive dental environment to quantify its comforting effects for children with ASD.

Beyond sensing affect in interactions, physiological sensors can further help individuals with ASD to better understand and express emotions. Saadatzi et al. (2013) developed an affect-sensitive feedback system using a robot to teach social media skills. Bekele et al. (2013) used a virtual reality emotional expression presentation system to explore new teaching paradigms related to emotion identification. Leite et al. (2013) examined the variation of physiological patterns with respect to different supportive behaviors elicited by a robot and their association to a users' subjective experience. Finally, CaptureMyEmotion is a mobile application designed to help children with Autism identify and express their emotions by relating the contextual information of audio, videos, and photos imported by the user to recorded arousal levels (Leijdekkers et al. 2013).

Signal-processing technologies can provide unique opportunities for analyzing and interpreting physiological data in relation to affective states.

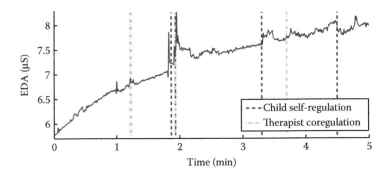

Figure 15.10 EDA plotted with child and therapist regulation events during a therapy session. (From Chaspari, T. et al. 2014. *IEEE Int. Conf. Acoustics, Speech Signal Process.* 39:1611–5.)

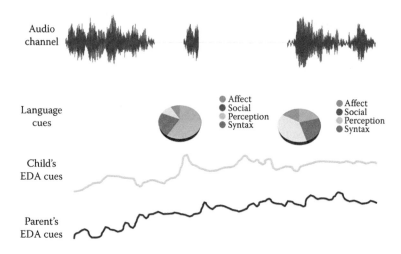

Figure 15.11 Modeling verbal response latencies of children with ASD using physiology and language cues during child–parent–computer interactions. (From Chaspari, T. et al. 2013. *IEEE Int. Conf. Acoust., Speech Signal Process.* 38:3702–6.)

Physiological measures can help caregivers and therapists to better understand and more effectively support individuals with ASD, as well as aiding self-awareness and self-manipulation of emotions. These measures can also provide valuable data to the research community in order to more effectively explore and address questions related to ASD. However, it is important to be aware of limitations of physiological data capture mechanisms and signal-processing technologies; researchers need to develop noise-robust, easily interpretable, and individualized physiological indices. The latter also relates to appropriate physiological baseline methodologies. Last, another important research domain is the translation of data analysis techniques to accessible user-friendly applications.

15.5 Meta-data processing with machine learning

The field is currently overwhelmed with various behavioral modeling tools that rely on qualitative behavioral observation for diagnosis and intervention (i.e., ADOS, ADI, SRS, BOSC-C, CGI, etc.), all of which contain partial information about the child. This behavioral battery is sure to continue to grow with new and more precise behavioral measures, including those computed objectively through signal data. In a diagnostic protocol, clinicians typically perform a subset of instrumental assessments selected depending on time, clinical training, and monetary constraints; then the clinician pools all available information to make a best-estimate clinical (BEC) decision. But to what degree do clinicians within sites or across sites perform this informational aggregation (i.e., different instruments and personal observation) the same? Do experienced clinicians rely more on their own observations and opinions and rely less on a standardized instrument's thresholds? These are areas in which machine learning is primed for translational application. The role of machine learning becomes even more important when considering new behavioral measures that can be generated through direct signal-based methods; for example, some measures may only hold value for specific sub-populations with ASD, and these algorithms can make such deductions.

Machine learning offers objective methods to optimize a given objective function. Many machine-learning methods are based on traditional statistical techniques, but old techniques have been generalized and new ones created to handle a diverse set of problems. Take, for example, the case of designing an algorithm and setting thresholds for a standardized instrument like the ADOS. Previously, this has been accomplished with correlational-based statistical analysis and some hand-selected design based on domain expertise. However, if we have expert best estimates made, independent of the ADOS algorithm, then we can potentially use machine learning to optimize exactly the function of interest; specifically, a researcher may want to optimize sensitivity and specificity jointly, but with slightly higher weight on sensitivity. Computational methods can even estimate how well a result will generalize, and is not simply "fitting" the observed data.

Machine learning has numerous methods that work robustly with high-dimensional ("big") data. But alongside this tremendous promise come potential troubles. We have previously discussed at length the potential pitfalls that certain studies have succumbed to in both the conceptual framework (i.e., lack of instrument knowledge) and technical framework (i.e., inappropriate practices with machine learning); such concerns are critical in this domain since translational applications may affect many thousands of lives (Bone et al. 2015b). More recently, we have concentrated on the promise of machine learning for developing more effective and efficient diagnostic algorithms for the ADI–R and the SRS, as well the potential gains from fusion (Bone et al. 2015c). While machine learning is gaining appeal, it remains an underutilized, powerful tool for aiding modeling of this heterogeneous disorder.

15.6 Conclusion

ASD research is at an exciting epoch, with researchers from diverse fields intimately working together toward understanding and treating this complex disorder. Novel advances in signal processing and devices that measure human behavior stand to contribute to this collaborative effort by creating objective, dimensional metrics that are sensitive to behavior change. Moreover, machine learning is a powerful tool with emerging domain applications; it can be used for fusing information from multiple behavioral signals, or even directly applied to instrument design. There is great potential for behavioral sensing to have a profound translational impact.

References

Abrahams, B. S. and D. H. Geschwind. 2010. Connecting genes to brain in the autism spectrum disorders. *Arch. Neurol.* 67:395–9.

Álvarez, R. A., A. J. M. Penín, and X. Antón Vila Sobrino. 2013. A comparison of three QRS detection algorithms over a public database. *Procedia Technol.* 9:1159–65.

Arzeno, N. M., Deng, Zhi-De, and Poon, Chi-Sang. 2008. Analysis of first-derivative based QRS detection algorithms. *IEEE Trans. Biomed. Eng.* 55:478–84.

Bach, D. R., J. Daunizeau, N. Kuelzow, K. J. Friston, and R. J. Dolan. 2011. Dynamic causal modeling of spontaneous fluctuations in skin conductance. *Psychophysiology* 48:252–7.

Bach, D. R., K. J. Friston, and R. J. Dolan. 2013. An improved algorithm for model-based analysis of evoked skin conductance responses. *Biol. Psychol.* 94:490–7.

Baltaxe, C., J. Q. Simmons, and E. Zee. 1984. Intonation patterns in normal, autistic and aphasic children. *Proc. Int. Congr. Phonetic Sci.* 10:713–8.

Baron-Cohen, S., A. M. Leslie, and U. Frith. 1985. Does the autistic child have a 'theory of mind'? *Cognition* 21:37–46.

Bekele, E., Z. Zhi, S. Amy, C. Julie, W. Zachary, and S. Nilanjan. 2013. Understanding how adolescents with autism respond to facial expressions in virtual reality environments. *IEEE Trans. Visual. Comput. Graph.* 19:711–20.

Benedek, M. and C. Kaernbach. 2010. Decomposition of skin conductance data by means of nonnegative deconvolution. *Psychophysiology* 47:647–58.

Benitez, D. S., P. A. Gaydecki, A. Zaidi, and A. P. Fitzpatrick. 2000. A new QRS detection algorithm based on the Hilbert transform. *Comput. Cardiol.* 27:379–82.

Bentler, R. A., Y. H. Wu, J. B. Tomblin, and M. P. Moeller. 2010. Acoustic considerations in LENA protocols. *First LENA Users Conference.* Denver, CO, April.

Berntson, G. G., J. T. Bigger, D. L. Eckberg et al. 1997. Heart rate variability: Origins, methods, and interpretive caveats. *Psychophysiology* 34:623–48.

Berntson, G. G. and J. T. Cacioppo. 2004. Heart rate variability: Stress and psychiatric conditions. In *Dynamic Electrocardiography*, eds. M. Malik and A. J. Camm, 57–64. New York: Wiley.

Black, M., D. Bone, M. E. Williams, P. Gorrindo, P. Levitt, and S. S. Narayanan. 2011. The USC CARE Corpus: Child-psychologist interactions of children with autism spectrum disorders. *Proceedings of INTERSPEECH* 1497–1500.

Bone, D., M. P. Black, C.-C. Lee, M. E. Williams, P. Levitt, S. Lee, and S. Narayanan. 2012. Spontaneous-speech acoustic-prosodic features of children with autism and the interacting psychologist. *Proc. Interspeech* 13:1043–6.

Bone, D., M. P. Black, A. Ramakrishna, R. B. Grossman, and S. Narayanan. 2015a. Acoustic-prosodic correlates of "awkward" prosody in story retellings from adolescents with autism. *Proc. Interspeech* 16:1616–20.

Bone, D., S. Bishop, M. P. Black, C. Lord, and S. Narayanan. 2016. Use of machine learning to improve autism screening and diagnostic instruments: Effectiveness, efficiency, and multi-instrument fusion. *J. Child Psychol. Psychiatry* 57(8):927–37.

Bone, D., M. S. Goodwin, M. P. Black, C.-C. Lee, K. Audhkhasi, and S. Narayanan. 2015b. Applying machine learning to facilitate autism diagnostics: Pitfalls and promises. *J. Autism Dev. Disord.* 45:1121–36.

Bone, D., C.-C. Lee, M. P. Black, M. E. Williams, S. Lee, P. Levitt, and S. Narayanan. 2014a. The psychologist as an interlocutor in autism spectrum disorder assessment: Insights from a study of spontaneous prosody. *J. Speech, Language, Hearing Res.* 57:1162–77.

Bone, D., C.-C. Lee, T. Chaspari, M. P. Black, M. E. Williams, S. Lee, P. Levitt, and S. Narayanan. 2013. Acoustic-prosodic, turn-taking, and language cues in child-psychologist interactions for varying social demand. *Proc. Interspeech* 14:2400–4.

Bone, D., C.-C. Lee, and S. Narayanan. 2014b. Robust unsupervised arousal rating: A rule-based framework with knowledge-inspired vocal features. *IEEE Trans. Affective Comput.* 5:201–13.

Bone, D., C.-C. Lee, A. Potamianos, and S. Narayanan. 2014c. An investigation of vocal arousal dynamics in child-psychologist interactions using synchrony measures and a conversation-based model. *Proc. Interspeech* 15:218–22.

Boucsein, W. 2012. *Electrodermal Activity.* New York: Springer Science & Business Media.

Burns, A., B. R. Greene, M. J. McGrath, T. J. O'Shea, B. Kuris, S. M. Ayer, F. Stroiescu, and V. Cionca. 2010. SHIMMER™—A wireless sensor platform for noninvasive biomedical research. *IEEE Sensors J.* 10:1527–34.

Busso, C., Z. Deng, S. Yildirim, M. Bulut, C. M. Lee, A. Kazemzadeh, S. Lee, U. Neumann, and S. Narayanan. 2004. Analysis of emotion recognition using facial expressions, speech and multimodal information. *Proc. Int. Conf. Multimodal Interfaces* 6:205–11.

Celani, G., M. W. Battacchi, and L. Arcidiacono. 1999. The understanding of the emotional meaning of facial expressions in people with autism. *J. Autism Dev. Disord.* 29:57–66.

Cermak, S. A., L. I. Stein Duker, M. E. Williams, M. E. Dawson, C. J. Lane, and J. C. Polido. 2015. Sensory adapted dental environments to enhance oral care for children with autism spectrum disorders: A randomized controlled pilot study. *J. Autism Dev. Disord.* 45:2876–88.

Chaspari, T., D. Bone, J. Gibson, C.-C. Lee, and S. Narayanan. 2013. Using physiology and language cues for modeling verbal response latencies of children with ASD. *IEEE Int. Conf. Acoust., Speech Signal Process.* 38:3702–6.

Chaspari, T., M. Goodwin, O. Wilder-Smith, A. Gulsrud, C. Mucchetti, C. Kasari, and S. Narayanan. 2014. A non-homogeneous Poisson process model of skin conductance responses integrated with observed regulatory behaviors for Autism intervention. *IEEE Int. Conf. Acoustics, Speech Signal Process.* 39:1611–5.

Chaspari, T., A. Tsiartas, L. Stein, S. Cermak, and S. S. Narayanan. 2015. Sparse representation of electrodermal activity with knowledge-driven dictionaries. *IEEE Trans. Biomed. Eng.* 62:960–71.

Chellali, R. and S. Hennig. 2013. Is it time to rethink motion artifacts? Temporal relationships between electrodermal activity and body movements in real-life conditions. *Humaine Assoc. Conf. Affect. Comput. Intell. Interaction* 5:330–5.

Dawson, G., S. J. Webb, L. Carver, H. Panagiotides, and J. McPartland. 2004. Young children with autism show atypical brain responses to fearful versus neutral facial expressions of emotion. *Dev. Sci.* 7:340–59.

Dawson, M. E., A. M. Schell, and D. L. Filion. 2007. The electrodermal system. In *Handbook of Psychophysiology*, 3rd ed., eds. J. T. Cacioppo, L. G. Tassinary, and G. Berntson, 157–581. Cambridge: Cambridge University Press.

Diehl, J. J., D. Watson, L. Bennetto, J. Mcdonough, and C. Gunlogson. 2009. An acoustic analysis of prosody in high-functioning autism. *Appl. Psycholinguist* 30:385–404.

Franco, J. H., R. L. Lang, M. F. O'Reilly, J. M. Chan, J. Sigafoos, and M. Rispoli. 2009. Functional analysis and treatment of inappropriate vocalizations using a speech-generating device for a child with autism. *Focus Autism Other Dev. Disabilities* 24:146–55.

Franklin, B., A. S. Warlaumont, D. Messinger, E. Bene, S. Nathani Iyer, C.-C. Lee, B. Lambert, and D. K. Oller. 2014. Effects of parental interaction on infant vocalization rate, variability and vocal type. *Language Learning Dev.* 10:279–96.

Gacek, A. 2012. An introduction to ECG signal processing and analysis. In *ECG Signal Processing, Classification and Interpretation*, eds. A. Gacek and W. Pedrycz, 21–46. London: Springer.

Goldberger, A. L., L. A. N. Amaral, L. Glass, J. M. Hausdorff, P. Ch. Ivanov, R. G. Mark, J. E. Mietus, G. B. Moody, C.-K. Peng, and H. E. Stanley. 2000. Physiobank, physiotoolkit, and physionet components of a new research resource for complex physiologic signals. *Circulation* 101:e215–20.

Goodwin, M. S. 2008. *Telemetric Assessment of Stereotypical Motor Movements in Children with Autism Spectrum Disorder.* Kingston: University of Rhode Island. http://digitalcommons.uri.edu/dissertations/AAI3314456

Goodwin, M. S., J. Groden, W. F. Velicer, L. P. Lipsitt, M. G. Baron, S. G. Hofmann, and G. Groden. 2006. Cardiovascular arousal in individuals with autism. *Focus Autism Other Dev. Disabilities* 21:100–23.

Grossman, R. B., L. R. Edelson, and H. Tager-Flusberg. 2013. Emotional facial and vocal expressions during story retelling by children and adolescents with high-functioning autism. *J. Speech, Language, Hearing Res.* 56:1035–44.

Guha, T., Z. Yang, A. Ramakrishna, R. B. Grossman, D. Hedley, S. Lee, and S. S. Narayanan. 2015. On quantifying facial expression-related atypicality of children with autism spectrum disorder. *IEEE Int. Conf. Acoustics, Speech Signal Process.* 40:803–7.

Hamilton, P. S. and W. J. Tompkins. 1986. Quantitative investigation of QRS detection rules using the MIT/BIH arrhythmia database. *IEEE Trans. Biomed. Eng.* 12:1157–65.

Hedman, E., L. Miller, S. Schoen, D. Nielsen, M. Goodwin, and R. W. Picard. 2012. Measuring autonomic arousal during therapy. *Proc. Int. Design Emotion Conf.* 8:11–4.

Heeman, P. A., R. Lunsford, E. Selfridge, L. Black, and J. Van Santen. 2010. Autism and interactional aspects of dialogue. *In Proceedings of the Special Interest Group on Discourse and Dialogue* 249–252.

Hernandez, J., I. Riobo, A. Rozga, G. D. Abowd, and R. W. Picard. 2014. Using electrodermal activity to recognize ease of engagement in children during social interactions. *ACM Int. Joint Conf. Pervasive Ubiquitous Comput.* 16:307–17.

Hirstein, W., P. Iversen, and V. S. Ramachandran. Autonomic responses of autistic children to people and objects. 2001. *Proc. Royal Soc. London B: Biol. Sci.* 268:1883–8.

Jaimovich, J. and R. B. Knapp. 2015. Creating biosignal algorithms for musical applications from an extensive physiological database. *Proceedings of the 2015 Conference on New Interfaces for Musical Expression* Baton Rouge, LA. 15:1–4.

Joshi, S. L., R. A. Vatti, and R. V. Tornekar. 2013. A survey on ECG signal denoising techniques. *Int. Conf. Commun. Systems Network Technol.* 2013:60–4.

Kabir, M.d. A. and C. Shahnaz. 2012. Denoising of ECG signals based on noise reduction algorithms in EMD and wavelet domains. *Biomed. Signal Process. Control* 7:481–9.

Kushki, A., E. Drumm, M. P. Mobarak, N. Tanel, A. Dupuis, T. Chau, and E. Anagnostou. 2013. Investigating the autonomic nervous system response to anxiety in children with autism spectrum disorders. *PLoS One* 8:e59730.

Lee, C.-C., A. Katsamanis, M. P. Black, B. R. Baucom, A. Christensen, P. G. Georgiou, and S. S. Narayanan. 2014. Computing vocal entrainment: A signal-derived PCA-based quantification scheme with application to affect analysis in married couple interactions. *Comput. Speech Lang.* 28:518–39.

Lee, C. C., Mower, E., Busso, C., Lee, S., and Narayanan, S. 2011. Emotion recognition using a hierarchical binary decision tree approach. *Speech Communication* 53(9):1162–1171.

Lee, C. M. and S. S. Narayanan. 2005. Toward detecting emotions in spoken dialogs. *IEEE transactions on speech and audio processing* 13(2):293–303.

Lee, C. M., S. Narayanan, and R. Pieraccini. 2001. Recognition of negative emotions from the speech signal. *Proceedings of the IEEE Workshop on Automatic Speech Recognition and Understanding* 240–243.

Lee, S., A. Potamianos, and S. Narayanan. 1999. Acoustics of children's speech: Developmental changes of temporal and spectral parameters. *The Journal of the Acoustical Society of America* 105(3):1455–1468.

Lee, Y., B. Lee, and M. Lee. 2010. Wearable sensor glove based on conducting fabric using electrodermal activity and pulse-wave sensors for e-health application. *Telemed. e-Health* 16:209–17.

Leijdekkers, P., V. Gay, and F. Wong. 2013. CaptureMyEmotion: A mobile app to improve emotion learning for autistic children using sensors. *Int. Symp. Comput. Based Med. Systems* 26:381–4.

Leite, I., R. Henriques, C. Martinho, and A. Paiva. 2013. Sensors in the wild: Exploring electrodermal activity in child-robot interaction. *Proc. ACM/IEEE Int. Conf. Human-Robot Interaction* 2013:41–8.

Lim, C. L., C. Rennie, R. J. Barry, H. Bahramali, I. Lazzaro, B. Manor, and E. Gordon. 1997. Decomposing skin conductance into tonic and phasic components. *Int. J. Psychophysiol.* 25:97–109.

Liu, C., K. Conn, N. Sarkar, and W. Stone. 2008. Online affect detection and robot behavior adaptation for intervention of children with autism. *IEEE Trans. Robot.* 24:883–96.

Lobodzinski, S. S. and M. M. Laks. 2012. New devices for very long-term ECG monitoring. *Cardiol. J.* 19:210–4.

Lord, C. and R. M. Jones. 2012. Annual research review: Re-thinking the classification of autism spectrum disorders. *J. Child Psychol. Psychiatry* 53:490–509.

Lord, C., S. Risi, L. Lambrecht, E. H. Cook Jr, B. L. Leventhal, P. C. DiLavore, A. Pickles, and M. Rutter. 2000. The Autism Diagnostic Observation Schedule—Generic: A standard measure of social and communication deficits associated with the spectrum of autism. *J. Autism Dev. Disord.* 30:205–23.

Lucani, D., G. Cataldo, J. Cruz, G. Villegas, and S. Wong. 2006. A portable ECG monitoring device with Bluetooth and Holter capabilities for telemedicine applications. *Int. Conf. IEEE Eng. Med. Biol. Soc.* 28:5244–7.

Martínez, A., R. Alcaraz, and J. Joaquín Rieta. 2010. Application of the phasor transform for automatic delineation of single-lead ECG fiducial points. *Physiol. Meas.* 31:1467–85.

McCann, J. and S. Peppé. 2003. Prosody in autism spectrum disorders: A critical review. *Int. J. Lang. Commun. Disord.* 38:325–50.

Mendes, W. B. 2009. Assessing autonomic nervous system activity. In *Methods in Social Neuroscience*, eds. E. Harmon-Jones and J. S. Beer, 118–47. New York: Guilford Press.

Messinger, D. S., M. H. Mahoor, S.-M. Chow, and J. F. Cohn. 2009. Automated measurement of facial expression in infant–mother interaction: A pilot study. *Infancy* 14:285–305.

Mower, E., M. P. Black, E. Flores, M. Williams, and S. Narayanan. 2011. Rachel: Design of an emotionally targeted interactive agent for children with autism. *IEEE Int. Conf. Multimedia Expo* 2011:1–6.

Narayanan, S. and P. G. Georgiou. 2013. Behavioral signal processing: Deriving human behavioral informatics from speech and language. *Proc. IEEE* 101:1203–33.

Oweis, R. J. and B. O. Al-Tabbaa. 2014. QRS detection and heart rate variability analysis: A survey. *Biomed. Sci. Eng.* 2:13–34.

Pan, J. and W. J. Tompkins. 1985. A real-time QRS detection algorithm. *IEEE Trans. Biomed. Eng.* 3:230–236.

Paul, R., A. Augustyn, A. Klin, and F. R. Volkmar. 2005. Perception and production of prosody by speakers with autism spectrum disorders. *J. Autism Dev. Disord.* 35:205–20.

Peppé, S., J. McCann, F. Gibbon, A. O'Hare, and M. Rutherford. 2007. Receptive and expressive prosodic ability in children with high-functioning autism. *J. Speech, Language, Hearing Res.* 50(4):1015–28.

Picard, R. W. 2009. Future affective technology for autism and emotion communication. *Philos. Trans. Royal Soc. B: Biol. Sci.* 364:3575–84.

Poh, M.Z., N. C. Swenson, and R. W. Picard. 2010. A wearable sensor for unobtrusive, long-term assessment of electrodermal activity. *IEEE Trans. Biomed. Eng.* 57:1243–52.

Pronovost, W., M. P. Wakstein, and D. J. Wakstein. 1966. A longitudinal study of the speech behavior and language comprehension of fourteen children diagnosed atypical or autistic. *Exceptional Children* 33:19–26.

Ranogajec, S. and G. Geršak. 2014. Measuring site dependency when measuring skin conductance. *Int. Electrotechn. Comput. Sci. Conf.* 23:155–8.

Rehg, J. M., G. D. Abowd, A. Rozga, M. Romero, M. Clements, S. Sclaroff, I. Essa et al. 2013. Decoding children's social behavior. *IEEE Conf. Comput. Vision Pattern Recogn.* 2013:3414–21.

Saadatzi, M. N., K. N. Welch, R. Pennington, and J. Graham. 2013. Towards an affective computing feedback system to benefit underserved individuals: An example teaching social media skills. In *Universal Access in Human-Computer Interaction: User and Context Diversity*, eds. C. Stephanidis and M. Antona, 504–13. Berlin: Springer.

Schuller, B., E. Marchi, S. Baron-Cohen, H. O'Reilly, D. Pigat, P. Robinson, and I. Daves. 2014. The state of play of ASC-Inclusion: An integrated Internet-based environment for social inclusion of children with autism spectrum conditions. arXiv preprint arXiv:1403.5912.

Shriberg, L. D., J. Kwiatkowski, C. Rasmussen, G. L. Lof, and J. F. Miller. 1992. *The Prosody-Voice Screening Profile (PVSP): Psychometric Data and Reference Information for Children*. Phonology Project technical report no. 1. Madison: Waisman Center.

Shriberg, L. D., R. Paul, J. L. McSweeny, A. Klin, D. J. Cohen, and F. R. Volkmar. 2001. Speech and prosody characteristics of adolescents and adults with high-functioning autism and Asperger syndrome. *J. Speech, Language, Hearing Res.* 44:1097–115.

Shriberg, L. D., R. Paul, L. M. Black, and J. P. Van Santen. 2011. The hypothesis of apraxia of speech in children with autism spectrum disorder. *J. Autism Dev. Disord.* 41:405–26.

Taylor, S., N. Jaques, W. Chen, S. Fedor, A. Sano, and R. Picard. 2015. Automatic identification of artifacts in electrodermal activity data. *Int. Conf. IEEE Eng. Med. Biol. Soc.* 37:1934–7.

Van Dooren, M. and J. H. Janssen. 2012. Emotional sweating across the body: Comparing 16 different skin conductance measurement locations. *Physiol. Behav.* 106:298–304.

Van Santen, J. P.H, E. T. Prud'hommeaux, L. M. Black, and M. Mitchell. 2010. Computational prosodic markers for autism. *Autism* 14:215–36.

Wang, Y., S. Doleschel, R. Wunderlich, and S. Heinen. 2015. A wearable wireless ECG monitoring system with dynamic transmission power control for long-term homecare. *J. Med. Systems* 39:35.

Warren, S. F., J. Gilkerson, J. A. Richards, D. K. Oller, D. Xu, U. Yapanel, and S. Gray. 2010. What automated vocal analysis reveals about the vocal production and language learning environment of young children with autism. *J. Autism Dev. Disord.* 40:555–69.

Wasilewski, J. and L. Poloński. 2012. An introduction to ECG interpretation. In *ECG Signal Processing, Classification and Interpretation*, eds. A. Gacek and W. Pedrycz, 1–20. London: Springer.

Welch, K. C.. 2012. Physiological signals of autistic children can be useful. *IEEE Instrum. Meas. Mag.* 15:28–32.

Ye, Z., Y. Li, Y. Liu, C. Bridges, A. Rozga, and J. M. Rehg. 2015. Detecting bids for eye contact using a wearable camera. *IEEE Int. Conf. Workshops Automatic Face Gesture Recogn.* 11. doi: 10.1109/FG.2015.7163095.

Chapter 16 Behavior Imaging®
Innovative technology to enable remote autism diagnosis

N. Nazneen, Agata Rozga,
Gregory D. Abowd,
Christopher J. Smith,
Ron Oberleitner,
Rosa I. Arriaga, and
Jasjit S. Suri

Contents

Abstract 345
16.1 Introduction 346
16.2 Naturalistic Observation Diagnostic Assessment. 346
    16.2.1 NODA SmartCapture 347
    16.2.2 NODA Connect. 347
16.3 In-field evaluation 350
16.4 Proposed workflow model for field adoption 352
Acknowledgments 352
References 353

Abstract

This chapter presents a behavior imaging solution, NODA® (Naturalistic Observation Diagnostic Assessment), which supports remote diagnosis of autism using in-home videos. The design of the system is informed by a series of studies conducted with parents and clinicians of children with autism. A pilot feasibility study in the field demonstrates that the system allows:

1. Parents to easily record in-home video evidence of their child's behavior that are clinically useful for conducting an autism diagnosis.

2. Diagnosticians to complete a diagnostic assessment for autism consistent with diagnosis in the child's medical record, and to do so with a high level of confidence.

16.1 Introduction

The best-practice guidelines for diagnosing conditions like autism suggest that direct observation of the child in the natural environment, such as the home or school, is optimal to obtain an accurate and comprehensive assessment of a child's behavior (Siegel 2008; Matson 2011; McLeod et al. 2013) but in practice it is mostly limited to direct observation in clinics. Another key obstacle with respect to autism diagnosis is that there is significant time lag of about 20–60 months between the age at which parents first become concerned about their child's development and the age at which the child finally gets a diagnosis (Howlin and Asgharian 1999; Sivberg 2003; Wiggins et al. 2006). Lower socioeconomic status (SES) communities and rural areas have lack of access to autism-specific services, whereas in urban areas the long waiting lists at autism centers and clinics hinder timely diagnosis. Delay in diagnosis leads to delay in early intervention and hence, could impact a child's future learning capabilities and developmental outcomes (McEachin et al. 1993; Siegel 2008; Matson 2011; Rattazzi 2014). We posit that a telehealth behavior imaging solution can connect parents and clinicians to enable timely remote diagnostic assessment of autism based on naturalistic evidence of behaviors. NODA is a novel behavior imaging solution which supports remote diagnosis of autism using in-home videos (Nazneen et al. 2015). In this chapter, we present the design of NODA and summarize results from an in-field feasibility study. We conclude this chapter with a proposed potential model for large-scale field adoption of NODA.

16.2 Naturalistic Observation Diagnostic Assessment

NODA implementation consists of:

1. NODA SmartCapture: A smartphone-based application for parents to easily record clinically valid in-home behavior evidence of their child as per given prescription, and
2. NODA Connect: HIPAA-conforming Web portal for diagnosticians to guide in-home evidence collection process and to conduct remote diagnostic assessment for autism using in-home videos, brief developmental history, and their clinical judgment.

NODA was designed through an iterative design process. The initial prototype was informed by feedback from interviews conducted with 11 clinicians and 6 parents of children with autism as well as our previous research (Smith et al. 2009; Nazneen et al. 2010). Initial design of NODA SmartCapture was iteratively revised based on experience of families of children with autism using it in a controlled home-like setting (Kidd et al. 1999). Whereas, NODA Connect was iteratively revised through a participatory design process involving a collaborating diagnostician with more than 20 years of experience in autism diagnosis and an autism domain expert.

16.2.1 NODA SmartCapture

NODA SmartCapture is a smartphone-based application for parents to easily record clinically valid in-home behavior evidence of their child as per given prescription. See Figure 16.1 for selected screenshots of NODA SmartCapture. It guides parents to record and upload four 10-min NODA scenarios. These scenarios were chosen based on our previous research on video-based diagnostic assessment of autism (Smith et al. 2009). NODA scenarios include the child playing alone, the child playing with a peer, a family mealtime, and any behavior that is of concern to the parent.

One prime design goal was that NODA SmartCapture should be simple and visual so parents can easily use it. The other major design goal was that NODA SmartCapture should enable parents to collect video evidence that are clinically meaningful and useful for diagnosis of autism. Therefore, for each scenario, exact recording instructions for parents about how to stage the recordings (e.g., "Make sure the child's face is facing the camera," "relevant toy(s) and the person the child is interacting with is in the field of view") and how to structure the interaction (social presses e.g., "call the child's name and see if child responds") along with a sample video (BehaviorConnect 2014a–d) were embedded as a prescription within NODA SmartCapture. The collaborating diagnostician and autism domain expert finalized these instructions and sample videos after analyzing videos recorded by parents in the controlled home-like setting.

16.2.2 NODA Connect

NODA Connect is a HIPAA-compliant Web portal for diagnosticians to conduct a remote diagnostic assessment based on parent-collected in-home videos, a brief developmental history and their clinical judgment. Through NODA Connect the diagnostician can view uploaded videos and if required can send notifications to parents with specific recording instructions (Figure 16.2). For example, the diagnostician can ask parents to rerecord "play alone" scenario while holding a toy away in order to assess how child requests.

Once diagnosticians receive some or all videos as per given prescription, they can start tagging them with behaviors relevant to diagnosing autism

347

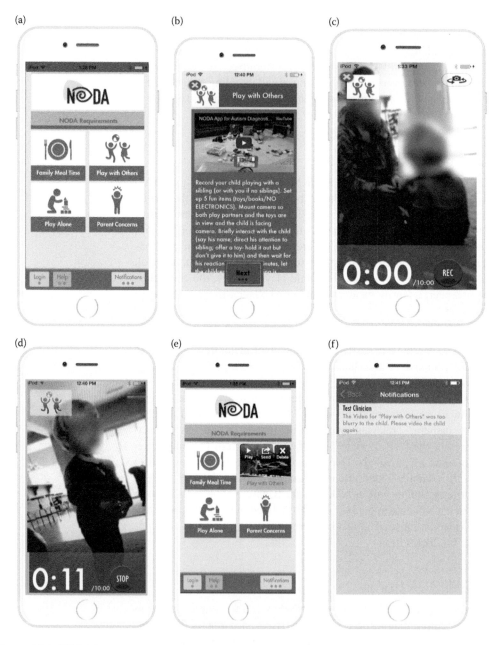

Figure 16.1 NODA SmartCapture. (a) The home screen has four NODA scenarios. (b) Each scenario has an embedded prescription including a sample video and recording instructions. Pressing "Next" proceeds to recording interface. (c) Recording mode has a clear time elapsed status, progress bar, and a green boundry reinforcing recording mode. (d) Recording can be stopped any time or will auto-stop after 10 min. (e) Home screen showing NODA scenarios and a completed recording to view video and either upload it or delete a not yet uploaded video. (f) Notifications for parents from diagnosticians.

(a)

(b)

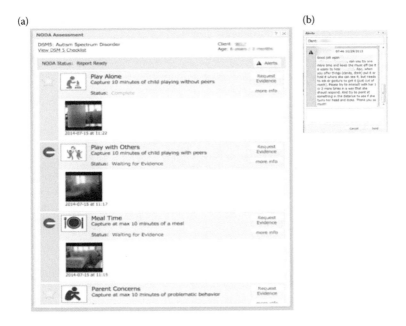

Figure 16.2 NODA Connect: For the selected family, the diagnostician can view videos uploaded by families (a) and if required can send notifications to parents (b) with specific recording instructions.

(Figure 16.3). NODA Connect has a predefined list of tags as behavior markers, for example, no eye contact, no facial expression. These tags were extracted from the standard autism diagnostic criteria known as *Diagnostic and Statistical Manual of Mental Disorders* (DSM-V, American Psychiatric Association 2013). The list of tags was compiled by the collaborating diagnosticians and an autism domain expert, and

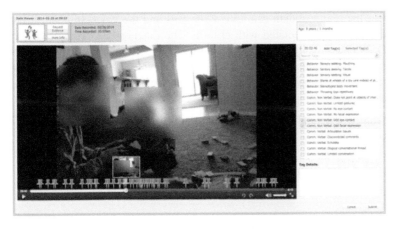

Figure 16.3 NODA Connect: During video observation when a specific behavior is noticed, the diagnostician can pause the video and add a suitable tag(s) from the predefined list.

349

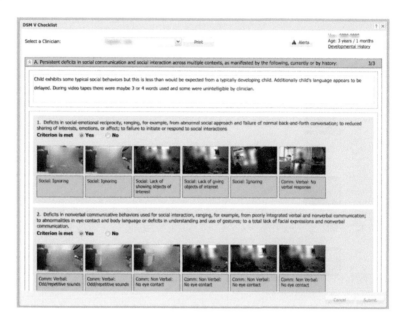

Figure 16.4 NODA Connect: Each tag inserted into a video is automatically linked by the system to the associated DSM-V criteria. During review of the DSM-V checklist, the diagnostician reviews the tags and decides if a criterion has been met or not.

was reviewed by an additional clinical expert. In total there were 66 tags in NODA Connect including both typical behavior tags (representing typical development) as well as atypical behavior tags (representing atypical development).

Each tag inserted into a video is automatically linked by the system to the associated DSM-V criteria. During review of the DSM-V checklist, the diagnostician can review the tags and the video snippet of the assigned tag associated with criteria. The diagnostician completes the DSM checklist by indicating whether each individual criterion has been met or not (Figure 16.4). NODA Connect provides diagnosticians access to the child's brief developmental history provided by parents by filling an online form during in-home video collection.

Finally, a diagnostic report is generated that summarizes the evidence supporting each DSM criterion and the diagnostician's clinical judgment. The report can be shared with the parent and the referring pediatrician. See Figure 16.5 for the report layout.

16.3 In-field evaluation

During the in-field feasibility study, five families of 2- to 6-year-old children (four children diagnosed with autism; one child developing

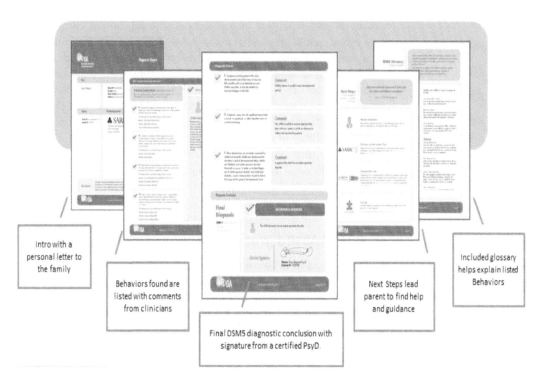

Figure 16.5 NODA Connect: A diagnostic report summarizes a remote diagnostic assessment.

typically) participated and completed in-home recordings under the remote guidance of the collaborating diagnostician. Three additional diagnosticians were recruited to complete remote diagnostic assessment. For each participant family, two participant diagnosticians, blind to the child's previous diagnostic status, independently completed a diagnostic assessment for autism. Results of this in-field evolution show that without any prior training, parents were able to record videos and rated NODA SmartCapture as easy to use (average rating of 4 on a scale from 1—very difficult to use to 5—very easy to use). In addition, 96% of the videos recorded by parents in the study were rated to be clinically useful for autism diagnostic assessment by the collaborating diagnostician. The three participant diagnosticians also rated parent-collected videos useful for conducting autism diagnosis (average rating 4 on a scale from 1—not useful to 5—very useful) once they completed remote diagnostic diagnosis. Furthermore, for four children (three children with autism; one typically developing child) both diagnosticians independently arrived at the same diagnosis, which was also consistent with the child's previous diagnostic status in the medical record. For the fifth family, one diagnostician matched the diagnosis in the child's record but the second did not, though the latter indicated with high confidence that the child was not typically developing. A third diagnostician also reviewed this case via NODA Connect, and confirmed the diagnosis in the child's medical record. Overall, of all the assessments conducted, in 91% cases (10 out of 11 assessments) diagnosticians were able to arrive at a diagnostic outcome that matches the diagnosis in the child's medical record, and did so with a high level of confidence (average rating of 4.5 on a scale from 1—not confident to 5—highly confident). A large-scale clinical study, consisting of 40 families seeking an ASD evaluation for their child and 11 families of typically developing children, demonstrated the clinical utility and validity of diagnostic outcome of NODA (Smith et al. 2016). Results from this clinical study shows that the diagnostic agreement between NODA and the in-person diagnosis was 88.2% (K = 0.75) in the full sample (Smith et al. 2016).

16.4 Proposed workflow model for field adoption

In our proposed workflow model for NODA field adoption, first the pediatrician puts a referral for a remote diagnostic assessment for a child showing early signs of autism. Next, a diagnostician at an affiliated diagnostic center guides in-home behavior collection process. At the early stages of in-home collection a less experienced clinician can guide parents, and once good quality video evidence is collected, an experienced diagnostician (a more expensive resource) can perform the remote diagnostic assessment. Once parents collect all video evidence as per given prescription, the diagnostician completes the diagnostic assessment for autism through NODA Connect and shares final assessment report with the pediatrician, who then subsequently shares it with the parents.

This workflow model has two potential benefits. First, it engages pediatricians who usually see children at regular intervals during the early years of development and hence are in the best position to notice early warning signs of developmental delay and take appropriate timely action. Research suggests that pediatrician involvement in the referral and diagnostic process can result in more timely diagnosis (Hart-Hester and Noble 1999; American Academy of Pediatrics 2001; Swanson et al. 2013; Zuckerman et al. 2013). Second, it will allow autism diagnostic centers that usually have a long waiting list to expedite the process of diagnosis by remotely completing diagnostic assessment. Children whose diagnostic outcome is not clear through this remote diagnostic procedure can be seen in person for a more comprehensive diagnostic assessment.

Acknowledgments

This work is based on collaboration among Georgia Institute of Technology, Behavior Imaging Solutions, Inc. (BIS) and the Southwest Autism Research and Resource Center (SARRC). Behavior Imaging Solutions is working on the commercialization of NODA. This work is funded by NIH.

References

American Academy of Pediatrics. 2001. The pediatrician's role in the diagnosis and management of autistic spectrum disorder in children. *Pediatrics* 107:1221–6.

American Psychiatric Association. 2013. *Diagnostic and Statistical Manual of Mental Disorders*, 5th ed. (*DSM-5®*). Washington, DC: American Psychiatric Publishing.

BehaviorConnect. 2014a. NODA app for autism diagnostic assessment: Meal time. https://www.youtube.com/watch?v=d40_rDAqprg Archived at: http://www.webcitation.org/6XFePxJHyBehaviorConnect. 2014b. NODA app for autism diagnostic assessment: Play alone. https://www.youtube.com/watch?v=4Clh027Zyo0 Archived at: http://www.webcitation.org/6XFea6T6x.

BehaviorConnect. 2014c. NODA app for autism diagnostic assessment: Play with others. https://www.youtube.com/watch?v=z3oKRoGOlac Archived at: http://www.webcitation.org/6XFegPR5P.

BehaviorConnect. 2014d. NODA app for autism diagnostic assessment: Problem time. https://www.youtube.com/watch?v=nAyw6GOUMlc Archived at: http://www.webcitation.org/6XFeku3Qj.

Hart-Hester, S. and S. L. Noble. 1999. Recognition and treatment of autism: The role of the family physician. *J. Miss. State Med. Assoc.* 40:377–83.

Howlin, P. and A. Asgharian. 1999. The diagnosis of autism and Asperger syndrome: Findings from a survey of 770 families. *Dev. Med. Child Neurol.* 41:834–9.

Kidd, C. D., R. Orr, G. D. Abowd, C. G. Atkeson, I. A. Essa, B. MacIntyre, E. Mynatt, T. E. Starner, and W. Newstetter. 1999. The Aware Home: A living laboratory for ubiquitous computing research. *Lecture Notes Comput. Sci.* 1670:191–8.

Matson, J. L. 2011. *Clinical Assessment and Intervention for Autism Spectrum Disorders.* Amsterdam: Academic Press.

McEachin, J. J., T. Smith, and O. I. Lovaas. 1993. Long-term outcome for children with autism who received early intensive behavioral treatment. *Am. J. Ment. Retard.* 97:359–72.

McLeod, B. D., A. J. Doss, and T. H. Ollendick. 2013. *Diagnostic and Behavioral Assessment in Children and Adolescents: A Clinical Guide.* New York: Guilford Press.

Nazneen, A. Rozga, M. Romero, A. J. Findley, N. A. Call, and R. I. Arriaga. 2010. Supporting parents for in-home capture of problem behaviors of children with developmental disabilities. *Pers Ubiquitous Comput.* 16:193–207.

Nazneen, N., A. Rozga, C. J. Smith, R. Oberleitner, G. D. Abowd, and R. I. Arriaga. 2015. A novel system for supporting autism diagnosis using home videos: Iterative development and evaluation of system design. *JMIR mHealth and uHealth* 3(2):e68.

Rattazzi, A. 2014. The importance of early detection and early intervention for children with autism spectrum conditions. *Vertex* 25:290–4.

Siegel, B. 2008. *Getting the Best for Your Child with Autism, An Expert's Guide to Treatment.* New York: Guilford Press.

Sivberg, B. 2003. Parents' detection of early signs in their children having an autistic spectrum disorder. *J. Pediatr. Nurs.* 18:433–9.

Smith, C. J., S. E. Ober-Reynolds, K. Treulich, R. McIntosh, and R. Melmed. 2009. Using a behavioral imaging platform to develop a Naturalistic Observational Diagnostic Assessment for autism. *IMFAR Abstract Book* 119.25.

Smith, C. J., A. Rozga, N. Matthews, R. Oberleitner, N. Nazneen, and G. Abowd. 2016. Investigating the accuracy of a novel telehealth diagnostic approach for autism spectrum disorder. *Psychological Assessment.* PMID: 27196689.

Swanson, A. R., Z. E. Warren, W. L. Stone, A. C. Vehorn, E. Dohrmann, and Q. Humberd. 2013. The diagnosis of autism in community pediatric settings: Does advanced training facilitate practice change? *Autism* 18:555–61.

Wiggins, L. D., J. Baio, and C. Rice. 2006. Examination of the time between first evaluation and first autism spectrum diagnosis in a population-based sample. *J. Dev. Behav. Pediatr.* 27(2 suppl):S79–87.

Zuckerman, K. E., K. Mattox, K. Donelan, O. Batbayar, A. Baghaee, and C. Bethell. 2013. Pediatrician identification of Latino children at risk for autism spectrum disorder. *Pediatrics* 132:445–53.

Chapter 17 Behavior Imaging®
Resolving assessment challenges for autism spectrum disorder in pharmaceutical trials

Ron Oberleitner,
Uwe Reischl, Kamilla G.
Gazieva, N. Nazneen,
Jasjit S. Suri, and
Christopher J. Smith

Contents

Abstract 356
17.1   Introduction 356
17.2   Background 356
17.3   Technology platform 357
17.4   Behavior Imaging for research. 357
17.5   Behavior Capture™ 359
17.6   Behavior Connect™ 360
17.7   Pharmaceutical R&D. 360
17.8   Data quality challenges 361
17.9   Recent technology applications 362
17.10   Pharmaceutical trials 363
17.11   Retrospective evaluation of archived video data 365
17.12   Behavior Imaging in natural settings. 367
17.13   Conclusions 367
Acknowledgment. 368
References 368

Abstract

Behavior Imaging® was incorporated into an NIMH-funded multisite pharmaceutical trial to remotely document clinical rater reliability within a standardized observer evaluation protocol. Behavior Imaging provided a centralized telehealth system capable of documenting observer agreement. Interviewer–observer training and ongoing maintenance of assessment quality was performed efficiently. Behavior Imaging provided an important new quality control tool previously not available for such multisite research studies. The results indicate the potential for successful applications also to retrospective studies of archived video data and the evaluation of recorded data obtained in natural settings.

17.1 Introduction

An effective treatment for the autism spectrum disorders (ASD) has been elusive despite many years of clinical research nationally and internationally. Pharmaceutical trials addressing ASD have been especially challenging, expensive, and time-consuming because the symptoms associated with the neurodevelopmental disorder are complex and varied. To provide a new impetus into the improvement of the assessment and management of ASD symptoms, the National Institutes of Health (NIH) funded the so-called Fast-Fail Trials–Autism (FAST-AS) initiative in 2012. FAST promotes the testing of new therapeutic compounds that may be able to provide the basis for further large-scale trials at a later time (NIH 2012). As part of this initiative, Behavior Imaging (BI) was included in this program to provide improved measurement and documentation of research outcomes for multiple clinical sites. In this chapter, the key features of the Behavior Imaging platform are described, including an overview of the current applications and challenges associated with the use of this technology platform.

17.2 Background

The founders of Behavior Imaging Solutions, Inc. were challenged in 2007 to address the absence of professional resources available to provide timely ASD assessments. A legacy version of the Behavior Imaging platform (see below) was, therefore, deployed to determine whether inter-rater reliability among ASD healthcare providers, diagnosticians, and therapists could be as effective as "in-person" second opinions for assessments carried out remotely. This issue was considered to be critical because access to professionals capable of evaluating the functional performance of children with autism in a timely fashion was delaying the educational progress of children with autism both locally and regionally.

17.3 Technology platform

A new behavior-image platform was developed for use by healthcare providers to allow diagnostic assessments of ASD symptoms remotely. To ascertain the efficacy of this approach, the inter-rater reliability using this technology platform for scoring discrete trial functional performance tasks in children was studied. The video capture system was used to simultaneously record children and their in-person evaluators during discrete trial sessions, a common teaching technique used in Applied Behavior Analysis therapy. Ten children with an autism spectrum disorder diagnosis, each performing 10 discrete trials, were scored by their teacher, as well as an independent onsite evaluator. The onsite evaluator also used Behavior Capture to record the sessions, and these video recordings were then transmitted to a secure Web platform for review by 10 "external" raters. The reviewers rated each of the 100 video clips independently. Their scores provided the basis for an inter-rater reliability estimate. A comparison between the in-person evaluator and the external evaluator scores allowed an assessment of the overall effectiveness of the behavior capture methodology. A comparison of the external evaluator scores to the independent evaluator and among each other was used to determine the efficacy and inter-rater reliability of the system. A comparison of the in-person evaluator scores with the external evaluator scores also yielded insight into potential observational discrepancies. A high correlation between the on-site evaluators and the remote evaluators, as well as a high inter-rater reliability for the external evaluators, indicated that the new behavior-image technology platform can be used effectively in the remote evaluation of functional performance tests of children with autism (Reischl et al. 2007).

From this experience, other studies to use Behavior Imaging for inter-rater-reliability arose. The Behavior Imaging platform was enhanced for facilitating a large pharmaceutical trial. The components of the new technology platform are illustrated in Figure 17.1.

17.4 Behavior Imaging for research

There is an increasing demand by researchers to include behavior information in the assessment and treatment of neurodevelopmental disorders. To address this demand, academic and industry partners joined together to develop a new imaging technology called Behavior Imaging (BI). This technology allows a comprehensive documentation of patient behaviors in naturalistic and clinical environments. This is important because behavior information needs to be obtained not only in clinical settings but also in a person's home, or in a classroom. The Behavior Imaging system features video capture capability, clinical annotation tools, and integration into a personal health record platform. Once behavior information is collected, the data can be securely shared among

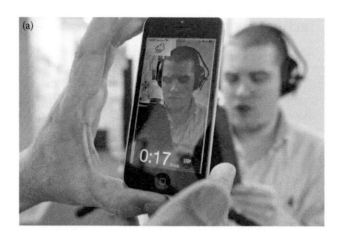

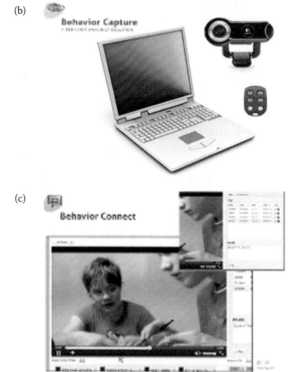

Figure 17.1 Illustration of the key components of the new technology platform: (a) App options to enable video capture for smartphones, (b) laptops, and (c) associated online clinical assessment interface.

a patient, their caregivers and/or providers, and researchers. This can be done globally without regard for the stakeholders' geographic location (Oberleitner et al. 2010). In the area of pharmaceutical trials, BI provides researchers a Web-based platform to document inter-rater reliability, conduct effective interviewer-observer training, and perform ongoing assessment of reporting reliability. The Behavior Imaging technology is delivered through Behavior Capture™ and Behavior Connect™.

17.5 Behavior Capture™

Behavior Capture was developed at the Georgia Institute of Technology's College of Computing. Behavior Capture consists of a video recording application on a PC, smartphone, or iPad, which can be used in a home or in an institutional environment. When a user selects a "Behavior" setting, Behavior Capture features a unique video buffering capability that documents relevant events occurring before, during, and after a specific behavior. This "After-the-Fact™" feature can provide an insight into the causes or "triggers" of certain observed behaviors. Behavior Capture records this data before and after activation using a small wireless remote control device referred to as "select archiving." The camera/computer system continuously captures videos but does not commit it to memory until the remote control is pressed. For example, a provider can set the system to record events that occurred before the remote is activated. This application eliminates the need for a stand-alone camera, eliminates time-consuming transfers of video data from the camera to a computer, and prevents remote sharing of confidential information via nonsecure channels such as e-mail or organizational networks. Behavior Capture also provides an "Interview" or "Assessment" setting, which allows an observer to begin and to end video recording via a hand-held remote control. This feature was used in the FAST-AS pharmaceutical trial. A schematic illustration of Behavior Capture is shown in Figure 17.2.

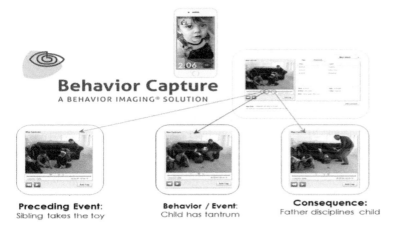

Preceding Event:
Sibling takes the toy

Behavior / Event:
Child has tantrum

Consequence:
Father disciplines child

Figure 17.2 Schematic illustration of Behavior Capture using an After-the-Fact recording feature that enables a caregiver to create a video clip of behaviors containing "before," "during," and "after" event behaviors observed in natural settings, that is, the home environment. Resultant video clip permits "tagging" of behaviors that a caregiver or a health professional can later annotate.

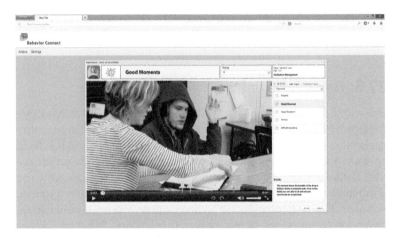

Figure 17.3 Behavior Connect platform used by researchers to rate (or tag) specific behaviors observed on a special data viewer.

17.6 Behavior Connect™

Behavior Connect is a secure, Web-based health record platform that allows clinicians to organize, analyze, and share documents and videos with patients, other healthcare providers, teachers, and therapists. To date, applications of Behavior Connect include autism spectrum disorder behavior assessments, diagnostic evaluations, Web-based supervision of staff working with autistic children, evaluation and therapeutic documentation, and assessment of inter-rater reliability in multisite pharmaceutical trials. The key components of the Behavior Connect system are illustrated in Figure 17.3.

17.7 Pharmaceutical R&D

In spite of growing investments in the biomedical sciences, there is a significant decline in new drug development (FDA 2004). There has also been a significant decline in overall pharmaceutical clinical research (Woodcock 2013). In a report by the President's Council of Advisors on Science and Technology (PCAST) titled "Propelling Innovation in Drug Discovery, Development and Evaluation," the key factors were identified that are known to contribute to this decline including the following:

1. High failure rates: A new medical compound is estimated to have only 8% chance of reaching the market (Mahajan and Gupta 2010).
2. High costs of development: The cost of development for a successfully marketed drug is estimated to be $1 billion (Adams and Brantner 2010).
3. Long development time: The average time required for the development of a new drug is about 9 years (Mahajan and Gupta 2010).
4. Substantial regulatory uncertainty (Woodcock 2013).

In 2004, the U.S. Food and Drug Administration (FDA) recommended steps to reverse this trend. One of the key recommendations was to develop better evaluation tools such as biomarkers (The FDA 2004). The National Institutes of Health (NIH) addressed this goal by supporting the concept of "Fast-Fail Trials" (FAST). FAST trials are different from standard clinical trials by requiring fewer test subjects (only 10 to 30 patients), and requiring shorter time periods in conducting the clinical trials. This strategy is expected to reduce drug development costs significantly—$9 million vs $500 million (UCLA 2012).

FAST trials require two or more clinical sites and all of the sites must follow a common treatment and data collection protocol. One of the sites is charged with accruing, processing, and analyzing the data obtained by all of the sites (Kraemer 2000). These multisite trials provide opportunities to answer questions regarding efficacy of treatment and also allow the recruitment of relatively large heterogeneous populations. FAST trials can generate large sample sizes which lead to greater statistical power and are, therefore, more generalizable.

17.8 Data quality challenges

While multisite trials offer advantages, they also present disadvantages including the risk of poor data quality, heterogeneity of results, and poor interview quality (Del Boca et al. 1994; Keefe and Harvey 2008). Spirito et al. (2009) reported significant differences in the reported drug efficacies in a multisite clinical trial because of sampling discrepancies and treatment protocol discrepancies. Multisite clinical trials can increase the variability in treatment, variability in diagnostic observations, and an overall decrease in the likelihood of detecting a difference between groups (Scahill and Lord 2004). It has also been noted that improvements in social function were found only in patients who had the same examiner throughout the trial or who had an IQ higher than 70 (Kaufman 2014). If all subjects had the same rater, the positive outcomes might have been higher. Assessment tools, which are dependent on an examiner's judgment only, could, therefore, benefit from use of two blinded raters or benefit from centralized scoring. BI technology allows a blind analysis of video-recorded assessments using two or more evaluators and also allows documentation of inter-rater reliability between these evaluators. Arnold et al. (2000) outlined the limitations associated with ratings based on the judgment of one clinician. Researchers use different standards to define changes in symptoms when compared to a control group. Widely accepted outcome measures such as the Clinical Global Impression rating scale (CGI) rely on the clinician's "gut" sense (Busner and Targum 2007). This approach leaves room for significant uncertainty (Arnold et al. 2000). To address this challenge, Arnold et al. added a parent's rating to the child's Irritability subscale. However, the disadvantage of including a parent's measures is that the parent may not fully understand the intent of the rating scale. Such measures are also vulnerable to the expectations of a parent (Scahill and Lord 2004).

17.9 Recent technology applications

While quality issues in multisite pharmaceutical clinical trials may be addressed statistically, systematic errors resulting from interviewer discrepancies across clinical sites cannot be resolved statistically (Keefe and Harvey 2008). However, specific approaches can be used to enhance the inter-rater reliability. These include the following:

1. *Rater training and use of video recordings* (Arnold et al. 2000). Advantages of rater training with the use of videos include improved quality of interviews and improved data collection. However, video recordings can be time-consuming and expensive because the findings must be transferred onto paper-based assessment forms (Scahill and Lord 2004). Demitrack et al. (1998) identified these issues as significant factors contributing to poor study results. He evaluated these challenges by conducting a series of inter-rater reliability training sessions. The 17-item Hamilton Depression Rating Scale was used at the start of a Phase II multisite clinical drug trial. The findings of this study "underscored the magnitude of error present in such a test setting and provided preliminary evidence of an effect of this problem on the detection of clinical change" (Demitrack et al. 1998). In a report by Schnurr et al. (2005), the use of video-taped recordings to provide feedback to therapists for the purpose of ensuring adherence to a specified treatment protocol during the clinical trial was found to be highly beneficial.

2. *Centralized scoring* (Williams et al. 2012). Findings in this study suggested "that remote centralized raters may reduce a primary risk of study failure in clinical trials by decreasing a placebo response as a result of their blinded baseline scoring."

3. *Video recording.* Video recordings are "objective" and are less vulnerable to misinterpretations based on the expectations of an evaluator. Use of video-recorded data has been shown to "minimize selective bias and provide the opportunity to employ more rigorous strategies for ensuring reliability" (Caldwell and Atwal 2005). Baranek et al. (2005) conducted a naturalistic investigation of object-based play skills in infants with autism ages 9–12 months. The study demonstrated the feasibility of using a computer-based coding technology for the purpose of a retrospective video analysis. It must be recognized, however, that the evaluation of video recorded interviews and observations may be influenced by the quality of the video data obtained. Also, coding of videotapes can be time-consuming and expensive. Also, it

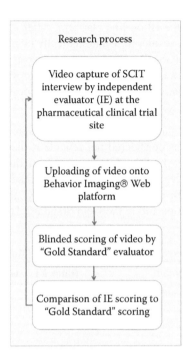

Figure 17.4 Illustration of the research workflow for multiple sites collaborating via the Behavior Imaging platform.

may be difficult to achieve good inter-rater reliability in multisite studies if centralized scoring is not employed (Scahill 2004). The workflow for multiple collaborating research sites collaborating using the video capture technology is illustrated in Figure 17.4.

17.10 Pharmaceutical trials

Behavior Imaging was employed to improve inter-rater reliability and the data collection process for multiple clinical sites used in a pharmaceutical trial. The technology platform facilitated the training of independent raters and provided an automated measure of the inter-rater reliability. The system was based on a "store-and-forward" method. The objective of the study was to document rater reliability outcomes for two interview protocols including the Autism Diagnostic Observation Schedule (ADOS) and the Social Communication Interaction Test (SCIT). Attention was placed on identifying items in both of the diagnostic tests that contributed to inconsistencies in ratings between raters and the "Gold Standard" (GS). This feedback allowed targeted training of the raters to improve inter-rater reliability.

Methods: The study was conducted by four medical research institutions. Rater reliability checks were established at the beginning of the study. Raters viewed prerecorded interviews and were asked to score their observations using the BI on-line platform. After each rater completed the scoring task, the results were automatically tabulated and compared to a Gold Standard (GS). Discrepancies in the scoring in relation to the GS were identified and recommendations for improving the rater's accuracy were made. Raters were then required to repeat their scoring tasks until they were able to match the GS scores.

Results: Table 17.1 summarizes the training exercise using the SCIT protocol. A rater was considered not reliable if there was a difference of more than 1 for each of the domains and more than 10% for the total score. The summaries show that Rater #1 matched the Gold Standard in the domains A, B, E, and F, while domains C and D were different by one point in relationship to the Gold Standard. However, none of the

Table 17.1 Summary of Rater Responses for an Initial Training Session

	Domain	Rater #1	Gold Standard	Δ
A	Social awareness and nonverbal responsiveness to others	2	2	0
B	Awareness and verbal responsiveness to others	4	4	0
C	Intentions of communication	5	4	1
D	Conversational turn-taking	3	4	1
E	Appropriateness of interaction	3	3	0
F	Insight and ability to describe emotion	3	3	0
	Total Score	20	20	0%
	Domain	**Rater #2**	**Gold Standard**	**Δ**
A	Social awareness and nonverbal responsiveness to others	2	2	0
B	Awareness and verbal responsiveness to others	4	4	0
C	Intentions of communication	4	4	0
D	Conversational turn-taking	4	4	0
E	Appropriateness of interaction	4	3	1
F	Insight and ability to describe emotion	3	3	0
	Total Score	21	20	4.8%
	Domain	**Rater #4**	**Gold Standard**	**Δ**
A	Social awareness and nonverbal responsiveness to others	2	2	0
B	Awareness and verbal responsiveness to others	3	4	1
C	Intentions of communication	3	4	1
D	Conversational turn-taking	2	4	2
E	Appropriateness of interaction	2	3	1
F	Insight and ability to describe emotion	3	3	0
	Total Score	15	20	25%

differences were greater than "1" and the total score was the same as that for the Gold Standard. Therefore, Rater #1 was considered "Reliable." Rater #4 met the Gold Standard for domains A and F. Domain D was off by 2 points and domain E was off by 1 point. The difference between the Gold Standard and Rater #4 was off by 25% and was, therefore, not considered "Reliable."

The study demonstrated the practicality of using the BI technology to document inter-rater reliability throughout the duration of a multisite pharmacological study, conducting effective interviewer-observer training, and performing ongoing maintenance of assessment reliability. Behavior Imaging can provide important functions in support of multisite clinical research trials such as:

- Provide training for researchers at different sites to ensure consistency in observations.
- Provide timely and quality feedback regarding assessment quality and consistency.
- Provide documentation capture for repeated assessment at a later time.

The ability to reanalyze video-recorded observations at a later time is important. With current methods, a rater's subjective narrative is the only piece of data that is stored. Use of the Behavior Imaging technology and Behavior Connect system allows the creation, sharing, analysis, and storage of video evidence for later review if needed. Also, it is known that research subjects and patients do not present their underlying pathologies in a clinical environment in the same way that they do at home—being in a clinical environment can change a person's behavior that can mask the actual symptoms they exhibit at home. To more accurately document changes in behavior, the use of Behavior Imaging allows the recording of a person's behavior within a natural, nonclinical, environment.

17.11 Retrospective evaluation of archived video data

In pharmacological management of autism spectrum disorder, a desired outcome measure is usually defined in terms of changes in specific behavior domains. Since ASD patients are known to exhibit a wide range of symptoms, it is not uncommon for subjects to show improvement in altogether different domains. Subsequently, study results become inconsistent and the outcomes are hard to interpret. Traditionally, clinical researchers have only paper assessments and rater notes available to review the outcomes. However, video-behavior data allows researchers to refine and expand their analysis at a later time and potentially identify differences between treatment protocols that cannot be observed immediately using traditional paper-and-pencil methods.

365

Using Behavior Connect, researchers can now store and share video data while Behavior Imaging helps quantify the specific social behaviors found in both clinical environments and in natural settings. This is important since changes in social functioning are defined as specific target outcome measures in autism spectrum disorder treatment studies (Frye 2014). With Behavior Connect, clinicians look for particular behaviors in the video that define social functioning, tag these behaviors, and then describe them with qualifiers. The system prepares a tally of the tagged behaviors. This will then allow the clinician to make a determination with regard to the social functioning status of the patient. In addition, the videos can be analyzed blindly by multiple clinicians providing a measure of reliability. The researchers/clinicians can then work together from different geographical locations, have access to the same data, and analyze videos independently.

A feasibility study was conducted to determine whether or not additional value could be gained by reassessing interviews captured by Behavior Imaging, and using revised scoring criteria using Behavior Connect. Figure 17.5a illustrates a partial list of behavioral terms (tags) that were used in the feasibility study, and Figure 17.5b depicts the different outcome scores for the selected behaviors at three different time periods.

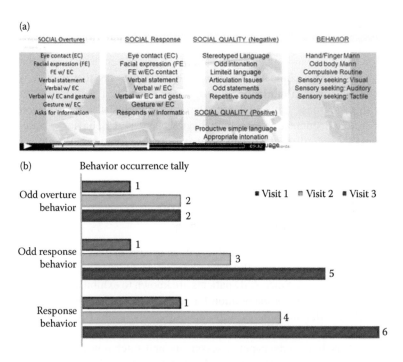

Figure 17.5 (a) Behavioral terms (tags) presented to the Behavior Imaging platform viewer. (b) Summary of outcome scores for the selected behaviors at three different time periods.

17.12 Behavior Imaging in natural settings

Based on research showing that caregivers are able to successfully collect and share behavioral data via Behavior Imaging (Nazneen et al. 2015; Matthews et al. 2015), a feasibility study has been initiated to train ASD patients and their at-home caregivers to collect socially relevant behavioral data via video clips and to then share these clips with their healthcare providers and researchers. This approach may help transform the communication process between patients and caregivers and potentially accelerate future pharmaceutical trials of ASD.

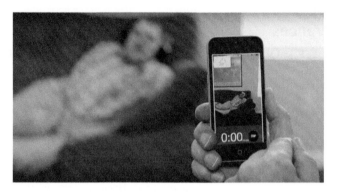

17.13 Conclusions

In support of efforts to find new approaches for the management of ASD, review of archived research video-data via Behavior Connect can reduce redundancies in autism research and foster more collaboration among researchers internationally. Multiple assessment instruments can be evaluated by using video-recorded behaviors of patients in clinical or natural environments. This approach will cut the cost and time in the recruitment of subjects and the collection of data.

The effective use of Behavior Imaging was demonstrated in the FAST multisite pharmaceutical trial where Behavior Connect was able to eliminate data management concerns and facilitated the sharing of information among the research teams. The system allowed ongoing assessment of inter-rater reliability and supported the training of raters to insure rater consistency.

The development of Behavior Connect is ongoing. Anticipated improvements include the following:

- Inclusion of additional assessment instruments
- A more streamlined reporting system
- Use in research of other mental and behavioral disorders where outcome measures must be based on the multiple rater assessments

The proposed innovations will allow the research community to further address challenges and opportunities in pharmaceutical trials that focus on the diagnosis, treatment, and management of autism spectrum disorder.

Acknowledgment

Support for this research study was possible due to NIMH 9R44MH099035.

References

Adams, C. P. and V. V. Brantner. 2010. Spending on new drug development. *Health Econ.* 19(2):130–141.

Arnold, L. E., M. G. Aman, A. Martin, A. Collier-Crespin, B. Vitiello, E. Tierney, R. Asarnow, and F. Vokmar. 2000. Assessment in multisite randomized clinical trials of patients with autistic disorder: The autism RUPP network. *J. Autism Dev. Disord.* 30(2):99–111.

Baranek, G. T., C. R. Barnett, E. M. Adams, N. A. Wolcott, L. R. Watson, and E. R. Crais, 2005. Object play in infants with autism: Methodological issues in retrospective video analysis. *Am. J. Occup.* 59:1.

Busner, J. and S. D. Targum. 2007. The clinical global impressions scale: Applying a research tool in clinical practice. *Psychiatry (Edgmont)*, 4(7):28–37.

Caldwell, K. and A. Atwal. 2005. Non-participant observation: Using video tapes to collect data in nursing research. *Nurse Res.* 13(2):42–54.

Del Boca, F. K., T. F. Babor, and B. McRee. 1994. Reliability enhancement and estimation in multisite clinical trials. *J. Stud. Alcohol Suppl.* 12:130–6.

Demitrack, M. A., D. Faries, J. M. Herrera, D. DeBrota, and W. Z. Potter. 1998. The problem of measurement error in multisite clinical trials. *Psychopharmacol Bull.* 34(1):19–24.

Food and Drug Administration. 2004. Innovation or stagnation: Challenge and opportunity on the critical path to new medical products. Retrieved http://www.fda.gov/ScienceResearch/SpecialTopics/CriticalPathInitiative/CriticalPathOpportunitiesReports/ucm077262.htm

Frye, R. 2014. Clinical potential, safety, and tolerability of arbaclofen in the treatment of autism spectrum disorder. *Drug, Healthcare Patient Safety* 6:69–76.

Kaufman, W. 2014. Autism clinical trials are ripe for improvement. Retrieved from http://vectorblog.org/2014/03/autism-clinical-trials-are-ripe-for-improvement/

Keefe, R. S. E. and P. D. Harvey. 2008. Implementation considerations for multisite clinical trials with cognitive neuroscience tasks. *Schizophrenia Bull.* 34(4):656–663.

Kraemer, H. C. 2000. Pitfalls of multisite randomized clinical trials of efficacy and effectiveness. *Schizophrenia Bull.* 26(3):533–541.

Mahajan, R. and K. Gupta. 2010. Food and drug administration's critical path initiative and innovations in drug development paradigm: Challenges, progress, and controversies. *J. Pharmacy Bioallied Sci.* 2:4.

Matthews, N., C. J. Smith, Nazneen, R. Oberleitner, A. Rozga, G. Abowd, and R. I. Irriaga. 2015. Analysis of parent responses to using a remote autism diagnostic assessment system, *14th Annual International Meeting for Autism Research (IMFAR)*, Salt Lake City, UT.

National Institutes of Health. 2012. Accelerating the pace of psychiatric drug discovery. Retrieved from http://www.nimh.nih.gov/research-priorities/research-initiatives/fast-fast-fail-trials.shtml

Nazneen, A. Rozga, C. J. Smith, R. Oberleitner, G. Abowd, and R. Arriaga, 2015. A Novel System for Supporting Autism Diagnosis using Home Videos: Iterative Development and Evaluation of System Design. *JMIR mHealth and uHealth*, 3(2):e68.

Oberleitner, R., U. Reischl, T. Lacy, M. Goodwin, and J. Spitalnick. 2010. *Emerging use of Behavior Imaging for Autism.* Commun Med Care Compunetics. Berlin: Springer-Verlag.

Reischl, U., J. Ball, G. Abowd, R. Oberleitner, P. Elison-Bowers, and S. Lockwood. Inter-rater Reliability Using a Behavior Imaging Web Platform, *6th Annual International Meeting for Autism Research (IMFAR)*, Seattle, WA, May 2007.

Scahill, L. and C. Lord. 2004. Subject selection and characterization in clinical trials in children with autism. *CNS Spectrums* 9(01):22–32.

Schnurr, P. P., M. J. Friedman, C. C. Engel, E. B. Foa, M. T. Shea, P. M. Resick, K. E. James, and B. K. Chow. 2005. Issues in the design of multisite clinical trials of psychotherapy: VA Cooperative Study No. 494 as an example. *Contemporary Clin. Trials,* 26(6):626–36.

Spirito, A., K. Z. Abebe, S. Iyengar, D. Brent, B. Vitiello, G. Clarke, K. D. Wagner, and M. Keller. January 01, 2009. Sources of site differences in the efficacy of a multisite clinical trial: The treatment of SSRI-Resistant Depression in Adolescents. *J. Consult. Clin. Psychol.* 77(3):439–50.

University of California, Los Angeles. 2012. UCLA researcher receives $9-million NIMH contract for "FAST FAIL" studies of autism drug. Retrieved from https://www.ctsi.ucla.edu/news/item?item_id=88520

Williams, J.B.W., J. Dunn, K. Kobak, E. Giller, L. Curry, P. Wilson et al. 2012. Placebo response assessed by site and remote blinded centralized raters in a GAD trial, *NCDEU Annual Meeting*, Boca Raton, FL.

Woodcock, J. 2013. The PCAST report on pharmaceutical innovation: Implications for the FDA. *Clin. Pharmacol. Therap. St Louis* 94(3):297–300.

Chapter 18 Virtual reality with psychophysio-logical monitoring as an approach to evaluate emotional reactivity, social skills, and joint attention in autism spectrum disorder

Estate M. Sokhadze,
Manuel F. Casanova,
Desmond L. Kelly,
Guela E. Sokhadze,
Yi Li, Adel S. Elmaghraby,
and Ayman S. El-Baz

Contents

Abstract 372
18.1   Background. 373
18.2   Review of the state of the art of VR application in autism. . . 375

18.3   Suggested directions of future research using VR in ASD . . 376
18.4   Emotional state detection and differentiation using
       psychophysiological measures 378
18.5   Autonomic balance dysfunctions in autism 380
       18.5.1 Heart-rate variability and phasic HR responses. 380
       18.5.2 Electrodermal activity and sympathetic
               overarousal in autism 381
18.6   Importance of autonomic control assessment in
       understanding social deficits in autism. 382
18.7   Phasic and tonic heart-rate responses as indicators of
       attention and emotion processes. 383
18.8   Social engagement deficits in autism and HRV 383
18.9   Pilot data of psychophysiological reactivity of children
       with ASD to emotional stimuli. 384
       18.9.1 Introduction 384
       18.9.2 Measurement of the ANS-dependent variables 384
               18.9.2.1 Experiments 1–2. 384
               18.9.2.2 Experiments 3–4 385
               18.9.2.3 Experiment 5 385
       18.9.3 Results. 385
               18.9.3.1 Experiment 1 385
               18.9.3.2 Experiment 2 386
               18.9.3.3 Experiment 3 386
               18.9.3.4 Experiment 4 386
               18.9.3.5 Experiment 5 387
18.10 Discussion and conclusions 388
References 391

Abstract

Impairments in social communication skills and deficient social and emotional competence are thought to be core deficits in children with autism spectrum disorder (ASD). In recent years, several assistive technologies, particularly virtual reality (VR), have been proposed as therapeutic devices that promote social interactions in autism. Furthermore, the application of psychophysiological monitoring during VR exposure captures real-time response to VR interaction allowing customized assessment of emotional reactivity, social competence, and social skills. Subjective reports, parental and clinicians' evaluations, behavioral performance scores, and psychophysiological monitoring can be effectively used to document the effects of VR within a realistic and dynamic three-dimensional (3D) context matched to the specifics of autism research queries. We propose that the integration of VR and applied psychophysiology methods holds the promise of enhancing social and emotional competence in autism. The major objective of the review is to consider a strong rationale to assess emotional reactivity, social competence, and joint attention in high-functioning children with ASD during exposure to a VR environment with concurrent psychophysiological monitoring. Furthermore, the chapter aims to examine whether there are possible ways to develop VR-based methods of training emotional reactivity, social skills, and joint attention initiation and responsiveness in individuals with ASD. The application of VR and psychophysiology monitoring-based emotional and social skills assessment and potentially also social skills training courses may significantly improve the generalization of acquired skills. The application of psychophysiology-informed VR systems could be adjusted for use not only in laboratory settings but also in more natural settings such as outpatient clinics and school and home settings. An additional important component of the innovation of the proposed line of research is that VR with concurrent real-time psychophysiological monitoring can be converted into a far more advanced novel solution where VR scenarios might be modified using physiological activity inputs, that is, operate in biofeedback mode.

18.1 Background

Impairments in social communication skills and deficient social and emotional competence are thought to be core deficits in children with autism spectrum disorder (Downs and Smith 2004; Begeer et al. 2008; APA 2013). In recent years, several assistive technologies, particularly virtual reality (VR), have been proposed to be used to assess communication skills and promote social interactions in this population (Parsons et al. 2002, 2004; Goodwin 2008; Ehrlich and Miller 2009; Bellani et al. 2011). Adaptation of VR technology to support customized evaluation of emotional reactivity and social skills training has a very promising potential for application in autism research and treatment. Furthermore, the application of portable psychophysiological monitoring systems during VR exposure for measurement of physiological activity to capture real-time response to VR social interaction scenes and ability to better adapt VR environment to psychophysiological pattern has even more perspectives (Côté and Bouchard 2005; Wiederhold and Rizzo 2005). VR technology has undergone a transition in the past few years after the emergence of new inexpensive systems such as Oculus Rift (Oculus 2015) and similar VR units, and now has all chances to transform from an "expensive toy" for entertainment into a functional technology for clinical research in the autism area. VR systems have huge potential as a viable tool for a wide range of clinical and research applications that are not limited only to exposure applications (e.g., for phobias treatment, Rothbaum et al. 1995; Garcia-Palacios et al. 2002). The rights for Oculus Rift VR system was recently acquired by Facebook and soon it will be in a mass production and widely available to prospective users for a very affordable price.

There is a rather strong rationale for the integration of VR with real-time psychophysiological monitoring for advanced cognitive and affective neuroscience research and relevant clinical applications in autism. In the psychophysiology area, the technology for noninvasive recording of physiological activity is used to investigate and understand correlates of cognitive processes and emotional states. The use of VR now allows for the measurement of interaction within more realistic dynamic three-dimensional (3D) content using precise emotional and socially meaningful stimulus delivery within more naturalistic scenarios well matched for the specifics of autism research questions.

There is a need to begin establishing VR as a useful tool for conducting controlled experimental trials where precise stimuli can be delivered to participants with ASD, while perceptual, attentional, and emotional responses can be objectively recorded using psychophysiological measures such as skin conductance level (SCL), heart-rate variability (HRV) indices, respiration rate, electromyogram (EMG), eye tracking, and other similar peripheral variables, and potentially also electroencephalogram (EEG) and event-related potentials (ERP).

The major objective of this chapter is to review and to evaluate the feasibility of an approach that is aimed to assess basic emotional reactivity, social competence, and joint attention in high-functioning children with autism (HFA) during exposure to VR environment with concurrent psychophysiological monitoring. It is tempting as well to consider and examine the possibility whether training emotional reactivity, social skills, and joint attention initiation and responsiveness in VR-based course has the potential to improve the above skills. Based on the existing literature (e.g., Blocher and Picard 2002; Cobb et al. 2002; Parsons et al. 2002, 2004; Moore et al. 2005; Herrera et al. 2006, 2008; Bailenson et al., 2008; Naoi et al. 2008; Josman et al. 2011; Jarrold et al. 2013), our pilot studies on children using exposure to two-dimensional (2D) and VR emotional scripts (Sokhadze et al. 2012a,b; Dombroski et al. 2013; Li and Elmaghraby 2014; Li et al. 2015), and studies on autonomic activity alterations in ASD (van Engeland 1984; van Engeland et al. 1991; Porges, 1995, 2003; Althaus et al. 1999, 2004; Hirstein et al. 2001; Ming et al. 2005, 2011; Toichi and Camio 2003; Patriquin et al. 2013; Schaaf et al. 2015) we propose that the well-documented deficits in joint attention, social competence, and emotional responsiveness will manifest in individuals with ASD compared with typically developing children in terms of weaker social communication skills, poorer performance on social skills tests, and less differentiated and altered emotional reactivity to affective stimulation in VR assessed using psychophysiological biomarkers.

Unlike other therapeutic test options, such as role-playing, VR represents more realistic experiences in a safe, controllable manner that allow for repeated practice and exposure, which is a key element in any training or occupational treatment. The flexibility of the VR environment, without the stress of face-to-face interactions with an instructor, may be very appealing to many individuals with ASD. All the above-stated advantages of VR-based psychophysiological profiling system suggest that VR may prove to be a more effective platform for the functional assessment of social skills, social cognition, and emotional and social reciprocity in children with ASD compared to other diagnostic tools. This requires a careful examination and review of the current state of VR applications in autism research and treatment.

18.2 Review of the state of the art of VR application in autism

Only few VR studies in individuals with ASD have been reported (for review, see Bellani et al. 2011). Earlier studies have found that VR can be utilized by children with ASD as a learning tool (Strickland 1997), to teach safety skills (Josman et al. 2011), to engage their interest (Cobb et al. 2002), to monitor eye gaze (Lahiri et al. 2011, 2015), to aid learning of pretend play (Herrera et al. 2006, 2008), and to more accurately interpret emotions of VR avatars (Moore et al. 2005; Cheng and Ye 2010). It should be noted that VR applications were also used in the past as therapeutic tools to help people with autism to recognize emotions and improve their mentalizing (theory-of-mind) skills (Cobb et al. 2002; Picard 2009; Palmen et al. 2012; Kandalaft et al. 2013).

Previous studies reported preliminary findings using social scenes of a virtual café and/or virtual bus ride situation in children with ASD. The VR software provided users an opportunity to maneuver an avatar and engage in simplified interactions, such as finding a place to sit, placing order to a waiter, and so on. Parsons et al. (2002, 2004) investigated the use of the virtual café in teenagers with ASD having only mild impairments. When compared to the matched controls, the ASD group had difficulties maneuvering avatars. The ASD children were reported to engage in the virtual environment as a representation of reality. A qualitative case study of two adolescents was conducted to further investigate the use of VR in ASD interventions (Parsons et al. 2004) and results indicated that the ASD adolescents interpreted VR as lifelike, while enjoying the task and discussions with the real-life facilitator seated next to them. A subsequent study utilized trained raters to quantify social judgment and reasoning in six adolescents using Likert scales at three time points. These preliminary studies have demonstrated that individuals with ASD can use, appropriately understand, enjoy, and practice social interactions in VR settings.

While these previous VR studies showed some promise and perspective, they were limited in several ways. First, the VR software in these studies incorporated using keyboard, mouse, or joystick to click on the screen to activate feedback on programmed social decisions. Second, the measurement of social performance over time was limited to few experimental measures and raters' evaluations. The measurement of social skills and social competence behavior is difficult, especially since few social measures are published or standardized. A further complication is the lack of sensitive measures of physiological responses to emotional stimuli and social cues. The need for reliable and valid tools to measure social cognition and functioning remains a challenge, particularly for adolescents and young adults with ASD. Another, and probably the most important, limitation of the prior studies was the absence of any psychophysiological measurement, reduced flexibility of the skills training programs, and inability of dynamic interaction guided by the emotional status of participants. Majority of the VR social skills training studies were limited to children and used simplistic VR scripts. Only a few were conducted on adolescents and young adults with ASD, a population that might benefit the most from the ability to use VR for evaluation and training of more advanced social skills. In addition to the listed limitations, it must be specifically noted that some of the studies cited above were "virtual simulators" on regular 2D screen computers, rather than actual immersive helmet-based VR studies, and such studies cannot even qualify to use VR terminology in their titles.

18.3 Suggested directions of future research using VR in ASD

Our suggestions of research directions are more oriented at creating a basis for research in VR platform and social skills and social cognition testing utilizing technology that uses ongoing physiological activity changes during exposure to VR for mapping facial expression, vocal prompts, and/or movement on the avatar in VR and modifications in the VR environment. This will allow more naturalistic real-time facial affect and bodily gestures to be projected onto an avatar in the VR scene, thus decreasing the loss of social information from real life to VR, and creating deeper immersion and presence feeling in children and adolescents with ASD. Among the important advantageous features of the VR system with psychophysiological monitoring can be listed a possibility to create environments where children can learn rules and repeat the tasks, while experimenters may concurrently monitor participants' vital functions (e.g., heart rate and skin conductance and temperature) and further correlate their emotional states during exposure to emotional and social challenges. Furthermore, interacting with avatars in VR, where social situations are replicated and explained in detail, will enable ASD patients to work on these situations and find more flexible and socially appropriate solutions of these situations, and to show less signs of emotional overreactivity and anxiety.

The proposed future technology trend should make it possible to create avatars or more real-looking characters and environments to enable participants with autism to work on facial emotional expressions and recognize them while also creating controlled environments to make them feel safe and not feel stressful pressure. Therefore, this technology can provide clear advantages as a functional diagnostics tool and even as a support tool in social communication skills training. In addition to environment and facial and bodily emotional cues, it can be enhanced by verbal and gesture-based interaction in VR environments, achieving even more effective social communication imitations in children with ASD.

This means that virtual environment may represent a novel adequate instrument to work on social skills, emotional reciprocity, social and emotional competence assessment, and even probably also training of these skills in ASD population. Some reviews, positive preliminary results, and case studies were already reported in the literature (Cobb et al. 1997; Strickland 1997; Moore et al. 2005; Herrera et al. 2006, 2008; Ehrlich and Miller 2009; Cheng and Ye 2010; Schwartz et al. 2010; Bellani et al. 2011; Jarrold et al. 2013; Kandalaft et al. 2013). For instance, Josman et al. (2011) developed a safe environment using VR technology, which enabled persons with ASD to learn how to cross the street. Six children with ASD formed the experimental group and six children with neurotypical development formed the control group. The researchers concluded that persons with ASD learned the skills needed to make the right decisions when crossing the street in a virtual environment and thus, the knowledge acquired could be applied to real situations. Virtual environments have also been studied to help learn skills such as playing. Herrera et al. (2006, 2008) conducted two case studies on children with autism in which they evaluated this skill with virtual environments. The findings showed improvement in play skills following the intervention. Ehrlich and Miller (2009) developed a 3D virtual world called Animated Visual Supports for Social Skills (AViSSS). This system enabled patients with Asperger's syndrome to work on social skills training using different environments and situations. Participants had to choose how to behave or select objects. This platform afforded them the opportunity to practice different social situations without the tension or anxiety involved in the real world. However, during the initial tests, the authors concluded that the students with ASD did not respond well to the virtual teacher, due to the fact that they appeared to perceive teachers as being uninterested, impatient to deal with them.

A growing number of studies are investigating applications of advanced interactive technologies such as VR environments for social communication-related intervention. Nevertheless, only few studies have measured not only observable behavioral signs of the engagement of individuals with ASD with these tasks but also psychophysiological engagement indices (as expressed through phasic heart rate deceleration, skin conductance response [SCR], gaze direction, etc.). The research reported in Lahiri et al. (2011, 2015) combined a simulation-based conversational learning system with physiological measures of predicted engagement to determine if there are possibilities for improvement in learning trajectories of people with ASD when the quasi-VR (nonimmersive) system responds to the participants considering their engagement levels in addition to their performance on the task.

Actual VR systems can offer the benefit of representing abstract concepts through visual means (e.g., thought bubbles with text descriptions of a virtual character's thoughts, changes of colors, shading, and brightness) and allow for fast or gradual changes to the environment that may be impossible to accomplish in a real-world setting. VR can also depict various scenarios that may not be feasible in a "real-world" therapeutic setting, given naturalistic social constraints and resource challenges. Thus, VR is well suited for creating interactive skill training paradigms in core areas of impairment for individuals with ASD. As an important addition, profile of phasic and tonic physiological measures can be used as an important index of emotional experience, which can provide feedback regarding participant's engagement, learning, and intervention outcome.

Given the promise of VR-based social interaction and the usefulness of monitoring autonomic nervous system (ANS) activity in real time, novel VR and ANS-based dynamic interactive systems should be planned to be developed and tested in the near future. In more advanced versions of VR environments, participants with ASD will not merely observe virtual "avatars" in the VR environment but will also be able to interact with them during engagement into bidirectional communication. However, operationalization of "engagement" in such a prospective system should not be tied to a specific concrete emotional state, such as participant self-ratings of emotion or only behavioral observation. Rather, "engagement" should be assessed using a pattern of dynamical changes in specific physiological signals (e.g., simultaneous phasic heart rate deceleration and specific SCR in a given emotional context). Thus, the system of this type would uniquely combine VR with measurements of physiology pattern to develop an individualized adaptive capability in VR-based autism intervention technology. In this regard, it is extremely important to have the ability to recognize behavioral or emotional state using psychophysiological indices.

Prior pilot findings and theoretical consideration provide support for a utility of VR as a tool of engagement for children who participate in intervention aimed at improving social engagement and emotional communication skills. The current perspective of the directions of VR for ASD population specifically emphasizes the important role of the autonomic system in supporting social engagement behaviors and the need of combining VR exposure with concurrent event-synchronized psychophysiological monitoring.

18.4 Emotional state detection and differentiation using psychophysiological measures

Emotional state detection, recognition, and strength assessment using psychophysiological measures is one of the greatest challenges in affective neuroscience research (Ekman et al. 1983; Stemmler 1989, 1992; Levenson 1992, 1994; Collet et al. 1997; Adolphs 2001; Kim et al. 2004; Bachevalier and Loveland 2006; Kreibig 2010; Gouizi et al. 2011; Khezri et al. 2015). Accurate emotion recognition would allow psychophysiological monitoring systems with relevant applications to recognize emotion occurrence and therefore react accordingly by changing the VR environment. Most promising should be an approach for emotion recognition that will be based on physiological (mostly autonomic) signals profile or pattern analysis (Stern and Sison 1990; Sohn et al. 2001; Sokhadze 2007; Jang et al. 2015).

The emotions can be readily induced through the presentation of VR scenes to the subjects. The more important issue is the selection of sufficiently affect-sensitive psychophysiological measures and their combination from recorded electrophysiological signals. The physiological signals of interest in this analysis will be focused on electromyogram, respiratory volume (RV), skin temperature (SKT), electrodermal activity (EDA) including skin conductance level, skin conductance response, frequency of nonspecific SCR (NS.SCR), photoplethysmogram (PPG) or electrocardiogram (ECG) for heart rate (HR), and HR variability (HRV, in both time and frequency domains). The electrophysiological signals (EMG, ECG, EDA) and derivate measures (e.g., HR, HRV, SCR, NS.SCR, and pulse volume [PV]) are selected to extract characteristic parameters and their combination, which could be used to detect emotional response, to evaluate the strength of induced emotion, and for classifying the emotions. The focus on autonomic measures sounds quite justified considering their role in the detection of emotions.

Identification and differentiation of emotions by autonomic manifestations can be guided by the following conceptual and methodological approaches. First, there is a need of identification of the pattern of autonomic variables' characteristic to the onset (occurrence) of the basic emotions under study (happiness, sadness, anger, etc.). In a similar manner, it might be focused not on individual emotions from the list of basic emotions but on an identification of the patterns specific to a particular group of emotions classified according to their position in two-dimensional affective space (positive–negative valence, high–low arousal). Second, there is a need to develop signatures (i.e., emotion-specific profiles) using electrodermal, vascular, and cardiorespiratory measures. Selection of the measures differentially sensitive to specific aspects of emotional manifestations, including those that are biomarkers of emotion onset, the time course of emotional manifestation, and termination of emotional state is needed. Short-term pulse volume decrease, positive direction of phasic HR change (acceleration), flattening of HR (decreased HRV), decrease of temperature, and high amplitude of specific (orienting) SCR is a pattern of anger onset, while the magnitude of SCR, tonic SCL change over time, NS.SCR frequency and magnitude of HR change, and tonic HR level can serve as a pattern describing the intensity of experienced anger. Similar

379

constructs can be developed for each emotion (or class of emotions using dimensional affective space measures) incorporating both qualitative and quantitative methods of assessment of emotion-related physiological responses. Third, there is a need of identification of normative values of basic parameters (dependent on age and gender) and normative reactivity measures (response, nonresponse rate, floor–ceiling of parameters, virtual reality sensory modality specificity and VR situational contexts, age–gender deviations, etc.) for typical children, and for those with ASD diagnosis. Other important considerations include requirements of identification of individual differences (personality traits, temperament, etc.), which affect the emotional reactivity and concomitant psychophysiological profiles of responses within a given emotional context (Stemmler 1989, 1992; Witvliet and Vrana 1995). One more objective should be development of sufficiently effective rules for the classification of children under study according to their preferential reactivity channel (e.g., mostly sympathetic reactivity in ASD) and general lability of particular monitored responses (e.g., low lability of parasympathetic system in ASD). Resolving the crucial needs of the VR system listed above with psychophysiological monitoring would be helpful in the creation of the template and decision-making rules for the algorithm for the classification of emotions by their physiological manifestations, further reliable differentiation of particular emotions (or their belonging to particular type of emotions), and labeling their relative strength.

18.5 Autonomic balance dysfunctions in autism

18.5.1 Heart-rate variability and phasic HR responses

Several types of autonomic dysfunctions have been reported in autism, including increased basal sympathetic tone, as well as reduced baseline parasympathetic activity in association with increased baseline sympathetic tone (Palkovitz and Wiesenfeld 1980; Porges 1995; Corona et al. 1998; Hirstein et al. 2001; Julu et al. 2001; Porges 2003; Althaus et al. 2004; Ming et al. 2005, 2011; Kylliäinen et al. 2006; Sokhadze et al. 2012a,b; Dombroski et al. 2013; Hensley et al. 2013; Casanova et al. 2014, 2015; Schaaf et al. 2015; Wang et al. 2016). Heart-rate variability measures are widely used in psychopathology research (Berntson et al. 1997, 1998) for the assessment of phasic and tonic cardiac autonomic control, including the task of emotional response differentiation (Collet et al. 1997; Sohn et al. 2001; Kim et al. 2004; Gouizi et al. 2011; Jang et al. 2015). Reduced HRV, specifically the attenuated power of the high frequency (HF, usually calculated as the spectral power in the 0.15–0.4 Hz range) component of the HRV (also called "respiratory sinus arrhythmia" [RSA]), is an indicator of limited psychophysiological flexibility (Thayer and Lane 2000, 2005).

Several studies have shown that typical children suppressed the HF in HRV more than autistic children, and autistic children have unusually small deceleratory HR responses to stimuli (Hirstein et al. 2001; Ming et al. 2005, 2011; Porges 2003; Althaus et al. 2004; Patriquin et al. 2013; Li and Elmaghraby 2014; Li et al. 2015; Schaaf et al. 2015). The vagus nerve activity deficits may also affect the ability of children with autism to engage in social communication (Porges 2003). Dysfunctions in the parasympathetic system negatively affect social behavior in infants and young children with ASD by impacting heart rate modulation. The inhibitory parasympathetic vagus nerve acts as a brake and slows the heart rate (Porges et al. 1996; Porges 2003). Functionally, the vagal "brake," which modulates HR, enables rapid engagement and disengagement with objects and people, a skill important for promoting social behaviors (Porges 1995, 2003).

Heart-rate variability represents a measure that has already started to be intensively used in psychopathology research (Thayer and Friedman 2002) for the assessment of cardiac autonomic control (Berntson et al. 1997). Deficits in the modulation of the HRV in HF range in different social tasks have been found in autism. Typical children suppressed the HF in HRV more than children with autism (Hutt et al. 1975; Althaus et al. 1999). Analysis of the HRV, and specifically the HF of HRV, and short-term (phasic) HR responses associated with dynamic parasympathetic activity may provide very important information about the autonomic dysfunctions in autism. The HRV measures along with other autonomic measures (e.g., SCR) can be used for the detection of emotional response occurrence and even for the differentiation between several basic emotions (Sohn et al. 2001; Kim et al. 2004; Kreibig 2010) and labeling the strength of evoked emotions.

18.5.2 Electrodermal activity and sympathetic overarousal in autism

Studies of the ANS in autism have demonstrated several manifestations of abnormal sympathetic functions. Skin conductance response studies in autism have shown a lack of the normal habituation in the SCR to the same stimulus over time (van Engeland 1984; van Engeland et al. 1991). Children with autism had blunted HR and SCR responses to visual or auditory social stimuli (Palkovitz and Wisenfeld 1980; Hirstein et al. 2001). Higher basal tonic electrodermal activity as well as larger SCRs to sounds were observed in autistic children compared to controls. All these findings are indications of increased basal sympathetic tone in autism (Hirstein et al. 2001). Stereotyped and repetitive motor behavior, which is one of the core features of autism, has been proposed as a response to reduce hyperresponsive sympathetic activity (Toichi and Kamio 2003). Furthermore, several of our own pilot studies (Sokhadze et al. 2012a,b; Dombroski et al. 2013; Hensley et al. 2013; Casanova et al. 2014; Li and

Elmaghraby 2014; Li et al. 2015) also support excessive but less differentiated SCR to affective audio, visual, and audiovisual stimuli. Since SCL is controlled solely by sympathetic inputs (Boucsein 2012), the above effects are indications of high sympathetic tone and low selectivity of autonomic responses in autism. Other informative electrodermal measures include number of nonspecific SCR (NS.SCR) and amplitude and latency of specific SCR to known stimulus (Boucsein 2012). The importance of autonomic dysfunctions should be considered in more detail given the role of autonomic control in social interaction context.

18.6 Importance of autonomic control assessment in understanding social deficits in autism

Many studies have shown that poor control of HR, vulnerability to tachycardia, and flat HRV curve are negative consequences of chronic increased sympathetic activity paired with decreased vagal tone (Berntson et al. 1998). In a study of Althaus et al. (2004), children with autistic-type difficulties in social adjustment showed a decrease in central vagal tone during task performance as compared to typical children. High vagal tone enhances cardiac control in terms of beat-to-beat adjustments to environmental demands. Low vagal tone, in contrast, is associated with a more rigid and inflexible system vulnerable to dysregulated responses to stressors and situational demands (Thayer and Friedman 2002). High levels of baseline vagal tone have been described to be associated with greater awareness and reactivity to the environment (Porges et al. 1996; Althaus et al. 1999; Porges 2003). Poorer modulation for vagal tone, on the other hand, has been associated with greater social anxiety, while lower vagal tone was associated with greater defensiveness and lower behavioral activation sensitivity (Movius and Allen 2005).

Cardiac vagal tone has been proposed as a stable biological marker for the ability to sustain attention and regulate emotions, and can be used as a predictor of behavioral and emotional dispositional tendencies (Porges 1995; Movius and Allen 2005). The ability to suppress vagal tone was related to fewer behavioral problems in preschool, greater sustained attention, and better behavior regulation (Suess et al. 1994; Porges et al. 1996; Calkins 1997). From the neurovisceral integration perspective (Thayer and Lane 2000; Thayer and Friedman 2002), the baseline sympathetic arousal found in ASD may be a condition of disinhibition, resulting from compromised baseline parasympathetic inhibition. Transient suppressions of vagal cardiac control and its reinstatement for self-regulation necessarily involve both subcortical and prefrontal cortical structures. Thus, cardiac activity regulation is a critical biological function, which interfaces involuntary responses and automatic behaviors with learned, inhibitory, and executive cognitive and attentional capacities.

18.7 Phasic and tonic heart-rate responses as indicators of attention and emotion processes

Heart rate is known as a traditional measure in developmental psycho-physiology (Porges 1991). The parameters of HR include directional changes (HR deceleration and acceleration) and the magnitude of HR changes in response to particular emotion-eliciting stimulus, social communication cue, or social interaction situation (Fox and Calkins 1993). With respect to patterns of HR changes, Laceys showed HR acceleration in "environmental rejection" situations in which the stimulation is aversive and requires the mobilization of internal resources for a response, and HR deceleration in "environmental intake" situations requiring the taking in information (Lacey and Lacey 1970; Stern and Sison 1990). It has been suggested that the various types of HR changes (i.e., tonic shifts in level, decelerative and accelerative phasic changes, and short latency variations in the duration of individual cardiac cycles) are manifestations of motor and perceptual preparatory responses and of information-processing activities. Therefore, the measures of cardiac activity can be useful as indirect indices of cognitive processing of stimulus in social context. Parasympathetic inputs are assumed to play a leading role in the mediation of dynamic HR changes, especially when immediate engagement of attention is required (Porges 1995). The evoked HR responses, often used to monitor cognitive activity and affect (Graham et al. 1970; Porges 1991, 1995), are controlled by the sympathetic and parasympathetic nervous systems. Heart rate acceleration is assumed to be a manifestation of excitatory sympathetic influences, and heart rate deceleration to be a manifestation of the inhibitory parasympathetic influences via the vagus. However, in virtually every situation in developmental research, the phasic HR changes are primarily mediated by the vagus (Porges and Fox 1986). Thus, although the mean HR is determined by the additive input of the tonic sympathetic and parasympathetic systems, the evoked HR response in children is determined primarily by the changing vagal tone (Porges and Fox 1986; Porges 1991, 1995).

18.8 Social engagement deficits in autism and HRV

It was shown that children with serious problems in communication and interaction with others are featured with significantly less cardiac responsiveness to the demands of attention task, and show greater limitation in behavioral control of attention than do healthy children (Althaus et al. 1999). In other studies, the HRV measures were related to performance on attention task and appeared to correlate with several measures of the children's observable behavior (Jennings 1986; Jennings et al. 1997). There are also other studies suggesting that lower executive control of behavior is associated with decreased vagal modulation of cardiac responses and generally attenuated autonomic responsiveness to task-related information processing in individuals with autism (Zahn and Kruesi 1993). Most of these studies have found that children with ASD are less capable of flexible allocation of energy to cope with task requirements. Thus, deficient vagal responses in autistic subjects are probably reflecting a reduced ability to mobilize processing resources appropriately and may result in a flattened affect and general detachment from the environment (Zahn and Kruesi 1993; Porges et al. 1996). Besides decreased vagal tone and reduced ability to timely access task-related processing resources, Althaus et al. (2004) suggested that the resulting decreased peripheral feedback (e.g., via vagal afferents) may fail to form coherent somatic representations (so-called somatic markers, Damasio 1996) required for the development of mental representations of somatic states. Therefore, reduced autonomic feedback may represent yet another functional aspect of unbalanced autonomic responsiveness in autism, which may negatively affect the normal development of social communication skills.

18.9 Pilot data of psychophysiological reactivity of children with ASD to emotional stimuli

18.9.1 Introduction

In order to gain more data of physiological responses of children with ASD to affective stimulation, a series of experiments were conducted by our research team. These experiments were aimed to analyze emotions induced by affective audio, facial expression pictures, videos, and 3D VR scenarios. Some of the experiments were conducted for other affect reactivity-related projects, but all experiments included children with ASD as subjects. Children with ASD often suffer from emotional impairment, and thus the "standard" emotional responses of autism group were expected to be different from typically developed persons.

18.9.2 Measurement of the ANS-dependent variables

18.9.2.1 Experiments 1–2   Electrocardiogram, electromyogram from the dominant hand, pneumogram (PNG), and electrodermal activity were acquired by a NeXus-10 wireless system (Mind Media, B.V., the Netherlands) with BioTrace+ software. Three Ag/AgCl electrodes were attached for the measurement of Lead II ECG, and PNG was recorded with a strain gauge transducer. EDA was recorded by Ag/AgCl electrodes attached to the distal phalanx of the index and middle fingers to measure skin conductance level, skin conductance response, and a number of nonspecific SCRs per min (NS.SCR). *Cardiovascular activity*: Average heart rate; the standard deviation of the HR (SDHR); power of high frequency (HF), low frequency (LF), very-low-frequency (VLF) components; % power of LF (%LF [of VLF + LF + HF]) and of HF (%); and the ratio of the LF over the HF (LF/HF ratio is used as an indirect autonomic balance index) of HRV were calculated as cardiac activity measures. Artifact-corrected 3 min long recording epochs were analyzed with the fast Fourier transform (FFT) to assess HRV. Integrals of the spectrum in 0.003–0.04 Hz (VLF of HRV), 0.04–0.15 Hz (LF of HRV), and 0.15–0.40 Hz (HF of HRV) bands were measured (in ms^2). Furthermore, all HR data were analyzed offline using Kubios HRV software (Finland). *Respiratory activity*: Respiration rate (RESP) on per minute basis, inspiration wave amplitude (IA), and peak respiration frequency (PFRQ) were calculated. These measures are used to control HF peak in HRV related to respiratory frequencies in HRV. *Electrodermal activity*: Skin conductance level (in μS) and amplitude of the SCR, defined as fluctuation with more than 0.02 μS increment, and NS.SCR—number of nonspecific SCR (per minute)—were calculated. The magnitude of SCR and NS.SCR corresponds to the strength of the emotion and can be used as an indicator of quantitative aspects of emotional arousal and reactivity (Sohn et al. 2001; Boucsein 2012). *EMG*: Integrated EMG measures were used for muscle tension assessment and detection of gross movements.

18.9.2.2 Experiments 3–4 The recording in Experiments 3–4 was conducted using C2 monitor of J&J Engineering Inc. (Poulsbo, Washington) with USE software and Physiodata applications. ECG was recorded using three Ag/AgCl electrodes (Lead I), EDA was recorded by dry Ag/AgCl electrodes attached to the distal phalanx of the index and middle fingers, and EMG was recorded from the right hand.

18.9.2.3 Experiment 5 The autonomic nervous system variables in Experiment 5 included heart rate recorded using photoplethysmogram, heart-rate variability indices (LF, HF, LF/HF ratio, etc.), skin conductance response, and pulse volume (PV), and so on. The sensors were from ProComp Infiniti, and the software to collect and store data was the BioGraph Infiniti produced by Thought Technology Ltd (Montreal, Quebec, Canada).

18.9.3 Results

18.9.3.1 Experiment 1 Baseline level of autonomic activity was investigated in 19 children with ASD (mean age 12.9 ± 1.8 years) and 21 typically developing subjects (16.8 ± 5.2 years). Analysis of autonomic measures during 5 min long resting baseline revealed higher HR (93.5 beats per minute [bpm] in ASD versus 80.4 bpm in controls, $F = 5.95$, $p = 0.019$), higher SCL (7.3 μS versus 4.4 μS in controls, $F = 4.74$, $p = 0.036$), and a tendency ($F = 3.93$, $p = 0.056$) to lower power of HF component of HRV in autism. High basal tonic SCL and accelerated HR in association with lower HRV index found in children with autism are indicators of excessive sympathetic and reduced parasympathetic activation in ASD.

18.9.3.2 Experiment 2 We used affective sounds chosen from the International Affective Digitized Sound (IADS, Bradley and Lang 1999) database that provides international affective digitized sounds. The effects of affective sounds were investigated in eight children with ASD (12.5 years) and six age-matched controls. Children with ASD showed higher HR in response to both emotional and neutral 6 s long sounds (e.g., negative, 96.8 in ASD versus 67.4 bpm in controls, $F = 13.75$, $p = 0.004$; neutral, 97.4 versus 66.7 bpm in controls, $p = 0.003$), and higher SCL (positive, 8.05 μS in ASD versus 4.4 μS in controls, $F = 5.43$, $p = 0.04$; negative, 8.21 μS versus 4.48 μS, $F = 5.34$, $p = 0.04$; neutral, 8.04 μS versus 4.2 μS, $F = 6.15$, $p = 0.03$). The children with ASD showed less pronounced phasic HR deceleration (4 s poststimulus versus baseline) in response to sounds than controls. Though HRV variability measures did not show significant statistical differences, the HF component of HRV in the autism group was lower and nonreactive to stimulation, thus demonstrating decreased responsiveness of the parasympathetic control of HR in this group.

18.9.3.3 Experiment 3 The same group of children participated in the autonomic reactivity test for facial stimuli. Forty-eight facial expression stimuli were selected from Matsumoto and Ekman (2004) and presented on a monitor. The order of presentation was as follows: positive, negative, and neutral. Affective facial stimuli were presented in blocks with eight images of the same emotional content per block. Typical children demonstrated a marginal trend to higher phasic HR deceleration across negative facial expressions than children with autism (mean 2.76 ± 0.38 bpm versus −0.61 ± 1.3 bpm, $p = 0.057$). Most pronounced between-group differences in a form of Emotion × Group interaction were found in HRV measures: LF ($F = 4.92$, $p = 0.03$) and HF ($F = 15.21$, $p < 0.01$). Effect (i.e., power of HF component of HRV) can be described as a lower and emotion-irresponsive cardiac parasympathetic response (i.e., respiratory sinus arrhythmia) in the autistic group, and higher but less differentiated sympathetic response to negative facial images in the autistic group. Therefore, the group of children with autism demonstrated lower parasympathetic and higher basal sympathetic tone during visual affective stimulation in this facial emotion test.

18.9.3.4 Experiment 4 This experiment used video clips to induce emotion in children with ASD. In 18 children with ASD (13.9 years, 5 females) and 8 age-matched typical children, emotional reactivity to episodes from *The Lion King* (Disney) was investigated using autonomic measures. All children were exposed to 8 min of the movie. Children with ASD showed higher HR as compared to controls

(94.6 ± 16.1 bpm versus 78.1 ± 8.5 bpm, $F = 6.57$, $p = 0.017$), with higher power of the LF component of HRV ($F = 5.34$, $p = 0.032$). Skin conductance level, another measure of sympathetic arousal, also tended to be higher in ASD (14.8 ± 7.4 μS versus 10.2 ± 6.2 μS, $F = 3.74$, $p = 0.066$, n.s.).

18.9.3.5 Experiment 5 This experiment used a virtual reality setting to evoke emotional responses. Three emotionally laden VR scenarios were designed and chosen specifically to induce emotion states in neutral, negative, and positive context. The scenarios were chosen based on the experience of the above research studies, and were generally divided into three categories: (1) "neutral" scenario was simply exploring VR environment (underwater, with fishes around user), (2) "negative" scenario used affective audio sounds and a series of events (bees, spiders, dinosaurs entering classroom, etc.) that causes fear, disgust, and other uncomfortable experiences, and (3) "positive" scenario was a collection of happy scenes, including interesting bright-colored toys and smiling people, with harmonious music. The hardware to host VR was an Oculus Rift Development Kit 2, and the software platform was Unity 4.6 Pro by Unity Technologies (San Francisco, California) with C++ as the developing language. Autonomic nervous system variables were measured and recorded by sensors attached to subjects simultaneously with exposure to the above VR scenes. The neutral scenario served as an introduction of VR and baseline, in order to eliminate the variation of first exposure to immersive environment. Each scenario took around 3 min for subjects to explore; one session requires exploration of all three scenes, which took 20 min in total, including configuration and mount time. Investigators were able to monitor the scenario by streaming the screen of Oculus to a working computer, in order to take actions when needed.

Then the recorded data were analyzed along with the synchronized events and triggers from the VR scenes. The subjects consisted of a group of four high-functioning children and adolescents with ASD between the ages of 9 and 14 years. As a control group and for general data collection, 20 typically developed individuals (children and undergraduate-level students, 9–19 year range) were recruited to take the same sessions to record the series of ANS data. The common pattern as expected was SCL being low for neutral scenarios, and high for negative scenarios. The major difference was that the autism group showed higher responses across all three scenarios. Nonspecific SCR frequency variables allowed to distinguish negative emotions from neutral and positive emotions ($F = 7.79$, $p = 0.032$), while neutral and positive emotions were not significantly different from each other. On the other hand, using HRV, it was possible to differentiate neutral and positive emotions. In addition, the trend for responses to positive and negative themes was different between the two groups. The common pattern as expected was SCL being low for neutral scenarios and high for negative scenarios.

18.10 Discussion and conclusions

Computer-simulated reality, also called virtual reality, is a multimedia experience that allows users to immerse themselves and interact via different sensors in a safe but realistic environment. The simulated environment creates lifelike experiences to individuals of all ages and it is presently widely used as a means of exposure therapy in anxiety disorders. The technique is of special interest as a therapeutic intervention for individuals with autism spectrum disorder as many of them feel uncomfortable in real-world social interactions and suffer difficulties in communication. Adaptation of VR for emotional competence and social skills testing and assessment in ASD is one of the most appealing possibilities. VR offers the potential to create unique systems for functional testing and, in future developments, even training environments that allow for the precise control of complex and dynamic stimulus presentations.

Subjective reports, behavioral performance, and physiological monitoring can be effectively used to document effects of VR and, in future developments, even affect scenery using feedback. It can be proposed that the integration of VR and applied psychophysiology methods shows promise in controlled autism research studies aimed at the functional assessment of social competence, communication reciprocity, and emotional reactivity in autism. Psychophysiology allows one to systematically monitor the response of ASD participants undergoing VR exposure. Furthermore, physiological feedback (i.e., or so-called physiology-informed and emotional state-driven VR environment modulation) can be used to improve the efficacy of VR immersion and emotionality testing in autism. In addition, during the development of VR worlds specific to this particular neurodevelopmental disorder's symptoms (e.g., emotional cues recognition deficits, poor social communication skills, joint attention abnormalities in autism), psychophysiology may provide objective measurements for assuring that appropriate affective cues included in the VR presentation during test procedure are adequately designed for this population.

All diagnostic manuals (e.g., DSM-IV-TR, DSM-V, ICD-10, ADI–R, and ADOS) include qualitative impairments in emotional competence in autism. However, as Begeer et al. (2008) noted, emotional competence should be acknowledged along with social competence. Diagnostic manuals define emotional and social impairments as marked deficits in using nonverbal behaviors, such as eye contact, gestures, facial expression, postures to enhance social interaction, along with impairments in joint attention expressed in a lack of seeking of sharing or pointing to objects of interests, nor sharing joy, and in general lack of both emotional and social reciprocity. It is not surprising, therefore, that social skills and joint attention targeting interventions are very popular training procedures in individuals with ASD (Mundy 1995; Blocher and Picard 2002; Baron-Cohen and Belmonte 2005; Jones et al. 2006; Kozima et al. 2007; Mundy and Newell 2007; Williams-White et al. 2007; Naoi et al. 2008;

Jones 2009; Mathai and Ruble 2009; Mundy et al. 2009; Palmen et al. 2012). However, the majority of these interventions have been group social skills based, which may limit the amount of practice of social skills and the time spent interacting with others outside those with ASD, that is, with typically developing peers. These interventions may also be somewhat limited by the impacted imagination, which has been frequently noted in this population (Herrera et al. 2008). This lack of naturalistic training may hinder the generalization of social skills training effects. The application of VR-based emotional and social communication skills training may significantly improve the generalization of acquired skills.

Though the initial focus of the review is aimed at targeting the rationale of the development of adequate VR and psychophysiology-based tools for social interaction only of children with ASD, it is reasonable to extrapolate the methodology and procedures on the VR platform developed in the course of this ASD-centered research review perspectives to applications for tests of other neurodevelopmental disorders (e.g., ADHD, dyslexia, and learning disorder). These applications could be adjusted for the use not only in lab settings but also in more natural environments such as outpatient clinics and school and home settings.

Prior reports of our group (Li and Elmaghraby 2014; Li et al. 2015) described several projects under development and plans to develop and evaluate the application of a novel physiologically responsive virtual reality-based technological system for joint attention and social communication skills evaluation in children and adolescents with ASD. The system will alter components of VR and the avatar's behavior based on (1) the performance alone of the subject (correctness of recognition of emotional context or facial expression of emotion) and/or (2) the composite index of physiological metrics of behavioral engagement (e.g., heart rate slowing, SCR, and holding respiration). We propose that psychophysiologically informed VR technologies may have the potential of being very effective tools in the hands of clinical psychologists aiming to improve the quantitative evaluation of social skills in ASD population.

The methodology that uses more realistic stimulation has definite novelty features, as VR is a platform that provides opportunities to practice dynamic and real-life social interactions, which is a computer-based simulation of reality in which visual representations, based on everyday life settings, are presented on a screen of VR helmet. Furthermore, an additional important component of VR might be concurrent real-time physiological activity monitoring that might even be converted into a far more advanced novel solution where VR scenarios are modified using physiological activity inputs. So far, right now, there are no VR-based psychophysiological monitoring systems and no application specifically aimed to test emotional reactivity and joint attention, let alone those that are specifically designed to be used in children with autism.

The main underlying rationale for using VR in children with autism links cardiac underreactivity in socially engaging situations to dysfunctions in autonomic regulation in autism, which results in a reduced attentional capacity to attend socially relevant stimuli critical for effective communication with peers. This outlines an important role of the autonomic nervous system, which is intimately involved in manifestations of affect, emotional expression, facial gestures, vocal communication, and other social behavior. Poor control of HR and vulnerability to tachycardia is an important consequence of chronic increased sympathetic activity and decreased vagal tone. Electrodermal activity measures in autism (SCL, SCR, NS.SCR) both in rest and in response to exposure to emotional cues were reported as showing clear signs of sympathetic overactivation. The baseline sympathetic arousal found in autism may be a condition of disinhibition, resulting from compromised baseline parasympathetic inhibition. Reduced fronto-limbic connectivity and poor prefrontal tonic inhibitory control over limbic system might be one of the reasons of excessive excitation of sympathetic system in ASD.

Changes in HR can be a rich source of information concerning attention processing and their changes in neurodevelopmental disorders. Thus, developmental changes in cardiovascular reactivity seem to be more dependent on cardiac vagal tone and the HRV analysis can contribute to the understanding the specific role of parasympathetic system in social engagement responses in children. Developmental pathology of autonomic control may exert a negative impact on the ability of young children to attend social stimuli and adequately process information in social context.

The application of VR technology enhanced by physiological monitoring means for emotional competence and social skills assessment and enhancement training in children with autism has the potential to result in the development of very unique systems for functional testing, training, manipulation, and precise control of the VR environments. Psychophysiological indices (or pattern of several indices) are sufficiently sensitive to allow the real-time monitoring of emotional state and biomarkers of attentive engagement of participants during VR immersion. Feedback based on psychophysiological indices (i.e., biofeedback or so-called psychophysiology-informed and psychophysiology-driven VR environment modulation) can be used to further improve the efficacy of VR-based autism research and treatment. During the development of VR environments specific to autism spectrum disorder, psychophysiology provides objective measures (mostly using indices of autonomic activity) for assuring that appropriate affective scripts and scenarios are included in testing and social skills training procedures.

The major goal of this chapter was to elaborate the rationale to develop and use VR systems with concurrent psychophysiological monitoring to assess emotional reactivity, social competence, and joint attention in high-functioning children with autism. In addition, the review examined the possibility that training of emotional reactivity, social skills, and joint attention initiation and responsiveness using VR-based training course may improve these skills and their generalization in everyday life.

References

Adolphs, R. 2001. The neurobiology of social cognition. *Curr. Opin. Neurobiol.* 11:231–9.

Althaus, M., L. J. Mulder, G. Mulder, C. C. Aarnoudse, and R. Minderaa. 1999. Cardiac adaptivity to attention-demanding tasks in children with a pervasive developmental disorder not otherwise specified (PDD-NOS). *Biol. Psychiatry* 46:799–809.

Althaus, M., A. M. Van Roon, L. Mulder, G. Mulder, C. Aarnoudse, and R. Minderaa. 2004. Autonomic response patterns observed during the performance of an attention-demanding task in two groups of children with autistic-type difficulties in social adjustment. *Psychophysiology* 41:893–904.

American Psychiatric Association. 2013. *Diagnostic and Statistical Manual of Mental Disorders*, 5th ed. Washington, D.C.: American Psychiatric Press.

Bachevalier, J. and K. A. Loveland. 2006. The orbitofrontal-amygdala circuit and self-regulation of social-emotional behavior in autism. *Neurosci. Biobehav. Rev.* 30:97–117.

Bailenson, J. N., N. Yee, J. Blascovich, A. C. Beall, N. Lundblad, and M. Jin. 2008. The use of immersive virtual reality in the learning sciences: Digital transformations of teachers, students and social context. *J. Learn. Sci.* 17:102–41.

Baron-Cohen, S. and M. K. Belmonte. 2005. Autism: A window onto the development of the social and the analytic brain. *Annu. Rev. Neurosci.* 28:109–26.

Begeer, S., H. Koot, C. Rieffe, M. M. Terwogt, and H. Stegge. 2008. Emotional competence in children with autism: Diagnostic criteria and empirical evidence. *Dev. Rev.* 28:342–69.

Bellani, M., L. Fornasari, L. Chittaro, and P. Brambilla. 2011. Virtual reality in autism: State of the art. *Epidemiol. Psychiatry Sci.* 20:235–8.

Berntson, G. G., J. T. Bigger Jr., D. L. Eckberg, P. Grossman, P. G. Kaufmann, and M. Malik. 1997. Heart rate variability: Origins, methods and interpretive caveates. *Psychophysiology* 34:623–48.

Berntson, G., M. Sarter, and J. T. Cacioppo. 1998. Anxiety and cardiovascular reactivity: The basal forebrain cholinergic link. *Behav. Brain Res.* 94:225–48.

Blocher, K. and R. W. Picard. 2002. Affective social quest: Emotion recognition therapy for autistic children. In *Socially Intelligent Agents: Creating Relationships with Computers and Robots*, eds. K. Dautenhahn, A. H. Bond, L. Canamero, and B. Edmonds, 133–40. Dordrecht: Kluwer Academic Publishers.

Boucsein, W. 2012. *Electrodermal Activity*, 2nd ed. New York: Springer.

Bradley, M. and P. Lang. 1999. The international affective digitized sounds (IADS): Stimuli, instruction manual and affective ratings. NIMH Center for the Study of Emotion and Attention.

Calkins, S. D. 1997. Cardiac vagal tone indices of temperamental reactivity and behavioral regulation in young children. *Dev. Psychobiol.* 31:125–35.

Casanova, M. F., M. K. Hensley, E. M. Sokhadze, A. S. El-Baz, Y. Wang, X. Li, and L. Sears. 2014. Effects of weekly low-frequency rTMS on autonomic measures in children with autism spectrum disorder. *Front. Hum. Neurosci.* 8:851. doi: 10.3389/fnhum.2014.00851.

Casanova, M. F., E. Sokhadze, I. Opris, Y. Wang, and X. Li. 2015. Autism spectrum disorders: Linking neuropathological findings to treatment with transcranial magnetic stimulation. *Acta Paediatr.* 104:346–55.

Cheng, Y. and J. Ye. 2010. Exploring the social competence of students with autism spectrum conditions in a collaborative virtual learning environment—The pilot study. *Comput. Educ.* 54:1068–77.

Cobb, S., L. Beardon, R. Eastgate et al. 2002. Applied virtual environments to support learning of social interaction skills in users with Asperger's Syndrome. *Digit. Creativity* 13:11–22.

Collet, C., E. Vernet-Maury, G. Delhomme, and A. Dittmar. 1997. Autonomic nervous system response patterns specificity to basic emotions. *J. Auton. Nerv. Syst.* 62:45–57.

Corona, R., C. Dissanayake, S. Arbelle, P. Wellington, and M. Sigman. 1998. Is affect aversive to young children with autism? Behavioral and cardiac responses to experimenter distress. *Child Dev.* 69:1494–502.

Côté S. and S. Bouchard. 2005. Documenting the efficacy of virtual reality exposure with psychophysiological and information processing measures. *Appl. Psychophysiol. Biofeedback* 30:217–32.

Damasio, A. R. 1996. The somatic marker hypothesis and the possible functions of the prefrontal cortex. *Philos. Trans. R. Soc. Lond. B Biol. Sci.* 351:1413–20.

Dombroski, B., M. Kaplan, B. Kotsamanidis, S. M. Edelson, G. Sokhadze, M. F. Casanova, and E. Sokhadze. 2013. Ambient lenses and visuomotor exercise effects on autonomic reactivity in autism. *Appl. Psychophysiol. Biofeedback* 38:235.

Downs, A. and T. Smith. 2004. Emotional understanding, cooperation, and social behavior in high-functioning children with autism. *J. Autism Dev. Disord.* 34:625–35.

Ehrlich, J. A. and J. R. Miller. 2009. A virtual environment for teaching social skills: AViSSS. *IEEE Comput. Graphics Appl.* 29:10–6.

Ekman, P., R. W. Levenson, and W. V. Friesen. 1983. Autonomic nervous system activity distinguishes among emotions. *Science* 221:1208–10.

Fox, N. and S. Calkins. 1993. Multiple-measure approaches to the study of infant emotion. In *Handbook of Emotions*, eds. M. Lewis and J. M. Haviland, 167–84. New York: Guilford Press.

Garcia-Palacios, A., H. Hoffman, A. Carlin, T. A. Furness, and C. Botella. 2002. Virtual reality in the treatment of spider phobia: A controlled study. *Behav. Res. Ther.* 40:983–93.

Graham, F. K., K. M. Berg, W. K. Berg, J. C. Jackson, H. M. Hatton, and S. R. Kantrowitz. 1970. Cardiac orienting response as a function of age. *Psychon. Sci.* 19:363–5.

Goodwin, M. S. 2008. Enhancing and accelerating the pace of autism research and treatment: The promise of developing innovative technology. *Focus Autism Other Dev. Disabil.* 23:125–8.

Gouizi, K., F. Bereksi Reguig, and C. Maaoui. 2011. Emotion recognition from physiological signals. *J. Med. Eng. Technol.* 35:300–7.

Hensley, M., A. El-Baz, M. F. Casanova, and E. Sokhadze. 2013. Heart rate variability and cardiac autonomic measures changes during rTMS course in autism. *Appl. Psychophysiol. Biofeedback* 38:238.

Herrera, G., F. Alcantud, R. Jordan, A. Blanquer, G. Labajo, and C. De Pablo. 2008. Development of symbolic play through the use of virtual reality tools in children with autistic spectrum disorders: Two case studies. *Autism* 12:143–57.

Herrera, G., R. Jordan, and L. Vera. 2006. Abstract concept and imagination teaching through virtual reality in people with autism spectrum disorders. *Technol. Disabil.* 18:173–8.

Hirstein, W., P. Iversen, and V. S. Ramachandran. 2001. Autonomic responses of autistic children to people and objects. *Proc. Biol. Sci. R. Soc.* 268:1883–8.

Hutt, C., S. J. Forrest, and J. Richer. 1975. Cardiac arrhythmia and behavior in autistic children. *Acta Psychiatr. Scand.* 51:361–72.

Jang, E. H., B. Park, M. S. Park, S. H. Kim, and J. H. Sohn. 2015. Analysis of physiological signals for recognition of boredom, pain, and surprise emotions. *J. Physiol. Anthropol.* 34:25.

Jennings, J. R. 1986. Bodily changes during attending. In *Psychophysiology: Systems, Processes and Applications*, eds. M. G. Coles, E. Donchin, and S. W. Porges, 268–89. New York: Guilford Press.

Jennings, J. R., M. W. van der Molen, W. Pelham, K. B. Debski, and B. Hoza. 1997. Inhibition in boys with attention deficit disorder as indexed by heart rate changes. *Dev. Psychol.* 33:308–18.

Jarrold, W., P. Mundy, M. Gwaltney et al. 2013. Social attention in a virtual public speaking task in higher functioning children with autism. *Autism Res.* 6:393–410.

Jones, E. A. 2009. Establishing response and stimulus classes for initiating joint attention in children with autism. *Res. Autism Spectr. Disord.* 3:375–89.

Jones, E. A., E. G. Carr, and K. M. Feeley. 2006. Multiple effects of joint attention intervention for children with autism. *Behav. Modif.* 30:782–834.

Josman, N., H. M. Ben-Chaim, S. Friedrich, and P. L. Weiss. 2011. Effectiveness of virtual reality for teaching street-crossing skills to children and adolescents with autism. *Int. J. Disabil. Hum. Dev.* 7:49–56.

Julu, P. O., A. M. Kerr, F. Apartipoulos et al. 2001. Characterisation of breathing and associated central autonomic dysfunction in the Rett disorder. *Arch. Dis. Childhood* 85:29–37.

Kandalaft, M. R., N. Didehbani, D. Krawczyk, T. T. Allen, and S. B. Chapman. 2013. Virtual reality social cognition training for young adults with high-functioning autism. *J. Autism Dev. Disord.* 43:34–44.

Khezri, M., M. Firoozabadi, and A. R. Sharafat. 2015. Reliable emotion recognition system based on dynamic adaptive fusion of forehead biopotentials and physiological signals. *Comput. Methods Programs Biomed.* 122:149–64.

Kim, K. H., S. W. Bang, and S. R. Kim. 2004. Emotion recognition system using short-term monitoring of physiological signals. *Med. Biol. Eng. Comput.* 42:419–27.

Kozima, H., C. Nakagawa, and Y. Yasuda. 2007. Children-robot interaction: A pilot study in autism therapy. *Progr. Brain Res.* 164:385–400.

Kreibig, S. D. 2010. Autonomic nervous system activity in emotion: A review. *Biol. Psychol.* 84:394–421.

Kylliäinen, A. and J. K. Hietanen. 2006. Skin conductance responses to another person's gaze in children with autism. *J. Autism Dev. Disord.* 36:517–25.

Lacey, J. L. and B. C. Lacey. 1970. Some autonomic-central nervous system interrelationships. In *Physiological Correlates of Emotion*, ed. P. Black, 205–27. New York: Academic Press.

Lahiri, U., Z. Warren, and N. Sarkar. 2011. Design of a gaze-sensitive virtual social interactive system for children with autism. *IEEE Trans. Neural Syst. Rehabil. Eng.* 19:443–52.

Lahiri, U., E. Bekele, E. Dohrmann, Z. Warren, and N. Sarkar. 2015. A physiologically informed virtual reality based social communication system for individuals with autism. *J. Autism Dev. Disord.* 45:919–31.

Levenson, R. W. 1992. Autonomic nervous system differences among emotions: Patterning in emotion. *Psychol. Sci.* 3:23–7.

Levenson, R. W. 1994. The search for autonomic specificity. In *The Nature of Emotion: Fundamental Questions*, eds. P. Ekman and R. J. Davidson, 252–7. New York: Oxford University Press.

Li, Y. and A. S. Elmaghraby. 2014. A framework for using games for behavioral analysis of autistic children. *Computer Games: AI, Animation, Mobile, Multimedia, Educational and Serious Games. The 19th International Conference on Computer Games (CGAMES 2014).* Louisville, KY, 1–4.

Li, Y., A. S. Elmaghraby, and E. M. Sokhadze. 2015. Designing immersive affective environments with biofeedback. *The 20th International Conference on Computer Games (CGAMES 2015)*. Louisville, KY, 73–7.

Mathai, G. and L. Ruble. 2009. Implementing a social skills group for children with autism spectrum disorders. *J. Psychol. Pract.* 15:135–56.

Matsumoto, D. and P. Ekman. 2004. *Japanese and Caucasian Expressions of Emotion (jacfee) and Neutral Faces (jacneuf)*. Berkeley, CA.

Ming, X., P. O. Julu, M. Brimacombe, S. Connor, and M. L. Daniels. 2005. Reduced cardiac parasympathetic activity in children with autism. *Brain Dev.* 27:509–16.

Ming, X., J. Bain, D. Smith, M. Brimacombe, G. Gold von-Simson, and F. B. Axelrod. 2011. Assessing autonomic dysfunction symptoms in children: A pilot study. *J. Child Neurol.* 26:420–7.

Moore, D., Y. Cheng, P. McGrath, and N. J. Powell. 2005. Collaborative virtual environment technology for people with autism. *Focus Autism Other Dev. Disabil.* 20:231–43.

Movius, H. L. and J. J. Allen. 2005. Cardiac vagal tone, defensiveness, and motivational style. *Biol. Psychol.* 68:147–62.

Mundy, P. 1995. Joint attention and social-emotional approach behavior in children with autism. *Dev. Psychopathol.* 7:63–82.

Mundy, P. and L. Newell. 2007. Attention, joint attention, and social cognition. *Curr. Direct. Psychol. Sci.* 16:269–74.

Mundy, P., L. Sullivan, and A. M. Mastergeorge. 2009. A parallel and distributed-processing model of joint attention, social cognition and autism. *Autism Res.* 2:2–21.

Naoi, N., R. Tsuchiya, J. Yamamoto, and K. Nakamura. 2008. Functional training for initiating joint attention in children with autism. *Res. Dev. Disabil.* 29:595–609.

Oculus, VR. 2015. Oculus Rift. Available from: http://www.oculusvr.com/rift

Palmen, A., R. Didden, and R. Lang. 2012. A systematic review of behavioral intervention research on adaptive skills building in high-functioning young adults with autism spectrum disorder. *Res. Autism Spectr. Disord.* 6:602–17.

Palkovitz, R. J. and A. R. Wiesenfeld. 1980. Differential autonomic responses of autistic and normal children. *J. Autism Dev. Disord.* 10:347–60.

Parsons, S., P. Mitchell, and A. Leonard. 2004. The use and understanding of virtual environments by adolescents with autistic spectrum disorders. *J. Autism Dev. Disord.* 34:449–66.

Parsons, S. and P. Mitchell. 2002. The potential of virtual reality in social skills training for people with autistic spectrum disorders. *J. Intellect. Disabil. Res.* 46:430–43.

Patriquin, M. A., A. Scarpa, B. H. Friedman, and S. W. Porges. 2013. Respiratory sinus arrhythmia: A marker for positive social functioning and receptive language skills in children with autism spectrum disorders. *Dev. Psychobiol.* 55:101–12.

Picard, R. W. 2009. Future affective technology for autism and emotion communication. *Philos. Trans. R. Soc. Lond. B Biol. Sci.* 364:3575–84.

Porges, S. W. 1991. Vagal tone: an autonomic mediator of affect. In *The Development of Emotion Regulation and Dysregulation*, eds. J. Garber and K. A. Dodge, 111–28. Cambridge: Cambridge University Press.

Porges, S. W. 1995. Orienting in a defensive world: mammalian modifications of our evolutionary heritage. A polyvagal theory. *Psychophysiology* 32:301–18.

Porges, S. W. 2003. The polyvagal theory: Phylogenetic contributions to social behavior. *Physiol. Behav.* 79:503–13.

Porges, S. W., J. A. Daussard-Roosevelt, A. L. Portales, and S. I. Greenspan. 1996. Infant regulation of the vagal "brake" predicts child behavioral problems: A psychobiological model of social behavior. *Dev. Psychobiol.* 29:697–712.

Porges, S. W. and N. A. Fox. 1986. Developmental psychophysiology. In *Psychophysiology: Systems, Processes and Applications*, eds. M. G. H. Coles, E. Donchin, and S. W. Porges, 611–25. New York: Guilford Press.

Rothbaum, B. O., L. F. Hodges, R. Kooper, D. Opdyke, J. S. Williford, and M. North. 1995. Virtual reality graded exposure in the treatment of acrophobia: A case report. *Behav. Ther.* 26:547–54.

Schwartz, C., G. Bente, A. Gawronski, L. Schilbach, and K. Vogeley. 2010. Responses to nonverbal behavior of dynamic virtual characters in high-functioning autism. *J. Autism Dev. Disord.* 40:100–11.

Schaaf, R. C., T. W. Benevides, B. E. Leiby, and J. A. Sendecki. 2015. Autonomic dysregulation during sensory stimulation in children with autism spectrum disorder. *J. Autism Dev. Disord.* 45:461–72.

Sohn, J. H., E. Sokhadze, and S. Watanuki. 2001. Electrodermal and cardiovascular manifestations of emotions in children. *J. Physiol. Anthropol. Appl. Hum. Sci.* 20:55–64.

Sokhadze, G., M. Kaplan, S. M. Edelson, E. Sokhadze, A. El-Baz, M. Hensley, and M. F. Casanova. 2012a. Effects of ambient prism lenses on autonomic reactivity to emotional stimuli in autism. *Appl. Psychophysiol. Biofeedback* 37:303.

Sokhadze, E. M., M. Kaplan, S. M. Edelson et al. 2012b. Ambient prism lenses affect autonomic reactivity and attention to audio-visual stimuli in autism. *Psychophysiology* 49:S40.

Sokhadze, E. 2007. Effects of music on the recovery of autonomic and electrocortical activity after stress induced by aversive visual stimuli. *Appl. Psychophysiol. Biofeedback* 32:31–50.

Stemmler, G. 1989. The autonomic differentiation of emotions revisited: Convergent and discriminant validation. *Psychophysiology* 26:617–32.

Stemmler, G. 1992. The vagueness of specificity: Models of peripheral physiological emotion specificity in emotion theories and their experimental discriminability. *J. Psychophysiol.* 6:17–28.

Stern, R. M. and C. E. Sison. 1990. Response patterning. In *Principles of Psychophysiology: Physical, Social, and Inferential Elements*, eds. J. T. Cacioppo and L. G. Tassinary, 193–215. New York: Cambridge University Press.

Strickland, D. 1997. Virtual reality for the treatment of autism. In *Virtual Reality in Neuropsychophysiology*, ed. G. Riva, 81–6. Amsterdam: IOS Press.

Suess, P. E., S. W. Porges, and D. J. Plude. 1994. Cardiac vagal tone and sustained attention in school-age children. *Psychophysiology* 31:17–22.

Toichi, M. and Y. Kamio. 2003. Paradoxical autonomic response to mental task in autism. *J. Autism Dev. Disord.* 33:417–26.

Thayer, J. F. and R. D. Lane. 2005. The importance of inhibition in dynamical systems models of emotion and neurobiology. *Brain Behav. Sci.* 28:218–9.

Thayer, J. F. and B. H. Friedman. 2002. Stop that! Inhibition, sensitization, and their neurovisceral concomitants. *Scand. J. Psychol.* 43:123–30.

Thayer, J. F. and R. D. Lane. 2000. A model of neurovisceral integration in emotion regulation and dysregulation. *J. Affect. Disord.* 61:201–16.

van Engeland, H. 1984. The electrodermal orienting response to auditive stimuli in autistic children, normal children, mentally retarded children, and child psychiatric patients. *J. Autism Dev. Dis.* 14:261–79.

van Engeland, H., J. W. Roelofs, M. N. Verbaten, and J. L. Slangen. 1991. Abnormal electrodermal reactivity to novel visual stimuli in autistic children. *Psychiatry Res.* 38:27–38.

Wang, Y., M. K. Hensley, A. Tasman, L. Sears, M. F. Casanova, and E. M. Sokhadze. 2016. Heart rate variability and skin conductance during repetitive TMS course in children with autism. *Appl. Psychophysiol. Biofeedback* 41:47–60.

Wiederhold, B. K. and A. Rizzo. 2005. Virtual reality and applied psychophysiology. *Appl. Psychophysiol. Biofeedback* 30:183–5.

Williams-White, S., K. Keonig, and L. Scahill. 2007. Social skills development in children with autism spectrum disorders: A review of the intervention research. *J. Autism Dev. Disord.* 37:1858–68.

Witvliet, C. V. and C. R. Vrana. 1995. Psychophysiological responses as indices of affective dimensions. *Psychophysiology* 32:436–43.

Zahn, T. P. and M. J. Kruesi. 1993. Autonomic activity in boys with disruptive behavior disorders. *Psychophysiology* 30:605–14.

Chapter 19 The impact of robots on children with autism spectrum disorder

Zhi Zheng, Esubalew
Bekele, Amy Swanson,
Amy Weitlauf,
Zachary Warren, and
Nilanjan Sarkar

Contents

Abstract 398
19.1 Introduction 398
    19.1.1 Robotic platform development 399
    19.1.2 Patterns of robot–children interactions 401
19.2 Representative robot-mediated skill training for children
    with ASD 402
    19.2.1 Robot-mediated joint attention training 402
        19.2.1.1 System development 402
        19.2.1.2 User study results 405
        19.2.1.3 Habituation study 406
    19.2.2 Imitation learning 408
        19.2.2.1 System development 408
        19.2.2.2 User study 410
        19.2.2.3 User study results 410
19.3 Discussion 412
    19.3.1 Increasing the autonomous level of the
        robotic systems 412
    19.3.2 Unrestricted interaction environment 413
    19.3.3 Large group study 413
    19.3.4 Robot-mediated intervention generalization 413
Acknowledgments 414
References 414

Abstract

Robot-mediated intervention for children with autism spectrum disorder (ASD) has been investigated for decades, building tremendous momentum toward further technical development and psychological understanding. The developed robotic platforms for children with ASD possess more and more advanced hardware design and interaction patterns. In this chapter, we review representative robotic studies that have been conducted to help children with ASD. It has been shown that robots can catch and hold the attention of children with ASD, and be used to teach them social communication skills. In addition, we provide detailed examples to illustrate the design and development of effective robot-mediated intervention systems that have been applied to teach children with ASD joint attention and imitation skills. Finally, we discuss a few important research directions that need further exploration.

19.1 Introduction

Autism spectrum disorder (ASD) is a pervasive developmental disorder whose core deficits include impairments in social communication and repetitive abnormal behaviors. In recent years, modern technology has been broadly applied to the study of psychological and neurodevelopmental disorders such as virtual reality environment (Blascovich et al. 2002), computer-assisted intervention (Liu et al. 2008b), and robotic technology (Scassellati et al. 2012). In particular, robotic technology is gaining momentum as an intervention platform for children with ASD. Robots have several advantages over traditional human-led interactions, including precise control of intervention modality, robust consistency, simplified features, autonomous operation, and potential cost effectiveness. Since 1976, when Weir and Emanuel (Weir and Emanuel 1976) found that robots could improve social interaction for children with ASD, a plethora of works have been published that have demonstrated the effectiveness of robotic interventions for children with ASD. This includes exploring children with ASD's response to robot-like characteristics; eliciting specific behaviors; modeling, teaching, and practicing skills; as well as providing feedback and encouragement during interactions (Ricks and Colton 2010; Diehl et al. 2012). In this chapter, we will review representative publications, describe current state-of-the-art research, and explore future directions for the field.

There is significant heterogeneity in studies conducted to date regarding sample size, interaction type, and ages of participants that creates challenges when summarizing the literature. The age range of participants stretches from preschoolers (Ioannou et al. 2015) to teenagers (Pierno et al. 2008). The user group ranges in size from one (Costa et al. 2011) to dozens (Anzalone et al. 2014; Costescu et al. 2015) to hundreds (Scassellati 2005). The interaction patterns mainly included free interactions (Feil-Seifer and Mataric 2011) as well as task-specific interactions (Greczek et al. 2014; Zheng et al. 2014). There were both longitudinal, multisession studies (Costa et al. 2011) and short-term, single-session studies. The results in many multisession studies showed that the children's performance and attention on the robot progressed across sessions (Costa et al. 2011; Zheng et al. 2013). Because ASD is four times more prevalent in males than females, the majority of participants were males, with some exceptions that included equal numbers of both sexes (Pierno et al. 2008). Although most studies conclude that their findings need more extensive testing in the future, this did not often happen, as testing beyond a pilot study is a time-, cost-, and labor-intensive process.

19.1.1 Robotic platform development

There are three main categories of robots that have been utilized with children with ASD. The first category is a traditional machine-like robot. Costa et al. (2011) used a LEGO robot to help a child with ASD learn how to share objects and fulfill orders. Pierno et al. (2008) used a robot arm to study the imitation behavior of children with ASD. Liu et al. (2008a) developed an interactive basketball-playing robot, which could adapt its behavior based on the participant's emotional state. None of these robots resembled living creatures.

The second category is an animal-like robot. Several studies have found that robots with animal features can elicit social behaviors from children with ASD. For example, Stanton et al. (2008) tested the interaction between a robotic dog AIBO and children with ASD. The results showed that the participants were engaged and showed fewer autism symptoms such as verbal engagement and reciprocal interaction. Dickstein-Fischer et al. (2011) built a robotic penguin for the same purpose. Kim et al. (2013) studied how a robotic dinosaur Pleo could elicit social behaviors for children with ASD. Even though the outward appearances were very different, each of these different animalistic designs showed promise for social intervention purposes.

The third category is a humanoid robot, which currently is the most comprehensively designed and widely used robot for ASD-related studies with robots. Even though the appearances of most of the humanoid robots are kept relatively simpler than a real person, their functionalities have been dramatically improved in recent years. Pioggia et al. (2007) developed a robotic face (called FACE) to interact with participants based on their facial expressions, body gestures, and psychophysical signals. Goodrich et al. (2011) developed a robot with two arms and a flat screen face, which presented different facial expressions. Kozima and Yano (2001) developed an upper-body humanoid robot, Infanoid, to investigate its ability to affect social intentionality, identification, and communication as part of ASD intervention. Some researchers created full-body robots as well. Fujimoto et al. (2011) used a full-body humanoid robot to teach children with ASD to imitate arm gestural skills. Wainer, Dautenhahn, Robins, and Amirabdollahian (Dautenhahn et al. 2009; Amirabdollahian et al. 2011; Wainer et al. 2014) developed a full-body child-like robot, KASPAR (Wainer et al. 2014), which is capable of eliciting different social communication behaviors such as joint attention, imitation, tactile exploring, and collaborative game playing. Furthermore, other researchers have used full-body robots within modifiable environments, such as when Feil-Seifer and Mataric (2011) set a humanoid robot on top of a mobile robot and used it to measure children's interaction pattern with respect to distance-based features.

Each of these robots was developed within research labs. However, there are also commercial robotic platforms that have been broadly applied to work with children with ASD, such as the full-body humanoid robots NAO (Bekele et al. 2013; Greczek et al. 2014) and Zeno (Torres et al. 2012; Ranatunga et al. 2013). An advantage of using commercial robots is that a design based on them can be easily reproduced and improved by different groups. However, a general robot platform may not be as flexible and cost effective as a task-customized robot developed as part of research.

During a robot-mediated intervention, the robot usually serves as a game mediator and promoter (Costa et al. 2011), and many functionalities are targeted as such. For example, a primary parameter when designing a robot for ASD intervention is the motion flexibility, which depends on the intervention needs (and the robot's role). A simple robot with only a few degrees of freedom such as "Keepon" (Kozima et al. 2005) is enough to catch children's attention, while a more complex robot-like NAO (Rilling and Insel 1999) is necessary for explicit imitation training. Another parameter is the need for including other peripheral sensing technologies to track the participant's behavior. For example, Boccanfuso et al. developed a doll-like robot CHARLIE (Boccanfuso and O'Kane 2011) with computer vision-based hand and face-tracking functions. Chuah et al. developed a robot LILI (Chuah et al. 2014) that had embedded functionalities, including gesture recognition and speech recognition. Finally, Ravindra et al. (2009) developed a robot with gaze-tracking function for training joint attention skills for children with ASD.

As seen from the above discussion, given the wide range of designs, functions, and capabilities, it is very important to consider a robot's role within an intervention when deciding on its ability to move, catch, and direct a child's attention, and gather data about children with ASD they are helping to treat. It may be more appropriate for certain features to be important in some intervention designs (e.g., the prominence of FACE for promoting facial expressions) than others (e.g., the hand-tracking abilities of CHARLIE). Although all of these technologies have their own limitations in terms of detection accuracy, robustness, and detection range, they represent the general movement of the field toward ideal robotic platforms for different environments and treatment goals.

19.1.2 Patterns of robot–children interactions

A primary question raised regarding using robotic technology for children with ASD is whether the children will accept the robots and interact with them as opposed to humans, due to the differences in the robots' physical appearance, voice, and behavior. In 2005, Robins et al. (2005) conducted a study where the same person interacted with children with ASD in two ways, first while dressing and acting like a robot and then while dressing and acting normally. Similar to other works (Dautenhahn and Werry 2004; Kim et al. 2013; Zheng et al. 2013), their results showed that children with ASD interacted more with the person when he had a simplified robotic appearance. Indeed, children with ASD are interested in robots with a simple appearance. For example, a very simple small yellow snowman-like robot "Keepon" developed by Kozima et al. (2005) was successful in eliciting positive responses from children with ASD. The most obvious appearance features of Keepon are simply an elastic body, two eyes, and one nose. However, the robot successfully elicited positive responses from children with ASD such as playful behaviors with Keepon and induced relaxed mood. Even today, the design principle for robot appearance in many studies still follows the principle of simplicity (Costa et al. 2014).

Currently, data collection on social interactions for robot-mediated intervention is performed using a combination of manual video coding as well as by autonomous methods within the system. In the early days of robotic intervention work, most studies were forced to utilize manual video coding to analyze data, most of which consisted of gaze pattern, tactile pattern, gestures, speech, and other interaction-specific behaviors (Pierno et al. 2008; Stanton et al. 2008; Amirabdollahian et al. 2011; Costa et al. 2011). Later on, as autonomous technologies have improved dramatically, more and more children's behaviors and responses can be tracked and recorded automatically. This laid the groundwork for the development of closed-loop, adaptive interaction systems using increasingly complex, integrated technologies. This includes tracking participants' movements within the test environment. For example, in Pierno et al. (2008), the participant's arm motion was recorded in 3D space by using infrared (IR) cameras that tracked passive markers put on the participants' arms. Bekele et al. (2013) applied a camera-based head-tracking system to approximate children's gaze direction. Greczek et al. (2014) used Microsoft Kinect to track the motion of the participants.

Both manual and automated data-recording methods have their own advantages and disadvantages. The manual video coding method can be used for any visual measurable parameter that cannot be effectively and automatically detected by current technology. However, video coding is impacted by the personal bias of the coder, and it is also labor and time intensive. Technology-based data-recording methods reduce labor time and costs, and avoid personal biases, such as the coder's attention and habits. However, the signals that can be detected automatically are still limited. For instance, camera-based methods are sensitive to illumination and occlusion. Limited tracking rules may not be flexible enough to accommodate different types of participants and for complex interaction recognition. Even so, the development of these technologies represents a primary push of future research trends, and we are optimistic based upon recent advancement that more and more methods will be developed to ameliorate these current limitations.

Scassellati et al. (2012) concluded in a review article that a robot in imitative games should possess three important features, and those can be generalized to other kinds of robot-mediated interactions: (1) the robot must be either controlled remotely or programmed to autonomously observe physical behavior; (2) the robot must know when to begin and sense the child's response with sufficient accuracy; and (3) the robot must be able to map those responses to its own, potentially limited, effectors in order to replicate the behavior as closely as possible, in a recognizable fashion. Based on those principles, we will discuss two of our own works in the next section as examples of building robotic interaction platforms and conducting pilot user studies based on those developed platforms. The first example describes robot-mediated joint attention training, and the second describes robot-mediated imitation training. We present these two examples since joint attention and imitation are two of the most important foundational skills in children's early social communication development, and are among the core deficits in ASD (Boucenna et al. 2014).

19.2 Representative robot-mediated skill training for children with ASD

19.2.1 Robot-mediated joint attention training

Bekele et al. (2013) proposed an adaptive and individualized robot-mediated system, ARIA, for training joint attention skills to children with ASD. The system was composed of the humanoid robot NAO (Rilling and Insel 1999) with its vision augmented by a network of cameras for real-time head pose tracking. Based on the child's head movement, the robot intelligently adapted itself to generate prompts and reinforcements to promote joint attention skills, one of the core deficits of early social orienting for children with ASD. A pilot study of six children with ASD and a control group of six typically developing (TD) children was conducted to validate the proposed system.

19.2.1.1 System development The system arranged in the experiment room is shown in Figure 19.1. The system had two 24-inch computer monitors fixed on the left and right walls in the experiment room, which provided visual and auditory stimuli such as static pictures, audios, and videos. Specific sounds or videos were used as enhanced triggering if a participant did not respond to the robot NAO. These stimuli were

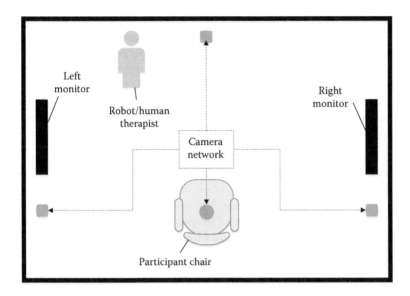

Figure 19.1 ARIA system arrangement in the experiment room.

changed adaptively to provide different joint attention prompt levels and rewards based on the participant's response. The humanoid robot NAO is a child-like humanoid robot with 25 degrees of freedom. It is 58 cm high and weighs approximately 4.3 kg. In this work, NAO's vision was extended using a distributed network of external IR cameras to track the participant's head pose for closed-loop interaction. The robot worked as the prompting agent that guided the participant's attention to speech and gesture stimuli. Figure 19.2 shows the image of the robot pointing toward a target monitor, which was showing a cartoon video.

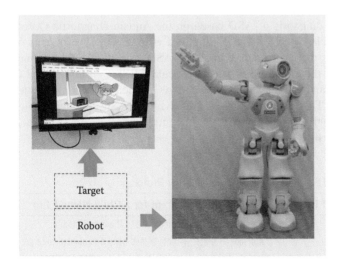

Figure 19.2 Robot NAO and attention stimulus.

A participant's gaze was approximated by the head's frontal orientation. The participant wore a baseball hat modified in-house with an array of infrared light-emitting diodes (LEDs) on its top and sides in straight lines. Those lines could be detected by the IR cameras to indicate the head pose. The frontal head orientation was approximated as the gaze, and was fed back to the robot. ARIA could also be used with human therapist who replaced the humanoid robot but with all other components in place.

To test and verify the ARIA system, a user study was designed based on common paradigms for indexing early joint attention capacity. A behavior protocol was developed based on the least-to-most prompt (LTM) hierarchy (Demchak 1990), which essentially provides support to the learner only when needed. The LTM approach allowed us to identify the lowest level of prompts needed by each child to look at the target monitor (target hit). Each participant took part in an experiment, which consisted of two human therapist-administered and two robot-administrated subsessions interwoven together. Each subsession was 2–4 min long. There were four trials in each subsession, where each trial consisted of 3–5 s of prompt followed by 3–5 s used to monitor the response of a participant.

The hierarchical prompt protocol in a trial is shown in Table 19.1. The administrator first cued the participant to look at a specific picture displayed on one of the two computer monitors. The next higher prompt level added a pointing gesture to the target by the administrator. The next higher prompt level added an audio prompt at the target, with the pointing gesture cue and the verbal cue. The final level added a video in addition to the last level. If the participant hit the target, the robot would say, "Good job!" and a rewarding video was displayed on the monitor. Otherwise, the robot issued the next level of prompt.

The participants were between 2 and 5 years old, and had an established diagnosis of ASD based on the Autism Diagnostic Observation Schedule Generic (ADOS-G) (Lord et al. 2000). The parents of both groups of participants completed ASD screening/symptom measurements: the Social Responsiveness Scale (SRS) (Constantino and Gruber 2002) and the Social Communication Questionnaire (SCQ) (Rutter et al. 2010). The TD participants did not evidence ASD-specific impairments. The study was approved by the Institutional Review Board of Vanderbilt University.

Table 19.1 Levels of the Hierarchical Protocol

Prompt Levels	Robot Prompt for a Child Named Jim
1 and 2	"Jim, look!" + robot turned head to the target monitor
3 and 4	"Jim, look at that!" + robot turned head and pointed to target monitor
5	Prompt level 4 + audio displayed at the target monitor
6	Prompt level 5 and then video onset for 30 s

Table 19.2 Profile of the Participants in ARIA User Study

	Age	ADOS-G	ADOS CSS	ADOS-G RJA	SRS	SCQ	IQ
ASD_M	4.70	16.0	7.33	1.17	70.33	13.33	71.5
ASD_SD	0.70	6.58	1.97	1.07	12.24	5.91	22.65
TD_M	4.26	NA	NA	NA	45.50	3.83	NA
TD_SD	1.05	NA	NA	NA	3.30	3.53	NA

NA: not applicable.

Initially, 18 participants (10 with ASD and 8 TD) were recruited. Six TD and six ASD participants successfully completed the study. Among the children who did not participate, three out of the four subjects with ASD withdrew because they could not tolerate the hat. One was distressed during the interaction and as such the session was discontinued. Two typically developing children were not willing to participate after parent consent. These difficulties reflect the need for the development of nonwearable technology and underscore that robotic therapies may not be for every child. The details of the TD and ASD group who completed the study are given in Table 19.2.

19.2.1.2 User study results As Figure 19.3 shows, the group with ASD looked at the robot for 52.76% of the robot subsession time in average. By comparison, they looked at the human therapist for 25.11% of the subsession time. *t*-test was used for statistical analysis. The group with ASD looked at the robot therapist 27.65% longer than the human therapist ($p < 0.005$). The TD group looked at the robot therapist for 54.27% of the robot subsession, while they looked at the human therapist for 33.64% of the human subsession. As such, the TD group looked at the robot for 20.63% longer than the human therapist ($p < 0.005$). The results indicated a statistically significant preferential orientation toward the robot as compared to the human therapist for both groups. This difference was most pronounced for the group with ASD than that of the TD group. These findings are similar to another work (Duquette et al. 2008), which found that children with ASD pay more attention to robots than human therapists.

In the robot subsessions, 95.83% trials of the group with ASD and 97.92% trials of the TD group resulted in target hit. The human therapist was able to achieve 100% success for both groups. Taken together with preferential looking data, the robot was able to perform the task with success rates similar to that of the human therapist. As shown in Figure 19.4, the group with ASD required 0.9 more levels of prompt in the robot subsessions than that in the human subsessions. The TD group required 0.6 more levels of prompt in the robot subsessions than that in the human therapist subsessions. Both these differences for the two groups were statistically significant ($p < 0.05$). The TD group required fewer prompt levels for success in general than the group with ASD. In

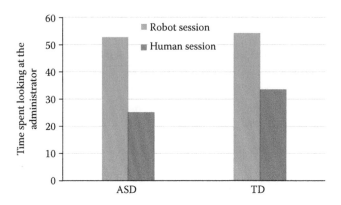

Figure 19.3 Time spent looking at the administrator.

the robot subsession, the TD group required 0.7 fewer prompt levels than the group with ASD while they required 0.4 fewer prompt levels than the ASD group on average in the human therapist subsession.

Generally, children in the group with ASD attended more to the robot and were less attracted by the targets than their TD counterparts. The relatively higher number of prompt levels required for children with ASD might be best attributed to their attention bias for the robot than the nature of the disorder itself.

19.2.1.3 Habituation study The work of ARIA compared a robot versus a human therapist and the potential difference between children with ASD and TD children. Later on, Warren et al. (2015) conducted a habituation study based on this work to explore (1) whether repeated interactions with the robot would impact the children's performance, and (2) whether the initial attentional preference to the robot would hold over time.

The original head-tracking method using a hat described in our previous work was not tolerated by at least 30% of the participants with ASD.

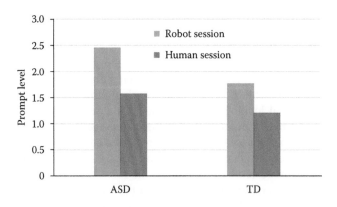

Figure 19.4 Prompt level needed for target hit.

Table 19.3 Diagnoses of the Participants with ASD

	ADOS Raw Score	ADOS Severity Score	SRS-2 Raw Score	SRS-2 T Score	SCQ Lifetime Total Score	IQ	Age
Mean	20.83	8.67	96.17	71.00	17.00	73.67	3.46
Std	5.15	1.86	24.23	9.38	6.32	20.29	0.73

Therefore, in this study, a commercial eye tracker was used for evaluating the participants' attention toward the robot, and a therapist monitored the participant's response in the experiment. Once the participant looked at the target monitor, the therapist pressed a button to inform the robot. Six 2- to 5-year-old children with ASD were recruited for this study. Their characteristics are listed in Table 19.3.

Each of the participants completed four sessions, and each session included eight trials. The trial setup was the same as before except that the video clips were shortened to 10 s to ensure that children would not get used to looking at a particular monitor.

Across all sessions, 99.48% of the trials ended with a target hit. Figure 19.5 displays how the participants' performance improved from session 1 to session 4. In session 1, the average target hit prompt level was 2.17. As children completed sessions and became more familiar with the "game," the target hit prompt level went lower, falling to 1.44 by session 4. Two-sided Wilcoxon rank-sum test was used for this study. The difference between session 1 and session 4 was statistically significant ($p < 0.005$).

We defined the "robot attention region" as a box of 76 cm × 58 cm, which covered the body and arm movement of NAO. We defined this region to quantitatively estimate how much attention a participant paid to the robot by looking within this region in space. Examining looking times across all participants and sessions, the average time that the participants looked at the robot was 14.75%. As shown in Figure 19.6, from session 1 to session 4, participants looked at the robot for 14.88%, 15.17%, 17.94%, and 11.02% of the session time in average, respectively. However, the differences in looking time among all sessions were not statistically significant. This indicates that the initial interest that the participants showed toward the robot did not change significantly with repeated exposure.

This small study indicated that the children with ASD documented sustained interest with the humanoid robot NAO over several sessions and demonstrated improved performance within system regarding joint attention skills. Together, these findings provide support for both robotic system capabilities and potential relevance of application. Robotic systems endowed with enhancements for successfully pushing toward correct orientation to target, with either systematically faded prompting or potentially embedding coordinated action with human partners, might be further capable of taking advantage of baseline enhancements in

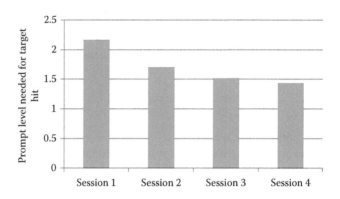

Figure 19.5 Average prompt level needed for target hit.

nonsocial attention preference (Klin et al. 2009; Annaz et al. 2012) in order to meaningfully enhance skills related to coordinated attention.

19.2.2 Imitation learning

Another example of the application of robotics for children with ASD is imitation skill training. Here, we summarize a relevant work conducted by Warren et al. (2015).

19.2.2.1 System development The imitation skill learning system was embedded with the robot NAO and a Microsoft Kinect. Figure 19.7 shows the system arrangement in the experiment room (Mann 1982). The Kinect was placed in front of the participant to track his/her body movement, and the tracked data were sent to a gesture recognition module to compute imitation performance in real time. The distance between the participant and the Kinect was approximately 1.5 m, and the distance between the participant and the robot or human therapist was about 2 m. The robot first showed a target gesture to the child. Then, the child was

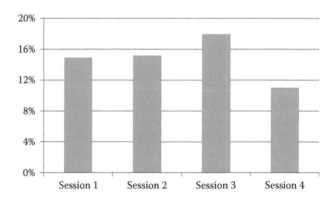

Figure 19.6 Average time spent looking at the robot.

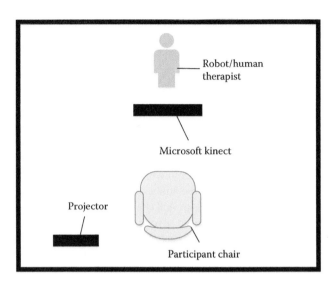

Figure 19.7 Imitation training system arrangement in experiment room.

asked by the robot to imitate the gesture. Based on the performance, the robot either moved toward another gesture or aided the child with reinforced gesture demonstration within their motor movements. The robot gave appropriate rewards and encouragement when the child imitated a gesture correctly. The Kinect 3D face tracking provided robust head pose estimation. The frontal head orientation was used to approximate the participant's attention on the gesture prompting administrator. We used a 85.77 cm × 102.42 cm box around the robot and the upper body of the human therapist as the target attention region. Figure 19.8 illustrates the main components of the system as discussed.

Four gestures were selected for this study: (1) raising one hand, (2) raising two hands, (3) waving, and (4) reaching arms out to the side. These four gestures were simple enough to target the participant's imitation skills rather than gross motor abilities.

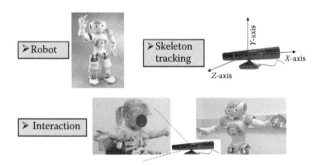

Figure 19.8 Imitation training system demonstration.

Table 19.4 Participant Group Characteristics

	ADOS-G	MSEL	SRS-2 T Score	SCQ	Age
ASD_M	7.63	64.75	75.29	17.88	3.83
ASD_SD	1.69	22.11	12.62	6.58	0.54
TD_M	NA	NA	42.75	3.88	3.61
TD_SD	NA	NA	10.08	2.95	0.64

NA: not applicable.

19.2.2.2 User study   Eight children with ASD and eight typically developing children participated in the study. All children in the ASD group had received a clinical diagnosis of ASD based on DSM-IV-TR (Buldyrev et al. 2000) criteria from a licensed psychologist, met the spectrum cutoff of the Autism Diagnostic Observation Schedule (ADOS) (Lord et al. 2000) and had existing data regarding cognitive abilities from the Mullen Scales of Early Learning (Mullen 1995). Parents of children in the ASD and non-ASD group completed both the Social Communication Questionnaire (Rutter et al. 2010) and the Social Responsiveness Scale (Constantino and Gruber 2002) to index current ASD symptoms (see Table 19.4). The study was approved by Vanderbilt Institutional Review Board.

Each participant had two human-administered subsessions and two robot-administered subsessions. All four gestures were exhaustively tested in a randomized order. We compared participants' performance between the robot sessions and the human sessions regarding imitation of the gestures. We also computed how much attention a participant paid toward the robot and the human administrator.

Prior to the demonstration of each gesture, the robot and human administrator imitated the child's movements for 15 s followed by the verbal prompt, "Let's play! I will copy you!" A trial was started after the gesture mirroring. The administrator (robot or human) first gave the verbal prompt, "Okay! Now you copy me. Look at what I am doing!" and then demonstrated a gesture twice and said, "You do it!" If correct, the child was presented with praise and asked to imitate the gesture again. If incorrect, the system copied the child's movements and then transferred from this position to the correct gestural movement. The robot then asked the child to imitate the presented gesture again. In the human therapist-administered subsessions, the human replicated robot-administered trials. The control flow was computed by the system and the human therapist followed instructions projected on the wall behind the participant. Therefore, the human therapist could fully match what would happen in robot-administered trials, while still maintaining eye contact with the participant.

19.2.2.3 User study results   Attention to the administrator was used as a marker for engagement within intervention paradigms, which is shown in Figures 19.9 and 19.10.

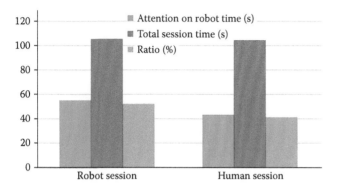

Figure 19.9 Attention of children with ASD.

Regarding the percentage of time that the participants looked at each administrator, the group with ASD looked at the robot 11% longer compared with that of the human therapist, while the TD group paid similar attention to robot and human therapists. The group with ASD required a similar amount of time to complete the tasks in both robot and human sessions, while the TD group spent more time to complete the robot session. However, two-sided Wilcoxon rank-sum test results showed that the difference between attention paid to the robot and the human therapist for both groups was not significant.

Next we examined the participants' demonstrated imitation skills between the human and robot administrator conditions. Each gesture performed by the participants was scored along a scale from 0 to 10, and the average results across all the trials were computed. Figure 19.11 shows the group performance between ASD and TD. Given that impairments in imitation represent a core symptom of ASD, the TD group was more successful than the group with ASD across both conditions and did not demonstrate much difference in performance between the robot and human sessions. Within the group with ASD, children were far more successful imitating the target gestures in the robot session than that in

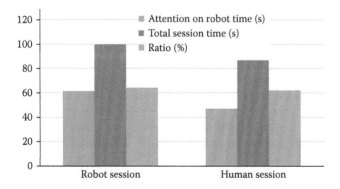

Figure 19.10 Attention of children with TD.

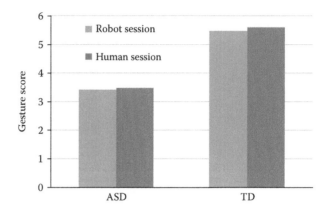

Figure 19.11 Average gesture score of both groups.

the human session. Regarding the attentional preference results, there was no statistically significant difference between performance in the robot session and the human session although the ASD group was closer to having a statistical difference.

19.3 Discussion

Robot-mediated intervention for children with ASD has been developed for decades, building tremendous momentum toward further technical development and psychological understanding. From simple to complex, from general to specific, the developed robots for children with ASD possess more and more advanced hardware design and interaction patterns. However, as we can see from the development of this field in recent years, several future goals for exploration and development still remain.

19.3.1 Increasing the autonomous level of the robotic systems

The ultimate goal of robot-mediated intervention is to make the robot work on its own to help children with ASD as much as possible, reducing the workload of human therapists and, potentially, the cost to families and system. Although there are still some systems that use the Wizard of Oz operation, where a human experimenter fills in for a technology behind the scene when a participant conducts a task (Kelley 1984), researchers are still working toward fully autonomous systems. The automatic detection of children's behavior is critical for any system in this field. Although there are techniques such as face tracking, gesture estimation, gaze tracking, speech recognition, and so on that have been developed already, there is no end to pursuing higher accuracy, robustness, and real-time computation ability. Natural and smooth interaction between robots and children depends on intelligent system control. Early systems such as basic rule-based systems are simple and rigid. If we take advantage of artificial intelligence, machine learning, and pattern recognition techniques, more adaptive, individualized, and anthropomorphic robotic systems can be invented.

19.3.2 Unrestricted interaction environment

As many of the robot prototypes are fragile or not safe for children to use independently, interacting with robots usually requires adult supervision. For example, some robots may become unbalanced or even fall down if pushed by a child. Some sensors on a robot may not endure patting or pushing, which are common behaviors as children explore a new object or environment. The camera used for tracking the participant's behavior usually has a limited view, needs to be put under particular illumination conditions, and on specific geometric position with respect to the robot or participant. On the other hand, keeping the children safe is always the priority. Some mechanical parts of a robot may pinch the children's finger if not placed properly. A heavy and unbalanced robot may injure a child in movement. The power supply of a robot also needs to be safe and easy to handle. Since children's behavior is not always predictable, it is important to pay attention to these safety issues when thinking about designing technological interventions.

19.3.3 Large group study

Most of the technical publications reviewed talked about the limitation of a pilot study with a few children, and pointed out that larger group studies are necessary. Small participant groups may not cover enough situations and lead to statistically significant results. We have seen that in spite of the difficulties of expanding beyond pilot work, as already discussed, researchers are working hard to conduct more experiments (Anzalone et al. 2014; Costescu et al. 2015). Although many different robots have been developed, the majority of them have common features such as similar mechanical structure, application area, and intervention pattern. Therefore, a standard testing method needs to be established to regulate and synthesize different studies, as this can be helpful to unify the results of discrete small studies into a general conclusion.

19.3.4 Robot-mediated intervention generalization

At this time, the impact of robotic interventions on children with ASD is mainly academic in application and exploration. It will be important for future work to disseminate these technologies more broadly, as with other medical robots, to test their application and usability.

413

Commercialization of a mature robot platform could make robots standardized, less expensive, and able to be used in rehabilitation centers as well as at homes. The development of robust technologies with minimum operation requirements is critical, so that therapists and parents may operate them at home and hospital. Even though the question of whether robots can be formally involved in clinical intervention is still a topic of debate (Diehl et al. 2012), researchers have been making great efforts toward this direction over the past decades, with many promising avenues for future work.

Acknowledgments

We would like to thank all the participants and their families for their help. This study was supported in part by the following grants: a grant from the Vanderbilt Kennedy Center (Hobbs Grant), a Vanderbilt University Innovation and Discovery in Engineering and Science (IDEAS) grant, National Science Foundation Grant 1264462, and the National Institute of Health Grants 1R01MH091102-01A1 and 5R21MH103518-02. This work also includes core support from NICHD (P30HD15052) and NCATS (UL1TR000445-06).

References

Amirabdollahian, F., B. Robins, K. Dautenhahn, and Z. Ji. 2011. Investigating tactile event recognition in child-robot interaction for use in autism therapy. *2011 Annual International Conference of the IEEE Engineering in Medicine and Biology Society*, pp. 5347–51. IEEE.

Annaz, D., R. Campbell, M. Coleman, E. Milne, and J. Swettenham. 2012. Young children with autism spectrum disorder do not preferentially attend to biological motion. *J. Autism Dev. Disord.* 42:401–8.

Anzalone, S. M., E. Tilmont, S. Boucenna, J. Xavier, A.-L. Jouen, N. Bodeau, K. Maharatna, M. Chetouani, D. Cohen, and M. S. Group. 2014. How children with autism spectrum disorder behave and explore the 4-dimensional (spatial 3D+ time) environment during a joint attention induction task with a robot. *Res. Autism Spectr. Disord.* 8:814–26.

Bekele, E. T., U. Lahiri, A. R. Swanson, J. A. Crittendon, Z. E. Warren, and N. Sarkar. 2013. A step towards developing adaptive robot-mediated intervention architecture (ARIA) for children with autism. *IEEE Trans. Neural Syst. Rehabil. Eng.* 21:289–99.

Blascovich, J., J. Loomis, A. C. Beall, K. R. Swinth, C. L. Hoyt, and J. N. Bailenson. 2002. Immersive virtual environment technology as a methodological tool for social psychology. *Psychol. Inq.* 13:103–24.

Boccanfuso, L. and J. M. O'Kane. 2011. CHARLIE: An adaptive robot design with hand and face tracking for use in autism therapy. *Int. J. Soc. Robot.* 3:337–47.

Boucenna, S., A. Narzisi, E. Tilmont, F. Muratori, G. Pioggia, D. Cohen, and M. Chetouani. 2014. Interactive technologies for autistic children: A review. *Cogn. Comput.* 6:722–40.

Buldyrev, S. V., L. R. C. Cruz, T. Gomez-Isla, E. Gomez-Tortosa, S. Havlin, R. Le, H. E. Stanley, B. Urbanc, and B. T. Hyman. 2000. Description of microcolumnar ensembles in association cortex and their disruption in Alzheimer and Lewy body dementias. *Proc. Natl. Acad. Sci. USA* 97:5039–43.

Chuah, M. C., D. Coombe, C. Garman, C. Guerrero, and J. Spletzer. 2014. Lehigh Instrument for Learning Interaction (LILI): An interactive robot to aid development of social skills for autistic children. *2014 IEEE 11th International Conference on Mobile Ad Hoc and Sensor Systems*, pp. 731–6, IEEE.

Constantino, J. N. and C. P. Gruber. 2002. *The Social Responsiveness Scale*. Los Angeles: Western Psychological Services.

Costa, S., H. Lehmann, K. Dautenhahn, B. Robins, and F. Soares. 2014. Using a humanoid robot to elicit body awareness and appropriate physical interaction in children with autism. *Int. J. Soc. Robot.* 1–14.

Costa, S., F. Soares, C. Santos, M. J. Ferreira, F. Moreira, A. P. Pereira, and F. Cunha. 2011. An approach to promote social and communication behaviors in children with autism spectrum disorders: Robot based intervention. *2011 RO-MAN*, pp. 101–6, IEEE.

Costescu, C. A., B. Vanderborght, and D. O. David. 2015. Reversal learning task in children with autism spectrum disorder: A robot-based approach. *J. Autism Dev. Disord.* 45(11):3715–25.

Dautenhahn, K., C. L. Nehaniv, M. L. Walters, B. Robins, H. Kose-Bagci, N. A. Mirza, and M. Blow. 2009. KASPAR—A minimally expressive humanoid robot for human–robot interaction research. *Applied Bionics and Biomechanics* 6(3–4):369–97.

Dautenhahn, K. and I. Werry. 2004. Towards interactive robots in autism therapy: Background, motivation and challenges. *Pragm. Cogn.* 12:1–35.

De Silva, R. S., K. Tadano, A. Saito, M. Higashi, and S. G. Lambacher. 2009. Therapeutic-assisted robot for children with autism. *IEEE/RSJ International Conference on Intelligent Robots and Systems, 2009. IROS 2009*, pp. 3561–7. IEEE.

Demchak, M. 1990. Response prompting and fading methods: A review. *Am. J. Ment. Retard.* 94(6):603–15.

Dickstein-Fischer, L., E. Alexander, X. Yan, H. Su, K. Harrington, and G. S. Fischer. 2011. An affordable compact humanoid robot for autism spectrum disorder interventions in children. *2011 Annual International Conference of the IEEE Engineering in Medicine and Biology Society*, 5319–22. IEEE.

Diehl, J. J., L. M. Schmitt, M. Villano, and C. R. Crowell. 2012. The clinical use of robots for individuals with autism spectrum disorders: A critical review. *Res. Autism Spectr. Disord.* 6:249–62.

Duquette, A., F. Michaud, and H. Mercier. 2008. Exploring the use of a mobile robot as an imitation agent with children with low-functioning autism. *Auton. Robots* 24:147–57.

Feil-Seifer, D. and M. Mataric. 2011. Automated detection and classification of positive vs. negative robot interactions with children with autism using distance-based features. In *Proceedings of the 6th International Conference (ACM/IEEE) on Human–Robot Interaction*, 323–30. New York, NY: ACM Press.

Fujimoto, I., T. Matsumoto, P. R. S. De Silva, M. Kobayashi, and M. Higashi. 2011. Mimicking and evaluating human motion to improve the imitation skill of children with autism through a robot. *Int. J. Soc. Robot.* 3:349–57.

Goodrich, M. A., M. A. Colton, B. Brinton, and M. Fujiki. 2011. A case for low-dose robotics in autism therapy. *Proceedings of the 6th International Conference on Human–Robot Interaction (HRI)*. 143–4. ACM.

Greczek, J., E. Kaszubski, A. Atrash, and M. J. Matarić. 2014. Graded cueing feedback in robot-mediated imitation practice for children with autism spectrum disorders. *Proceedings of the 23rd IEEE International Symposium on Robot and Human Interactive Communication (RO-MAN 2014)*. pp. 561–6. IEEE.

Ioannou, A., E. Andreou, and M. Christofi. 2015. Pre-schoolers' interest and caring behaviour around a humanoid robot. *TechTrends* 59:23–6.

Kelley, J. F. 1984. An iterative design methodology for user-friendly natural language office information applications. *ACM Trans. Inf. Syst. (TOIS)* 2:26–41.

Kim, E. S., L. D. Berkovits, E. P. Bernier, D. Leyzberg, F. Shic, R. Paul, and B. Scassellati. 2013. Social robots as embedded reinforcers of social behavior in children with autism. *J. Autism Dev. Disord.* 43(5):1038–49.

Klin, A., D. J. Lin, P. Gorrindo, G. Ramsay, and W. Jones. 2009. Two-year-olds with autism orient to nonsocial contingencies rather than biological motion. *Nature* 459:257–61.

Kozima, H., C. Nakagawa, and Y. Yasuda. 2005. Interactive robots for communication-care: A case-study in autism therapy. *IEEE International Workshop on Robot and Human Interactive Communication, 2005. ROMAN 2005*, pp. 341–6, IEEE.

Kozima, H. and H. Yano. 2001. A robot that learns to communicate with human caregivers. *Proceedings of the First International Workshop on Epigenetic Robotics*, pp. 47–52.

Liu, C., K. Conn, N. Sarkar, and W. Stone. 2008a. Online affect detection and robot behavior adaptation for intervention of children with autism. *IEEE Trans. Robot.* 24:883–96.

Liu, C., K. Conn, N. Sarkar, and W. Stone. 2008b. Physiology-based affect recognition for computer-assisted intervention of children with autism spectrum disorder. *Int. J. Hum. Comput. Stud.* 66:662–77.

Lord, C., S. Risi, L. Lambrecht, E. H. Cook, B. L. Leventhal, P. C. DiLavore, A. Pickles, and M. Rutter. 2000. The Autism Diagnostic Observation Schedule—Generic: A standard measure of social and communication deficits associated with the spectrum of autism. *J. Autism Dev. Disord.* 30:205–23.

Mann, D. M. A. 1982. Nerve cell protein metabolism and degenerative disease. *Neuropathol. Appl. Neurobiol.* 8:161–76.

Mullen, E. M. 1995. *Mullen Scales of Early Learning: AGS Edition.* Circle Pines, MN: American Guidance Service.

Pierno, A. C., M. Mari, D. Lusher, and U. Castiello. 2008. Robotic movement elicits visuomotor priming in children with autism. *Neuropsychologia* 46:448–54.

Pioggia, G., M. L. Sica, M. Ferro, R. Igliozzi, F. Muratori, A. Ahluwalia, and D. De Rossi. 2007. Human-robot interaction in autism: FACE, an android-based social therapy. *The 16th IEEE International Symposium on Robot and Human Interactive Communication, 2007. RO-MAN 2007*, pp. 605–12. IEEE.

Ranatunga, I., M. Beltran, N. A. Torres, N. Bugnariu, R. M. Patterson, C. Garver, and D. O. Popa. 2013. Human-robot upper body gesture imitation analysis for autism spectrum disorders. In *Social Robotics*, pp. 218–28. Springer International Publishing.

Ricks, D. J. and M. B. Colton. 2010. Trends and considerations in robot-assisted autism therapy. *2010 IEEE International Conference on Robotics and Automation (ICRA)*, pp. 4354–9. IEEE.

Rilling, J. K. and T. R. Insel. 1999. The primate neocortex in comparative perspective using magnetic resonance imaging. *J. Hum. Evol.* 37:191–223.

Robins, B., K. Dautenhahn, R. Te Boekhorst, and A. Billard. 2005. Robotic assistants in therapy and education of children with autism: Can a small humanoid robot help encourage social interaction skills? *Univ. Access Inf. Soc.* 4:105–20.

Rutter, M., A. Bailey, and C. Lord. 2010. *The Social Communication Questionnaire.* Los Angeles, CA: Western Psychological Services.

Scassellati, B. 2005. Quantitative metrics of social response for autism diagnosis. *IEEE International Workshop on Robot and Human Interactive Communication, 2005. ROMAN 2005*, pp. 585–90. IEEE.

Scassellati, B., H. Admoni, and M. Mataric. 2012. Robots for use in autism research. *Annu. Rev. Biomed. Eng.* 14:275–94.

Stanton, C. M., P. H. Kahn, R. L. Severson, J. H. Ruckert, and B. T. Gill. 2008. Robotic animals might aid in the social development of children with autism. *2008 3rd ACM/IEEE International Conference on Human–Robot Interaction (HRI)*, pp. 271–8, IEEE.

Torres, N. A., N. Clark, I. Ranatunga, and D. Popa. 2012. Implementation of interactive arm playback behaviors of social robot Zeno for autism spectrum disorder therapy. *Proceedings of the 5th International Conference on Pervasive Technologies Related to Assistive Environments*, p. 21. ACM.

Wainer, J., K. Dautenhahn, B. Robins, and F. Amirabdollahian. 2014. A pilot study with a novel setup for collaborative play of the humanoid robot KASPAR with children with autism. *Int. J. Soc. Robot.* 6:45–65.

Warren, Z., Z. Zheng, S. Das, E. M. Young, A. Swanson, A. Weitlauf, and N. Sarkar. 2015. Brief report: Development of a robotic intervention platform for young children with ASD. *J. Autism Dev. Disord.* 45(12):3870–6.

Warren, Z. E., Z. Zheng, A. R. Swanson, E. Bekele, L. Zhang, J. A. Crittendon, A. F. Weitlauf, and N. Sarkar. 2015. Can robotic interaction improve joint attention skills? *J. Autism Dev. Disord.* 45(11):3726–34.

Weir, S. and R. Emanuel. 1976. *Using LOGO to Catalyse Communication in an Autistic Child.* Department of Artificial Intelligence, University of Edinburgh.

Zheng, Z., S. Das, E. M. Young, A. Swanson, Z. Warren, and N. Sarkar. 2014. Autonomous robot-mediated imitation learning for children with autism. *2014 IEEE International Conference on Robotics and Automation (ICRA)*, pp. 2707–12. IEEE.

Zheng, Z., L. Zhang, E. Bekele, A. Swanson, J. Crittendon, Z. Warren, and N. Sarkar. 2013. Impact of robot-mediated interaction system on joint attention skills for children with autism. *2013 IEEE International Conference on Rehabilitation Robotics (ICORR)*, pp. 1–8. Seattle, Washington: IEEE.

Chapter 20 Using an ecological systems approach to target technology development for autism research and beyond

Rosa I. Arriaga

Contents

Abstract 419
20.1 Introduction 420
20.2 Design by any other name: The role of design in HCI and
     psychology research 421
20.3 Theory in practice: Building a new bridge between
     psychology and HCI 422
20.4 EST for autism: Targeting research 425
20.5 Conclusion 434
References 435

Abstract

This chapter considers the role of theory in design and how it can be used to better support technology to improve quality of life for individuals with autism and their caregivers. It also provides a review how theory has been used by human computer interaction (HCI) researchers from the beginning of the discipline to now. Finally, Urie Bronfenbrenner's Ecological Systems Theory is proposed as another theory that can be used by HCI researchers. A set of examples are provided that show how this theory can be used to aid design.

20.1 Introduction

The promise of technology is that it can scale human effort over time and space. This is just what caregivers of individuals with autism want to hear that there are technologies that can help automate current treatment, monitoring, and management practices. Further, these technologies can fortify all aspects of support for both the individual with autism and his caregivers. In this chapter, I will introduce Urie Bronfenbrenner's (1977, 1979) ecological systems theory (EST) as a tool researchers can use as they consider where they can target their technological intervention such that the entire ecology of the individual with autism is served. The chapter starts with a forced distinction between methods used in psychology and the computer science field of human–computer interaction (HCI). This will lead to a set of definitions about the role of design in both of these fields. Once this framework has been laid out, the role that theory plays in HCI research will be considered. After this, an outline will be proposed for how the EST fits within the taxonomy of theories in HCI. Finally, an example of how research has been guided by the EST will be provided.

Psychology is the study of human thought, perception, and behavior. Science is the method of choice. Psychologists systematically make observations, make predictions from what they observe, and then test these hypothesis. Psychologists of a certain disposition use this cycle to develop interventions to improve the human condition. Computer scientists who study human computer interaction (HCI) do all of the above in the context of understanding how to build "better" technological systems. Where "better" means that the systems are more useful and usable by the intended user. Experimental studies play a more limited role in HCI compared to psychology. Instead, HCI researchers use a variety of ethnographic methodologies to better understand how the individual ("user") engages in a task with a given technological interface.

Ethnography is the in-depth study of group interactions in their natural settings (Lazzar et al. 2010). Burke and Kirk (2001) go on to state that in HCI the goal of ethnography is to find problems in the way a system is currently used and thus, to improve the system in a way that is also culturally relevant.

One might ask where else, besides methodologies, do HCI and psychology meet? In computer science, technology provides a way to scale human effort over time and space. An oversimplification is that psychologists can meet one client at a time but technology can reach many people. Thus, technology can be used to deliver psychological interventions that can have multiplicative impact. This is especially important in the context of ubiquitous technology such as mobile phones, social media, and the Web. Psychology, on the other hand, has offered HCI theories to facilitate understanding human behavior and cognition that can lead to "better" system design. In this chapter, one additional theory that HCI researchers can use in their methodological tool kit, Urie Bronfenbrenner's (1977, 1979) ecological systems theory will be presented. It is argued that this theory can be used as a way to systematically consider the "context" that envelops a user and this in turn can help researchers consider where else to "target" system design.

20.2 Design by any other name: The role of design in HCI and psychology research

Before moving on to how the EST can be used by HCI researchers, it is helpful to define three important terms: design, system, and interface. Dix et al. (2004) define design as "achieving goals within constraints" and interface as the "mediation of the user's task and the systems core functions." They argue that the goal of design is to understand the system's purpose. Here a system is technological solution that will allow the user to complete a desired task. Constraints are related to the users contexts for example, how should the system be implemented, what interface will be easiest for the user to navigate, what affordances should the interface have? Rogers et al. (2011) enumerate over 20 types of interfaces from mobile, to speech, to robotics, to brain-computer. A mundane example of a task a user may want to achieve is to sweep the house. In the not so distant future, it may be easy enough to tell (speech input) our Roomba (interface) which rug needs to be cleaned (output). Or we may be able to simply use our phone to communicate the desired output. Dix et al. (2004) go on to state that there is a golden rule to designing systems, "know they user"; also to assume that they are probably "not like you" (i.e., the designer). As mentioned earlier, the HCI researcher will use many ethnographic tools: interviews, focus groups, surveys, participatory design, and contextual inquiry. Likewise, they urge researchers to not just find out what the user does but why he does it (Figure 20.1).

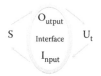

Figure 20.1 The user's task (U_t) is carried out via the system's input (I) channels and provides desired output (O).

A psychologist tasked with designing a system would probably conduct a broad range of quantitative studies. In the descriptive stage of identifying the problem, it would look similar to the HCI researcher's consisting of observational studies. Then she would likely try to cross validate what she saw with a slew of "observed" variables and preexisting measures on the given topic. This would allow her to conduct correlational studies. Finally, in order to get to the best design, she might conduct some experiments to ascertain which features are more effective leading to the highest participant satisfaction. Additionally, she might call on theories to drive her design. The idea being that rather than contextualizing what the participant is doing—the participant is first and foremost a human and there are theories that can help us solve the problem.

20.3 Theory in practice: Building a new bridge between psychology and HCI

Theory also plays an important role in HCI.[*] Rogers (2012) argues that in HCI, unlike psychology, theory has a less restricted role. It not only aims to adhere to the scientific conceptualization of a theory but is more eclectic. It helps them conceptualize, frame, prescribe, and inform their work. Rogers goes on to summarize the history of utilization of theories within HCI into three eras: classical, modern, and contemporary. In the classical era, theories were directly imported from cognitive psychology and were focused on how information processing would affect HCI design. Another significant contribution to HCI methodology came from cognitive psychology's method that modeled people's goals and how they were met. This work went on in lab settings.

In order to gain a better understanding of the role that the environment played in how users engaged in completing tasks, HCI research moved into the wild. Here the classic theories and data collection measures had limited use. Thus, this ushered the modern theories era in HCI. Now along with cognitive theories that tried to elucidate the role that external representation had for users (i.e., distributed cognition), there were also theories that were more closely aligned with anthropological and sociological (e.g., situated action) methods that were being utilized. According to Rogers, we are now in the contemporary era of theory utilization in HCI. This is characterized by theories that take into account different value-driven agendas. These are exemplified by the focus on a variety of human experiences beyond mainstream euro-centric and broadened its vision to include feminism, multiculturalism, and critical theory. According to Rogers, this shows a shift away from what had previously been seen as the goal of HCI: efficiency and productivity. She states, "Indeed, a new set of concepts, tools and methods is beginning to appear that are intended to address the wider range of human values, rather than well versed human needs (e.g., computers should be easy to learn, easy to use, etc.)," p. 66. Rogers then describes a number of "turns" that characterize the new wave of contemporary theories, these include: turn to design, turn to culture, turn to the wild, and turn to embodiment.

Roger's treatment of the role of theory in HCI provides a good backdrop to the introduction of Uri Bronfenbrenner's ecological systems theory[†] (1977, 1979) and what it can offer to designers in HCI and beyond. Uri Bronfenbrenner was a developmental psychologist. Developmental psychologists study how time affects the individual not only in childhood but throughout the life span. Time is important for two reasons:

---

[*] See Rogers (2012) for an excellent treatment of the topic.

[†] Note that in this chapter, I focus only on Bronfenbrenner's characterization of time and space as essential for studying the individual's "ecological systems." I do not take into consideration his complete theory (bio-ecological) which describes the process-person-context time. This is a valid practice according to Tudge et al. (2009).

first the historical context affects development (as in the common notion of generation gaps) and at the individual level, a 5-year period in childhood would have marked differences than a 5-year period in adulthood. Bronfenbrenner believed that in order to understand an individual you needed to study the interaction of that person in time (chronosystem) and space with other individuals (Tudge 2009; Figure 20.2). Bronfenbrenner's theory is "ecological" in that it emphasized the interrelatedness of the person-context (Tudge et al. 2009). He operationalized "proximal processes" as the activities that individuals engaged in every day and the interpersonal interactions that happened during a given activity. Proximal processes are the drivers of development because they are interactions that occur in the environment on a regular basis (Bronfenbrenner 1977, 1979). The spatial context is defined as a set of four nested layers that envelop the child. First is the microsystem level, which is where the child spends most time. Once again, if we think about activities, these include spending time with parents within a given neighborhood, going to school, and engaging with other children and adults. Mesosystems refer to how the various microsystems interact. For example, the child's home life as reflected within her household will affect her school life. If there are few resources at home, the child may go to school hungry and thus be unable to concentrate on learning.

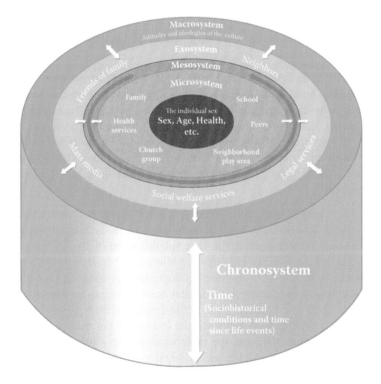

Figure 20.2 Bronfenbrenner's conceptualization of an individual's ecological context.

Whereas the microsystem and mesosystem are experienced directly by the child, the third and fourth layers are not. The exosystem and macrosystem are experienced indirectly. The exosystem takes into account the interactions at the microsystem. For example, in a school district where school funding is based on local taxes and there is a low tax base, there are poorly funded schools. The child experiences the burden of dilapidated buildings or teachers that are stressed because of large class sizes. The macrosystem can be construed as the cultural layer, being made up of people who have shared identity, values, and access to resources. However, this layer is also fluid because an individual may have a stake in more than one macrosystem. A child born in East Los Angeles may identify as both Mexican and American and hold both the collective and individualistic values representative of both cultures.

Bronfenbrenner may have never considered the role of technology in an individual's life or how technology can be used to navigate and facilitate interactions among individuals at the various contextual layers yet his conceptualization of time and space can be an important tool for HCI designers. The EST has the ability to provide prescriptive support (Bederson and Shneiderman, cited in Rogers 2012). Specifically, a designer can use the various ecological layers to get guidance of where technology can be targeted (Figure 20.3). The next section provides a description of how this approach has been used in the context of autism. However, this approach has also been proposed in the context of designing at the intersection of technology and asthma (Jeung and Arriaga 2009).

Bronfenbrenner's theory clearly fits into Roger's HCI theory taxonomy in the contemporary section. First, it can be conceptualized to be concerned with understanding the role of technology beyond one user and one device. Second, the contextualization of the user's experience and how he interacts with the technology as a part of a mediated experience with others is also central. Finally, this theory forces designers to consider the broader cultural values that influence the effect the use of technology.

The EST's spatial layers were reconceptualized in order to make it easier for designers to use. The various layers are now instantiated in each of the nested rings (Figure 20.3). This simplification of the EST allows designers to more easily visualize the interaction between the different contexts. In this version, the microsystem layers include the individual and the family, the mesosystem includes member of the community that the individual could interact with, while the exosystem represents members of society that may influence the individual but that he may not come into contact with and the macrosystem layer embodies both the cultural environment and the natural environment. The addition of the natural environment is considered important because some individuals with chronic conditions (e.g., asthma) are highly affected by pollen and smog. The chronosystem layer is embedded in the use of technology

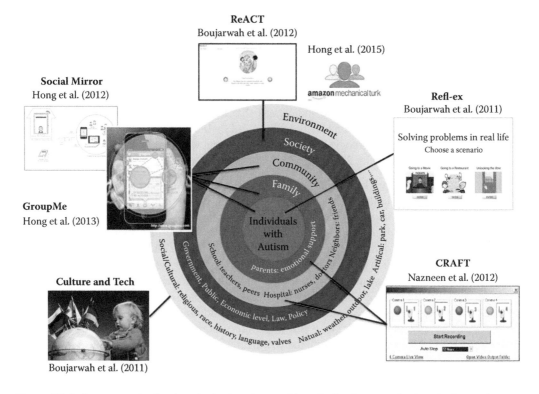

Figure 20.3 A reconceptualized ecological system and how technology can be targeted at various layers.

since technology would necessarily have to be adaptive to be of most use to the individuals using the technology. In the following section, examples are presented for how technology for autism can be targeted at each of the layers.

20.4 EST for autism: Targeting research

Bronfenbrenner understood the essential role that personality and biology have on an individual's development. This drove the reconceptualization of his theory to be called the bio-ecological system theory (Rosa and Tudge 2013). Autism spectrum disorder is a set of developmental disabilities that is characterized by significant social, communicative, and behavioral challenges (CDC 2014). Individuals with autism have cognitive profiles that range from low IQ and no language to high IQ and "normal" language development. The latter are often referred to as having high-functioning autism spectrum disorder (HFASD; Lake et al. 2014). Despite their lack of intellectual impairment, these individuals with HFA have social and communicative impairment that effect their interactions with other individuals. Using Bronfenbrenner's terminology,

425

the individual's proximal processes are disrupted. Further because of the impairments that people with HFASD have, their ability to obtain independence from their caregivers is also hampered. In this section, one perspective on how technology can be used to support individuals with HFASD and their caregivers[*] is presented. There is a paucity of research that includes adolescents and young adults with HFASD, but there are indications that they respond well to computer-assisted instruction (Williams et al. 2002). Indeed there is a general call for more technologies that specifically target social skills training (Putnam and Chang 2008).

Adolescents and young adults with HFASD are a heterogeneous population with a wide range of needs and abilities. Social skills deficits, however, are generally considered defining characteristics of HFASD. Deficits in socialization interfere with the educational experience and quality of life of individuals with HFASD. They require explicit instruction to help them acquire age-appropriate social skills. One of the quintessential deficits is their inability to form what Schank and Abelson (1977) called scripts, or standard event sequences. Scripts enable individuals to know what to expect and how to behave in a given situation. A number of social skills interventions have been developed to help aid individuals with these difficulties. Perhaps the most famous is social stories (Gray 1995). This intervention requires that the therapist identify the sequence of a given event (e.g., waiting in line for the water fountain) and present them in a standardized manner. This therapy is usually implemented in a paper form.

Boujarwah et al. (2011) expanded on an existing proof of concept system called Re-Flex (Gillesen et al. 2009). The goal of this system was to provide individuals with a loop of experiencing and reflecting on a variety of social tasks. It was targeted at the "individual layer" of the EST (Figure 20.4). The Re-Flex system was meant to engage the individual with HFASD in one of the three scenarios (going to a new restaurant, unlocking the door, and going to a movie) and the unexpected events that arise along the way. This system differed from social stories in that it had more of a "choose your own adventure" quality. The individual would choose a path from a set of options (in two decision points) and these would necessarily take him to a final outcome. Each scenario had two main components, an experience section and a reflection section. The results were based on log data from the system. It indicated that all eight participants were able to successfully complete all three scenarios. This supports the idea that the software was able to provide the scaffolding necessary to enable even the participants who struggled with the "paper-based" testing to be successful during the software intervention. The analysis of the thinking time provided an

---

[*] For a comprehensive review of technology that has been developed for autism, see Kientz et al. (2013).

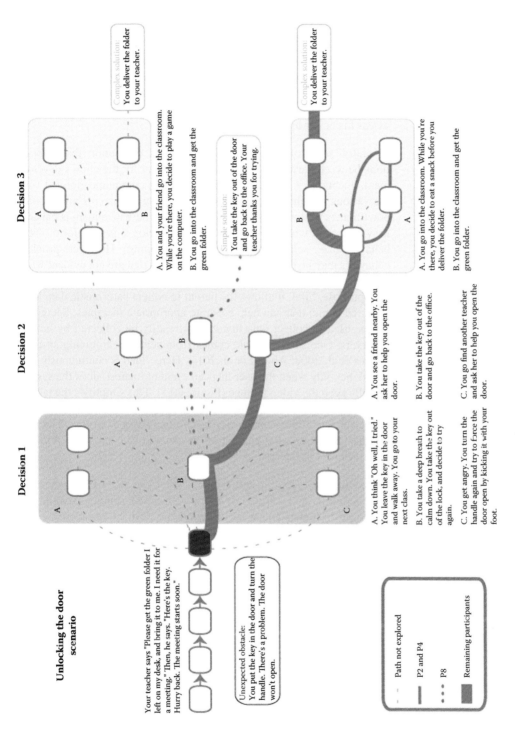

Figure 20.4 The various paths taken by the eight participants to solve the unlocking door scenario.

additional means to observe differences between participants, and the processing time required at the point in which the unexpected obstacle is introduced, and at the two major decision points. This data showed that the thinking time varied within participants, between participants, and across scenarios. This data could be used in the future to further facilitate the customization of the software for each participant, and to assess his or her learning.

A central tenet of Bronfenbrenner's EST is the notion that interactions between various caretakers are important for the child's development. Technology can be used to mediate the communication between the various stakeholders. In autism, the ability for parents and clinical practitioners to share information about the child with autism is particularly important when there is the need to develop a therapy for problem behavior (e.g., self-injurious, aggressive, eloping). However, problem behaviors may be triggered by contextual cues that are not evident when the child is in a clinical setting. At this point, technology can serve a dual purpose. First, it allows the parent to collect naturalistic data (e.g., from the home) that can help generate appropriate therapies. Second, it can be used to collect data that cannot readily be collected by human observers. One such example comes from selective archiving systems (Hayes et al. 2008; Abowd et al. 2014). Here video is continuously collected, but only when the user flags an event of interest, does the system actually keep the video footage (Figure 20.5). This simplifies the task of reviewing video because rather than watching hours and hours of video the researcher or user can simply watch the "flagged" events. The user can also designate what amount of data should be captured before and after the event of interest.

The continuous recording and flagging technology (CRAFT) system targets the family and community layers of the EST (Figure 20.3). It was developed to understand what behaviors are deemed "problematic" by parents and to ascertain which of the behaviors the parents flagged meet the clinical criteria for problem behaviors by professionals (Nazneen et al. 2012). Thus, parents and caregivers can communicate more effectively. Problem behavior can occur anywhere in the home thus, a functional requirement for CRAFT is to support robust and continuous capture from multiple synchronized cameras as well as time-stamped events triggered by the human via a small wireless device. Parents used the wireless device to flag the onset of their child's problem behavior. Behavior analysts had access to continuous video recording, which allowed them to view continuous footage and identify "problem behavior" that the parent may have missed. The result from a deployment in the home of eight different families showed that parents were able to successfully capture at least one instance of problem behavior. The authors note that this in-home system holds promise for streamlining a whole host of processes that could better serve children with autism and their parents. This includes collecting home data to facilitate or expedite

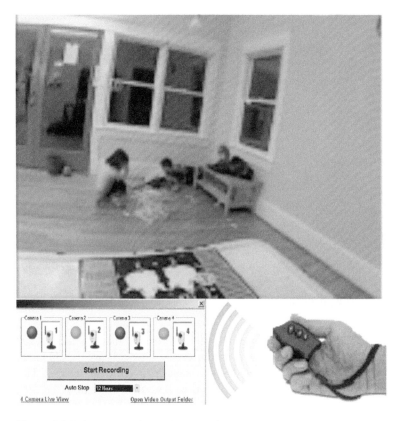

Figure 20.5 Parents activate the recording system when they see a behavior of interest.

the intake process at clinics, or collect evidence that the parent is able to carry out a therapy at home, that was learned in the clinic.

The previous two systems that were described separately targeted the layers that include the individual with autism (Re-Flex) and the parents and therapists (CRAFT). Engaging the community layer (people that may be known to the individual with autism) is important because it may provide an extended care network for the individual with autism (Muller et al. 2008; Taylor and Seltzer 2011). At the same time, having an expanded support network for the person with autism can also ease the burden felt by many primary caregivers (e.g., parents) of individuals with autism (Krauss et al. 2005). In two studies, Hong et al. (2012, 2013) designed and carried out an evaluation using a specialized social network that engaged the individuals with autism, their caregivers, and friends of their families (Figure 20.3).

Hong et al. (2012) engaged 12 adults with HFASD and 16 of their caregivers both parents and teachers in a design exercise to understand what technological would support increased independence for the individual

(a)   (b)

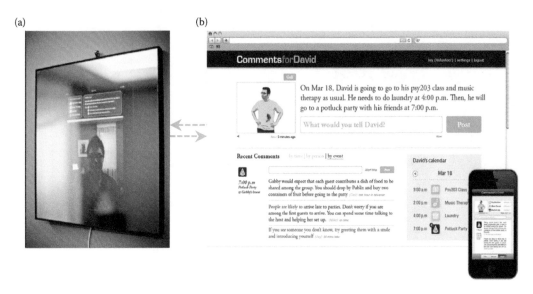

Figure 20.6 Social Mirror in the home (a) and online (b).

with HFASD. The results of the study indicated that the technology would have to support three main objectives. It would have to help motivate the individual with HFASD to engage in self-help activity. The system would have to embed advice from the social network in the context of everyday events. Finally, the system would have to leverage the natural network of caregivers. The latter issue was related to engaging members of the community that knew the individual with HFASD and that could be trusted with personal information.

The technology prototype that Hong et al. developed was called Social Mirror. The main features of this prototypic system were a controlled access social network, a mirror (that would facilitate daily photo updates, a shared calendar that allowed contextualized text messaging (Figure 20.6). The prevailing scenario was that Social Mirror would allow individuals with HFASD to tap an extended support network to help with everyday tasks.* For example, the network could access the shared calendar and thus remind the individual with HFASD that there was an upcoming exam or what appropriate attire is for a job interview. A chat system would also allow the individual with HFASD to reach out to his network with queries.

Developing Social Mirror led Hong et al. (2013) to consider how an actual specialized social network could be designed. They opted to appropriate a preexisting service, GroupMe. Three individuals and their care network were asked to use this system over a 1-month period. The

---

* A video of the prototype can be found here: https://www.youtube.com/watch?v=nGs1464Epwg

results indicated that the individuals with HFASD had a positive experience with the system. Specifically, they mentioned being able to monitor how "typical" individuals used the service allowed them to practice appropriate social engagement skills on the service. Second, they noted that being on the social network opened up rich interactions with the community members that they did not know well. The online interaction actually led to real world outings. The system also allowed for immediate responses when the individual with HFASD had questions. It also allowed the individual with HFASD to voice needs that the primary caregivers had overlooked. There were a number of challenges with this type of specialized social network. First, some of the community members were overwhelmed with the amount of messages that were sent via the system. Second, there was tension as to who would allow different community members to join the social network. For this study, it was the parents that asked the community members to join; thus, they felt that these individuals were responsible. However, parents feared that the individuals with HFASD may allow community members that did not share their values on to the network and that these members would provide inappropriate answers. In all, the participants in the study had positive experiences with the specialized social network and noted that it did foster independence in the person with HFASD and did alleviate the need for the primary caregivers to be constantly monitoring the needs of their child.

The Social Mirror and GroupMe studies highlighted the communication and interactions that could be prompted by introducing technology into the lives of individuals with HFASD but an open question was what happens in natural settings? In the reconceptualized Bronfenbrennerian ecosystem, the society layer can be thought of as the community at large, that is, those people that the individual with HFASD may normally not come into contact with. Once again, technology bridges this gap in time in space. Now individuals with HFASD have a variety of forums where they can meet other like-minded individuals (e.g., WrongPlanet). These are individuals that they may not meet under normal circumstances (may live in different parts of the country or the world). The EST's notion of interconnection (between the layers) and the argument in this paper that the EST can drive design of technology (targeted to help individuals with autism and their caregivers), leads to the hypothesis that there are interventions that can leverage society at large.

One of the pressing problems for individuals with autism both at the lower and higher end of the spectrum is a problem with social skills acquisitions. As mentioned earlier, social stories (Gray 1995) require that a teacher or therapist develop easily digestible sequences of events to deal with an everyday task. The second requirement is that the teacher takes into account the individual's with autism's unique needs (e.g., sensitivity to florescent lights) and incorporating coping strategies for this issue into the social story. In considering these two requirements, it

431

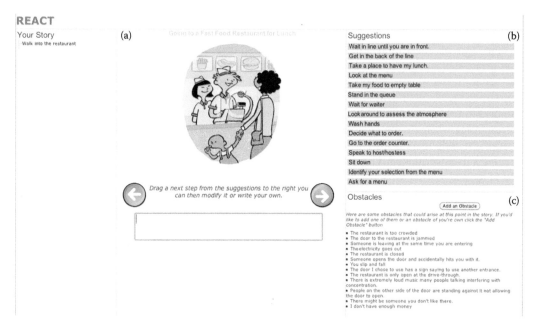

Figure 20.7 Therapist can enter their own steps (a) or use the suggestions provided by the crowd (b, c).

becomes obvious that the part of this kind of social skills training that can be automated is the script portion. This is the case because developing a sequence of events related to an everyday task (e.g., going to a fast food restaurant) is something that is easily accomplished by individuals with normal cognitive functioning. This led to the realization that the "society" layer could be called on to automate the process of script development.

In social computing, the "crowd" has been used to solve a number of tasks that are easy for humans but not for computers to solve; thus, Boujarwah et al. (2012) were able to use the crowdsourced platform Amazon Turk* workers to build these script sequences. Capitalizing on what they had learned about skills training from Re-Flex, they also were able to get the crowd to provide a set of obstacles and solutions at each of the step of the sequence of events for the task of going to a fast food restaurant. The information provided by the crowd was then used in an interface that the therapist could use (Figure 20.7) to develop a social skills training therapy. They called this system REACT (Refl-Ex Authoring and Critiquing Tool) because the teacher, therapist, or even parent could author social skills modules. The author would then be able to focus her/his attention on customizing the steps to reflect the unique characteristics of the individual with autism. For example, this could be done by introducing

---

* A crowdsourcing Internet marketplace that individuals and business can do human-subject tasks, https://www.mturk.com/mturk/welcome.

an "obstacle" and a "solution" that was specific to that individual (e.g., encountering and dealing with florescent lights, respectively).

REACT used the society layer in the EST to help the caregivers automate the task of social skills training module development. Can the society layer be used to help the individual himself? As previously discussed, individuals with HFASD have developed forums where they can voice their opinion and questions on a number of topics. In a new set of studies, Arriaga and her colleagues have shown that much of the communication in this forum is centered around asking question about everyday events (Hong et al. 2015a). In a second study, Arriaga and colleagues (Hong et al. 2015b) addressed the question, can the crowd provide answers to questions posed on these forums and how do they compare with those provided by other members? The results indicated that answers from the crowd were more direct, more concise, and prescriptive (included steps to be taken to address the problem) but had an empathic quality similar to that of the forum members. The goal of future studies is to design systems that could offer the members of the forum an opportunity to get answers from the crowd. A future interface can also be developed to help the forum members craft better questions and minimize the sensitive information that is disclosed.

The two studies described above (Boujarwah et al., 2010; Hong et al., 2015b) evidence that technology can be designed to leverage the society layer of the EST. The last layer of the EST takes into account the individual's environment. This is different from society because a designer must consider the values that are held in a given place and time. Here the environment layer acts as a reminder that the technology that is designed in one cultural environment may not work in another. Arriaga and her colleagues conducted a survey of individuals in America, Korea, Pakistan, and Kuwait to understand how each of these cultures perceived individuals with developmental disabilities. Also, to understand how a variety of technologies developed in the United States would be perceived in these four different cultures. As expected, the values for what constitutes appropriate therapies for individuals was quite different among the four cohorts. Some of the interesting findings were related to how religious views effect people's perception of individuals with disabilities. For example, among some Muslims, individuals with disabilities are considered "angles" and the goal is to keep them content. In this context, engaging therapies that require too much effort from the disabled individual would not be valued. Likewise, in some Muslim households, women's presentation in public and in the home is different (e.g., wearing headscarves). Thus capture and access systems that have video footage that may be viewed by outside stakeholders would be unacceptable. Economics and infrastructure also played an important role in the kind of training that would be desirable for individuals with ASD. In countries like Korea and the United States, with more prevalent views of autonomy,

433

independence was valued, but in Pakistan and Kuwait, it was desirable to have the individual at home indefinitely (the same was true for typical individuals).

20.5 Conclusion

Autism and other developmental disabilities affect the individual and those around him. Both psychologists and computer scientists are motivated to design interventions to help them. In this chapter, design was considered from both a psychology and a human–computer interaction (HCI) perspective. Psychologists who work directly with individuals with autism and their families can use technology to scale their efforts. HCI researchers with their mantra of developing useful and usable systems can leverage offerings from psychology. In this chapter, it is argued that Urie Bronfenbrenner's ecological systems theory (EST) is a developmental theory that has much to offer to HCI. We have now shown that it can just as easily be applied to developing technology for autism as it was for asthma (Jeong and Arriaga 2009).

The EST is a psychosocial theory that operationalizes the various interactions that define an individual's development. It provides a systematic manner to consider the ripple effect of interactions that individuals with autism have by operationalizing the various layers that envelop the individual. The EST starts with the individual and moves to the family, community (those around the individual), society (those individuals beyond the immediate community), and the environment (which includes place in time and culture). In making the connection between the individual and the outer layers (society and culture), the EST falls in the category of modern theories according to Roger's classification.

In this chapter, a series of examples showed how the EST can help researchers conceptualize how to design interventions that target the individuals with autism's ecosystem. Also, it showed that in using the EST the notion of caregiver can be broadened to include people that the individual with autism had never met. In fact, Hong et al. (2013) have called for developing a network of e-volunteers, trusted strangers, who can be called upon to aid the individual with autism and his primary caregivers. The idea is that while researchers can pay the crowd, there are those that would do it for free. Crowd workers can move from Mechanical Turk to donating their time on "Philantropic Turk." This opens a broad range of questions about what motivates individuals to volunteer online. How to develop reward schemes that maximize volunteer work and how to assure that they are reliable and can provide information for the individual with autism and his/her primary caregivers will be both useful and usable. These set of questions open yet another frontier for psychologists and HCI researchers to investigate.

References

Abowd, G. D., J. A. Kientz, G. R. Hayes, R. I. Arriaga, and Nazneen. 2014. Tools to support simplified capture activities in natural environments. *Technology Tools for Students with Autism: Innovations that Enhance Independence and Learning.* eds. K. L. Boser, M. S. Goodwin, and S. C. Wayland, Baltimore, MD: Brookes Publishing.

Boujarwah, F. A., G. D. Abowd, and R. I. Arriaga. 2012. Socially computed scripts to support social problem solving skills. In *Proceedings of the SIGCHI Conference on Human Factors in Computing Systems (CHI '12),* 1987–96. New York: ACM. doi: http://dx.doi.org/10.1145/2207676.2208343.

Boujarwah, F. A., H. Hong, G. D. Abowd, and R. I. Arriaga. 2011. Towards a framework to situate assistive technology design in the context of culture. In *The Proceedings of the 13th International ACM SIGACCESS Conference on Computers and Accessibility (ASSETS '11),* 19–26. New York: ACM. doi: http://dx.doi.org/10.1145/2049536.2049542.

Bronfenbrenner, U. 1977. Toward an experimental ecology of human development. *Am. Psychol.* 32:515–31.

Bronfenbrenner, U. 1979. *The Ecology of Human Development: Experiments by Nature and by Design.* Cambridge: Harvard University Press.

Burke, J. and A. Kirk. 2001. *Ethnographic Methods.* College Park: University of Maryland. http://lte-projects.umd.edu/charm/ethno.html (accessed March 1, 2016).

CDC. 2014. Autism spectrum disorder (ASD). http://www.cdc.gov/ncbddd/autism/index.html (accessed March 1, 2016).

Dix, I., J. Finlay, G. D. Abowd, and R. Beale. 2004. *Human-Computer Interaction,* 3rd ed. Englewood Cliffs, NJ: Prentice Hall.

Gillesen, J., H. Hong, and R. I. Arriaga. 2009. Refl-ex: Towards designing an interactive and intelligent tool for social skill development of individuals with HFASD/AS. *Proceedings of Designing Pleasurable Products and Interfaces,* Compienge, France, October 13–16.

Gray, C. A. 1995. Teaching children with autism to "read" social situations. In *Teaching Children with Autism: Strategies to Enhance Communication and Socialization,* ed. K. Quill, 219–42. New York: Delmar.

Hayes, G. R., L. M. Gardere, G. D. Abowd, and K. N. Truong. 2008. CareLog: A selective archiving tool for behavior management in schools. In *Proceedings of the SIGCHI Conference on Human Factors in Computing Systems (CHI '08),* 685–94. New York: ACM. doi: http://dx.doi.org/10.1145/1357054.1357164.

Hong, H., S. Yarosh, J. G. Kim, G. D. Abowd, and R. I. Arriaga. 2012. Designing a social network to support the independence of young adults with autism. In *Proceedings of the ACM 2012 Conference on Computer Supported Cooperative Work (CSCW '12),* 627–36. New York: ACM. doi: http://dx.doi.org/10.1145/2145204.2145300.

Hong, H., S. Yarosh, J. G. Kim, G. D. Abowd, and R. I. Arriaga. 2013. Investigating the use of circles in social networks to support independence of individuals with autism. In *Proceedings of the SIGCHI Conference on Human Factors in Computing Systems (CHI '13),* 3207–16. New York: ACM. doi: http://dx.doi.org/10.1145/2470654.2466439.

Hong, H., G. D. Abowd, and R. I. Arriaga. 2015a. Towards designing social question-and-answer systems for behavioral support of individuals with autism. *2015 9th International Conference on Pervasive Computing Technologies for Healthcare (PervasiveHealth),* 17–24. Istanbul. doi: 10.4108/icst.pervasivehealth.2015.259282.

Hong, H., E. Gilbert, G. D. Abowd, and R. I. Arriaga. 2015b. In-group questions and out-group answers: Crowdsourcing daily living advice for individuals with autism. In *Proceedings of the 33rd Annual ACM Conference on Human*

Factors in Computing Systems (CHI '15). 777–86. New York: ACM. doi: http://dx.doi.org/10.1145/2702123.2702402.

Jeong, H. Y. and R. I. Arriaga. 2009. Using an ecological framework to design mobile technologies for pediatric asthma management. *Proceedings of the 11th International Conference on Human-Computer Interaction with Mobile Devices and Services.* doi: 10.1145/1613858.1613880.

Kientz, J. A., M. Goodwin, G. R. Hayes, and G. D. Abowd. 2013. Interactive technologies for autism. *Synth. Lect. Assist. Rehabil. Health Preserv. Technol.* 2(2):1–177.

Krauss, M. W., M. M. Seltzer, and H. T. Jacobson. 2005. Adults with autism living at home or in non-family settings: Positive and negative aspects of residential status. *J. Intellect. Disabil. Res.* 49:111–24.

Lake, J. K., A. Perry, and Y. Lunsky. 2014. Mental health services for individuals with high functioning autism spectrum disorder. *Autism Res. Treat.* 2014:502420. doi: 10.1155/2014/502420.

Lazzar, J., H. J. Feng, and H. Hochheiser. 2010. *Research Methods in Human Computer Interaction.* New York: Wiley.

Muller, E., A. Schuler, and G. B. Yates. 2008. Social challenges and supports from the perspective of individuals with Asperger syndrome and other autism spectrum disabilities. *Autism* 12:173–90.

Nazneen, A., M. Rozga, A. J. Romero et al. 2012. Supporting parents for in-home capture of problem behaviors of children with developmental disabilities. *J. Pers. Ubiquitous Comput.* 16:193–207.

Putnam, C. and L. Chong. 2008. Software and technologies designed for people with autism: What do users want? In *Proceedings of the 10th International ACM SIGACCESS Conference on Computers and Accessibility (Assets '08),* 3–10. New York: ACM. doi: http://dx.doi.org/10.1145/1414471.1414475.

Rogers, Y. 2012. *HCI Theory: Classical, Modern and Contemporary. Synthesis Lectures on Human-Centered Informatics,* 1st ed. San Rafael, CA: Morgan and Claypool Publishers.

Rogers, Y., H. Sharp, and J. Preece. 2011. *Interaction Design: Beyond Human Computer Interaction,* 3rd ed. New York: Wiley.

Rosa, E. M. and J. R. Tudge. 2013. Urie Bronfenbrenner's theory of human development: Its evolution from ecology to bioecology. *J. Family Theory Rev.* 5(6):243–58.

Schank, R. C. and R. P. Abelson. 1977. *Scripts, Plans, Goals, and Understanding: An Inquiry into Human Knowledge Structures.* Hillsdale, NJ: Erlbaum.

Taylor, J. L. and M. M. Seltzer. 2011. Employment and post-secondary educational activities for young adults with autism spectrum disorders during the transition to adulthood. *J. Autism Dev. Disord.* 41(5):566–74.

Tudge, J. R. H. 2009. Social contextual theories. In *The Child: An Encyclopedic Companion.* eds. R. A. Shweder, T. R. Bidell, A. C. Dailey, S. D. Dixon, P. J. Miller, and J. Modell, 268–71. Chicago, IL: University of Chicago Press.

Tudge, J. R. H., I. Mokrova, B. E. Hatfield, and R. B. Karnick. 2009. Uses and misuses of Bronfenbrenner's bioecological theory of human development. *J. Family Theory Rev.* 1:198–210.

Williams, C., B. Wright, G. Callaghan, and B. Coughlan. 2002. Do children with autism learn to read more readily by computer assisted instruction or traditional book methods? *Autism* 6:71–91.

Chapter 21 Electrophysiology of error processing in individuals with autism spectrum disorder
A meta-analysis

Wen-Pin Chang

Contents

Abstract 437
21.1 Introduction 438
21.2 Methods 441
    21.2.1 Literature search. 441
    21.2.2 Inclusion criteria. 441
    21.2.3 Meta-analysis procedure and data analysis 441
21.3 Results. 441
    21.3.1 Error-related negativity. 444
    21.3.2 Error positivity 444
21.4 Discussion. 449
    21.4.1 Error-related negativity and error positivity. 449
    21.4.2 Implication for the theory of executive dysfunction
          in ASD 452
    21.4.3 Limitations 452
References 453

Abstract

Error processing is indispensable for efficient goal-directed performance of human behavior. Deficient error processing can lead to per-
severative responding and stereotyped repetitive behaviors, which are
features that tend to be manifested in individuals with autism spectrum
disorder (ASD). In addition, previous research has suggested that social–
emotional and social–cognitive impairments in ASD are associated with

deficient error processing. Consequently, studies have examined differences in error-related negativity (ERN or Ne) and error positivity (Pe), two electrophysiological indices of error processing, between healthy controls and ASD. This meta-analysis sought to determine whether there is reliable evidence of diminished error processing in ASD based on current available published studies. The analysis of the DerSimonian and Laird random-effects model showed an overall significant pooled effect size d of 0.63 with 95% confidence interval (CI) of 0.26–1.00, $p < 0.001$ for the ERN amplitude. The result of heterogeneity of the single effects was significant, Cochrane $Q = 13.76$, $p = 0.032$. For the Pe amplitude, the result showed an overall significant pooled effect size d of 0.38 with the 95% CI of 0.06–0.70, $p < 0.01$. The result of heterogeneity of the single effects was not significant, Cochrane $Q = 4.22$, $p = 0.38$. These results indicate prominent reduced ERN and slightly altered Pe in ASD as compared to healthy controls and support the idea that a general impairment in error processing underlies social–cognitive disturbance in individuals with ASD.

21.1 Introduction

Autism spectrum disorder (ASD) is a pervasive developmental disorder that includes Asperger's disorder, autistic disorder, childhood disintegrative disorder, and pervasive developmental disorder not otherwise specified (PDD-NOS). Individuals with ASD commonly demonstrate developmental delays in social communication ability and restricted and repetitive behaviors (American Psychiatric Association [APA], 2013). According to the *Diagnostic and Statistical Manual of Mental Disorders* (5th ed.; DSM-V; APA 2013), persistent deficits in social communication ability consist of deficits in social-emotional reciprocity, nonverbal communicative behaviors used for social interaction, and developing and maintaining relationships. Restricted and repetitive behaviors are manifested such as excessive adherence to routines, ritualized patterns of verbal or nonverbal behavior, or excessive resistance to change, and highly restricted, fixated interests that are abnormal in intensity or focus (DSM-V; APA 2013).

According to Autism and Developmental Disabilities Monitoring Network surveillance year 2008, the estimated prevalence of ASD in the United States was 1 in 88 children aged 8 years (Centers for Disease Control and Prevention [CDC] 2012). The prevalence of ASD has recently increased to about 1 in 68 children aged 8 years (CDC 2014). Previous research has revealed that the ASD diagnosis in boys is four times higher than that in girls. In the absence of intellectual impairment, the ASD diagnosis in boys becomes 10 times higher than that in girls. Yet, girls with ASD are more likely to have significant intellectual impairment when compared to boys with ASD (see Rivet and Matson 2011 for review). With the effect of changes of diagnostic criteria to the

DSM-V, the number of individuals with ASD will decrease (Kulage et al. 2014); however, the societal burden of the effect of ASD remains.

Several cognitive theories have been developed to elucidate the causes and mechanisms of social interaction and behavior issues in individuals with ASD (see Rajendran and Mitchell 2007 for review). Among these theories, theory of mind (ToM), weak central coherence (WCC) theory, and theory of executive dysfunction are the most common ones. Per ToM, individuals with autism or ASD fail to "impute mental states to themselves and others" (Premack and Woodruv 1978, p. 515), that is, fail to understand and represent other people's mental states (Baron-Cohen et al. 1985; Frith et al. 1991). Social features of ASD have been related to deficits in ToM (Happé and Ronald 2008). According to WCC theory, individuals with ASD tend to process information in a specific perceptual-cognitive style that is detail-focused, limiting their ability to understand context or to "see the big picture" (Frith and Happé 1994; Happé 1999). This theory posits that as a result of the detailed-focused processing, global processing abilities that are important in social interaction are affected, leading to impairments such as face and emotion recognition and social communication (Happé and Frith 2006). This theory explains why some individuals with ASD demonstrate superior performance in tasks or subjects demanding detailed-focused processing such as mathematics and engineering (Rajendran and Mitchell 2007).

The theory of executive dysfunction provides an alternative account to shed light on symptoms of ASD that are not easily explained by the ToM and WCC theory (Rajendran and Mitchell 2007). Executive function (EF) is intrinsically domain-general while the ToM is domain-specific (Rajendran and Mitchell 2007). In general, EF is important for cognitive flexibility, goal-directed planning, and decision making (Pennington and Ozonoff 1996). Restricted, repetitive, and stereotyped patterns of behavior in individuals with ASD have been linked to EF deficits (Turner 1999). However, the global impairments in EF are not unveiled in ASD and multiple studies reveal differences in the specific component areas of EF deficit (see O'Hearn et al. 2008 for review). This leads to the need for further research to delineate potential specific cognitive patterns of EF in ASD with a different perspective.

One particular perspective is to discern performance monitoring, which is a type of EF abilities that is the ability to continuously monitor the optimization of performance and future behavior by reaching action goals (Stuss et al. 1995). Performance monitoring comprises of error processing, which includes error detection and error awareness (Ullsperger and von Cramon 2001). Behavioral studies have shown that individuals with ASD fail to either correct their errors (Russell and Jarrold 1998) or exhibit posterror slowing (Bogte et al. 2007). A specific theory-informed error processing is reinforcement learning (RL). "A central assumption of the RL theory of error processing is that a similar dip in midbrain DA neuron firing occurs in humans upon commission of a response error, or very generally, when negative feedback is received" (Ullsperger et al. 2014, p. 47). The RL theory of error processing indicates that the dorsal (cognitive) region of the anterior cingulate cortex (ACC) uses reward prediction error signals (Holroyd and Coles 2002), and error information, that is, internally generated response errors and negative environmental feedback, activates the dorsal ACC (Holroyd et al. 2004).

Mundy (2003) argued that social behavior disturbances in autism are due to deficits in cognitive functions of the dorsal ACC. Structural and functional abnormalities in the ACC in ASD have been reported (Haznedar et al. 2000; Ohnishi et al. 2000; Levitt et al. 2003; Di Martino et al. 2009; Simms et al. 2009). The role of dorsal ACC has been linked to social orienting (Dawson et al. 1998), joint attention (Mundy et al. 2000; Henderson et al. 2002), developing representations of the self (Craik et al. 1999), and relating the self to others (Frith and Frith 2001). All of these have been implicated in individuals with ASD.

One common neuroimaging technique used to study error processing in relation to ACC is the event-related potential (ERP) during the electroencephalography recordings. Two ERP components that index error processing are the error-related negativity (ERN or Ne) and the error positivity (Pe; e.g., Falkenstein et al. 1991, 2000; Simons 2010). The ERN is a large negative response-locked ERP component that reaches its maximum at the frontocentral site (FCz) and peaks in the time period 50–100 ms after an erroneous response commission (Falkenstein et al. 1991; Gehring et al. 1993). It represents a rapid internal detection of neural system that is crucial for adaptive and goal-directed actions (Ridderinkhof et al. 2004). The Pe is a slow positivity that follows the ERN and peaks its maximum in the time period 200–400 ms (Falkenstein et al. 2000). It represents a signature of conscious awareness or reflection of committing an error (Yordanova et al. 2004; O'Connell et al. 2007) or the connotation of the error to an individual (Overbeek et al. 2005).

Henderson et al. (2006) published the first ERP study of error processing in ASD; they found that the ERN amplitude related to impairment in social interaction in individuals with high-functioning ASD. Since then, there has been an increase, but sparse studies in the electrophysiology of error processing in ASD and the findings among the studies are mixed. In order to better characterize the error processing in individuals with ASD, this preliminary meta-analytical appraisal focuses on determining the extent of potentially deficient error processing in this population indexed by the amplitude of ERN and Pe through gathering the evidence to obtain an overall conclusion considering the data published to date. The purpose of this meta-analysis, therefore, aims to improve on the current state of the literature by presenting a quantitative report on the magnitude of the differences in error processing between neurotypical individuals and individuals with ASD that can serve as an up-to-date reference for ongoing efforts to eventually help refine the theory of executive dysfunction in ASD.

21.2 Methods

21.2.1 Literature search

Studies were searched from the PubMed and PsychINFO databases as well as from Science Direct and Google Scholar up to September 2014. The keyword phrases and the combination used in the search were as follows: "error negativity AND autism," "error negativity AND autism spectrum disorder," "error-related negativity AND autism," and "error-related negativity AND autism spectrum disorder." Only studies published in English were considered. After removing the duplicates, there were nine potential studies to be analyzed before subsequent review for inclusion.

21.2.2 Inclusion criteria

To be included, the studies must report the number of participants in each of the autism or ASD and neurotypical control groups and report the mean and standard deviation (SD) of the ERN and or Pe amplitudes in each group. If the studies did not report the mean and SD, but reported t and p values, they would be included in the analysis. After carefully reviewing the studies based on these criteria, seven out of nine studies were included in this meta-analysis.

21.2.3 Meta-analysis procedure and data analysis

Prior to effect size calculation, reported standard errors of mean (if any) were converted to SD. The effect size calculations were using Cohen's d, that is, standard mean difference. This was computed by estimating the difference between the mean of the neurotypical group and the mean of the ASD group divided by the pooled SD. Furthermore, weighted random-effects models of meta-analysis were carried out using the method of DerSimonian and Laird (1986). The rationale of choosing random-effects model was the assumption that true effect size from a population of studies examined is normally distributed. The homogeneity of the effect sizes was tested with the Q statistic, quantifying by I^2. The MetaEasy software (Kontopantelis and Reeves 2009) was used to conduct these analyses. Furthermore, publication bias was examined using (a) fail-safe N (Orwin 1983), that is, calculating the number of unpublished studies to obtain a small effect size ($d = 0.2$; Cohen 1988), (b) funnel plots, and (c) Egger's regression test.

21.3 Results

Table 21.1 presents the seven studies included in the meta-analysis with an overview of sample characteristics, task, and result of group comparison between ASD and neurotypical control. In these seven studies, six studies focused on children and one study examined adults. There were a total of 148 individuals with ASD aged 8–51 years and a total of 130

Table 21.1 Individual Studies Included in the Meta-Analysis with Information on Sample Characteristics, Tasks, and Findings

Study	Participants	Task	Group Difference Neurotypical vs. ASD
Henderson et al. (2015)	38 High-functioning autism (HFA) and 36 control without autism Age HFA: 13.16 ± 2.49, range: 8.58–16.75; control: 12.61 ± 2.39, range: 8.83–16.75 Verbal IQ HFA: 104.5 ± 12.11; control: 108.61 ± 10.72 Social communication score HFA: 21.22 ± 5.71, control: 4.94 ± 3.83 Autism symptom severity score HFA: 28.00 ± 9.84, control: 3.16 ± 9.84 (p. 551)	A modified Eriksen flanker task Compatible: >>>>> or <<<<< Incompatible: >><<> or <><<< Three blocks of 96 trials with equal compatible and incompatible trials (p. 552)	No direct comparison between HFA and control in ERN at FCz site
Henderson et al. (2006)	24 HFA and 17 control without autism Age (in months) HFA: 136.6 ± 24.7; control: 136.8 ± 22.3, WISC-VCI HFA: 100.1 ± 14.5; control: 106.21 ± 12.9 WISC-PRI HFA: 9.1 ± 14.6; control: 106.1 ± 10.4 Social communication score: HFA: 6.6 ± 1.7, control: 1.6 ± 1.5 Autism symptom severity score: HFA: 26.7 ± 8.3, control: 5.1 ± 4.9 (p. 99)	A modified Eriksen flanker task Compatible: >>>>> or <<<<< Incompatible: >><<> or <><<< Three blocks of 96 trials with equal compatible and incompatible trials (p. 100)	No direct comparison between HFA and control in ERN at FCz site
Santesso et al. (2011)	15 High-functioning adults with ASD and 16 control adults Age ASD: 36.0 ± 11.1, range: 18.8–51.6; control: 35.7 ± 10.6, range: 22.6–47.8 IQ ASD: 101.5 ± 14.4, range: 82–136; control: 103.4 ± 14.0, range: 76–121 Autism spectrum quotient ASD group has significantly higher scores on social skills, communication skills, and imagination than controls (p. 243)	Number Eriksen flanker task Congruent trial 333 or 444 Incongruent trial 343 or 434 Also close distance or far distance 8 blocks of 72 trials (p. 243)	ASD showed significantly smaller ERN than control, $t(27) = 2.28$, $p = .03$ as well as Pe, $t(27) = 2.38$, $p = 0.025$ (p. 245)
Sokhadze et al. (2010)	14 Children with ASD and 14 control Age ASD: 13.0 ± 2.5, range: 9–18; control: 14.1 ± 3.9, range: 9–21 Full IQ	A traditional visual three-stimuli oddball task with a total of 480 trials. Stimuli letters "X," "O," and novel distracters ("v," "∧," "∧," ">," and "<" signs)	ASD showed significantly smaller ERN than control, $F(1, 27) = 4.88$, $p = 0.036$, not Pe, $p = 0.14$, n.s. (p. 85)

(Continued)

Table 21.1 (*Continued*) Individual Studies Included in the Meta-Analysis with Information on Sample Characteristics, Tasks, and Findings

Study	Participants	Task	Group Difference Neurotypical vs. ASD
	ASD: 92.2 ± 15.3 Social responsiveness scale score Repetitive behavior: 27.79 ± 15.34 Social awareness: 83.00 ± 8.20 Irritability: 9.86 ± 6.16 Hyperactivity: 14.07 ± 8.25 (p. 84)	"0": 50% of the trials; the novel stimuli: 25% of the trials "X": the remaining 25% of the trials—the target (p. 84)	
Sokhadze et al. (2012)	16 Children with ASD and 16 control Age ASD: 12.6 ± 2.3, range: 9–17; control: 14.6 ± 3.9, range: 9–20 Full IQ ASD: 95.35 ± 19.11 ASD children have comorbidity and take medications (p. 17)	Three stimuli visual oddball with illusory Kanizsa figures (targets, 25% probability), Kanizsa triangles (rare non- target distracters, 25% probability), and non-Kanizsa figures (standards, 50% probability) (p. 18)	ASD showed significantly smaller ERN than control, p = 0.001, not Pe, p = 0.36, n.s. (p. 20)
South et al. (2010)	24 High-functioning children with ASD and 21 control Age ASD: 14.03 ± 2.40, range: 9–21; control: 14.23 ± 2.83, range: 8–18 Full IQ ASD: 109.71 ± 13.16, range: 87–132; control: 112.05 ± 14.44, range: 74–138 Performance IQ ASD: 107.62 ± 13.96, range: 89–139, control: 109.90 ± 9.69 range: 88–128 Social communication score ASD: 21.13 ± 4.77, range: 13–19 (p. 243)	A modified Eriksen flanker task Congruent: ##< or >## Incongruent: #<# or #># Two blocks of 200 trials: 60% are incongruent, 40% are congruent (p. 244)	ASD showed significantly smaller ERN than control, t(43) = 2.55, p = 0.02, d = 0.76 (p. 246)
Vlamings et al. (2008)	17 Children with ASD and 10 control Age ASD: 10.42 ± 2.04; control: 9.23 ± 20 Full IQ ASD: 94.5 ± 16.2, range: 61–120; control: 95.1 ± 12.5, range: 81–116 Performance IQ ASD: 99.19 ± 17.9, range: 59–129, control: 100.6 ± 14.3 range: 73–118 Verbal IQ ASD: 92.19 ± 15.3, range: 64–112; control: 90.8 ± 10.8, range: 77–114 (p. 400)	An auditory decision task A total of 140 trials: 68 trials of cat sound and 72 trials of non cat sound (easy task) In the hard task, the animal sounds were evenly divided Right-hand button: the sound was the same as the preceding sound Left-hand button: dissimilar sound (p. 400)	ASD showed significantly smaller ERN than control, t(25) = 3.11, p < 0.01 (p. 401)

neurotypical controls aged 8–47 years comparable according to age and intelligent quotient (IQ). The IQ of individuals with ASD ranged from 61 to 136, whereas it was ranged from 73 to 138 in the control participants. All participants with ASD in these studies were high functioning. Among the studies, some type of Eriksen flanker task was mostly used to determine error processing (Table 21.1).

For the calculation of the effect sizes of Cohen's d, the absolute numeric values of the ERN amplitudes at the frontocentral (FCz) site of the ASD group subtracted from that of the control group. The Pe amplitude at the parietocentral (Pz) site or the central (Cz) site was calculated with the same approach. The rationale was because the ASD group was hypothesized to demonstrate smaller amplitudes than the control group.

21.3.1 Error-related negativity

Table 21.2 presents the ERN amplitude, effect size, and 95% confidence interval (CI) of effect size of each included study. It was noted that each study employed a different method to measure and quantify the ERN amplitude. Among the seven studies, the ASD group displayed a smaller ERN amplitude than the control group in six studies. The effect size ranged from −0.33 to 1.17 and four studies had a large effect size based on Cohen's classification ($d > 0.8$; Cohen 1988); the 95% CI of effect size of five studies was greater than 0. Figure 21.1 presents the forest plot of the results of the individual and pooled effect sizes for the ERN amplitude for all seven studies.

The analysis of the DerSimonian and Laird random-effects model showed an overall significant pooled medium effect size of 0.63 with the 95% CI of 0.26–1.00, $p < 0.001$, indicating that individuals with ASD displayed a moderate reduced ERN amplitude when compared with the neurotypical controls. The result of heterogeneity of the single effects was Cochrane $Q = 13.76$, $p = 0.032$, $I^2 = 56.4\%$, $\tau^2 = 13.67\%$. The I^2 result showed that there was a moderate heterogeneity among these seven studies and the τ^2 result showed 13.67% of between-study variance for the true effect.

With regard to the publication bias, Egger's regression test of publication bias showed no bias, $\beta = 3.78$, 95% CI of β ranged from −3.83 to 11.40, $t = 1.28$, $p = 0.26$. The funnel plot (Figure 21.2) did not suggest a publication bias either. The result of Orwin's fail-safe N test revealed that 16 unpublished studies with a mean effect size of 0 would need to be included to reduce the observed medium effect size of 0.63 to 0.20.

21.3.2 Error positivity

Table 21.3 presents the Pe amplitude, effect size, and 95% CI of effect size of each included study. Similar to the ERN component, it was noted

Table 21.2 Results of ERN Component (Mean and Standard Deviation [SD] in µV) of Included Studies and Effect Sizes Obtained in the Meta-Analysis

Study	ERN Component	ASD Mean (SD)	Neurotypical Mean (SD)	Effect Size (d)	Lower 95% CI of d	Upper 95% CI of d	Error Bar of d
Henderson et al. (2015)	ERN mean amplitude	−2.59 (4.60)	−4.76 (6.35)	0.39	−0.06	0.85	0.46
Henderson et al. (2006)	ERN peak amplitude	−6.50 (6.70)	−4.40 (5.80)	−0.33	−0.95	0.29	0.62
South et al. (2010)	ERN mean amplitude	−1.73 (1.45)	−3.31 (2.62)	0.76	0.17	1.35	0.59
Santesso et al. (2011)	ERN peak amplitude	−3.97 (1.71)	−5.53 (1.93)	0.85	0.12	1.58	0.73
Sokhadze et al. (2010)	ERN adaptive mean amplitude	−0.29 (6.68)	−5.5 (5.76)	0.84	0.09	1.56	0.74
Sokhadze et al. (2012)	ERN adaptive mean amplitude	0.44 (7.29)	−5.81 (5.12)	0.99	0.30	1.69	0.69
Vlamings et al. (2008)	ERN mean area peak-to-peak amplitude	−3.01 (6.66)	−12.9 (10.99)	1.17	0.38	1.95	0.78

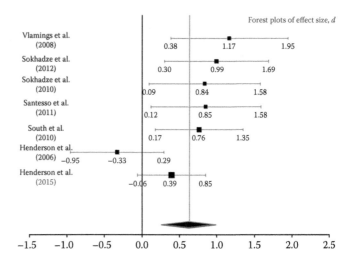

Figure 21.1 ERN amplitude: single effects and aggregated effects for the included studies. Each square was located at the estimate of the effect size with the size of the square proportional to the sample size. The blue horizontal lines indicated the 95% CI of the effect size for each comparison. The black line indicated the estimated effect size with its corresponding prediction interval.

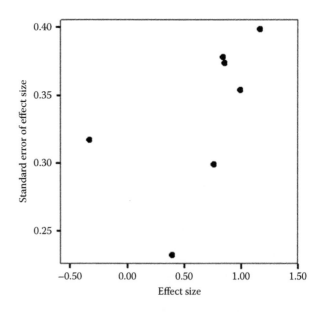

Figure 21.2 Funnel plot of effect size versus standard error (random-effects model). Funnel plot to examine publication bias in the ERN amplitude.

Table 21.3 Results of Pe Component of Included Studies and Effect Sizes Obtained in the Meta-Analysis

Study	Pe Component	ASD Mean (SD)	Neurotypical Mean (SD)	Effect Size (d)	Lower 95% CI of d	Upper 95% CI of d	Error Bar of d
South et al. (2010)	Pe mean amplitude	2.12 (1.69)	2.11 (1.97)	−0.05	−0.64	0.53	0.59
Santesso et al. (2011)	Pe peak amplitude	3.22 (2.34)	5.59 (2.90)	0.89	0.16	1.62	0.73
Sokhadze et al. (2010)[a]	Pe adaptive mean amplitude	NR	NR	0.56	−0.18	1.30	0.74
Sokhadze et al. (2012)[a]	Pe adaptive mean amplitude	NR	NR	0.32	−0.37	1.02	0.69
Vlamings et al. (2008)	Pe mean area peak-to-peak amplitude	4.66 (9.22)	12.55 (14.33)	0.40	−0.38	1.18	0.78

[a] The p value and df were used; NR = not reported; both Henderson et al. studies did not examine Pe.

that each study utilized a different method to measure and quantify the Pe amplitude. The ASD group displayed a smaller Pe amplitude than the control group in two studies. Two studies did not report the values of the Pe amplitude. The effect size ranged from −0.05 to 0.89 and only one study had a large effect size based on Cohen's classification ($d > 0.8$; Cohen 1988); the 95% CI of the effect size of only one study was greater than 0. Figure 21.3 presents the forest plot of the results of the individual and pooled effect sizes for the Pe amplitude for all five studies.

The analysis of the DerSimonian and Laird random-effects model showed an overall significant pooled effect size of 0.38 with the 95% CI of 0.06 to 0.70, $p < 0.01$, indicating that individuals with ASD displayed a decreased Pe amplitude as compared to the neurotypical controls. The result of heterogeneity of the single effects was Cochrane $Q = 4.22$, $p = 0.38$, $I^2 = 5.3\%$, $\tau^2 = 0.71\%$. The I^2 result showed that there was no heterogeneity among these studies and the τ^2 result showed only 0.71% of between-study variance for the true effect.

With regard to the publication bias, Egger's regression test of publication bias showed no bias, $\beta = 7.05$, 95% CI of β ranged from −2.94 to 17.04, $t = 2.25$, $p = 0.11$. The funnel plot (Figure 21.4) did not suggest a publication bias either. The result of Orwin's fail-safe N test revealed that five unpublished studies with a mean effect size of 0 would need to be included to reduce the observed medium effect size of 0.38 to 0.20.

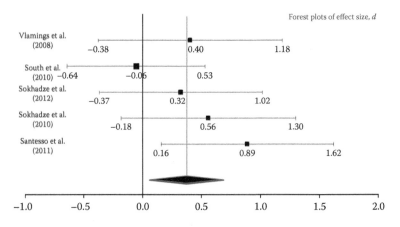

Figure 21.3 Pe amplitude: single effects and aggregated effects for the included studies. Each square was located at the estimate of the effect size with the size of the square proportional to the sample size. The blue horizontal lines indicated the 95% CI of the effect size for each comparison. The black line indicated the estimated effect size with its corresponding prediction interval.

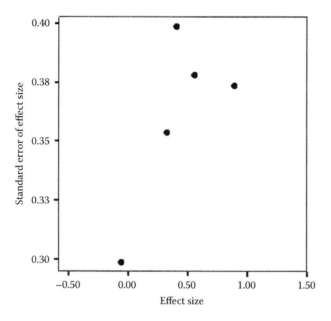

Figure 21.4 Funnel plot of effect size versus standard error (random-effects model). Funnel plot to examine publication bias in the Pe amplitude.

21.4 Discussion

To the best of my knowledge, this study is the first meta-analysis to determine diminished error processing in individuals with ASD as compared to neurotypical controls by evaluating the ERN and Pe ERP components. Although the data from available published studies were scarce and heterogeneous, the meta-analysis results revealed a salient and consistent reduction of the ERN amplitude in individuals with ASD. For the Pe, each of the five studies was capricious; nevertheless, the analysis of pooled effect size showed a notable reduction of the Pe amplitude in individuals with ASD. These results indicate a monitoring deficit as a fundamental feature of ASD as most participants in the meta-analysis are high-functioning ASD; and it is anticipated that individuals with more severe ASD symptoms will exhibit increased deficient error processing.

21.4.1 Error-related negativity and error positivity

Individuals with ASD have high interindividual variability in symptom presentation and developmental course. This has posed a critical and substantial challenge to the research of ASD (South et al. 2008). Therefore, identification of specific electrophysiological markers or profiles has been inconsistent or difficult across studies. In the research of error processing, Henderson et al. (2006) found an enhanced ERN amplitude in high verbal IQ ASD as compared to healthy controls whereas Groen et al. (2008) found no difference in the ERN amplitude between their ASD group and controls. Other studies included in this meta-analysis individually demonstrated medium-to-large difference in the reduction of the ERN amplitude in the ASD group than control group. Aggregately, this meta-analysis reveals that moderate ERN amplitude reduction can be a convinced electrophysiological profile for individuals with ASD.

The ERN is an index associated with the commission of errors, that is, early process of matching between an intended and executed response (Falkenstein et al. 2000), thought to be independent of conscious perception (Franken et al. 2007), and it appears to be impaired in individuals with ASD. Regardless of the heterogeneity of ASD symptoms and social functioning across the published studies included in this present study, such impaired early stage of error processing remains affected from childhood to adulthood of ASD. Previous ERP studies have uncovered that reduced ERN is associated with compromised social behavior (Dikman and Allen 2000; Santesso et al. 2005) and lack of empathy (Santesso and Segalowitz 2009). Low empathy has been found to be associated with ASD symptoms in numerous studies (e.g., Baron-Cohen et al. 2001; Baron-Cohen and Wheelwright 2004; Wheelwright et al. 2006; Lombardo et al. 2007). In addition, South et al. (2010) identified a relationship between the ERN amplitude and social behavior score and suggested that the social deficits in ASD are something unique and poor social behaviors may be associated with the ability to self-monitor in individuals with ASD. Thus, it is not surprising that the result of this meta-analysis collectively showed a reduction of ERN amplitude in individuals with ASD.

The neuronal generator region of the ERN has been source-localized to the dorsal ACC (see Taylor et al. 2007 for review). The ACC plays a crucial role in cognitive control on high-conflict and/or error trials (Carter and van Veen 2007) as well as action selection within a social context. In addition, the ACC plays a central role in self-monitoring that may contribute to social-emotional and social-cognitive development of individuals with autism or ASD (Mundy 2003). Three studies included in this meta-analysis (i.e., Vlamings et al. 2008; Sokhadze et al. 2010; Santesso et al. 2011) also source-localized the ERN generator to the ACC in individuals with ASD. Both Santesso et al. (2011) and Vlamings et al. (2008) specifically found that social skill deficits and severity of autism symptoms were related to ACC hypoactivity in their ASD groups. Santesso et al. (2011) further proposed that reduced ACC function (ACC hypoactivity) in ASD reflected in the ERN itself may indicate the disturbed error processing as a persistent or stable problem that could contribute to the severity of ASD symptoms and social impairments.

With regard to the Pe, few previous research studies identify a decreased Pe amplitude in individuals with ASD (Groen et al. 2008; Vlamings et al. 2008). In this present meta-analysis, however, based on effect size calculations, four studies did not show a true Pe amplitude reduction in individuals with ASD but only one study did. Nevertheless, this meta-analysis aggregately revealed a significant mild-to-moderate reduction of the Pe amplitude in individuals with ASD. This finding suggests that individuals with ASD demonstrate minor-to-moderate deficient error awareness and they are different from neurotypical controls in allocation of attention to errors. In contrast with the ERN (the early stage of error processing), the Pe (the later stage of error processing) appears to be less hampered in individuals with ASD.

The functionality of the Pe has been linked to conscious error recognition, adjustment of the response strategy, or subjective/emotional error assessment (e.g., Falkenstein et al. 2000; Van Veen and Cater 2002; Overbeek et al. 2005; Taylor et al. 2006). The Pe has been source-localized to the rostral ACC (rACC; Van Veen and Cater 2002). Thakkar et al. (2008) also reported exaggerated, abnormal rACC activation in individuals with ASD using functional magnetic resonance imaging (fMRI), linking abnormal error processing to restricted and repetitive behavior. Such abnormal signals in rACC may contribute to the affective or subjective/emotional salience of error assessment, which further supports the role of the Pe in motivational significance of errors (see Manoach and Agam 2013).

Overbeek et al. (2005) found that the Pe amplitude could be modulated by the motivational significance of errors. South et al. (2010) indicated that in contrast to the findings of both Groen et al. (2008) and Vlamings et al. (2008), their result of no reduced Pe amplitude in the ASD group could be due to the motivation factor of the experimental task employed in their study. However, the findings of this meta-analysis did not fully support this argument as individual studies included used a variety of tasks and only 95% CI of effect size of Santesso et al. (2011) did not contain 0, which was based on a number flanker task. Nevertheless, this meta-analysis shows that individuals with ASD, regardless of adolescents and adults, still manifest impairment in early error processing (ERN) and could not be compensated in the subsequent stage of error processing by consciously recognizing or monitoring their errors. This outcome results in attenuated Pe amplitude and does not depend on the task characteristics.

It should be noted that the amount of the attenuation of the Pe amplitude in individuals with ASD is less than that of the ERN amplitude. Geburek et al. (2013) explained that a smaller amount of attenuation in the Pe amplitude could be due to the fact that healthy individuals are more receptive to instruction or manipulation used in the task studying error processing, which may result in increased motor preparation obscuring the Pe due to an increased contingent negative variation (CNV). However, Geburek et al. (2013) indicated that this should be further tested.

21.4.2 Implication for the theory of executive dysfunction in ASD

The results of this meta-analysis provide support to refine executive dysfunction theory of ASD by embracing error processing (performance monitoring). As individuals with ASD demonstrate an "insensitivity to detect situations in which the chance of making errors is enhanced" (Vlamings et al. 2008, p. 399), the pattern of the ERN and Pe that emerged from the meta-analysis could be interpreted with respect to a lack of self-regulation competency in individuals with high-functioning ASD. Particularly, this meta-analysis produced consistent differences in both the ERN and the Pe between individuals with ASD and controls, indicating deficits in both error detection and conscious recognition of errors. However, the conscious recognition of errors appears to be less impaired as compared to error detection. This may suggest that if the efforts of compensation are exerted in the latter and more conscious process, the differences between individuals with ASD and controls may be reduced.

The results of this meta-analysis also suggest that interference control is a type of ability required in error monitoring/processing. Deficient monitoring and evaluating of errors to resolve interference in ASD might sustain second-order executive and self-regulatory dysfunctions. Such impairments in an ability to correctly and timely respond to errors and to learn from errors may lead to the persistence of rigid, repetitive, and stereotyped behaviors and deficits in adjustments of erratic behavior, which will result in consequent impairment in social interaction and/or communication.

In addition, the ERN and Pe can serve as bio-behavioral markers of cognitive processes that potentially moderate the development of individuals with ASD. Combing with other neuropsychological tests of executive functions, a more in-depth understanding of their nature in relation to other aspects of executive functions in individuals with ASD may result in better description of the role of error processing in the theory of executive dysfunction in ASD that will contribute to both developmental and behavioral phenotypic differences within this broad spectrum of pervasive developmental disorder.

21.4.3 Limitations

There are limitations in this meta-analysis. For example, data from only a few published studies are available. Because ASD is heterogeneous, this makes it difficult to conduct moderator analysis to examine the effect of age, gender, medication, and comorbid symptoms. Owing to a lack of the amount of reaction time differences in the posterror trials, the degree of posterror slowing (a behavioral index of error processing) difference between individuals with ASD and controls was undetermined in this meta-analysis. Adding such information will strengthen the findings of the ERN and Pe. In addition, only three studies included in this meta-analysis conducted source localization in ACC. It would be difficult to determine the aggregated precision of ACC source localization in this meta-analysis. However, adding such information to the findings of the ERN and Pe will be valuable.

In summary, this meta-analysis indicates prominent reduced ERN and slightly altered Pe in individuals with ASD when compared with neurotypical controls. This meta-analysis also provides evidence regarding the connotation of a general impairment in error monitoring that may underlie social-cognitive disturbances in ASD. However, more empirical studies are needed as this meta-analysis is only able to include seven studies.

References

American Psychiatric Association. 2013. *Diagnostic and Statistical Manual of Mental Disorders*, 5th ed. Washington, D.C.: American Psychiatric Association.

Baron-Cohen, S., A. M. Leslie, and U. Frith. 1985. Does the autistic child have a "theory of mind?" *Cognition* 21:37–46.

Baron-Cohen, S. and S. Wheelwright. 2004. The empathy quotient: An investigation of adults with Asperger syndrome or high functioning autism, and normal sex differences. *J. Autism Dev. Disord.* 34:163–75.

Baron-Cohen, S., S. Wheelwright, R. Skinner et al. 2001. The autism spectrum quotient (AQ): Evidence from Asperger syndrome/high functioning autism, males and females, scientists and mathematicians. *J. Autism Dev. Disord.* 31:5–17.

Bogte, H., B. Flammaa, J. van der Meere et al. 2007. Post-error adaptation in adults with high functioning autism. *Neuropsychologia* 45:1707–14.

Carter, C. S. and V. van Veen. 2007. Anterior cingulate cortex and conflict detection: An update of theory and data. *Cogn. Affective Behav. Neurosci.* 7:367–79.

Centers for Disease Control and Prevention. 2012. Prevalence of autism spectrum disorder among children aged 8 years—Autism and Developmental Disabilities Monitoring Network, 14 sites, United States, 2008. *MMWR* 61:3.

Centers for Disease Control and Prevention. 2014. Prevalence of autism spectrum disorder among children aged 8 years—Autism and Developmental Disabilities Monitoring Network, 11 sites, United States, 2010. *MMWR* 63:2.

Cohen, J. 1988. *Statistical Power Analysis for the Behavioral Sciences*, 2nd ed. New York: Routledge Academic.

Craik, F. I. M., T. M. Moroz, M. Moscovitch et al. 1999. In search of the self: A positron emission tomography study. *Psychol. Sci.* 10:26–34.

Dawson, G., A. N. Meltzoff, J. Osterling et al. 1998. Children with autism fail to orient to naturally-occurring social stimuli. *J. Autism Dev. Disord.* 28:479–85.

DerSimonian, R. and N. Laird. 1986. Meta-analysis in clinical trials. *Control. Clin. Trials* 7:177–88.

Dikman, Z. V. and J. J. B. Allen. 2000. Error monitoring during reward and avoidance learning in high- and low-socialized individuals. *Psychophysiology* 37:43–54.

Di Martino, A., K. Ross, L. Q. Uddin et al. 2009. Functional brain correlates of social and nonsocial processes in autism spectrum disorders: An activation likelihood estimation meta-analysis. *Biol. Psychiatry* 65:63–74.

Falkenstein, M., J. Hohnsbein, and J. Hoormann. 1991. Effects of crossmodal divided attention on late ERP components. II. Error processing in choice reaction tasks. *Electroencephalogr. Clin. Neurophysiol.* 78:447–55.

Falkenstein, M., J. Hoormann, S. Christ et al. 2000. ERP components on reaction errors and their functional significance: A tutorial. *Biol. Psychol.* 51:87–107.

Franken, I. H. A., J. W. van Striena, E. J. Franzek et al. 2007. Error-processing deficits in patients with cocaine dependence. *Biol. Psychol.* 75:45–51.

Frith, U. and C. Frith. 2001. The biological basis of social interaction. *Curr. Direct. Psychol. Sci.* 10:151–55.

Frith, U. and F. Happé. 1994. Autism: Beyond "theory of mind." *Cognition* 50:115–32.

Frith, U., J. Morton, and A. M. Leslie. 1991. The cognitive basis of a biological disorder: Autism. *Trends Neurosci.* 14:433–8.

Geburek, A. J., F. Rist, G. Gediga et al. 2013. Electrophysiological indices of error monitoring in juvenile and adult attention deficit hyperactivity disorder (ADHD)—A meta-analytic appraisal. *Int. J. Psychophysiol.* 87:349–62.

Gehring, W. J., B. Goss, M. G. H. Coles et al. 1993. A neural system for error detection and compensation. *Psychol. Sci.* 4:385–90.

Groen, Y., A. A. Wijers, L. J. M. Mulder et al. 2008. Error and feedback processing in children with ADHD and children with autistic spectrum disorder: A EEG event-related potential study. *Clin. Neurophysiol.* 119:2476–93.

Happé, F. 1999. Autism: Cognitive deficit or cognitive style? *Trends Cogn. Sci.* 3:216–22.

Happé, F. and U. Frith. 2006. The weak coherence account: Detail-focused cognitive style in autism spectrum disorders. *J. Autism Dev. Disord.* 36:5–25.

Happé, F. and A. Ronald. 2008. The "fractionable autism triad": A review of evidence from behavioural, genetic, cognitive and neural research. *Neuropsychol. Rev.* 18:287–304.

Haznedar, M. M., M. S. Buchsbaum, T.-C. Wei et al. 2000. Limbic circuitry in patients with autism spectrum disorders studied with positron emission tomography and magnetic resonance imaging. *Am. J. Psychiatry* 157:1994–2001.

Henderson, H. A., K. E. Ono, C. M. McMahon et al. 2015. The costs and benefits of self-monitoring for higher functioning children and adolescents with autism. *J. Autism Dev. Disord.* 45:548–59.

Henderson, H., C. Schwartz, P. Mundy et al. 2006. Response monitoring, the error-related negativity, and differences in social behavior in autism. *Brain Cogn.* 61:96–109.

Henderson, L. M., P. J. Yoderb, M. W. Yale et al. 2002. Getting the point: Electrophysiological correlates of protodeclarative pointing. *Int. J. Dev. Neurosci.* 20:449–58.

Holroyd, C. B. and M. G. H. Coles. 2002. The neural basis of human error processing: Reinforcement learning, dopamine and the error-related negativity. *Psychol. Rev.* 109:679–709.

Holroyd, C. B., S. Nieuwenhuis, N. Yeung et al. 2004. Dorsal anterior cingulate cortex shows fMRI response to internal and external error signals. *Nat. Neurosci.* 7:497–98.

Kontopantelis, E. and D. Reeves. 2009. MetaEasy: A meta-analysis add-in for Microsoft Excel. *J. Stat. Softw.* 30:1–25.

Kulage, K., A. Smaldone, and E. Cohn. 2014. How will DSM-5 affect autism diagnosis? A systematic literature review and meta-analysis. *J. Autism Dev. Disord.* 44:1918–32.

Levitt, J. G., J. O'Neill, R. E. Blanton et al. 2003. Proton magnetic resonance spectroscopic imaging of the brain in childhood autism. *Biol. Psychiatry* 54:1355–66.

Lombardo, M. V., J. L. Barnes, S. J. Wheelwright et al. 2007. Self-referential cognition and empathy in autism. *PLoS One* 2:e883.

Manoach, D. S. and Y. Agam. 2013. Neural markers of errors as endophenotypes in neuropsychiatric disorders. *Frontiers Hum. Neurosci.* 7:1–19.

Mundy, P. 2003. The neural basis of social impairments in autism: The role of the dorsal medial-frontal cortex and anterior cingulate system. *J. Child Psychol. Psychiatry* 44:793–809.

Mundy, P., J. Card, and N. Fox. 2000. EEG correlates of the development of infant joint attention skills. *Dev. Psychobiol.* 36:325–38.

O'Connell, R. G., P. M. Dockree, M. A. Bellgrove et al. 2007. The role of cingulate cortex in the detection of errors with and without awareness: A high-density electrical mapping study. *Eur. J. Neurosci.* 25:2571–9.

O'Hearn, K., M. Asatoa, S. Ordaz, and B. Luna. 2008. Neurodevelopment and executive function in autism. *Dev. Psychopathol.* 20:1103–32.

Ohnishi, T., H. Matsuda, T. Hashimoto et al. 2000. Abnormal regional cerebral blood flow in childhood autism. *Brain* 123:1838–44.

Orwin, R. G. 1983. A fail-safe *N* for effect size in meta-analysis. *J. Educ. Behav. Stat.* 8:157–9.

Overbeek, T. J. M., S. Nieuwenhuis, K. R. Ridderinkhof. 2005. Dissociable components of error processing: On the functional significance of the Pe vis-à-vis the ERN/Ne. *J. Psychophysiol.* 19:319–29.

Pennington, B. F. and S. Ozonoff. 1996. Executive functions and developmental psychopathology. *J. Child Psychol. Psychiatry* 37:51–87.

Premack, D. and G. Woodruv. 1978. Does the chimpanzee have a theory of mind? *Behav. Brain Sci.* 1:515–26.

Rajendran, G. and P. Mitchell. 2007. Cognitive theories of autism. *Dev. Rev.* 27:224–60.

Ridderinkhof, K. R., W. P. M. van den Wildenberga, S. J. Segalowitz et al. 2004. Neurocognitive mechanisms of cognitive control: The role of prefrontal cortex in action selection, response inhibition, performance monitoring, and reward-based learning. *Brain Cogn.* 56:129–40.

Rivet, T. T. and J. L. Matson. 2011. Review of gender differences in core symptomatology in autism spectrum disorders. *Res. Autism Spectr. Disord.* 5:957–76.

Russell, J. and C. Jarrold. 1998. Error-correction problems in autism: Evidence for a monitoring impairment? *J. Autism Dev. Disord.* 28:177–88.

Santesso, D. L., I. Drmic, M. K. Jetha et al. 2011. An event-related source localization study of response monitoring and social impairments in autism spectrum disorder. *Psychophysiology* 48:241–51.

Santesso, D. L. and S. J. Segalowitz. 2009. The error-related negativity is related to risk taking and empathy in young men. *Psychophysiology* 46:143–52.

Santesso, D. L., S. J. Segalowitz, and L. A. Schmidt. 2005. ERP correlates of error monitoring in 10-year-olds are related to socialization. *Biol. Psychol.* 70:79–87.

Simms, M. L., T. L. Kemper, C. M. Timbie et al. 2009. The anterior cingulate cortex in autism: Heterogeneity of qualitative and quantitative cytoarchitectonic features suggests possible subgroups. *Acta Neuropathol.* 118:673–84.

Simons, R. F. 2010. The way of our errors: Theme and variations. *Psychophysiology* 47:1–14.

Sokhadze, E. M., J. M. Baruth, A. El-Baz et al. 2010. Impaired error monitoring and correction function in autism. *J. Neurother.* 14:79–95.

Sokhadze, E. M., J. M. Baruth, L. Sears et al. 2012. Event-related potential study of attention regulation during illusory figure categorization task in ADHD, autism spectrum disorder, and typical children. *J. Neurother.* 16:12–31.

South, M., M. J. Larson, E. Krauskopf et al. 2010. Error processing in high-functioning autism spectrum disorders. *Biol. Psychol.* 85:242–51.

South, M., S. Ozonoff, Y. Suchy et al. 2008. Intact emotion facilitation for nonsocial stimuli in autism: Is amygdala impairment in autism specific for social information? *J. Int. Neuropsychol. Soc.* 14:42–54.

Stuss, D. T., T. Shallice, M. P. Alexander et al. 1995. A multidisciplinary approach to anterior attentional functions. *Ann. N. Y. Acad. Sci.* 769:191–212.

Taylor, S. F., B. Martis, K. D. Fitzgerald et al. 2006. Medial frontal cortex activity and loss-related responses to errors. *J. Neurosci.* 26:4063–70.

Taylor, S. F., E. R. Stern, and W. J. Gehring. 2007. Neural systems for error monitoring: Recent findings and theoretical perspectives. *Neuroscientist* 13:160–72.

Thakkar, K. N., F. E. Polli, R. M. Joseph et al. 2008. Response monitoring, repetitive behaviour and anterior cingulate abnormalities in autism spectrum disorders (ASD). *Brain* 131:2464–78.

Turner, M. A. 1999. Generating novel ideas: Fluency performance in high-functioning and learning disabled individuals with autism. *J. Child Psychol. Psychiatry* 40:189–201.

Ullsperger, M., C. Danielmeier, and G. Jocham. 2014. Neurophysiology of performance monitoring and adaptive behavior. *Physiol. Rev.* 94:35–79.

Ullsperger, M. and D. Y. von Cramon. 2001. Subprocesses of performance monitoring: A dissociation of error processing and response competition revealed by event-related fMRI and ERPs. *NeuroImage.* 14:1387–401.

Van Veen, V. and C. S. Cater. 2002. The timing of action-monitoring processes in the anterior cingulate cortex. *J. Cogn. Neurosci.* 14:593–602.

Vlamings, P. H. J. M., L. M. Jonkman, M. R. Hoeksma et al. 2008. Reduced error monitoring in children with autism spectrum disorder: An ERP study. *Eur. J. Neurosci.* 28:399–406.

Wheelwright, S., S. Baron-Cohen, N. Goldenfeld et al. 2006. Predicting autism-spectrum quotient (AQ) from the systemizing quotient-revised (SQ-R) and empathy quotient (EQ). *Brain Res.* 1079:47–56.

Yordanova, J., M. Falkenstein, J. Hohnsbein et al. 2004. Parallel systems of error processing in the brain. *NeuroImage* 22:590–602.

Chapter 22 Gamma abnormalities in autism spectrum disorders

Gina Rippon

Contents

Abstract 457
22.1 Introduction 458
22.2 Autism spectrum disorder. 459
    22.2.1 ASD characteristics 459
    22.2.2 Neurocognitive models of ASD 461
        22.2.2.1 Excitation–inhibition in autism 461
        22.2.2.2 Aberrant cortical connectivity in ASD 462
22.3 Gamma activity in the human brain. 463
    22.3.1 Measuring gamma 463
    22.3.2 Gamma metrics. 464
        22.3.2.1 Gamma frequencies. 464
        22.3.2.2 Task-related gamma. 466
        22.3.2.3 Task-free (resting-state) gamma. 471
    22.3.3 Gamma and connectivity measures 471
    22.3.4 GBA as a measure of GABA 473
    22.3.5 Functional significance of gamma oscillations 474
22.4 Gamma activity in autism. 474
    22.4.1 Visual gamma in ASD 475
    22.4.2 Auditory gamma in ASD 479
    22.4.3 Resting-state, "task-free" gamma activity 483
22.5 Summary 485
    22.5.1 Further refinements and future focus 486
References 487

Abstract

With the current emphasis on atypical patterns of connectivity in the brain hypothesized to be a core feature of autism spectrum disorders (ASDs), there has been a considerable focus over the last decade or so on high-frequency (gamma) band activity (GBA) in both the human and the non-human brain as a measure of connectivity. This chapter provides an overview of the measurement, analysis, and interpretation of GBA and links this to existing neurocognitive and neurophysiological models of ASD. A review of GBA research in ASD, particularly focussing on visual and auditory atypicalities, reveals some consistencies and some inconsistencies, generally arising from the application of different methodologies. It is concluded that, in parallel with emerging theoretical and analytical improvements, the study of GBA and GBA-related processes will continue to offer significant insights into ASD atypicalities at every level, additionally offering the possibility of identifying diagnostic biomarkers, serving as indices of therapeutic progress or contributing to the identification of endophenotypes.

22.1 Introduction

With the current emphasis on the understanding of the dynamics of brain function, there has been considerable focus on the role of gamma-band activity (GBA). This ranges from research at the fundamental level, where GBA is taken as an index of gamma-aminobutyric acid (GABA)-ergic cellular activity (Buzsáki and Wang 2012) and of neuronal excitation–inhibition balance (Rubenstein and Merzenich 2003; Bartos et al. 2007), through its roles in stimulus information coding (Herrmann et al. 2010), in the temporal synchronization or desynchronization of neuronal assemblies (Fries 2005, 2009; Lachaux et al. 2008) and the "binding" of sensory percepts (Rodriguez et al. 1999; Tallon-Baudry and Bertrand 1999; Engel and Singer 2001). It is accorded a central role in all modes of sensation and perception, for example, vision (Brunet et al. 2014), audition (Lakatos et al. 2005), somatosensory (Bauer et al. 2006), olfaction (Rojas Libano and Kay 2008), and in the orchestration of cortical connections underpinning higher-level cognitive functions (Fries 2005, 2009). These range from attention (Jensen et al. 2007) and attention-related modulation (Vidal et al. 2006; LaChaux et al. 2008); working memory (Morgan et al. 2011), memory, and memory matching (Herrmann et al. 2004); speech and language processing (Giraud and Poeppel 2012); face processing (Sato et al. 2012); and emotional processing (Jung et al. 2011; Maratos et al. 2012), right up to consciousness itself (Singer 2014) (see reviews by Herrmann et al. 2010; Rieder et al. 2011). The study of GBA thus offers the possibility of, on the one hand, insights into fundamental aspects of cortical function and, on the other, a potential cortical "fingerprint" of activation patterns associated with the full range of human behaviors, typical or atypical.

In a paper published in 2002, Brock et al. proposed that GBA, as a measure of temporal binding, could make a useful "candidate frequency" for the study of ASD. In an early dysfunctional connectivity model, it was proposed that the atypical perceptual behavior characteristic of

ASD might be linked to a failure in the integration of sensory information at the cortical level, caused by a reduction in the connectivity between specialized local neural networks in the brain and possibly associated with overconnectivity within isolated individual neural assemblies. As this process of information integration or "temporal binding" had been shown to be indexed by GBA (Tallon-Baudry and Bertrand 1999; Rodriguez et al. 1999), it was hypothesized that task-specific abnormalities in gamma would be found in ASD individuals, which could characterize the condition at the cortical level and which would inform modeling of atypical connectivity in the autistic brain (Brock et al. 2002; Rippon et al. 2007). It was proposed that a shift in focus from higher-level sociocognitive dysfunction such as "theory of mind" deficit (Baron-Cohen et al. 1985) to the study of lower-level anomalies in sensory and perceptual abilities could prove a fruitful field of investigation.

Developments in the last decade or so of research into brain oscillations have been characterized by increasing levels of sophistication in their measurement, modeling, and interpretation. The connectivity or "connectonomic" approach (Sporns 2011) has informed much research, with a focus on GBA. There has been increasing complexity in analytical techniques, beyond a focus on within-band evoked or induced power responses to cross-frequency models of phase–amplitude coupling (PAC) (Canolty and Knight 2010), together with quantification of gamma-based brain network properties (Stam and Reijneveld 2007). The examination of genetic factors in gamma brain oscillations (Hall et al. 2011; Van Pelt et al. 2012) and the identification of key developmental trajectories in GBA (Kitzbichler et al. 2015) offer further possibilities for refining the role of GBA research into ASD.

This chapter will review such theoretical and empirical advances in research into gamma activity in the human brain and the application of these advances into studying gamma abnormalities in ASD, and conclude with some discussion of the role this research is playing in furthering insights into this condition. These include the possibility that measures of GBA atypicalities could serve as diagnostic biomarkers or even endophenotypes, could index therapeutic progress, or even form the basis of a remedial process in its own right (Baruth et al. 2010; Casanova et al. 2015).

22.2 Autism spectrum disorder

22.2.1 ASD characteristics

Following recent changes in the classification of mental disorders, autism and autism-like disorders have been subsumed into a single spectrum of behaviors, autism spectrum disorder (ASD). The key characteristics are persistent deficits in social communication and social interaction across multiple contexts and restricted and repetitive patterns of behavior, interests, or activities (including hyper- or hyporeactivity to sensory input or unusual interests in sensory aspects of the environment) (APA 2013). Although atypical social behavior remains a primary characterization of ASD, the presence of sensory abnormalities has been given a more central role, consistent with reports that over 90% of ASD individuals have some form of sensory abnormality in multiple sensory domains, including touch, olfaction, and pain as well as auditory and visual (Leekam et al. 2007; Hazen et al. 2014).

Atypical perceptual abilities have also been the focus of research (e.g., Dakin and Frith 2005) with the associated development of theoretical models such as "weak central coherence" (Happé and Frith 2006) and "enhanced perceptual functioning" (Mottron et al. 2006). A key explanatory concept is the identification of a characteristic bias in ASD individuals toward a focus on local detail at the expense of global processing, something that Kanner identified as distinctive in autism in his original profiling, which included the inability to experience wholes without full attention to the constituent parts (Kanner 1943). This is the converse of the normal phases of typical perceptual processing, where stages are temporally organized so that they proceed from global structuring toward more and more fine-grained analysis. Superior processing of fine details can bring improved performance on tasks such as visual search (O'Riordan 2004). The associated imperviousness to the contextual aspects of perception could contribute to the alleged lack of susceptibility to illusory figures such as Kanizsa triangles or improved performance on Gestalt tasks (Bölte et al. 2007; Walter et al. 2009). It is also hypothesized as a basis for impaired face discrimination and recognition, due to the use of piecemeal feature processing rather than configural strategies (Behrmann et al. 2006). It has additionally been suggested that perceptual difficulties may underpin the restricted patterns of interests and activities typical of ASD and may even cascade into the characteristic social and behavioral deficits (Behrmann 2006; Kargas et al. 2015). An understanding of the origins of such difficulties could thus prove a fruitful focus for ASD research.

ASD is an extremely heterogeneous disorder (Jeste and Geschwind 2014), with, for example, intelligence quotient (IQ) scores from <70 to above average, and language abilities from nonverbal to normal. There is a high incidence of comorbidities such as ADHD and mounting criticism that it should not be considered as a single disorder, particularly in light of low levels of co-occurrence of the core impairments (Happé et al. 2006). ASD is highly heritable (Bailey et al. 1995) with a large range of candidate genes identified (Betancur 2011).

No common biological features have been identified, although there is a high incidence of epilepsy in ASD together with evidence of high levels of epileptiform cortical activity (Spence and Schneider 2009; see also Berg and Plioplys 2012), potentially linked to the findings of atypical high-frequency, gamma activity in ASD to be reviewed in this chapter. There have been consistent reports of atypical brain growth patterns in ASD, with measures of brain size, based on head circumference in young children, postmortem studies, and MRI data, indicating a rapid early overgrowth in ASD populations during the first 2 years of life, particularly in the frontal lobes, followed by an abnormal slowing (Redcay and Courchesne 2005; Courchesne et al. 2011). This is consistent with the very first observations of children with autism, who were noted as having unusually large heads, or macroencephaly (Kanner 1943). Early brain overgrowth has been interpreted as associated with atypical formation of cortical networks and network connections (Courchesne and Pierce 2005; Lewis and Elman 2008), which, as will be reviewed below, is consistently identified as the neural basis for many behavioral disorders, including ASD.

22.2.2 Neurocognitive models of ASD

22.2.2.1 Excitation–inhibition in autism   An early focus on abnormalities at the cellular level was on cortical minicolumns (Casanova et al. 2002; Rubenstein and Merzenich 2003). These are neuronal "microcircuits," which are distributed throughout the cortex, and comprise narrow radial columns of 80–100 neurons surrounded by GABA-containing interneurons, which act to segregate individual minicolumns, regulating their output and ensuring discrete channels of intracortical communication. Synchronization of these local systems is indexed by activity in the gamma frequency range (Whittington et al. 2011). Dysfunction in these local inhibitory neurons, indexed by abnormalities in GABA activity, could cause a generic disruption in the excitation–inhibition balance within the cortex, with associated increases in high-frequency or "noisy" activity in the brain, common in ASD (Spence and Schneider 2009). The resulting disorganization between local circuits could disrupt the synchronization necessary to ensure appropriate correlated coordination of response to stimulus input; this would be indexed by atypical sensory responses and abnormal gamma activity. Further, abnormalities in local circuits could impede the formation of long-distance connectivity between other parts of the cortex (Courchesne and Pierce 2005; Lewis and Elman 2008). As above, epileptiform activity is very common in ASD and, as this chapter will review, gamma/GABA anomalies are also common. The model is now being supported at the cytoarchitectural level (Casanova and Trippe 2009; Casanova et al. 2013; Stoner et al. 2014). As per the Brock et al. (2002) proposal, it is suggested that these minicolumn deficits would be associated with hyperactivity at the local level, possibly associated with heightened sensory experiences, but significant hypo- or underconnectivity cross-cortically, with subsequent deficits in higher cognitive processes (Casanova et al. 2002; Rubenstein and Merzenich 2003). This proposed excitation–inhibition imbalance therefore underpins the current focus on atypical patterns of

461

connectivity as the underlying neuronal cause of ASD, and links with translational models of autism identifying dysfunctional GABA-ergic mechanisms (see Section 22.3.4).

22.2.2.2 Aberrant cortical connectivity in ASD Disruption in neural synchrony or failures in dynamic network communication have been claimed as a potential unifying explanation for a wide range of behavioral and neurocognitive disorders and have been widely reviewed (e.g., Uhlhaas and Singer 2006; Menon 2011; Voytek and Knight 2015). A key aspect of the development of these models has been the major advances in techniques for studying connectivity (see Greicius and Seeley 2012). Earlier research employed functional magnetic resonance imaging (fMRI) techniques, with the fine spatial resolution enabling detailed mapping of network nodes and pathways, thus capturing the structural characteristics of hypothesized networks. Estimates of functional and/or effective connectivity between voxels or regions of interest (ROIs) were obtained using correlation or causal modeling metrics (Friston 2011). However, fMRI is less able to capture the proposed temporal dynamics of activated networks (Logothetis 2008) and cannot measure the spectral characteristics, especially GBA, which appear to be key indices of neural synchronization (Fries 2005, 2009). For this, the millisecond temporal resolution offered by electroencephalography (EEG) and magnetoencephalography (MEG) is required (e.g., da Silva 2013).

The study of neuronal circuit dysfunction specifically in ASD has formed a major part in connectivity research and has, similarly, been the subject of a number of reviews (Belmonte et al. 2004; Geschwind and Levitt 2007; Minshew and Williams 2007; Rippon et al. 2007; Wass 2011; Müller et al. 2011; Vissers et al. 2012; Port et al. 2014; Hahamy et al. 2015). The consensus from early findings of task-related activity was of accumulating evidence of long-distance structural and functional underconnectivity between specialized cortical regions underpinning a wide range of perceptual and cognitive processes (Just et al. 2004, 2007; Kana et al. 2007; Hughes 2007; Koshino et al. 2005). At this stage, the proposed "complementary" dysfunction of localized overconnectivity (Brock et al. 2002; Casanova et al. 2002; Belmonte et al. 2004) had received little support. However, it was noted that all of the early investigations had employed fMRI techniques, which would be less well suited to picking up the transient changes with specific spectral characteristics more likely to be a measure of localized activity (Thai et al. 2009). Müller et al. (2011) also noted that there were methodological differences between those fMRI studies whose findings supported a "general underconnectivity" hypothesis and those that did not. As will be shown below (see Section 22.4), subsequent studies using EEG and MEG have, indeed, identified patterns of GBA that would be consistent with an excitation–inhibition imbalance and localized hyperreactivity (Orekhova et al. 2008; Cornew et al. 2012) but equally, other studies report results consistent with reduced connectivity at the local as well as the long-distance level (Khan et al. 2013). One key issue to be considered is the validity of the spectral measures of connectivity being used, as inferences based on power measures alone can be inconsistent with more complex measures of coherence/phase-locking (Port et al. 2015) or of cross-frequency coupling (Canolty and Knight 2010) (see Section 22.4).

More recent fMRI studies using connectivity measures derived from resting-state measures report both under- (Dinstein et al. 2011) and over-connectivity (Keown et al. 2013; Supekar et al. 2013) or normal patterns (Tyszka et al. 2014). However, a recent review by Hahamy (2015) suggested that there are marked individual differences (or idiosyncrasies) shown by whole-brain analyses of connectivity and that closer attention to this source of variation may resolve some of the apparent contradictions. Developmental variations may also affect measures of connectivity—Dinstein et al. (2011) were studying toddlers with autism whereas Tyszka et al. (2014) were studying high-functioning adults. As discussed in Section 22.4.3, EEG/MEG resting-state measures of connectivity also show this varying pattern of results, which may also reflect developmental factors in GBA (Tierney et al. 2012) and also differences in the patterns of connectivity as revealed by different brain oscillation frequencies (von Stein and Sarnthein 2000; Kitzbichler et al. 2015).

22.3 Gamma activity in the human brain

Oscillatory activity in the brain arises from fluctuations in extracellular potentials in neuronal populations (Buzsáki and Wang 2012), which can be measured locally via local field potentials (LFPs), on the surface of the brain via subdural electrodes (electrocorticography, iEEG, or ECoG) or at the scalp via electroencephalographic (EEG) or magnetoencephalographic (MEG) techniques (see Da Silva 2009). High-frequency or gamma activity is commonly measured in stimulus-driven changes in network activation (Jia and Kohn 2011) and is associated with the activity of fast-spiking GABA-ergic inhibitory interneurons (Whittington et al. 1995).

The role of these inhibitory interneurons appears to be that of a bottom-up, feedforward regulatory mechanism, biasing neuronal excitability in pyramidal cortical cells and determining optimal response timing at the level of local networks (Jia and Kohn 2011; Whittington et al. 2011). The activity of these networks can be temporally linked or synchronized, both locally and also distally via long-range communication (Traub et al. 1996; see review by Whittington et al. 2011). This has been termed "communication through coherence" (Fries 2005).

22.3.1 Measuring gamma

Most studies of gamma activity in the human brain will use the noninvasive EEG or MEG techniques (e.g., da Silva 2009), although much has been learned in research into high-frequency cortical activity through the use of implanted electrodes (e.g., Jung et al. 2011). Both techniques have advantages and disadvantages with respect to measuring gamma per se. Given the small amplitude of the signal, measuring gamma at scalp level can be problematic for EEG techniques, although technical advances have considerably improved scalp distortion issues. As magnetic waves are minimally distorted by the skull, meninges, and so on, this is less of an issue, but MEG is claimed to have a problem with measuring deep sources, although, again, computational advances have at least partially overcome this (Hillebrand and Barnes 2002). Attention was recently drawn to the potentially contaminating effects of microsaccade artifacts in the measurement of visual evoked GBA using EEG (Yuval-Greenberg et al. 2008), but subsequent reports suggest that close attention to spatially relevant artifact rejection, possible use of some form of independent component analysis, as well as appropriate use of reference electrodes should avoid the problem (da Silva 2009). In MEG, the use of beamforming source localization techniques as well as ICA approaches also minimize artifact contamination of high-frequency data (Muthukumaraswamy 2013).

Electrode/sensor-level analyses can be carried out on both types of data but as the contemporary focus is on dynamic connectivity, particularly with respect to understanding cortical pathology, source-level analyses will be most informative. Perhaps a cautionary note should be sounded that, as there are potentially significant differences in head size between ASD and control groups, there should be minimal reliance on standardized head models for source localization of EEG signals and individual structural MRIs used whenever possible. It has been demonstrated that source localization using MEG is closely correlated with fMRI measures (Singh et al. 2002; Brookes et al. 2005), making it a particularly appropriate imaging modality of choice in research requiring both spatial and temporal accuracy. However, it should be noted that, particularly with low-functioning, possibly nonverbal and noncompliant, or just very young participants, it may be very challenging to use an MEG scanner or to acquire an MRI structural scan for source localization purposes (Thai et al. 2009), in which case sensor-level EEG data can still provide detailed and plausible insights into GBA, especially in young children (Elsabbagh et al. 2009).

22.3.2 Gamma metrics

22.3.2.1 Gamma frequencies   Original definitions of gamma rhythms based on electroencephalographic recordings cite a frequency range of 30–80 Hz, with a low amplitude of approximately 10–20 µV. With analog recording techniques, the cutoff point was determined by low-pass filters, set to screen out high-frequency artifacts such as electromyographic signals. Early studies of GBA in human behavior focused almost exclusively on its role in determining the binding together of separate sensory features to form a coherent percept, evident most clearly at or around 40 Hz (Singer and Gray 1995; Tallon-Baudry and Bertrand 1999).

More recently, with the advent of technical advances in cortical activation recording, such as broadband digital EEG, recording frequencies can now be extended up to 500 Hz and above (Buzsáki and Da Silva 2012), although it should be noted that SNR issues can still affect data quality. The wider use and efficiency of cortical implanted electrodes has allowed reliable recording of higher frequencies (Jacobs and Kahana 2009; Jerbi et al. 2009). "High" gamma is now similarly claimed to have a significant role in human behavior (Crone et al. 2011; Uhlhaas et al. 2011), with some studies demonstrating the higher levels of detail possible. Gaona et al. (2011), reporting ECoG findings from six patients carrying out single-word repetition tasks, showed spatially specific changes in the power, time course, and within-band frequency changes of GBA in the 60–500 Hz range, which discriminated between different task demands (speaking, reading, hearing) and were spatially specific to task-relevant cortical locations. Ossandón et al. (2011), similarly using implanted electrodes, noted that the temporal features (latency and duration) of desynchronous activity in high gamma band (60–140 Hz) power were closely correlated with task performance. Jung et al. (2011) used iEEG to investigate functional specificity within the orbitofrontal cortex. High-frequency (50–150 Hz) gamma activity distinguished between the processing of emotional faces (positive and negative) and of task feedback (positive and negative). This suggests that studies of high-frequency gamma could facilitate segregation of anatomical and functional underpinnings of the type of high-level visual-based cognitive processes where ASD deficits are characteristic.

Thus, gamma activity is now most commonly reported in terms of low (30–60 Hz) and high (60–120 Hz) frequencies, although some researchers include frequencies as high as 500 Hz in the upper gamma band (Crone et al. 2011). It should be noted that there are some inconsistencies in definitions of gamma employed by researchers, with some studies reporting GBA in terms of a single, broader range (e.g., Ohla et al. 2007 [25–100 Hz]; Mainy et al. 2007 [40–150 Hz]; Hoogenboom et al. 2006 [30–100 Hz]) and some with a narrow range that could "bridge" the newer definition of low and high gamma (e.g., Kim and Kim 2006 [35–90 Hz]). As it has now been suggested that there are potentially different spatial and functional significances for high and low gamma (Gaona et al. 2011; Uhlhaas et al. 2011), interpretation of GBA where it is reported as a single broadband or where it "bridges" the low- and high-range definitions should be viewed with caution, and might explain inconsistencies between studies (Rieder et al. 2011). This could particularly apply to studies of perception and gamma, of relevance to ASD research, where it has been shown, for example, that perceptual closure is associated with increases in high-frequency gamma (60–100 Hz) but decreases in low-frequency gamma (25–60 Hz) (Grützner et al. 2010).

Additionally, within the gamma band (however defined), differences in peak frequency have been associated with individual, heritable differences (Van Pelt et al. 2012), with differences in perceptual ability (Edden et al. 2009) and with stimulus characteristics (Hadjipapas et al. 2007). It has also been suggested that there is a positive correlation between white matter density and frequency of the visual evoked gamma band response, with the implication that higher-frequency responses were therefore associated with more efficient neuronal connectivity (Zaehle and Herrmann 2011). A recent paper by Başar et al. (2015) has proposed that GBA should be considered separately in frequency windows of 25–30 Hz, 30–35 Hz, and 40–48 Hz with evidence that these can separately distinguish sensory and cognitive processes. This is consistent with the Gaona et al. (2011) findings, reported above, that different subbands within a high gamma band (60–400 Hz) were spatially and temporally specific to different tasks. As it has also been recently suggested that gamma *frequency* may be a more stable and subtle measure of cortical responsivity than gamma *power* (Hadjipapas et al. 2015), it is clear that close attention should be paid to this metric in the designing and interpreting of research.

22.3.2.2 Task-related gamma   Poststimulus changes in gamma power can be depicted graphically (Figure 22.1a) or (more commonly) via time–frequency response (TFR) plots derived from continuous wavelet transforms, commonly Morlet (Le Van Quyen et al. 2001; Le Van Quyen and Bragin 2007) (Figure 22.1b). These are commonly used to identify a region of interest associated with peak response, and depict the amplitude changes within a prespecified frequency band.

More details can be provided by a TFR "envelope" giving additional measures of latency and duration. These profiles can be generated using an additional transform, the Hilbert transform (Le Van Quyen et al. 2001). This approach was utilized by Ossandon et al. (2011), tracking gamma band suppression during visual search (Figure 22.2).

The latter measure can be useful in studies of higher-level cognitive processes involving comparison of multiple areas over relatively longer timescales.

With respect to measures of task-related GBA power, a key distinction is the difference between *evoked* power, where the power changes are phase-locked to the eliciting event, and *induced* power, where changes are associated with but not phase-locked to the eliciting event and will show trial-by-trial variations. Evoked power is calculated by time-domain averaging across all trials before applying a wavelet transform, with induced power calculated by applying the transform to all EEG signals across each channel for each trial. Changes in induced power have also been referred to as event-related synchronization (ERS—increases) or desynchronization (ERD) or event-related perturbation (Pfurtscheller et al. 1999; Penny et al. 2004). As shown in Tallon-Baudry and Bertrand (1999), this distinction is

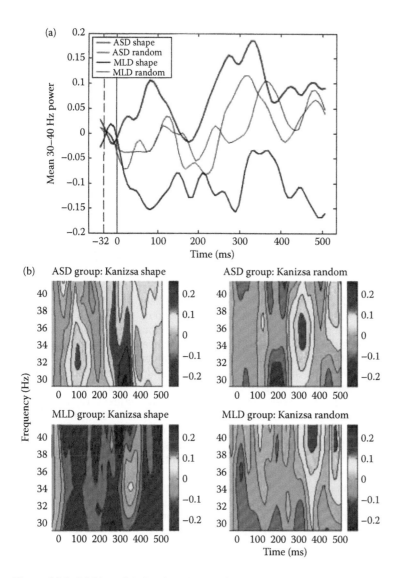

Figure 22.1 (a) Line plot showing changes in baseline-corrected mean gamma (30–40 Hz) activity summed over channels P1, 2, 3, 4 from 32 ms prior to until 512 ms after trial onset. Groups are participants with autism (ASD) and moderate learning difficulties (MLD) viewing Kanizsa triangles. (b) Spectrogram, derived using Morlet wavelet transform, showing power change in the frequency band 30–40 Hz over the first 500 ms of trial onset. Upper panels show recordings from children with autism (ASD group); lower panels show recordings from IQ-matched controls (MLD group); left-hand panels show recordings during Kanizsa shape condition; right-hand panels show recordings during Kanizsa random condition. Power increases are shown in red; power decreases are shown in blue. (Reprinted from Brown, C. et al. 2005. *Cortex* 41:364–76.)

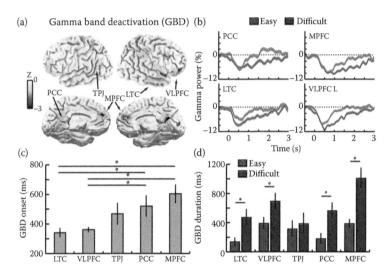

Figure 22.2 Brain-wide dynamics of gamma band power decrease, GBD, during visual search. (a) Anatomical distribution of statistically significant broadband gamma (60–140 Hz) suppression obtained by mapping depth electrode data in all subjects ($n = 14$) to a standard brain. Data snapshot at $t = 640$ ms following search array presentation (only power decreases are shown here). (b) GBD temporal profile during easy (blue) and difficult (red) search for four illustrative clusters: posterior cingulate cortex (Pcc), medial prefrontal cortex (MPFC), lateral temporal cortex (LTC), and ventrolateral prefrontal cortex (VLPFC) left (L). Time $t = 0$ ms indicates onset of search array display. (c) Mean GBD onset for each cluster. Values represent mean onset latency, that is, time sample at which deactivation reached statistical significance (group effect $F(4,98) = 6.817$, $p < 0.0001$; Tukey's HSD test [*] indicates $p < 0.05$). (d) Duration of GBD for easy (blue) and difficult (red) visual search conditions. Values represent mean duration of significant deactivation across all electrodes of each cluster (t test [*] indicates $t > 2.76$, $p < 0.01$). (Reprinted from Ossandón, T. et al. 2011. *J. Neurosci.* 31:14521–30.)

key where GBA is being used as a potential measure of temporal binding, as evoked changes will occur to any stimulus presentation whereas only induced power will distinguish coherent percepts, indicating the ongoing synchronizing process (Figure 22.3).

Early interpretations of induced power changes were taken as a measure of connectivity, with increases interpreted as increased or higher levels of connectivity and reductions as diminished or lower levels (e.g., Brown et al. 2005). However, as will be discussed below, a focus on power alone can be misleading.

One additional power-based measure in studies of sensory responsivity is the steady-state response (SSR), commonly measured to auditory or visual stimuli. The auditory SSR response is elicited by click trains or amplitude-modulated tones; the visual SSR response is elicited by flicker

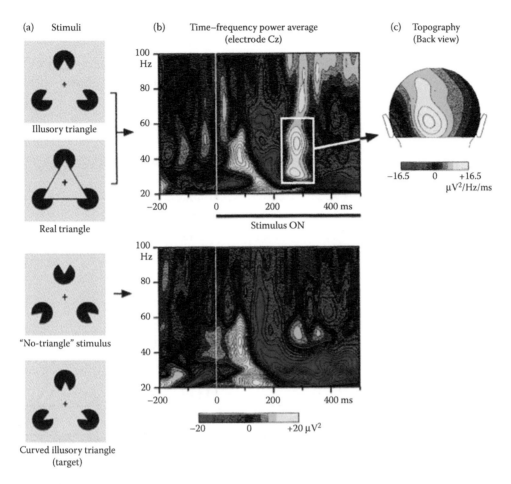

(a) Stimuli

Illusory triangle

Real triangle

"No-triangle" stimulus

Curved illusory triangle
(target)

(b) Time–frequency power average
(electrode Cz)

Stimulus ON

(c) Topography
(Back view)

−16.5   0   +16.5
μV²/Hz/ms

−20   0   +20 μV²

Figure 22.3 Induced gamma activity and visual bottom-up feature binding. (a) Subjects were presented with four different stimuli. Both the illusory (Kanizsa) and the real triangles were coherent stimuli, leading to a coherent percept through a bottom-up feature-binding process. The "no-triangle" stimulus served as control. Subjects had to silently count the occurrences of the target stimulus, a curved illusory triangle, and to report this number at the end of each recording block. This task, when correctly performed, ensured that subjects perceived correctly illusory triangles and remained attentive throughout the whole recording session. (b) Time–frequency power of the EEG at electrode Cz (overall average of eight subjects) in response to the illusory triangle (top) and to the no-triangle stimulus (bottom), the baseline level being taken in the prestimulus period. Two successive bursts of oscillatory activities were observed. A first burst occurred at about 100 ms and 40 Hz; it was an evoked response, phase-locked to stimulus onset, peaking at electrode Cz. It showed no difference between stimulus types, and thus cannot reflect the spatial feature-binding process required to perceive the triangles. The second burst, around 280 ms and between 30 and 60 Hz, was induced by the stimulus, and most prominent in response to coherent stimuli. There was no statistical difference in the gamma range between the responses to the illusory and real triangles. Induced gamma could thus reflect the spatial binding of the elementary features of the picture into a coherent representation of the triangle. It should be noted that no component of the evoked response discriminated between coherent and noncoherent stimuli. (c) Topography of the gamma power averaged between 250 and 350 ms and 30 and 60 Hz, in response to the illusory triangle. Maximum activity is observed at occipital electrodes. (Reprinted from Tallon-Baudry, C. and O. Bertrand. 1999. *Trends Cogn. Sci.* 3:151–62.)

or reversing checkerboard patterns and typically reflects the stimulus frequency and is sustained for the duration of the stimulus (Figure 22.4).

Responses within the gamma band range, at or around 40 Hz, have been shown to be associated with the greatest stimulus process efficiency.

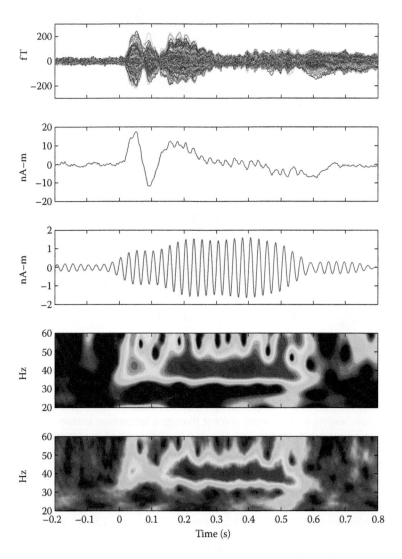

Figure 22.4 (a) Unfiltered time-domain average 248-sensor waveforms from single subject. (b) Unfiltered, averaged dipole waveform for right auditory cortex corresponding to data in (a). (c) Waveform in (b) filtered using a 35–45 Hz bandpass to emphasize gamma-band in time-domain. (d) Time–frequency representation of phase-locked, baseline-normalized evoked power from the same waveform in (b). (e) Time–frequency representation of phase-locking factor (PLF) corresponding to data in (b). (Reprinted from Rojas, D. C. et al. 2011. *Mol. Autism* 2:11.)

Failure to elicit an SSR or an SSR that does not closely reflect the stimulus frequency is taken as a measure of atypical cortical responsivity.

22.3.2.3 Task-free (resting-state) gamma fMRI studies of spontaneous activity in the awake, resting-state brain have provided evidence of different cortical networks acting as baseline, "default mode" networks and identified with consistent patterns of decrease in brain activation specific to generic task types such as vision, attention, language, etc. (Gusnard and Raichle 2001). These spectral characteristics of these networks have also been mapped with EEG (Mantini et al. 2007). This study showed that each network had a specific "neurophysiological signature," with gamma (30–50 Hz) activity associated with the network based around the ventromedial prefrontal cortex, generally associated with "self-reference" activities.

22.3.3 Gamma and connectivity measures

Given the hypothesized functional role of gamma in controlling the timing of cortical responsivity, both locally and distally, increasing attention is being paid to ways of quantifying *temporal synchronicity* in GBA. For example, based on a method developed by Lachaux et al. (1999), it is possible to measure synchronization between cortices of GBA phase, relatively independent of amplitude. This is known as the phase-locking factor (PLF), with values between 0 and 1 (with 1 as maximum synchrony) giving a measure of the percentage of measured signals in phase across trials or periods of measurement (Figure 22.5).

The term "phase-locking value" (PLV) can also be applied to measures of phase synchrony between pairs of signals for a given frequency (e.g., Martini et al. 2012). The resulting measures have been variously termed as InterTrial Coherence (ITC—Port et al. 2007), InterTrial Phase Coherence (ITPC—Sun et al. 2012), and Phase Synchrony (Isler et al. 2010). The similarity and sometimes apparent interchangeability of such terms is a potential cause of confusion, which is discussed in Burgess (2012). A key issue to note here is that phase synchrony can vary independently of power, so changes in power may not be a direct measure of synchronization (see, e.g., Port et al. 2015).

A newer, cross-frequency-based measure of connectivity is phase–amplitude coupling, where the phase of a lower-frequency signal can modulate the amplitude of higher-frequency activity, either at the level of a specific functional unit or across multiple cortical circuits (see review by Buzsáki and Wang 2012). The slower oscillations orchestrate long-range communication and can integrate the fast local processes associated with high-frequency activity. Such coupling has been shown to be correlated with task difficulty and task performance (Canolty and Knight 2010), with, for example, theta–gamma coupling closely linked to changes in memory state and memory performance (Lisman and Jensen 2013).

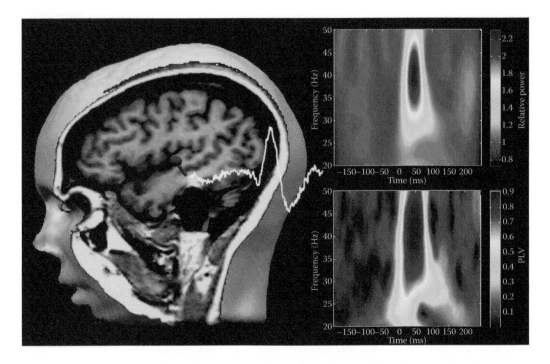

Figure 22.5 Source–space projection and time–frequency analysis. Left hemisphere data from a single participant are illustrated. A single equivalent current dipole was fit to the sensor data and is shown overlaid onto the coregistered MRI scan for the same individual (left). The yellow waveform is the unfiltered, source–space projected, phase-locked average waveform resulting from that dipole (the M50, M100, and M200 responses can be seen in the waveform). In the upper right panel, a time–frequency plot illustrates the transient gamma band response in terms of power relative to the prestimulus baseline. The lower right panel illustrates the PLF for the same data. Note the peak power and PLF centered around 50 ms poststimulus at 40 Hz. (Reprinted from Rojas, D. C. et al. 2008. *BMC Psychiatry* 8:66.)

Graph theory has been used to generate metrics that can characterize the structural and functional connectivity of brain networks (Sporns 2003; Stam and Reijneveld 2007). These can provide measures of the efficiency and stability of a network via measures such as path length and clustering coefficients respectively, together with measures of "synchronizability" of different networks. An assessment of the local processing power and global integration potential of any network can be measured, as can any deviation from the ideal of a "small world" network (Bassett and Bullmore 2006), with a local/global network compromise shown to be the most efficient configuration for rapid information transfer within and synchronization between networks. Originally applied to fMRI data, frequency-specific (including gamma) networks can be characterized using MEG and EEG techniques (Stam and Reijneveld 2007). This approach is clearly appropriate for the investigation of proposals of unusual cortical connectivity patterns in ASD and, as will be seen in Section 22.3.3, has already been applied to models of gamma connectivity.

22.3.4 GBA as a measure of GABA

Gamma rhythms in the brain are associated with pyramidal neurons and arise from recurrent phasic activity in a system of inhibitory interneurons, mediated by gamma-aminobutyric acid. There are several types of inhibitory interneurons; basket cells expressing the calcium-binding protein parvalbumin (PV+) are linked to the gamma-inducing inhibitory processes (Sohal et al. 2009). *In vitro* animal models have shown that GABA receptor activity is associated with specific aspects of GBA, with 40 Hz activity strongly linked to higher levels of receptor activity (Whittington et al. 2000).

Animal models of autism have demonstrated that *in utero* exposure to valproic acid (VPA) or targeted knock-out models will damage PV interneurons and produce a wide range of autism-like symptoms (Gogolla et al. 2009; Saunders et al. 2013). It has been proposed that the GABA-ergic dysfunction arising from PV+ disruption will affect the appropriate excitatory/inhibitory balance in developing neuronal circuits, accounting for both cortical and behavioral anomalies in ASD (Casanova et al. 2003; Rubenstein and Merzenich 2003; Pizzarelli and Cherubini 2011).

Measures of GABA and/or associated GBA abnormalities could therefore inform research into the neuronal underpinnings of ASD. Direct assessment of GABA activity in humans is limited due to technical difficulties although a few ASD studies have been reported, using magnetic resonance spectroscopy (MRS) or blood plasma measures. The results have been described as mainly inconclusive (Coghlan et al. 2012). However, a recent study by Gaetz et al. (2014) employed a newer MRS technique to study GABA concentrations in the motor, visual, and auditory areas of ASD brains, showing significant reductions in the auditory areas, and to a lesser extent in motor but not visual areas. Rojas et al. (2014) also report reduced GABA in the auditory cortex, in both ASD participants and their siblings.

As GBA is the outcome of this GABA-ergic system, it then should be possible to demonstrate that GBA measures reflect GABA activity. Muthukumaraswamy et al. (2009) combined MRS measures of resting GABA in the visual cortex with MEG measures of induced gamma responses to high-contrast grating stimuli, reliable inducers of gamma oscillations (Hadjipapas et al. 2007). The induced gamma response was sustained throughout the stimulus present with marked individual differences in the peak frequency (between 40 and 66 Hz). These individual differences in peak frequency were correlated with individual differences in GABA concentration, suggesting that variations in gamma peak frequency might be taken as a measure of variations in GABA activity and therefore provide useful indices of any atypicalities in ASD, interpretable as dysfunction in the PV+ inhibitory interneuron system (Pizzarelli and Cherubini 2011, 2013). However, a recent study by Cousijn et al. (2014) failed to replicate the gamma-GABA correlation.

473

So, although GABA measures alone are promising, a reliable proxy has not yet been found to overcome the challenges of assessing these *in vivo* in the human brain.

22.3.5 Functional significance of gamma oscillations

The synchronization of GBA serves as a "binding mechanism" to create and maintain the transient neuronal assemblies underpinning the integration of information necessary for perception (Singer and Gray 1995), both locally and distally to serve intercortical information transmission (Varela et al. 2001). The activity it signals serves to determine optimal neuronal response timing (Whittington et al. 2011; Buzsáki and Wang 2012) and ensure maximum accuracy in stimulus processing.

GBA has been described as the basis of a "temporal code" that can exactly specify stimulus features for memory-matching purposes (Herrmann et al. 2010), with synchronization or desynchronization serving to "sharpen" or more closely specify stimulus representation (Moldakarimov et al. 2010). Arnal and Giraud (2012) have proposed a model of sensory predictions based on patterns of cortical oscillations, with beta activity associated with the predicted timing of events and gamma activity with their nature. The resulting alignment of neuronal excitability can serve to reduce uncertainty and improve efficiency, with an adaptive reduction in unnecessary processing.

Clearly, any anomalies in this coding mechanism could have a significant impact on an individual's ability to process and make sense of their environment, with degrees of severity a function of the level of dysfunction in the system. Poor coding could render any input as apparently novel and potentially overwhelming for the system; inflexible or "overexact" coding could undermine the adaptive function of "approximation," allowing the incorporation of irrelevant mismatches into the anticipatory predictive code, and render an individual intolerant of novelty and change (Markram and Markram 2010; Gomot and Wicker 2012; Van de Cruys et al. 2014). If gamma activity is a measure of cortical predictive coding efficiencies (Arnal and Giraud 2012), then atypicalities of gamma could index this fundamental problem in ASD and link to many of the characteristic symptom patterns.

22.4 Gamma activity in autism

Earlier research into the role of GBA in ASD focused on sensory and perceptual task-related changes. Emergent theories of the role of GBA (at or around 40 Hz) in "temporal binding" or the formation of the coherent percepts essential for accurate information processing, indicated that gamma could be a useful "candidate" frequency for characterizing the cortical correlates of sensory and perceptual atypicalities (Brock et al. 2002). It should be noted that these earlier studies therefore use a frequency range that would now be classified as "low gamma." Additionally, findings are based on EEG sensor-level analysis and generally focus on task-related regions of interest rather than whole-brain measures.

22.4.1 Visual gamma in ASD

Early gamma studies in autism focused on the visual area where ASD anomalies are well documented (Dakin and Frith 2005). Grice et al. (2001) demonstrated that task-related induced GBA (32–48 Hz) from frontal regions in ASD participants was the same whether they were viewing upright or inverted faces, unlike a control group. No behavioral data were collected in order to assess whether the ASD group also responded in the same way to both types of orientation, but it was inferred that the failure to show the "face inversion" effect at the cortical level was consistent with reported deficits in face-processing characteristic of ASD. Inspection of these data also shows that the visual evoked potentials in the ASD group were smaller than the controls, as were the gamma bursts (Figure 22.6).

Brown et al. (2005), using Kanizsa triangles, demonstrated that although the ASD showed above 90% accuracy in identifying the presence or absence of illusory triangles, induced GBA (30–40 Hz) in the parietal region was markedly different from age- and IQ-matched controls. To "shape present" stimuli, the ASD group showed an early increase in GBA approximately 100 ms poststimulus and a further increase at approximately 300 ms markedly different from the control group. There were also similar increases in GBA to the "shape absent" stimuli, a failure to discriminate between stimulus conditions, consistent with the findings of Grice et al. (Figure 22.1).

Both studies interpreted their findings in terms of the atypical GBA indexing anomalous temporal binding, with Brown et al. (2005) additionally noting that the high levels of GBA increases poststimulus were consistent with deficits in neuronal excitation–inhibition balance. The localized nature of the increased GBA was also consistent with Brock et al.'s hypothesis of increased connectivity within *local* networks, possibly underpinning the perceptual hyperabilities identified as characteristic of some ASD individuals. Both studies reported there to be no significant difference in prestimulus baseline activity; in light of later analyses of whole-brain GBA, it is interesting to note the regional difference in GBA responsivity, with underactivity in the frontal areas in the Grice study and overactivity in the parietal areas in the Brown study.

These early studies inferred but did not measure connectivity differences. Isler et al. (2010) used a long-latency flash VEP task, measured coherence, and phase synchrony in a small group of young ASD children (5.5.–8.4 yo). It was hypothesized that interhemispheric synchrony between visual areas would be reduced in the ASD group; findings

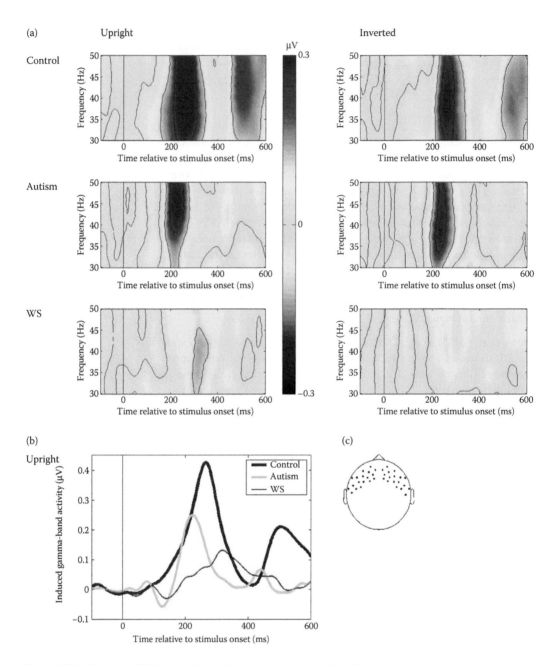

Figure 22.6 Gamma TFR to upright and inverted faces: (a) Time–frequency plots showing induced gamma-band activity by orientation for each group. (b) Graph shows averaged gamma-band activity over time for each group in the upright face condition. (c) Top-down view of the head with electrode locations used for analysis marked as black-filled circles. (Reprinted from Grice, S. J. et al. 2001. *Neuroreport* 12:2697–700.)

were reported in all frequency bands, with gamma defined as >25 Hz. Both coherence and phase synchrony were reduced in the ASD group at all frequencies, particularly those above theta. There was evidence of earlier and increased responsivity to the stimulus in the ASD group, consistent with the Brown et al. finding, but, in this case, in alpha/beta bands. This could be related to the differences in stimulus complexity. Other studies have similarly reported heightened levels of responsivity in lower-frequency bands (Coben et al. 2008).

A study by Sun et al. (2012) provides a good example of emerging analytical possibilities in the area, with the added benefit of using MEG. Using the perception of Mooney faces, a task reliably associated with gamma generation (Rodriguez et al. 1999), they examined whole-brain measures of power and intertrial coherence (phase-locking) at both the sensor and the source level and also considered GBA in terms of both low (25–60 Hz) and high (60–120 Hz) gamma. The ASD participants were high-functioning adults. Behaviorally, the ASD group performed worse than the control group, with longer reaction times and fewer correct identifications. Sensor-level analyses revealed an *increase* in both low and high gamma power over parieto-occipital channels in the control group as compared to a *decrease* in the ASD group. The control group also showed a reduction in low gamma power over the frontal areas, consistent with the earlier study by Grice et al. (2001). Intertrial coherence measures revealed reduced coherence in the ASD group over occipito-parietal areas, with greater intergroup differences in the lower-frequency band. Analyses of the GBA sources showed complex regional- and frequency-related differences in relative hyper- and hypoactivity in the two groups. In the low gamma band (25–60 Hz), the ASD group showed stronger activation in the face condition in frontal areas than the controls; in the high gamma band (60–125 Hz), there was stronger activation in posterior regions as compared to frontal areas in the ASD group; the control group showed greater activation in a frontoparietal network (Figure 22.7).

Correlations between behavioral measures and source power in the higher-frequency range revealed a different pattern in controls and in the ASD group, with faster reaction times associated with increased GBA in the lingual gyrus and insula (areas associated with face processing) in the control group as opposed to an association between faster reaction times and increased GBA in the medial temporal gyrus and cingulate gyrus (more posterior regions outside the normal face-processing network) in the ASD group.

Overall, this study demonstrates the range and complexity of potential insights that can be generated from the study of task-related GBA, but also the source of possible contradictions between studies. It is clearly important, where possible, to identify the source of any GBA differences rather than relying on sensor-level analyses, and also to note that different conclusions can be reached dependent on what gamma metric is being used. As outlined in Section 22.3.2.1, there is an emerging

(a)

(b)

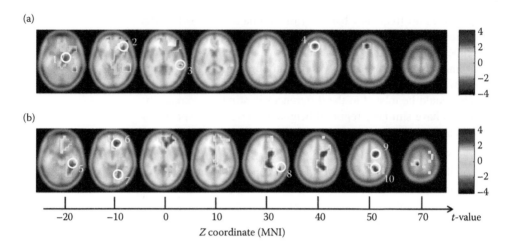

Figure 22.7 Source power in the high gamma band for the interaction between condition (face vs. no-face condition) and group (participants with ASD vs. controls). (a) Controls versus participants with ASD, face versus no-face, 25–60 Hz, (b) Controls versus participants with ASD, face versus no-face, 60–120 Hz. Red clusters represent stronger activation under the two conditions in controls, whereas blue clusters represent stronger activation under the two conditions in participants with ASD. Note that p values are calculated by cluster-based statistical analysis. (1) parahippocampal gyrus; (2) inferior frontal gyrus (IFG); (3) middle temporal gyrus (MTG); (4) medial frontal gyrus (MeFG); (5) parahippocampal gyrus; (6) MeFG; (7) lingual gyrus; (8) supramarginal gyrus; (9) middle frontal gyrus (2); (10) precuneus. (Reprinted from Sun, L. et al. 2012. *J. Neurosci.* 32:9563–73.)

interest in noting individual differences in the peak "operating" frequency in the gamma range as indicative of individual differences in processing efficiency, thus clearly relevant to the study of ASD. A recent study by Dickinson et al. (2015), employing a measure of peak gamma *frequency* within a standardized range (30–90 Hz) rather than gamma *power*, reported significant correlations between high levels of autistic personality traits as measured by the autism spectrum quotient (AQ) (Baron-Cohen et al. 2001), peak gamma frequency, and orientation discrimination thresholds. Those individuals best at discriminating between differently oriented visual stimuli had higher AQ scores and higher gamma peak frequencies (of the order of 77 Hz) as opposed to those with low AQ scores (54 Hz). The authors suggest that higher levels of peak gamma frequency are associated with higher levels of neuronal inhibition, thus, similar to Brown et al. (2005), implicating a disturbed excitation–inhibition balance but, in this instance, due to higher levels of inhibition rather than higher levels of excitation. As this study was of typically developing adults, it would clearly need replicating in an ASD population, but this approach could offer the possibility of addressing the issue of individual differences/heterogeneity, which can confound research in this area.

Where the interest in gamma is as a measure of cortical connectivity, the recent use of phase–amplitude coupling metrics has provided further insights. As outlined in Section 22.3.3, phase–amplitude coupling is the mechanism where the phase of a lower-frequency oscillation in one area (theta, alpha, beta) has been shown to modulate the amplitude of higher-frequency oscillations (commonly gamma) in other areas and the efficiency, or otherwise, of this coupling is taken as a measure of the functional connectivity between the various sources; both long- and short-range connectivity can be studied using this approach (Varela et al. 2001; Palva and Palva 2011). This method has therefore proved useful in the study of ASD populations. An MEG study by Khan et al. (2013) examined gamma power and alpha–gamma coupling in the fusiform face area (FFA) in young male ASD participants and matched controls in response to neutral or emotional faces as compared to houses. There were no group differences in evoked responses in either the alpha or gamma band. Long-range connectivity was measured using broadband (6–55 Hz) coherence and revealed lower levels in the ASD group. Alpha–gamma coupling measures revealed reductions in local functional connectivity in the fusiform face area in ASD, with the gamma effects in the high-frequency range (75–110 Hz) (Figure 22.8).

It is important to note that these PAC differences emerged despite the failure of both alpha and gamma power measures alone to distinguish between the groups and implicates the *timings* of any gamma-related changes rather than the power per se as potential distinguishing features. Additionally, the PAC measures were shown to be negatively correlated with ADOS scores, thus providing a useful biomarker for symptom severity, and also, using classifier techniques, successfully distinguishing the ASD and control group with 90% accuracy.

Studies of GBA and visual processing have therefore proved a useful testing ground for the application of different ways of measuring task-related GBA and linking this to hypothesized differences in cortical connectivity. Findings are complex but, on the whole, support models implicating greater reactivity in the early sensory processing stages combined with an apparent failure to "titrate" such reactivity as a function of the stimulus characteristics (e.g., upright vs. inverted faces, face vs. houses, presence or absence of illusory figures). A key aspect in assessing past studies and designing future ones is of the choice of gamma metric; it is clear that power measures alone are not sufficiently sensitive, differentiation between low and high gamma can be key, and attention to individual differences in peak frequency is important. In addition, where connectivity is an aspect of interpretation of GBA, measures of phase–amplitude coupling rather than simple coherence should be employed.

22.4.2 Auditory gamma in ASD

The study of GBA during auditory processing in ASD presents a slightly different picture, mainly because the focus has been on more fundamental aspects of sensory processing and because, from the outset, there

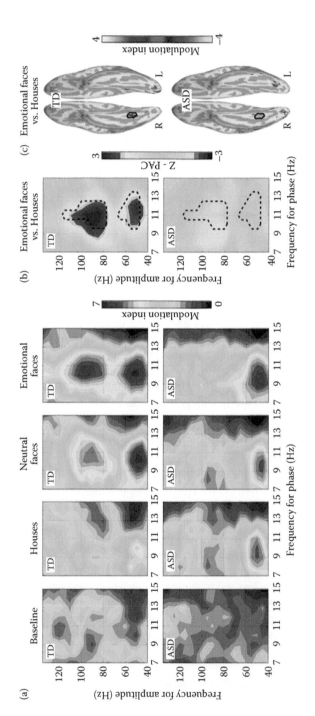

Figure 22.8 Phase–amplitude coupling (PAC) in the fusiform face area (FFA). (a) PAC in each condition for each group. (b) PAC for emotional faces normalized by PAC for houses (Z-PAC) for the TD group (upper) and ASD group (lower). Dotted lines indicate significant group differences in Z-PAC. (c) Z-PAC as in (b) but between alpha and high gamma only, computed over the entire cortex, for each group. The functionally determined FFA is outlined in bold. (Reproduced from Khan, S. et al. 2013. *Proc. Natl. Acad. Sci. USA* 110:3107–12.)

has been greater use of the fuller range of GBA measures. Abnormal auditory reactivity, both hypo- and hyperreactivity, has been observed in ASD (Leekam et al. 2007; Hazen et al. 2014) and has been linked with characteristic communication difficulties (Jeste and Nelson 2009) and therefore offers a fruitful arena for study.

Orekhova et al. (2008) examined auditory sensory gating in high- and low-functioning ASD children by comparing the P50 ERPs to click pairs. Normal sensory gating is associated with a significant reduction in the P50 response to the second click; this was significantly reduced in the low-functioning group. A measure of "spontaneous" gamma was acquired in parallel (during sustained attention tasks). The ASD group had higher levels of gamma power and a relationship between gamma power and poor sensory gating was demonstrated in the ASD groups, with higher gamma power correlating significantly with small or absent P50 suppression. This atypical sensory gating in the ASD group was interpreted as potentially indicating a deficit in central inhibitory circuits (Rubenstein and Merzenich 2003), reflected by the abnormal GBA. However, as there was no direct measure of GBA to auditory stimuli, this interpretation needed more supporting evidence.

In a more direct assessment of auditory GBA, Wilson et al. (2007), using MEG, measured steady-state responses to 500 ms, monaural click trains, amplitude-modulated at 40 cycles/s to elicit a steady-state response of increased 40 Hz power in the contralateral hemisphere. The controls and the ASD group showed similar patterns of responsivity in the right hemisphere, but the ASD group showed reduced left hemisphere power with no clear 40 Hz steady-state response. Roberts et al. (2010), also using MEG, also utilized auditory ERP differences as a distinguishing characteristic in ASD populations. In this case, the latency of the M100 auditory-evoked potential to 200, 300, 500, and 1000 Hz tones was examined. A marked delay to the 500 Hz tone in the *right* hemisphere in the ASD group was subjected to classifier analysis and had a positive predictive value of 86%. Gandal et al. (2010) measured gamma (30–50 Hz) power and synchronization in the same participants, with phase-locking factor as a measure of intertrial coherence. There was no significant difference in induced or evoked gamma power between the ASD and the control groups, but the ASD group showed significantly reduced gamma phase-locking. In parallel, this group also investigated auditory GBA in a VPA mouse model of ASD, reporting a similar delay in right hemisphere auditory ERPs, with reduced PLF significantly correlated with the severity of the behavioral deficits manifested in the rodents.

A follow-up study by Edgar et al. (2013) looked at low- as well as high-frequency responses to pure tones in a sample of 105 children with ASD, for whom there was also a measure of clinical symptoms such as core language functions. They showed higher levels of prestimulus power in *all* frequencies in this group, with smaller early-evoked gamma activity to all stimuli, and decreased left and right hemisphere intertrial coherence in the gamma band. The prestimulus abnormalities were most predictive of poststimulus abnormalities and of clinical symptoms.

The possibility that atypical auditory GBA might serve as an endophenotype for ASD was explored by Rojas et al. (2008), examining evoked and induced gamma power to a monaural, 200 ms 1 kHz sine-wave stimuli in children with autism and their parents. They reported that evoked gamma power was overall lower in the ASD group and their parents, but induced activity higher, consistent with a difference in GBA *timing*, confirmed by a significantly lower phase-locking factor score. This group subsequently investigated both evoked and steady-state responses in the parents of ASD probands (Rojas et al. 2011). Transient-evoked responses to 32, 40, and 48 Hz amplitude-modulated tones revealed an overall *right* hemisphere reduction in gamma power responses in the ASD parent group, driven by a significant difference at 48 Hz. It should be noted that this difference in right hemisphere-evoked power is inconsistent with the absence of power differences reported by Roberts et al. (2010); this could have been related to difference in stimulus characteristics or task demands, shown to be reflected by GBA (Nourski et al. 2015). Examination of steady-state responses also revealed a reduction in ASD parents, with the *left* hemisphere response the most reliable differentiator, consistent with the Wilson et al. (2007) finding.

These studies of auditory processing in ASD and ASD first-degree relatives show some consistency in their reports of reduction in *evoked* activity (ERP, GBA) (Orekhova et al. 2008; Rojas et al. 2011; Port et al. 2015) or SSR (Wilson et al. 2007; Rojas et al. 2011). This is in the context of less consensus over *induced* power, with Rojas et al. (2008) reporting higher levels of induced power as compared to no differences in other studies (Roberts et al. 2010; Rojas et al. 2011). These differences can be reconciled with the consistent reports of reduced phase-locking in ASD and ASD-related populations where this was also assessed, noting that reduced phase-locking will be associated with an imbalance between evoked and induced power (Rojas et al. 2011). This anomalous gamma and gamma-related activity in the auditory system could be consistent with a failure to establish accurate feedforward control of responsivity to ongoing auditory input and thus reduced efficiency in the processing of auditory information, resulting in anomalous auditory responsivity and also implications for language processing (Jochaut et al. 2015). Unfortunately, although there is some attempt to link the anomalous cortical responses to ASD symptomatology, there are no specific measures of auditory processing per se, perhaps via psychophysical techniques, which could have helped with the interpretation of these findings.

As noted above in the discussion of GBA and visual processing, the study of GBA has evolved to include measures of cross-frequency or phase–amplitude coupling. In auditory/speech models, it has been shown that auditory cortical responses to speech occur in the theta range, which then modulates gamma activity (Schroeder et al. 2008; Giraud and Poeppel 2012). Jochaut et al. (2015), using fMRI and EEG data, examined theta (4–7 Hz)–gamma (30–40 Hz) coupling in response to continuous speech in a heterogeneous group of ASD participants with IQ scores ranging from 35 to 124, and including dysphasic as well as linguistically normal participants. They noted that there were significantly higher prestimulus theta levels in the auditory cortex in the ASD group, which did not increase with speech stimulation. Subsequent examination of theta–gamma relationships demonstrated that theta activity in the left auditory cortex did not vary as a function of speech modulations and failed to downregulate gamma oscillations in the ASD group. This would be equivalent to the anomalous gamma activity described in the preceding studies, particularly those that reported higher levels of induced but not evoked gamma. Additionally, the theta–gamma measure predicted verbal ability in the ASD group ($r = 0.746$, $p = 0.008$) and was strongly tied to the general autism symptoms. Further, examining EEG–BOLD coupling allowed assessment of the connectivity between auditory cortex and speech areas and indicated reduced connectivity from A1 to Broca's area and the motor cortex, but not the other way round, suggesting the theta–gamma anomaly is primarily sensory. This provides an explanatory model for the sensory abnormalities in ASD and also is strong support for the notion that the origins of atypical ASD behavior may lie in more fundamental sensory and perceptual dysfunctions.

The findings in auditory gamma are rather more consistent than in the visual modality. Evoked activity in the form of the M100 of task-related GABA and steady-state responses are generally reduced, interpreted in terms of poorer synchronization of responses to auditory stimuli. Following the suggestion that GBA is associated with some form of "predictive coding" (Arnal and Giraud 2012), auditory deficits at this level could well have downstream consequences for higher-level language function, as indicated by Jochaut et al. (2015). The identification of unusual auditory GBA in first-degree relatives also offers the possibility of this measure serving as an endophenotype (Rojas et al. 2008, 2011).

22.4.3 Resting-state, "task-free" gamma activity

In addition to atypical sensory responsivity, consistent reports of high levels of epileptiform activity in ASD cortical activity as well as the high incidence of epilepsy (Berg and Plioplys 2012) suggest that there could be unusual levels of high-frequency activity in resting-state or spontaneous EEG/MEG activity in ASD populations. Some of the previous studies of task-related responsivity did report on prestimulus activity, but little consistency emerged, with some reporting no between-group prestimulus activity (Grice et al. 2001; Brown et al. 2005; Sun et al. 2012), whereas others report high levels of prestimulus or spontaneous activity (Orekhova et al. 2008; Rojas et al. 2008, 2011), with one study noting that the high levels of prestimulus power were predictive of anomalies in stimulus responsivity and also correlated with ASD clinical symptoms (Edgar et al. 2013).

As outlined in Section 22.3.2.3, the study of resting-state measures in typical cortical activity has often been in the context of studying cortical network connectivity, using simple coherence-based measures or more complex metrics based on graph theory, and also in the identification of "task-negative" or default mode networks (Gusnard and Raichle 2001). In ASD research, earlier studies, using EEG, reported anomalies in lower-frequency bands, such as high levels of theta activity and patterns of both inter- and intrahemispheric underconnectivity as measured by coherence (Murias et al. 2007; Coben et al. 2008). Later EEG studies employing more sophisticated technology and analytical approaches report on gamma anomalies in resting-state measures, with *reductions* in regional specific power (Maxwell et al. 2013) and coherence (Sheikhani et al. 2009) (see review by Billeci et al. 2013). MEG studies have also contributed to the debate, with Cornew et al. (2012) reporting regionally specific *increases* in high-frequency power (70–120 Hz), particularly in posterior brain regions. Other MEG studies using graph theory metrics applied to broadband frequencies report measures consistent with reduced efficiency, such as increased path length and clustering (Pollonini 2010; Tsiaras et al. 2011).

In a recent study by Kitzbichler et al. (2015), some attempt was made to reconcile the inconsistencies in the area. ASD participants comprised 15 males, ages ranging from 6 to 21 years. A key focus was on the importance of band-specific measures, including gamma (defined as 30–70 Hz). Whole-brain network properties in different frequency bands were characterized using graph theory metrics as measures of connectivity efficiency. The most powerful differences were in the gamma and beta bands. In the gamma band, the ASD group showed stronger and more efficiently connected networks, particularly in posterior regions, with many more connections *from* occipital areas to parietal, temporal, and frontal regions. The strength of this connectivity in the gamma band was positively correlated with ADOS scores, that is, with symptom severity. In the beta band, the ASD group was characterized by *less* efficiently connected networks, particularly those involving the frontal lobes, and these connectivity metrics were negatively correlated with ADOS scores, that is, the more severe symptoms were associated with reduced connectivity in the beta band. The authors interpret these differences as an imbalance between stimulus-induced feedforward mechanisms and frontally based regulatory feedback mechanisms.

Kitzbichler et al. also note group differences in age-related connectivity differences, with their (small) ASD group showing little evidence of connectivity changes with age, as compared to clear evidence of developmental changes in typically developing controls, particularly in those networks involving the frontal regions, where decreasing connectivity strength was shown in the lower-frequency bands, including beta. Of relevance to this, and indeed to all ASD studies using cohorts of different ages, is a report by Tierney et al. (2012) on resting EEG power, showing that the normal developmental trajectory of gamma decline in infancy is atypical in children at risk for ASD. High-risk infants show lower levels of gamma at 6 months than a low-risk group and an atypical rate of change between 6 and 24 months, a small *increase* of approximately 3.5% as compared to a *decline* of approximately 24% in low-risk infants. The overall result was persistently lower gamma power in high-risk infants; this was also found in alpha, whereas differences in other lower-frequency bands had disappeared by 24 months. Consideration of reported differences in brain growth in ASD populations, particularly involving the frontal lobes (Courchesne et al. 2011), in this very age range could well be relevant to understanding these connectivity differences as indexed by different frequencies; as these anomalies in developmental trajectory potentially persist into adulthood, as indicated by Kitzbichler's observations, they should be taken into consideration in the selection of participants and in the interpretation of findings.

Overall, resting-state measures offer a fruitful approach of the study of ASD, not least because they offer the opportunity of involving younger and/or lower-functioning participants. The possibility of characterizing the network connections using graph theory and demonstrating how these can be associated with symptom patterns (Kitzbichler et al. 2015) supports the suggestion that findings from studies of auditory gamma that GBA could serve as a potential biomarker for the condition.

22.5 Summary

Over the last decade or so, there have been considerable advances in the understanding of GBA mechanisms, via technological advances in measurement and the evolution of data metrics, modeling, and pattern analysis. This has revealed a greater potential for detailed profiling of gamma networks, detailed deconstruction of anatomical and task-related factors (Gaona et al. 2011; Jung et al. 2011), as well as individual differences in the patterns of gamma responsivity (Dickinson et al. 2015; Hadjipapas et al. 2015). Applications of classifier techniques have revealed the discriminatory power of well-specified gamma profiles (Roberts et al. 2010; Khan et al. 2013). A major focus on the human connectome and the assembling of large, multilab neuroimaging data sets such as ABIDE has supported these developments (Nielsen et al. 2013).

There is a greater awareness of the heterogeneity of ASD (Happé et al. 2006) and the importance of identifying subtypes as well as more detailed profiling of individual differences and cognitive phenotypes (Charman et al. 2011). There is a more detailed focus on atypicalities in fundamental sensory and perceptual processes and their possible downstream consequences for higher-level cognitive skills (e.g., Kargas et al. 2015). This accords well with the emerging predictive coding models of gamma's functional significance (Arnal and Giraud 2012), and makes a clearer link between the fundamental neurophysiology of gamma and the autism experience itself (Van de Cruys et al. 2014).

From the findings of GBA atypicalities reviewed here, together with the converging evidence that disorders of cortical connectivity underpin pathological conditions such as ASD, it is clear that the study of GBA and GBA-related processes will continue to offer significant insights into ASD pathology at every level, offering not only an understanding of specific aspects of the condition itself but also the potential to provide biomarkers or even endophenotypes (Rojas et al. 2008, 2011).

22.5.1 Further refinements and future focus

Research should aim for the refinement of the profiling of GBA and of gamma-related cortical networks, perhaps using graph theory metrics, with the aim of producing a GBA "fingerprint," which could characterize individual differences in degree of resting-state and/or sensory responsivity, and also in cortical connectivity characteristics.

There needs to be a greater focus in ASD cohorts on individual differences in symptom severity and symptom patterns, together with the inclusion of a different group more representative of different ages and levels of functioning. A clearer definition of the cognitive phenotype should inform task and participant selection, with subsequent detailed statistical mapping of the relationship between the atypical behavioral characteristics and the GBA profile. This could assist the development of more discriminatory ASD biomarkers, possibly identifying subtypes within the diagnostic category and/or endophenotypes and link to ongoing genetics research.

Additionally, translational work in this area offers the possibility of identifying potential pharmacological interventions with normalizing of GBA a measure of effectiveness (Tyzio et al. 2014; Nakamura et al. 2015). Direct manipulation of neurophysiological activity has been shown to be effective in modulating various aspects of ASD symptomatology (Baruth et al. 2010; Casanova et al. 2015). This aspect of gamma research, then, could take forward the possibility of developing interventions and thus contribute not only to a better understanding of the condition but also to its amelioration.

References

American Psychiatric Association. 2013. *Diagnostic and Statistical Manual of Mental Disorders*, 5th ed. Washington, D.C.: American Psychiatric Publishing.

Arnal, L. H. and A. L. Giraud. 2012. Cortical oscillations and sensory predictions. *Trends Cogn. Sci.* 16:390–8.

Bailey, A., A. Le Couteur, I. Gottesman, P. Bolton, E. Simonoff, E. Yuzda, and M. Rutter. 1995. Autism as a strongly genetic disorder: Evidence from a British twin study. *Psychol. Med.* 25:63–77.

Baron-Cohen, S., A. M. Leslie, and U. Frith. 1985. Does the autistic child have a "theory of mind"? *Cognition* 21:37–46.

Baron-Cohen, S., S. Wheelwright, R. Skinner, J. Martin, and E. Clubley. 2001. The autism-spectrum quotient (AQ): Evidence from asperger syndrome/high-functioning autism, malesand females, scientists and mathematicians. *J. Autism Dev. Disord.* 31(1):5–17.

Bartos, M., I. Vida, and P. Jonas. 2007. Synaptic mechanisms of synchronized gamma oscillations in inhibitory interneuron networks. *Nat. Rev. Neurosci.* 8:45–56.

Baruth, J. M., M. F. Casanova, A. El-Baz, T. Horrell, G. Mathai, L. Sears, and E. Sokhadze. 2010. Low-frequency repetitive transcranial magnetic stimulation modulates evoked-gamma frequency oscillations in autism spectrum disorder. *J. Neurother.* 14:179–94.

Başar, E., E. Tülay, and B. Güntekin. 2015. Multiple gamma oscillations in the brain: A new strategy to differentiate functional correlates and P300 dynamics. *Int. J. Psychophysiol.* 95:406–20.

Bassett, D. S. and E. D. Bullmore. 2006. Small-world brain networks. *Neuroscientist* 12:512–23.

Bauer, M., R. Oostenveld, M. Peeters, and P. Fries. 2006. Tactile spatial attention enhances gamma-band activity in somatosensory cortex and reduces low-frequency activity in parieto-occipital areas. *J. Neurosci.* 26:490–501.

Behrmann, M., G. Avidan, G. L. Leonard, R. Kimchi, B. Luna, K. Humphreys, and N. Minshew. 2006. Configural processing in autism and its relationship to face processing. *Neuropsychologia* 44:110–29.

Behrmann, M., C. Thomas, and K. Humphreys. 2006. Seeing it differently: Visual processing in autism. *Trends Cogn. Sci.* 10:258–64.

Belmonte, M. K., G. Allen, A. Beckel-Mitchener, L. M. Boulanger, R. A. Carper, and S. J. Webb. 2004. Autism and abnormal development of brain connectivity. *J. Neurosci.* 24:9228–31.

Berg, A. T. and S. Plioplys. 2012. Epilepsy and autism: Is there a special relationship? *Epilepsy Behav.* 23:193–8.

Betancur, C. 2011. Etiological heterogeneity in autism spectrum disorders: More than 100 genetic and genomic disorders and still counting. *Brain Res.* 1380:42–77.

Billeci, L., F. Sicca, K. Maharatna, F. Apicella, A. Narzisi, G. Campatelli, S. Calderoni, G. Pioggia, and F. Muratori. 2013. On the application of quantitative EEG for characterizing autistic brain: A systematic review. *Front. Hum. Neurosci.* 7:442.

Bölte, S., M. Holtmann, F. Poustka, A. Scheurich, and L. Schmidt. 2007. Gestalt perception and local-global processing in high-functioning autism. *J. Autism Dev. Disord.* 37:1493–504.

Brock, J., C. C. Brown, J. Boucher, and G. Rippon. 2002. The temporal binding deficit hypothesis of autism. *Dev. Psychopathol.* 14:209–24.

Brookes, M. J., A. M. Gibson, S. D. Hall et al. 2005. GLM-beamformer method demonstrates stationary field, alpha ERD and gamma ERS co-localisation with fMRI BOLD response in visual cortex. *NeuroImage* 26:302–8.

Brown, C., T. Gruber, J. Boucher, G. Rippon, and J. Brock. 2005. Gamma abnormalities during perception of illusory figures in autism. *Cortex* 41:364–76.

Brunet, N., M. Vinck, C. A. Bosman, W. Singer, and P. Fries. 2014. Gamma or no gamma, that is the question. *Trends Cogn. Sci.* 18:507–9.

Burgess, A. 2012. Towards a unified understanding of event-related changes in the EEG: The Firefly model of synchronization through cross-frequency phase modulation. *PLoS One* 7:e45630. doi: 10.1371/journal.pone.0045630.

Buzsáki, G. and F. L. da Silva. 2012. High frequency oscillations in the intact brain. *Progr. Neurobiol.* 98:241–9.

Buzsáki, G. and X. J. Wang. 2012. Mechanisms of gamma oscillations. *Annu. Rev. Neurosci.* 35:203–225.

Canolty, R. T. and R. T. Knight. 2010. The functional role of cross-frequency coupling. *Trends Cogn. Sci.* 14:506–15.

Casanova, M. and J. Trippe. 2009. Radial cytoarchitecture and patterns of cortical connectivity in autism. *Philos. Trans. R. Soc. B Biol. Sci.* 364:1433–6.

Casanova, M. F., D. P. Buxhoeveden, A. E. Switala, and E. Roy. 2002. Minicolumnar pathology in autism. *Neurology* 58:428–32.

Casanova, M. F., D. Buxhoeveden, and J. Gomez. 2003. Disruption in the inhibitory architecture of the cell minicolumn: Implications for autism. *Neuroscientist* 9:496–507.

Casanova, M. F., A. S. El-Baz, S. S. Kamat, B. A. Dombroski, F. Khalifa, A. Elnakib, and A. E. Switala. 2013. Focal cortical dysplasias in autism spectrum disorders. *Acta Neuropathol. Commun.* 1:67.

Casanova, M. F., E. Sokhadze, I. Opris, Y. Wang, and X. Li. 2015. Autism spectrum disorders: Linking neuropathological findings to treatment with transcranial magnetic stimulation. *Acta Paediatr.* 104:346–355.

Charman, T., C. R. Jones, A. Pickles, E. Simonoff, G. Baird, and F. Happé. 2011. Defining the cognitive phenotype of autism. *Brain Res.* 1380:10–21.

Coben, R., A. R. Clarke, W. Hudspeth, and R. J. Barry. 2008. EEG power and coherence in autistic spectrum disorder. *Clin. Neurophysiol.* 119:1002–9.

Coghlan, S., J. Horder, B. Inkster, M. A. Mendez, D. G. Murphy, and D. J. Nutt. 2012. GABA system dysfunction in autism and related disorders: From synapse to symptoms. *Neurosci. Biobehav. Rev.* 36:2044–55.

Cornew, L., T. P. Roberts, L. Blaskey, and J. C. Edgar. 2012. Resting-state oscillatory activity in autism spectrum disorders. *J. Autism Dev. Disord.* 42:1884–94.

Courchesne, E., K. Campbell, and S. Solso. 2011. Brain growth across the life span in autism: Age-specific changes in anatomical pathology. *Brain Res.* 1380:138–45.

Courchesne, E. and K. Pierce. 2005. Brain overgrowth in autism during a critical time in development: Implications for frontal pyramidal neuron and interneuron development and connectivity. *Int. J. Dev. Neurosci.* 23:153–70.

Cousijn, H., S. Haegens, G. Wallis, J. Near, M. G. Stokes, P. J. Harrison, and A. C. Nobre. 2014. Resting GABA and glutamate concentrations do not predict visual gamma frequency or amplitude. *Proc. Natl. Acad. Sci. USA.* 111:9301–6.

Crone, N. E., A. Korzeniewska, and P. J. Franaszczuk. 2011. Cortical gamma responses: Searching high and low. *Int. J. Psychophysiol.* 79:9–15.

da Silva, F. L. 2009. EEG: Origin and measurement. In EEG-fMRI. Springer, Berlin Heidelberg, pp. 19–38.

da Silva, F. L. 2013. EEG and MEG: Relevance to neuroscience. *Neuron* 80:1112–28.

Dakin, S. and U. Frith. 2005. Vagaries of visual perception in autism. *Neuron* 48:497–507.

Dickinson, A., M. Bruyns-Haylett, M. Jones, and E. Milne. 2015. Increased peak gamma frequency in individuals with higher levels of autistic traits. *Eur. J. Neurosci.* 41:1095–101.

Dinstein, I., K. Pierce, L. Eyler, S. Solso, R. Malach, M. Behrmann, and E. Courchesne. 2011. Disrupted neural synchronization in toddlers with autism. *Neuron* 70(6):1218–25.

Edden, R. A., S. D. Muthukumaraswamy, T. C. Freeman, and K. D. Singh. 2009. Orientation discrimination performance is predicted by GABA concentration and gamma oscillation frequency in human primary visual cortex. *J. Neurosci.* 29:15721–6.

Edgar, J. C., S. Y. Khan, L. Blaskey, V. Y. Chow, M. Rey, W. Gaetz, and T. P. Roberts. 2013. Neuromagnetic oscillations predict evoked-response latency delays and core language deficits in autism spectrum disorders. *J. Autism Dev. Disord.* 45:395–405.

Elsabbagh, M., A. Volein, G. Csibra, K. Holmboe, H. Garwood, L. Tucker, and M. H. Johnson. 2009. Neural correlates of eye gaze processing in the infant broader autism phenotype. *Biol. Psychiatry* 65:31–8.

Engel, A. K. and W. Singer. 2001. Temporal binding and the neural correlates of sensory awareness. *Trends Cogn. Sci.* 5:16–25.

Fries, P. 2005. A mechanism for cognitive dynamics: Neuronal communication through neuronal coherence. *Trends Cogn. Sci.* 9:474–80.

Fries, P. 2009. Neuronal gamma-band synchronization as a fundamental process in cortical computation. *Annu. Rev. Neurosci.* 32:209–224.

Friston, K. J. 2011. Functional and effective connectivity: A review. *Brain Connect.* 1:13–36.

Gaetz, W., L. Bloy, D. J. Wang, R. G. Port, L. Blaskey, S. E. Levy, and T. P. L. Roberts. 2014. GABA estimation in the brains of children on the autism spectrum: Measurement precision and regional cortical variation. *NeuroImage* 86:1–9.

Gandal, M. J., J. C. Edgar, R. S. Ehrlichman, M. Mehta, T. P. Roberts, and S. J. Siegel. 2010. Validating γ oscillations and delayed auditory responses as translational biomarkers of autism. *Biol. Psychiatry* 68:1100–6.

Gaona, C. M., M. Sharma, Z. V. Freudenburg, J. D. Breshears, D. T. Bundy, J. Roland, D. L. Barbour, G. Schalk, and E. C. Leuthardt. 2011. Nonuniform high-gamma (60–500 Hz) power changes dissociate cognitive task and anatomy in human cortex. *J. Neurosci.* 31:2091–100.

Geschwind, D. H. and P. Levitt. 2007. Autism spectrum disorders: Developmental disconnection syndromes. *Curr. Opin. Neurobiol.* 17:103–111.

Giraud, A. L. and D. Poeppel. 2012. Cortical oscillations and speech processing: Emerging computational principles and operations. *Nat. Neurosci.* 15:511–7.

Gogolla, N., J. J. LeBlanc, K. B. Quast, T. C. Südhof, M. Fagiolini, and T. K. Hensch. 2009. Common circuit defect of excitatory-inhibitory balance in mouse models of autism. *J. Neurodev. Disord.* 1:172–181.

Gomot, M. and B. Wicker. 2012. A challenging, unpredictable world for people with autism spectrum disorder. *Int. J. Psychophysiol.* 83:240–7.

Greicius, M. D. and W. W. Seeley. 2012. Introduction to the special issue on connectivity. *NeuroImage* 62:2181.

Grice, S. J., M. W. Spratling, A. Karmiloff-Smith, H. Halit, G. Csibra, M. de Haan, and M. H. Johnson. 2001. Disordered visual processing and oscillatory brain activity in autism and Williams syndrome. *Neuroreport* 12:2697–700.

Grützner, C., P. J. Uhlhaas, E. Genc, A. Kohler, W. Singer, and M. Wibral. 2010. Neuroelectromagnetic correlates of perceptual closure processes. *J. Neurosci.* 30:8342–352.

Gusnard, D. A. and M. E. Raichle. 2001. Searching for a baseline: Functional imaging and the resting human brain. *Nat. Rev. Neurosci.* 2:685–94.

Hadjipapas, A., P. Adjamian, J. B. Swettenham, I. E. Holliday, and G. R. Barnes. 2007. Stimuli of varying spatial scale induce gamma activity with distinct temporal characteristics in human visual cortex. *NeuroImage* 35:518–30.

Hadjipapas, A., E. Lowet, M. J. Roberts, A. Peter, and P. De Weerd. 2015. Parametric variation of gamma frequency and power with luminance contrast: A comparative study of human MEG and monkey LFP and spike responses. *NeuroImage* 112:327–340.

489

Hahamy, A., M. Behrmann, and R. Malach. 2015. The idiosyncratic brain: Distortion of spontaneous connectivity patterns in autism spectrum disorder. *Nat. Neurosci.* 18:302–9.

Hall, M. H., G. Taylor, P. Sham et al. 2011. The early auditory gamma-band response is heritable and a putative endophenotype of schizophrenia. *Schizophr. Bull.* 37:778–87.

Happé, F. and U. Frith. 2006. The weak coherence account: Detail-focused cognitive style in autism spectrum disorders. *J. Autism Dev. Disord.* 36:5–25.

Happé, F., A. Ronald, and R. Plomin. 2006. Time to give up on a single explanation for autism. *Nat. Neurosci.* 9:1218–20.

Hazen, E. P., J. L. Stornelli, J. A. O'Rourke, K. Koesterer, and C. J. McDougle. 2014. Sensory symptoms in autism spectrum disorders. *Harv. Rev. Psychiatry* 22:112–24.

Herrmann, C. S., I. Fründ, and D. Lenz. 2010. Human gamma-band activity: A review on cognitive and behavioral correlates and network models. *Neurosci. Biobehav. Rev.* 34:981–92.

Herrmann, C. S., M. H. Munk, and A. K. Engel. 2004. Cognitive functions of gamma-band activity: Memory match and utilization. *Trends Cogn. Sci.* 8:347–55.

Hillebrand, A. and G. R. Barnes. 2002. A quantitative assessment of the sensitivity of whole-head MEG to activity in the adult human cortex. *NeuroImage* 16:638–50.

Hoogenboom, N., J. M. Schoffelen, R. Oostenveld, L. M. Parkes, and P. Fries. 2006. Localizing human visual gamma-band activity in frequency, time and space. *NeuroImage* 29:764–73.

Hughes, J. R. 2007. Autism: The first firm finding = underconnectivity? *Epilepsy Behav.* 11:20–4.

Isler, J. R., K. M. Martien, P. G. Grieve, R. I. Stark, and M. R. Herbert. 2010. Reduced functional connectivity in visual evoked potentials in children with autism spectrum disorder. *Clin. Neurophysiol.* 121:2035–43.

Jacobs, J. and M. J. Kahana. 2009. Neural representations of individual stimuli in humans revealed by gamma-band electrocorticographic activity. *J. Neurosci.* 29:10203–14.

Jensen, O., J. Kaiser, and J. P. Lachaux. 2007. Human gamma-frequency oscillations associated with attention and memory. *Trends Neurosci.* 30:317–24.

Jerbi, K., T. Ossandon, C. M. Hamame et al. 2009. Task-related gamma-band dynamics from an intracerebral perspective: Review and implications for surface EEG and MEG. *Hum. Brain Mapp.* 30:1758–71.

Jeste, S. S. and C. A. Nelson. 2009. Event related potentials in the understanding of autism spectrum disorders: An analytical review. *J. Autism Dev. Disord.* 39:495–510.

Jeste, S. S. and D. H. Geschwind. 2014. Disentangling the heterogeneity of autism spectrum disorder through genetic findings. *Nat. Rev. Neurol.* 10:74–81.

Jia, X. and A. Kohn. 2011. Gamma rhythms in the brain. *PLoS Biol.* 9:e1001045.

Jochaut, D., K. Lehongre, A. Saitovitch, A. D. Devauchelle, I. Olasagasti, N. Chabane, M. Zilbovicius, and A. L. Giraud. 2015. Atypical coordination of cortical oscillations in response to speech in autism. *Front. Hum. Neurosci.* 9:171.

Jung, J., D. Bayle, K. Jerbi, J. R. Vidal, M. A. Hénaff, T. Ossandon, and J. P. Lachaux. 2011. Intracerebral gamma modulations reveal interaction between emotional processing and action outcome evaluation in the human orbitofrontal cortex. *Int. J. Psychophysiol.* 79:64–72.

Just, M. A., V. L. Cherkassky, T. A. Keller, and N. J. Minshew. 2004. Cortical activation and synchronization during sentence comprehension in high-functioning autism: Evidence of underconnectivity. *Brain* 127(8):1811–21.

Just, M. A., V. L. Cherkassky, T. A. Keller, R. K. Kana, and N. J. Minshew. 2007. Functional and anatomical cortical underconnectivity in autism: Evidence from an FMRI study of an executive function task and corpus callosum morphometry. *Cerebral Cortex* 17(4):951–61.

Kana, R. K., T. A. Keller, N. J. Minshew, and M. A. Just. 2007. Inhibitory control in high-functioning autism: Decreased activation and underconnectivity in inhibition networks. *Biological Psychiatry* 62(3):198–206.

Kanner, L. 1943. Autistic disturbances of affective contact. *Nervous Child* 2:217–50.

Kargas, N., B. López, V. Reddy, and P. Morris. 2015. The relationship between auditory processing and restricted, repetitive behaviors in adults with autism spectrum disorders. *J. Autism Dev. Disord.* 45:658–68.

Keown, C. L., P. Shih, A. Nair, N. Peterson, M. E. Mulvey, and R. A. Müller. 2013. Local functional overconnectivity in posterior brain regions is associated with symptom severity in autism spectrum disorders. *Cell Rep.* 5:567–72.

Khan, S., A. Gramfort, N. R. Shetty, M. G. Kitzbichler, S. Ganesan, J. M. Moran, and T. Kenet. 2013. Local and long-range functional connectivity is reduced in concert in autism spectrum disorders. *Proc. Natl. Acad. Sci. USA* 110:3107–12.

Kim, K. H. and J. H. Kim. 2006. Analysis of induced gamma-band activity in EEG during visual perception of Korean, English, Chinese words. *Neurosci. Lett.* 403:216–21.

Koshino, H., P. A. Carpenter, N. J. Minshew, V. L. Cherkassky, T. A. Keller, and M. A. Just. 2005. Functional connectivity in an fMRI working memory task in high-functioning autism. *Neuroimage* 24(3):810–21.

Lachaux, J. P., J. Jung, N. Mainy, J. C. Dreher, O. Bertrand, M. Baciu, and P. Kahane. 2008. Silence is golden: Transient neural deactivation in the prefrontal cortex during attentive reading. *Cereb. Cortex* 18:443–50.

Lachaux, J. P., E. Rodriguez, J. Martinerie, and F. J. Varela. 1999. Measuring phase synchrony in brain signals. *Human Brain Mapping* 8(4):194–208.

Lakatos, P., A. S. Shah, K. H. Knuth, I. Ulbert, G. Karmos, and C. E. Schroeder. 2005. An oscillatory hierarchy controlling neuronal excitability and stimulus processing in the auditory cortex. *J. Neurophysiol.* 94:1904–11.

Le Van Quyen, M. and A. Bragin. 2007. Analysis of dynamic brain oscillations: Methodological advances. *Trends Neurosci.* 30:365–73.

Le Van Quyen, M., J. Foucher, J. P. Lachaux, E. Rodriguez, A. Lutz, J. Martinerie, and F. J. Varela. 2001. Comparison of Hilbert transform and wavelet methods for the analysis of neuronal synchrony. *J. Neurosci. Methods* 111:83–98.

Leekam, S. R., C. Nieto, S. J. Libby, L. Wing, and J. Gould. 2007. Describing the sensory abnormalities of children and adults with autism. *J. Autism Dev. Disord.* 37:894–910.

Lewis, J. D. and J. L. Elman. 2008. Growth-related neural reorganization and the autism phenotype: A test of the hypothesis that altered brain growth leads to altered connectivity. *Dev. Sci.* 11:135–155.

Lisman, J. E. and O. Jensen. 2013. The theta-gamma neural code. *Neuron* 77:1002–16.

Logothetis, N. K. 2008. What we can do and what we cannot do with fMRI. *Nature* 453:869–78.

Mainy, N., P. Kahane, L. Minotti, D. Hoffmann, O. Bertrand, and J. P. Lachaux. 2007. Neural correlates of consolidation in working memory. *Hum. Brain Mapp.* 28:183–93.

Mantini, D., M. G. Perrucci, C. Del Gratta, G. L. Romani, and M. Corbetta. 2007. Electrophysiological signatures of resting state networks in the human brain. *Proc. Natl. Acad. Sci. USA* 104:13170–5.

Maratos, F. A., C. Senior, K. Mogg, B. P. Bradley, and G. Rippon. 2012. Early gamma-band activity as a function of threat processing in the extrastriate visual cortex. *Cogn. Neurosci.* 3:62–8.

Markram, K. and H. Markram. 2010. The intense world theory—A unifying theory of the neurobiology of autism. *Front. Hum. Neurosci.* 4:224.

Martini, N., D. Menicucci, L. Sebastiani, R. Bedini, A. Pingitore, N. Vanello, and A. Gemignani. 2012. The dynamics of EEG gamma responses to unpleasant visual stimuli: From local activity to functional connectivity. *NeuroImage* 60:922–32.

Maxwell, C. R., M. E. Villalobos, R. T. Schultz, B. Herpertz-Dahlmann, K. Konrad, and G. Kohls. 2013. Atypical laterality of resting gamma oscillations in autism spectrum disorders. *J. Autism Dev. Disord.* 45:292–7.

Menon, V. 2011. Large-scale brain networks and psychopathology: A unifying triple network model. *Trends Cogn. Sci.* 15:483–506.

Minshew, N. J. and D. L. Williams. 2007. The new neurobiology of autism: Cortex, connectivity, and neuronal organization. *Arch. Neurol.* 64:945–50.

Moldakarimov, S., M. Bazhenov, and T. J. Sejnowski. 2010. Perceptual priming leads to reduction of gamma frequency oscillations. *Proc. Natl. Acad. Sci. USA* 107:5640–5.

Morgan, H. M., S. D. Muthukumaraswamy, C. S. Hibbs, K. L. Shapiro, R. M. Bracewell, K. D. Singh, and D. E. Linden. 2011. Feature integration in visual working memory: Parietal gamma activity is related to cognitive coordination. *J. Neurophysiol.* 106:3185–94.

Mottron, L., M. Dawson, I. Soulieres, B. Hubert, and J. Burack. 2006. Enhanced perceptual functioning in autism: An update, and eight principles of autistic perception. *J. Autism Dev. Disord.* 36:27–43.

Müller, R. A., P. Shih, B. Keehn, J. Deyoe, K. Leyden, and D. Shukla. 2011. Underconnected but how? A survey of functional connectivity MRI studies in autism spectrum disorders. *Cereb. Cortex* 21:2233–43.

Murias, M., S. J. Webb, J. Greenson, and G. Dawson. 2007. Resting state cortical connectivity reflected in EEG coherence in individuals with autism. *Biological Psychiatry* 62(3):270–3.

Muthukumaraswamy, S. D. 2013. High-frequency brain activity and muscle artifacts in MEG/EEG: A review and recommendations. *Front. Hum. Neurosci.* 7:138.

Muthukumaraswamy, S. D., R. A. Edden, D. K. Jones, J. B. Swettenham, and K. D. Singh. 2009. Resting GABA concentration predicts peak gamma frequency and fMRI amplitude in response to visual stimulation in humans. *Proc. Natl. Acad. Sci. USA* 106:8356–61.

Nakamura, T., J. Matsumoto, Y. Takamura, Y. Ishii, M. Sasahara, T. Ono, and H. Nishijo. 2015. Relationships among parvalbumin-immunoreactive neuron density, phase-locked gamma oscillations, and autistic/schizophrenic symptoms in PDGFR-β knock-out and control mice. *PLoS One* 10:e0119258.

Nielsen, J. A., B. A. Zielinski, P. T. Fletcher, A. L. Alexander, N. Lange, E. D. Bigler, J. E. Lainhart, and J. S. Anderson. 2013. Multisite functional connectivity MRI classification of autism: ABIDE results. *Front. Hum. Neurosci.* 7:599.

Nourski, K. V., M. Steinschneider, H. Oya, H. Kawasaki, and M. A. Howard. 2015. Modulation of response patterns in human auditory cortex during a target detection task: An intracranial electrophysiology study. *Int. J. Psychophysiol.* 95:191–201.

Ohla, K., N. A. Busch, and C. S. Herrmann. 2007. Early electrophysiological markers of visual awareness in the human brain. *NeuroImage* 37:1329–37.

O'Riordan, M. A. 2004. Superior visual search in adults with autism. *Autism* 8:229–48.

Ossandón, T., K. Jerbi, J. R. Vidal, D. J. Bayle, M. A. Henaff, J. Jung, and J. P. Lachaux. 2011. Transient suppression of broadband gamma power in the default-mode network is correlated with task complexity and subject performance. *J. Neurosci.* 31:14521–30.

Palva, S. and J. M. Palva. 2011. Functional roles of alpha-band phase synchronization in local and large-scale cortical networks. *Front. Psychol.* 2:204.

Penny, W. D., K. E. Stephan, A. Mechelli, and K. J. Friston. 2004. Modelling functional integration: A comparison of structural equation and dynamic causal models. *NeuroImage* 23:264–74.

Pfurtscheller, G. and F. H. Lopes da Silva. 1999. Event-related EEG/MEG synchronisation and desynchronisation: Basic principles. *Clin. Neurophysiol.* 110:1842–57.

Pizzarelli, R. and E. Cherubini. 2011. Alterations of GABAergic signaling in autism spectrum disorders. *Neural Plast.* 2011:297153.

Pizzarelli, R. and E. Cherubini. 2013. GABA is essential for the construction of neuronal circuits early in development: Dysfunction in autism spectrum disorders. In *Neurobiology, Diagnosis and Treatment in Autism: An Update*, eds. D. Riva, S. Bulgheroni, and M. Zappella, 26–51. Montrouge: John Libbey Eurotext.

Pollonini, L., U. Patidar, N. Situ, R. Rezaie, A. C. Papanicolaou, and G. Zouridakis. 2010. Functional connectivity networks in the autistic and healthy brain assessed using Granger causality. *International Conference of the IEEE Engineering in Medicine and Biology Society* 32:1730–3.

Port, R. G., A. R. Anwar, M. Ku, G. C. Carlson, S. J. Siegel, and T. P. Roberts. 2015. Prospective MEG biomarkers in ASD: Pre-clinical evidence and clinical promise of electrophysiological signatures. *The Yale Journal of Biology and Medicine* 88(1):25–36.

Port, R. G., M. J. Gandal, T. P. Roberts, S. J. Siegel, and G. C. Carlson. 2007. Convergence of circuit dysfunction in ASD: A common bridge between diverse genetic and environmental risk factors and common clinical electrophysiology. *Neural and Synaptic Defects in Autism Spectrum Disorders* p. 162.

Port, R. G., M. J. Gandal, T. P. Roberts, S. J. Siegel, and G. C. Carlson. 2014. Convergence of circuit dysfunction in ASD: A common bridge between diverse genetic and environmental risk factors and common clinical electrophysiology. *Front. Cell. Neurosci.* 8:414. doi: 10.3389/fncel.2014.00414.

Redcay, E. and E. Courchesne. 2005. When is the brain enlarged in autism? A meta-analysis of all brain size reports. *Biol. Psychiatry* 58:1–9.

Rieder, M. K., B. Rahm, J. D. Williams, and J. Kaiser. 2011. Human gamma-band activity and behavior. *Int. J. Psychophysiol.* 79:39–48.

Rippon, G., J. Brock, C. Brown, and J. Boucher. 2007. Disordered connectivity in the autistic brain: Challenges for the "new psychophysiology." *Int. J. Psychophysiol.* 63:164–72.

Roberts, T. P., S. Y. Khan, M. Rey, J. F. Monroe, K. Cannon, L. Blaskey, and J. C. Edgar. 2010. MEG detection of delayed auditory evoked responses in autism spectrum disorders: Towards an imaging biomarker for autism. *Autism Res.* 3:8–18.

Rodriguez, E., N. George, J. P. Lachaux, J. Martinerie, B. Renault, and F. J. Varela. 1999. Perception's shadow: Long-distance synchronization of human brain activity. *Nature* 397:430–3.

Rojas, D. C., K. Maharajh, P. Teale, and S. J. Rogers. 2008. Reduced neural synchronization of gamma-band MEG oscillations in first-degree relatives of children with autism. *BMC Psychiatry* 8:66.

Rojas, D. C., D. Singel, S. Steinmetz, S. Hepburn, and M. S. Brown. 2014. Decreased left perisylvian GABA concentration in children with autism and unaffected siblings. *NeuroImage* 86:28–34.

Rojas, D. C., P. D. Teale, K. Maharajh, E. Kronberg, K. Youngpeter, L. B. Wilson, and S. Hepburn. 2011. Transient and steady-state auditory gamma-band responses in first-degree relatives of people with autism spectrum disorder. *Mol. Autism* 2:11.

Rojas-Líbano, D. and L. M. Kay. 2008. Olfactory system gamma oscillations: The physiological dissection of a cognitive neural system. *Cogn. Neurodyn.* 2:179–94.

Rubenstein, J. L. R. and M. M. Merzenich. 2003. Model of autism: Increased ratio of excitation/inhibition in key neural systems. *Genes Brain Behav.* 2:255–67.

Sato, W., T. Kochiyama, S. Uono, K. Matsuda, K. Usui, Y. Inoue, and M. Toichi. 2012. Temporal profile of amygdala gamma oscillations in response to faces. *J. Cogn. Neurosci.* 24:1420–33.

Saunders, J. A., V. M. Tatard-Leitman, J. Suh, E. N. Billingslea, T. P. Roberts, and S. J. Siegel. 2013. Knockout of NMDA receptors in parvalbumin interneurons recreates autism-like phenotypes. *Autism Res.* 6:69–77.

Schroeder, C. E., P. Lakatos, Y. Kajikawa, S. Partan, and A. Puce. 2008. Neuronal oscillations and visual amplification of speech. *Trends Cogn. Sci.* 12:106–13.

Sheikhani, A., H. Behnam, M. Noroozian, M. R. Mohammadi, and M. Mohammadi. 2009. Abnormalities of quantitative electroencephalography in children with Asperger disorder in various conditions. *Res. Autism Spectr. Disord.* 3:538–46.

Singer, W. 2014. How does the finding of a correlation between the three conscious states (REM dream, lucid dream, and waking) and 40 Hz power fit with your suggestion that 40 Hz is a substrate of consciousness? In *Dream Consciousness*, ed. N. Tranquillo, 201–3. Cham: Springer.

Singer, W. and C. M. Gray. 1995. Visual feature integration and the temporal correlation hypothesis. *Annu. Rev. Neurosci.* 18:555–86.

Singh, K. D., G. R. Barnes, A. Hillebrand, E. M. Forde, and A. L. Williams. 2002. Task-related changes in cortical synchronization are spatially coincident with the hemodynamic response. *NeuroImage* 16:103–14.

Sohal, V. S., F. Zhang, O. Yizhar, and K. Deisseroth. 2009. Parvalbumin neurons and gamma rhythms enhance cortical circuit performance. *Nature* 459:698–702.

Sun, L., C. Grützner, S. Bölte, M. Wibral, T. Tozman, S. Schlitt, F. Poustka, W. Singer, C. M. Freitag, and P. J. Uhlhaas. 2012. Impaired gamma-band activity during perceptual organization in adults with autism spectrum disorders: Evidence for dysfunctional network activity in frontal-posterior cortices. *J. Neurosci.* 32:9563–73.

Spence, S. J. and M. T. Schneider. 2009. The role of epilepsy and epileptiform EEGs in autism spectrum disorders. *Pediatr. Res.* 65:599–606.

Sporns, O. 2003. Graph theory methods for the analysis of neural connectivity patterns. In *Neuroscience Databases*, ed. R. Kötter, 171–85. New York: Springer.

Sporns, O. 2011. The human connectome: A complex network. *Ann. N. Y. Acad. Sci.* 1224:109–25.

Stam, C. J. and J. C. Reijneveld. 2007. Graph theoretical analysis of complex networks in the brain. *Nonlinear Biomed. Phys.* 1:3.

Stoner, R., M. L. Chow, M. P. Boyle, S. M. Sunkin, P. R. Mouton, S. Roy, A. Wynshaw-Boris, S. A. Colamarino, E. S. Lein, and E. Courchesne. 2014. Patches of disorganization in the neocortex of children with autism. *New Engl. J. Med.* 370:1209–19.

Sun, L., C. Grützner, S. Bölte, M. Wibral, T. Tozman, S. Schlitt, and P. J. Uhlhaas. 2012. Impaired gamma- activity during perceptual organization in adults with autism spectrum disorders: Evidence for dysfunctional network activity in frontal-posterior cortices. *J. Neurosci.* 32:9563–73.

Supekar, K., L. Q. Uddin, A. Khouzam, J. Phillips, W. D. Gaillard, L. E. Kenworthy, and V. Menon. 2013. Brain hyperconnectivity in children with autism and its links to social deficits. *Cell Rep.* 5:738–47.

Tallon-Baudry, C. and O. Bertrand. 1999. Oscillatory gamma activity in humans and its role in object representation. *Trends Cogn. Sci.* 3:151–62.

Thai, N. J., O. Longe, and G. Rippon. 2009. Disconnected brains: What is the role of fMRI in connectivity research? *Int. J. Psychophysiol.* 73:27–32.

Tierney, A. L., L. Gabard-Durnam, V. Vogel-Farley, H. Tager-Flusberg, and C. A. Nelson. 2012. Developmental trajectories of resting EEG power: An endophenotype of autism spectrum disorder. *PLoS One* 7:e39127.

Traub, R. D., M. A. Whittington, I. M. Stanford, and J. G. Jefferys. 1996. A mechanism for generation of long-range synchronous fast oscillations in the cortex. *Nature* 383:621–24.

Tsiaras, V., P. G. Simos, R. Rezaie, B. R. Sheth, E. Garyfallidis, E. M. Castillo, and A. C. Papanicolaou. 2011. Extracting biomarkers of autism from MEG resting-state functional connectivity networks. *Comput. Biol. Med.* 41:1166–77.

Tyzio, R., R. Nardou, D. C. Ferrari, T. Tsintsadze, A. Shahrokhi, S. Eftekhari, and Y. Ben-Ari. 2014. Oxytocin-mediated GABA inhibition during delivery attenuates autism pathogenesis in rodent offspring. *Science* 343:675–9.

Tyszka, J. M., D. P. Kennedy, L. K. Paul, and R. Adolphs. 2014. Largely typical patterns of resting-state functional connectivity in high-functioning adults with autism. *Cereb. Cortex* 24:1894–905.

Uhlhaas, P. J., G. Pipa, S. Neuenschwander, M. Wibral, and W. Singer. 2011. A new look at gamma? High- (>60 Hz) γ-band activity in cortical networks: Function, mechanisms and impairment. *Progr. Biophys. Mol. Biol.* 105:14–28.

Uhlhaas, P. J. and W. Singer. 2006. Neural synchrony in brain disorders: Relevance for cognitive dysfunctions and pathophysiology. *Neuron* 52:155–68.

Van de Cruys, S., K. Evers, R. Van der Hallen, L. Van Eylen, B. Boets, L. de-Wit, and J. Wagemans. 2014. Precise minds in uncertain worlds: Predictive coding in autism. *Psychol. Rev.* 121:649–675.

van Pelt, S., D. I. Boomsma, and P. Fries. 2012. Magnetoencephalography in twins reveals a strong genetic determination of the peak frequency of visually induced gamma-band synchronization. *J. Neurosci.* 32:3388–92.

Varela, F., J. P. Lachaux, E. Rodriguez, and J. Martinerie. 2001. The brainweb: Phase synchronization and large-scale integration. *Nat. Rev. Neurosci.* 2:229–39.

Vidal, J. R., M. Chaumon, J. K. O'Regan, and C. Tallon-Baudry. 2006. Visual grouping and the focusing of attention induce gamma-band oscillations at different frequencies in human magnetoencephalogram signals. *J. Cogn. Neurosci.* 18:1850–62.

Vissers, M. E., M. X. Cohen, and H. M. Geurts. 2012. Brain connectivity and high functioning autism: A promising path of research that needs refined models, methodological convergence, and stronger behavioral links. *Neurosci. Biobehav. Rev.* 36:604–25.

Von Stein, A. and J. Sarnthein. 2000. Different frequencies for different scales of cortical integration: From local gamma to long range alpha/theta synchronization. *Int. J. Psychophysiol.* 38:301–13.

Voytek, B. and R. T. Knight. 2015. Dynamic network communication as a unifying neural basis for cognition, development, aging, and disease. *Biol. Psychiatry* 77:1089–97.

Walter, E., P. Dassonville, and T. M. Bochsler. 2009. A specific autistic trait that modulates visuospatial illusion susceptibility. *J. Autism Dev. Disord.* 39:339–49.

Wass, S. 2011. Distortions and disconnections: Disrupted brain connectivity in autism. *Brain Cogn.* 75:18–28.

Whittington, M. A., M. O. Cunningham, F. E. N. LeBeau, C. Racca, and R. D. Traub. 2011. Multiple origins of the cortical gamma rhythm. *Dev. Neurobiol.* 71:92–106.

Whittington, M. A., R. D. Traub, and J. G. Jefferys. 1995. Synchronized oscillations in interneuron networks driven by metabotropic glutamate receptor activation. *Nature* 373:612–15.

Whittington, M. A., R. D. Traub, N. Kopell, B. Ermentrout, and E. H. Buhl. 2000. Inhibition-based rhythms: Experimental and mathematical observations on network dynamics. *Int. J. Psychophysiol.* 38:315–36.

Wilson, T. W., D. C. Rojas, M. L. Reite, P. D. Teale, and S. J. Rogers. 2007. Children and adolescents with autism exhibit reduced MEG steady-state gamma responses. *Biol. Psychiatry* 62:192–7.

Yuval-Greenberg, S., O. Tomer, A. S. Keren, I. Nelken, and L. Y. Deouell. 2008. Transient induced gamma-band response in EEG as a manifestation of miniature saccades. *Neuron* 58:429–41.

Zaehle, T. and C. S. Herrmann. 2011. Neural synchrony and white matter variations in the human brain—Relation between evoked gamma frequency and corpus callosum morphology. *Int. J. Psychophysiol.* 79:49–54.

Chapter 23 Repetitive transcranial magnetic stimulations (rTMS) effects on evoked and induced gamma frequency EEG oscillations in autism spectrum disorder

Estate M. Sokhadze, Ayman S. El-Baz, Allan Tasman, Guela E. Sokhadze, Heba Elsayed M. Farag, and Manuel F. Casanova

Contents

Abstract 498
23.1 Introduction 499
    23.1.1 Theoretical models of autism 499
23.2 Minicolumnar neuropathology model of autism and EEG
    gamma 500
23.3 Functional significance of gamma oscillations: General
    considerations 401
23.4 Review of gamma activity findings in autism 502
    23.4.1 Spontaneous, resting EEG gamma in autism 502

23.4.2 Investigation of evoked and induced gamma
responses in autism........................... 504
23.4.3 Cortical excitation/inhibition balance, GABA, and
gamma activity in autism 505
23.4.4 Investigation of evoked and induced gamma
oscillations using Kanizsa figures 507
23.5 Transcranial magnetic stimulation 512
23.6 Inhibition defects in autism and the potential role of TMS ... 515
23.7 Our studies in autism using rTMS 517
23.8 Discussion and conclusions 523
References 526

Abstract

Autism spectrum disorder (ASD) is characterized by severe disturbances in reciprocal social relations; varying degrees of language and
communication difficulty; and restricted, repetitive, and stereotyped
behavioral patterns. Additionally, another frequent symptom of ASD
is deficient executive functioning. Our group have proposed that super-
numerary minicolumns and reduced cell size of pyramidal cells bias
corticocortical connections in favor of short projections at the expense
of longer commissural ones. Furthermore, the abnormal width of minicolumns in autism reflects primarily a loss of the inhibitory tone of anatomical elements surrounding this modular structure. It is proposed that
this may result in higher excitation/inhibition ratio in autism. Majority
of electroencephalographic (EEG) studies presented findings of atypical resting-state oscillatory activity and abnormality of both evoked
and induced responses in the gamma frequency range in children with
ASD, suggesting that high-frequency oscillation anomalies are of possible clinical relevance, and support an imbalance of neural excitation/
inhibition as a potential ASD biomarker. Preliminary evidence suggests that ASD may be associated with changes in gamma-band oscillations. We proposed to use repetitive transcranial magnetic stimulation
(rTMS) that has been suggested as a therapeutic attempt at overcoming
lateral inhibitory minicolumnar deficits. In this chapter, we describe
this method of neurotherapy in autism treatment and EEG methods
aimed at the assessment of functional changes following rTMS-based
neuromodulation. The approach is meant to target the investigation of
rTMS-induced positive changes in electrophysiological activity (i.e.,
quantitative EEG and event-related potentials [ERPs] shown in our preliminary results) and to improve prefrontal executive functions in ASD
patients. The chapter will examine the effects of 6, 12, and 18 sessions
of low-frequency rTMS bilaterally over the dorsolateral prefrontal cortex (DLPFC) and post-TMS neurofeedback training on behavior, cognitive functions, and other behavioral clinical outcomes in children with
autism with the main focus on changes in evoked and induced gamma
oscillations.

23.1 Introduction

23.1.1 Theoretical models of autism

Autism is defined as a behavioral syndrome characterized by pervasive impairment in several areas of development: social interaction, communication skills, and repertoire of interests and activities. Thus far, there have been no neuropathological findings nor laboratory-based measures providing construct validity to the diagnosis of autism. In the absence of pathognomonic abnormalities, research in autism has been guided by a variety of ideologies and epistemological assumptions, each contributing to the development of explanatory models or "theories" such as executive functions (Ozonoff et al. 1994), "weak central coherence" (Frith and Happé 1994; Happé 1996), theory of mind (Baron-Cohen et al. 1985), and so on. Deficits in executive functioning skills are the salient feature of a model of autism that outlines the importance of prefrontal deficits in autism spectrum disorder (ASD) (Ozonoff 1997; Hill 2004). Other models of autism mainly emphasize impaired functional connectivity (Just et al. 2004; Welchew et al. 2005), which manifests as a cognitive deficit affecting the "binding together" of discrete features into a single, coherent object or concept. One of these theoretical models aimed to unify the existing knowledge on the etiology of autism focuses on abnormalities in neural connectivity (Belmonte et al. 2004a,b). The model states that autism might be characterized by functional disconnectivity of networks important for specific aspects of social cognition and emotional and behavioral control. One more model, proposed by Baron-Cohen et al. (1985), is the so-called theory of mind deficit in autism. This model suggests that the characteristic problems in social interaction observed in autistic patients arise from an inability to understand mental states in other people, for example, beliefs, desires, intentions, imagination, and emotions. There were other models, for instance, "mirror neurons system" (MNS) abnormalities and imitation deficit hypothesis that according to MNS and imitation role proponents might be responsible for a cascading effect resulting in lack of emotional responsiveness and empathy, deficient joint attention, theory of mind, and other self-other mapping impairments observed in autism (Williams et al. 2001; Rizzolatti and Craighero 2004; Ramachandran and Oberman 2006; Oberman and Ramachandran 2007; Oberman et al. 2008). Recently, the mirror neuron system and imitation deficit hypothesis were criticized on the grounds of numerous discrepancies, emphasizing that it cannot account for majority of the patterns of deficits observed in children with ASD and adult patients with autism (Mostofsky et al. 2006; Fan et al. 2010; Stieglitz Ham et al. 2011).

Recent attempts at deriving an overarching metatheory of autism have focused on a basic abnormality of neural connectivity (Belmonte et al. 2004a,b). This model is empirically based on lack of coordinated brain activity (functional imaging) and abnormal "binding" (EEG tracings) in the brains of autistic patients (Brock et al. 2002; Just et al. 2004; Brown

2005; Koshino et al. 2005). By themselves, these theories are incapable of accounting for all of the developmental, social, cognitive, and affective variables that define autistic psychopathology. One more current theory of autism takes a "minicolumnar" perspective and is based on the neuropathology of autism (Casanova et al. 2002a; Casanova 2006).

23.2 Minicolumnar neuropathology model of autism and EEG gamma

Recent studies by our group have characterized the neuropathology of autism as that of a minicolumnopathy. Postmortem studies using computerized image analysis of pyramidal cell arrays have found that the brains of autistic individuals have smaller minicolumns with most of the decrease stemming from a reduction in its peripheral neuropil space, with little, if any, reduction in their core space. This finding has been reproduced using different techniques (e.g., GLI index) and independent populations (Casanova et al. 2002a–c, 2006a,b). It is now known that minicolumnar width reduction in autism spans supragranular, granular, and infragranular layers (Casanova et al. 2010). The most parsimonious explanation for the findings is the possible abnormality of an anatomical element common to all layers. The peripheral neuropil space of minicolumns provides, among other things, for inhibitory elements distributed throughout all of its laminae. This is the so-called shower curtain of inhibition of the minicolumn described by Szentagothai and Arbib (1975). Our findings therefore suggest a deficit within the inhibitory elements that surround the cell minicolumn (Casanova et al. 2006b).

The anatomical disposition of inhibitory elements within the shower curtain of inhibition provides clues as to their function. While tangentially arrayed basket cells function, in part, to coordinate activity among remote neuronal ensembles, by contrast, radially oriented inhibitory interneurons prominently located in the peripheral neuropil space surrounding pyramidal cell columns likely function to segregate columns from interference, both from other minicolumns within an array and from fields of activity or inhibition in neighboring minicolumnar arrays (Casanova et al. 2003). The finding suggests a mechanistic explanation to the inhibitory/excitatory imbalance in autism and a possible explanation to the multifocal seizures often observed in this condition (Casanova et al. 2003).

Oscillations of pyramidal cells in minicolumns and across assemblies of minicolumns are maintained by networks of different species of inhibitory, GABA-expressing interneurons. In this regard, interneurons make a critical contribution to the generation of network oscillations, and help synchronize the activity of pyramidal cells during transient brain states (Mann and Paulsen 2007). Local excitatory–inhibitory interactions help shape neuronal representations of sensory, motor, and cognitive variables, and produce local gamma-band oscillations in the 30–80 Hz range (Donner and Siegel 2011). The excitatory–inhibitory bias caused by faulty pyramidal cell–interneuron dyads provides a receptive scenario to gamma frequency abnormalities in autism.

Gamma frequencies are closely associated with sensory processing, working memory, attention, and many other cognitive domains (Ward 2003; Jensen et al. 2007).

The brain's limited long-range wiring cannot directly sustain coordinated activity across arbitrary cortical locations, but it can convey patterns of synchronous activity as oscillatory neuronal fluxes, represented by local field potentials measured by EEG. Coordination of oscillations at varying interacting frequencies allows for relatively efficient and unconstrained segregation in varying forms and across hierarchical cortical levels. Disrupted patterns of coordinated oscillatory output in distributed minicolumnar networks might be associated with cortical "disconnection" in autism. More specifically, altered oscillatory activity in developing cortical circuits may contribute to impaired development of intra-areal and transcortical connections giving rise to a bias in short (e.g., arcuate) versus long corticocortical projections (e.g., commissural fibers) (Casanova et al. 2006a,b, 2009). The pervasive nature of abnormalities ingrained in this oscillatory activity bears significant analogy to the cognitive deficits observed in autism. It is therefore unsurprising that gamma oscillations have been claimed to be directly related to the pathophysiology of autism (Sohal 2012). To the authors' knowledge, every study on gamma frequencies in autism has been abnormal.

23.3 Functional significance of gamma oscillations: General considerations

Electroencephalography (EEG) has been used to decompose oscillatory patterns into several frequency bands: delta (0.5–4 Hz), theta (4–8 Hz), alpha (8–13 Hz), beta (13–30 Hz), and gamma (30–80 Hz). High-frequency gamma oscillations are most directly associated with entrainment of local networks. Strong evidence indicates that the gamma frequency activity is associated with binding of perceptual features in animals (Herrmann and Knight 2001). Human experiments have also found that induced gamma activity correlates with binding (Kaiser 2003). Binding of widely distributed cell assemblies by the synchronization of their gamma frequency activity is thought to underlie cohesive stimulus representation in the human brain (Keil et al. 1999; Rodriguez et al. 1999; von Stein et al. 1999; Bertrand and Tallon-Baudry 2000; Kahana 2006; Pavlova et al. 2006; Fries 2009). Increased gamma activity has been most widely associated with top-down attentional processing and object perception (Rodriguez et al. 1999; Gruber et al. 2001; Felli et al. 2003; Nakatani et al. 2005) subserving Gestalt pattern perception (von Stein et al. 1999; Herrmann and Mecklinger 2000).

Contemporary models of neural connectivity outline the role of integration and segregation of both local and distal networks, their phase synchronization, and large-scale integration of spontaneous, evoked, and induced neural activity (Tallon-Baudry et al. 1998, 2005; Varela et al. 2001; Tallon-Baudry 2003). Functional coupling and decoupling of neural assemblies could be analyzed within specific time and frequency windows of EEG activity. Gamma-band activity in response to stimulation can be divided into either evoked or induced: evoked gamma-band activity has been identified at a latency of around 100 ms after stimulus onset (Bertrand and Tallon-Baudry 2000; Herrmann and Mecklinger 2000) and is highly phase locked to the onset of the stimulus; induced gamma-band activity occurs later with a variable onset although it has been reported to start at around 250 ms (Brown et al. 2005). It has been proposed that evoked gamma-band activity reflects the early sensory processing and the binding of perceptual information within the same cortical area (i.e., intra-areal), whereas induced gamma-band activity reflects the binding of feedforward and feedback processing in a whole network of cortical areas (corticocortical) (Shibata et al. 1999; Müller et al. 2000; Brown et al. 2005). Variations of such activity have been termed event-related synchronization and desynchronization (ERS/ERD) (Pfurtscheller and Aranibar 1977) or event-related spectral perturbation (ERSP) and have been associated with the activation of task-relevant neuronal assemblies (Pfurtscheller and Lopes da Silva 1999; Rippon et al. 2007).

High-frequency EEG oscillations in the gamma range are intimately related to mental processes such as consciousness (Llinas and Ribary 1993), binding of sensory features into coherent percept (Tallon-Baudry et al. 1996; Engel and Singer 2001), object representation (Bertrand and Tallon-Baudry 2000), attention (Fell et al. 2001; Kahana 2006), and memory (Herrmann et al. 2004). Gamma oscillations are subdivided into spontaneous and stimulus related (steady-state, induced, and evoked oscillations), but these different classes of gamma oscillations may be generated in the same neural circuits (Herrmann and Knight 2001). High-frequency rhythms such as gamma are generated in neuronal networks involving excitatory pyramidal cells and inhibitory gamma-aminobutyric acid (GABA)-ergic interneurons (Whittington et al. 2000). Gamma oscillations are enhanced with arousal and attention or by stimulation of reticular formation (Rodriguez et al. 2004).

23.4 Review of gamma activity findings in autism

23.4.1 Spontaneous, resting EEG gamma in autism

Cantor et al. (1986) reported a high amount of slow rhythms in the EEG of children with ASD and mental retardation in a resting condition, which was interpreted as an indication of a developmental lag. Dawson et al.

(1995) in a visual task found normal beta activity power, but abnormally decreased EEG spectral power over frontal and temporal areas in the delta, theta, and alpha frequency ranges. In addition, an abnormal EEG hemispheric asymmetry was reported in a few studies (Cantor et al. 1986; Dawson et al. 1995; Lazarev et al. 2009). However, available EEG findings disagree even in respect to the directions of the altered hemispheric asymmetry in autism spectrum disorders (Ogawa et al. 1982; Dawson et al. 1995; Daoust et al. 2004). One of the distinctive features of spontaneous EEG oscillations, differentiating boys with autism from typically developing boys in a study by Stroganova et al. (2007), was an abnormal hemispheric asymmetry in children with ASD. The autism group demonstrated a broadband leftward EEG asymmetry at the temporal and some adjacent regions that was absent in controls. This feature was replicated in the two independent samples from different countries and clearly represents a reliable EEG marker of autism (Stroganova et al. 2007, 2012).

Gamma rhythm is normally defined as EEG activity in the frequency range between 30 and 80 Hz, although there is increasing awareness of a higher gamma range (>80 Hz). Our review mostly focuses on gamma activity within 35–45 Hz, or so-called 40 Hz-centered gamma activity (Galambos 1992). The interest in the investigation of gamma frequencies in autism research is understandable considering a role for them in cognitive activity and processes such as perceptual binding (Singer 1999; Belmonte et al. 2004a,b; Uhlhaas and Singer 2007; Uhlhaas 2011).

The mechanisms of spontaneous gamma oscillations in the cortex and hippocampus are well understood and described in the literature, especially in regard to the role of GABAergic interneurons results in recurrent inhibition of pyramidal cells, in turn synchronizing pyramidal cell output into the gamma-band range (Bartos et al. 2007; Hájos and Paulsen 2009). Reduced interneuron cell number is a common finding in autism (Casanova 2006; Gogolla et al. 2009). There is also human imaging evidence for reduced GABA concentration in frontal cortices (Harada et al. 2010).

Reported discrepancies and differences of findings regarding spontaneous gamma activity power in autism may stem from several sources. The first of all experimental conditions in previous studies were not similar in terms of the children's behavioral state. The considerations discussed by Stroganova et al. (2007) suggest that reported quantitative EEG differences between autism spectrum disorder and control groups may be both trait and state dependent. Another probable source of the differences in EEG profiles between ASD and typical children might be dependent on the age of children. In autism, age-related changes in EEG differ from normally developing children (Chugani et al. 1999; Courchesne et al. 2003; Ferri et al. 2003; Carper and Courchesne 2005; Hazlett et al. 2005; Sheikhani et al. 2009, 2012). Therefore, EEG abnormalities in autism may be age-specific and bias comparisons in resting conditions (Stroganova et al. 2007; Sun et al. 2012; Rojas and Wilson 2014).

23.4.2 Investigation of evoked and induced gamma responses in autism

Excitatory output of projection neurons is modulated and coordinated by oscillatory electrocortical activity of area-specific arrays of inhibitory interneurons. Phasic synchronization of these local oscillation patterns may provide a basis for functional integration across widely distributed cortical networks (Müller et al. 2000; Varela et al. 2001; Tallon-Baudry 2003; Tallon-Baudry et al. 2005). Visual and auditory perception anomalies as well as some features of language processing and social communication deficits, and executive dysfunctions associated with "weak central coherence" in autism (Frith and Happé 1994; Morgan et al. 2003; Mottron et al. 2003; Plaisted et al. 2003; Happé and Frith 2006) may be attributed to reduced gamma frequency synchronization and decreased temporal binding of activity between networks processing local features.

Disrupted visual perceptual congruence in individuals with autism is illustrated by a study (Brown 2005) in which subjects were presented with a visual shape illusion (Kanizsa 1976). The autistic individuals exhibited a burst of gamma activity in posterior areas at 300 ms, which was greater in power and duration than the corresponding gamma response in controls. In another study, Brown et al. (2005) could not find reaction time or accuracy differences between groups in a task of Kanizsa figure identification but they showed significant task-related differences in gamma activity. Control participants showed typical gamma-band activity over parietal regions at around 350 ms, while autistic participants showed overall increased activity, including an early 100 ms gamma peak and a late induced peak, occurring earlier than that shown by the control group. The authors interpreted the abnormal gamma activity to reflect decreased "signal to noise" due to decreased inhibitory processing.

Brock et al. (2002) described the parallels between the psychological model of "central coherence" in information processing (Frith and Happé 1994) and the neuroscience model of neural integration or "temporal binding." They proposed that autism is associated with abnormalities of information integration that is caused by a reduction in the connectivity between specialized local neural networks in the brain and possible overconnectivity within the isolated individual neural assemblies. This concept was further elaborated in an "impaired connectivity" hypothesis of autism (Rippon et al. 2007), which summarized theoretical and empirical advances in research implicating disordered connectivity in autism. The authors highlighted recent developments in the analysis of the temporal binding of information and the relevance of gamma activity to current models of structural and effective connectivity based on the balance between excitatory and inhibitory cortical activity (Casanova et al. 2002a–c; Rubenstein and Merzenich 2003; Belmonte et al. 2004a,b).

It has been proposed that "weak central coherence" (Frith and Happé 1994; Morgan et al. 2003; Mottron et al. 2003; Plaisted et al. 2003; Happé and Frith 2006; Murias et al. 2007) in autism could result from a reduction in the integration of specialized local networks in the brain caused by a deficit in temporal binding (Brock et al. 2002; Rippon et al. 2007). Audiovisual perception anomalies associated with weak central coherence may be attributed to a reduction in the synchronization of gamma activity between networks processing local features and can explain some of the features of language deficits, executive dysfunctions, and other impairments in social communication in autism. Excessive but not synchronized gamma can be linked to a reduction in the ability to focus attention. In autism, uninhibited gamma activity suggests that none of the circuits in the brain can come to dominance because too many of them are active simultaneously (Brown et al. 2005). A proposed "temporal binding deficit" hypothesis of autism (Grice et al. 2001; Brock et al. 2002; Rippon et al. 2007) suggests that many features of autism such as superiority in processing of detail (local processing) and disadvantage in global processing, necessitating integration of information either over space, time, or context can be explained by a failure of binding between cortical areas. Abnormal gamma activation would suggest disrupted neural signaling and would support the hypothesis of abnormal regional activation patterns.

23.4.3 Cortical excitation/inhibition balance, GABA, and gamma activity in autism

There are reports that suggest that increased fast frequency activity may be a characteristic EEG feature of autism. Another indication of a possible relation between fast EEG activity and autism comes from data on genetically mediated abnormalities in GABAergic and glutamatergic (Shuang et al. 2004) mediator systems in this disorder. The morphological integrity of GABAergic interneuron connections within cortical minicolumns is important for the generation of normal gamma oscillations (Whittington et al. 2000). Casanova et al. (2003) suggested that such abnormal minicolumn organization might result in a deficit of inhibitory GABAergic fiber projections, which in turn may facilitate the occurrence of epilepsy in autism. The presence of fast rhythms in EEG is usually considered as an electrophysiological index of cortical activation. Therefore, excess beta and gamma rhythms in EEG of children with autism would support the hypothesis of abnormally high excitation/inhibition ratio in cortical structures in this disorder (Rubenstein and Merzenich 2003).

There were only few EEG studies employing resting-state examinations in individuals with ASD and practically all report oscillatory anomalies. Specifically, eyes-open resting-state exams have shown greater relative delta and less relative alpha power in 4- to 12-year-old low-functioning children with ASD (Cantor et al. 1986), and greater 24–44 Hz power in 3- to 8-year-old boys with ASD (Orekhova et al. 2007). Eyes-closed exams have shown greater relative 3–6 Hz and 13–17 Hz power and less 9–10 Hz power in adults with ASD (Murias et al. 2007), and decreased delta and beta power, as well as increased theta power, in children with ASD (Coben et al. 2008). Although the aforementioned results implicate atypical oscillatory activity in ASD, findings are discrepant, and as it was noted probably due to between-study differences in age, level of functioning, and medication status of the ASD participants.

Cornew et al. (2012) showed that children with ASD exhibited regionally specific elevations in delta, theta, alpha, and high-frequency beta and gamma power, supporting an imbalance of neural excitation/inhibition as a neurobiological feature of ASD. Increased temporal and parietal alpha power was associated with greater symptom severity and thus is of particular interest. In the auditory domain, reduced entrainment to auditory stimulation at 40 Hz in participants with ASD has been demonstrated (Wilson et al. 2007). In contrast, during visual perception, there is evidence for both hyperactivity and hypoactivity of gamma-band oscillations (Grice et al. 2001; Brown et al. 2005; Milne et al. 2009; Isler et al. 2010; Stroganova et al. 2012), raising the question of the link between high-frequency oscillations (HFOs) and perceptual dysfunctions in the disorder. Orekhova et al. (2007) reported higher levels of EEG gamma-band activity in the 24–44 Hz range in children with ASD. Elevations in gamma were observed in anterior temporal, posterior temporal, and occipital sites using EEG (Cornew et al. 2012). Therefore, gamma-band abnormalities have been reported in many studies of autism spectrum disorders. Gamma-band activity is associated with perceptual and cognitive functions that are compromised in autism. The utility of gamma-band-related variables as diagnostic biomarkers is currently limited; there is still room for using gamma oscillation measures as functional markers of response to interventions such as rTMS-based neuromodulation or neurofeedback.

Based on current pathophysiological models of ASD that have discussed a dysfunction in the excitation–inhibition balance (E/I balance) (Rubenstein and Merzenich 2003) as well as atypical modulation in fronto-posterior networks (Minshew and Keller 2010), theoretically, it should be expected to have altered gamma-band power during perceptual processing in participants with ASD as well as abnormal modulation of high-frequency activity in frontal and parietal cortices. These findings highlight the contribution of impaired gamma-band activity toward complex visual processing in ASD, suggesting atypical modulation of high-frequency power in fronto-posterior networks.

It is well known that networks of inhibitory interneurons acting as GABA-gated pacemakers are critically involved in gamma oscillations (Grothe and Klump 2000; Whittington et al. 2000). Electrophysiological research has provided evidence that gamma activity is a physiological indicator of the coactivation of cortical cells engaged in processing visual stimuli (Singer and Gray 1995; Tallon-Baudry and Bertrand 1999; Keil et al. 2001) and integrating different features of a stimulus (Müller et al. 1996). The onset of a visual stimulus gives rise to a burst of gamma activity over occipital sites, and when more complex tasks are undertaken, discrete bursts of gamma activity have been identified overlying cortical regions thought to be engaged in those tasks (Brown et al. 2005). For example, tasks involving attention modulation or the top-down integration of features give rise to simultaneous bursts of gamma over frontal and occipitoparietal regions (Müller et al. 1996; Rodriguez et al. 1999; Müller and Gruber 2001).

In visual studies, the type of stimulus (for instance, face type stimuli vs. illusory nonface stimuli) may be important in determining whether gamma is lower (faces) or higher (nonfaces) in autism. In approximately half of resting gamma-band studies, reduced gamma is found in autism, while the remaining studies find increased gamma power in autism. Differences between resting gamma studies might be reconciled by attention to variables such as age, but also by careful attention to the state of alertness under which EEG data are acquired.

23.4.4 Investigation of evoked and induced gamma oscillations using Kanizsa figures

As it was noted above, Kanizsa illusory figures (Kanizsa 1976) have been shown to produce gamma oscillation bursts during visual cognitive tasks (Tallon-Baudry et al. 1996; Herrmann et al. 1999). Kanizsa stimuli consist of inducer disks of a shape feature and either constitute an illusory figure (square, triangle) or not (colinearity feature); in nonimpaired individuals, gamma activity has been shown to increase during "target-present" compared to "target-absent" trials (Müller et al. 1996; Tallon-Baudry et al. 1996; Brown et al. 2005). In several studies, Kanizsa figures were employed as stimuli in an oddball task paradigm to investigate the effects of target classification and discrimination between illusory stimulus features (Tallon-Baudry et al. 1998; Herrmann and Mecklinger 2000; Böttger et al. 2002; Brown 2005; Sokhadze et al. 2009a).

Kanizsa illusory figures require illusory perceptual closure and are easily evoking gamma activity. Several studies have investigated gamma-band activity during the perception of Kanizsa figures in autism (Brown 2005; Sokhadze et al. 2009a). While these three EEG studies utilized Kanizsa figures, the stimuli and tasks differed. Brown et al. (2005) utilized stimuli consisting of a rectangle of five circles by five circles with a missing 90° segment in each circle, which created stimuli with the presence or absence of a Kanizsa rectangle within the resulting pattern. Participants in this study, six adolescents with autism and eight adolescents with moderate learning difficulties, were required to press a button when they perceived the Kanizsa rectangle and another button when they did not. Our early study (Sokhadze et al. 2009a) utilized a modified oddball task consisting of Kanizsa square targets, Kanizsa triangle nontargets, and non-Kanizsa (both square and triangle) standards. Participants pressed buttons only for target stimuli. In the third study, Stroganova et al. (2012), 23 children with autism and 23 typically developing children passively viewed Kanizsa squares and non-Kanizsa squares.

Both the Brown et al. (2005) and Sokhadze et al. (2009a) studies reported increased induced gamma activity in adolescents with autism compared with control subjects. In contrast to these two studies, Stroganova et al. (2012) reported reductions of gamma activity in response to Kanizsa figures in children with autism. These findings were for evoked rather than induced activity, however. Further, the passive nature of the task may have reduced attention demands on participants. In the auditory domain, evoked gamma was reduced in autism.

In our study of gamma activity in autism (Sokhadze et al. 2009a; Baruth et al. 2010a; Casanova et al. 2012), we used a modification of such oddball test where subjects performed a visual discrimination task that required a response to target Kanizsa squares among nontarget Kanizsa triangles and non-Kanizsa figures. This task was used to examine gamma-band EEG activity and event-related potentials (ERPs). The power of induced gamma oscillations (at 12 left and right frontal, central, parietal, and occipital EEG sites, 30–80 Hz range, in μV^2) was analyzed using wavelet transformation. The density of induced power of gamma oscillations ($\mu V^2/Hz$) and the power density difference between gamma response to nontarget and target Kanizsa stimuli (target minus nontarget Kanizsa conditions) were also calculated and analyzed. The power of gamma oscillations in response to nontarget Kanizsa and non-Kanizsa standard stimuli was higher in the autism group at the left frontal (F1, F7), left and right parietal (P1, P2, P7, P8), and occipital (O1, O2) EEG channels.

Group (control, autism) differences in gamma oscillation power to nontarget and target Kanizsa stimuli were better expressed over the lateral frontal (F7, F8) and parietal (P7, P8) EEG sites. A *Stimulus* (target, nontarget) × *Group* (autism, control) interaction was highly significant for all recording sites, and described as higher gamma power to nontargets in the autism group compared to controls. We also found a *Hemisphere* × *Group* interaction across the lateral frontal and parietal sites, with difference between target and nontarget stimuli being more negative in the autism group at the right hemisphere. The most consistent finding was that gamma induced by the nontarget stimuli was globally higher in autistic subjects compared to controls at all sites. This interaction for *Stimulus* (nontarget, target) × *Topography* (frontal, parietal) × *Group* (autism, control) was significant. Power density differences to target and nontarget stimuli revealed significant and reproducible effect of higher response to nontargets rather than target Kanizsa figures in the autism group (Sokhadze et al. 2009a).

In a more recent study on 29 children with ASD and age- and gender-matched group of 29 typically developing children, we focused on evoked and induced 35–45 Hz range gamma activity and found significantly higher early gamma responses to nontarget (non-Kanizsa) standards, nontarget Kanizsa distracters, and target Kanizsa figures in children with autism as compared to typical children. These differences were more expressed at the parietal sites (e.g., P3 and P4, Figures 23.1 and 23.2), though they were statistically significant also at some frontal sites (e.g., F1, F2). Group differences were similar in the late (induced) gamma responses at the parietal sites. In addition, for nontarget and target illusory figures, we found *Stimulus × Hemisphere × Group* interaction, with differences being more pronounced for the nontarget stimuli at the left hemisphere in children with ASD.

Our findings of higher amplitude of ERP components (Sokhadze et al. 2009a,b; Casanova et al. 2012) and excessive gamma oscillations (Sokhadze et al. 2009a; Baruth et al. 2010a, 2011) in response to nontarget items are in agreement with other studies noting that neural systems in the brain of autistic patients are often inappropriately activated (Belmonte and Yurgelun-Todd 2003a). Kemner et al. (1994) also reported that the visual ERP components to novel distracters are larger when a person with autism is performing a task even when these novel stimuli are not relevant to the task in question. According to Belmonte and Yurgelun-Todd (2003a,b), perceptual filtering in autism occurs in an all-or-none manner with little specificity for the task relevance of the

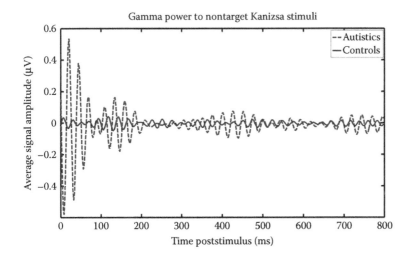

Figure 23.1 Evoked and induced gamma oscillations to nontarget Kanizsa figures in a visual oddball task with illusory figures. Grand averages of responses in 26 children with ASD and 26 age- and gender-matched typical children at the right parietal site (P4). The ASD group shows higher amplitude of the early-evoked gamma (around 120 ms poststimulus).

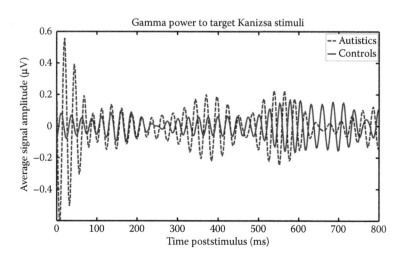

Figure 23.2 Evoked and induced gamma oscillations to target Kanizsa figures in a visual oddball task with illusory figures. Grand averages of responses in 26 children with ASD and 26 age- and gender-matched typical children at the right parietal site (P4). The ASD group shows higher amplitude of the late-induced gamma oscillations (within 300–400 ms poststimulus).

stimulus. Perceptual filtering may primarily depend on the control of general arousal rather than the activation of specific perceptual system. Since, in many tasks requiring attention, persons with autism perform at close to normal levels despite generally high arousal and low selectivity, some compensatory mechanisms may operate at a higher stage of processing to sort out relevant stimuli from poorly discriminated background. One candidate mechanism was suggested as an active inhibition of irrelevant distracters that have passed through earlier filtering (Belmonte and Yurgelun-Todd 2003b). It is unsurprising that increased ratio of excitation/inhibition in key neural systems and high "cortical noise" has been considered as a core abnormality of autism (Casanova et al. 2003; Rubenstein and Merzenich 2003).

Our study showed very similar gamma activation pattern both to "target" and "nontarget" Kanizsa stimuli (Sokhadze et al. 2009a; Baruth et al. 2010a,b, 2011). Furthermore, dipole source coherence analysis (BESA Coherence Module, Schreg 2005) of early evoked (40–150 ms) 40 Hz centered gamma responses to targets at the parietal sites (P3, P4) showed between three groups differences, specifically, higher hemispheric coherence coefficient values not only in typical children but also in attention deficit/hyperactivity disorder (ADHD) as compared to the autism group (e.g., 0.59 in ADHD vs. 0.38 in autism, $p = 0.003$).

The gamma frequencies, particularly those centered about 40 Hz, have been tied to visual, attentional, cognitive, and memory processes (Başar et al. 2001). As it was mentioned above, following a stimulus presentation during visual task, two gamma oscillations are typically noted: an early evoked oscillation and a late induced oscillation (Başar et al. 2001). The evoked gamma oscillations typically occur within the first 100 ms after the onset of a stimulus, and are locked in time from trial to trial. Because little variation is seen in the latency of the evoked gamma with changing stimulus type, it is believed that it may be a result of sensory processes. Conversely, induced gamma oscillations occur later, after 240 ms post-stimulus, and vary in latency from trial to trial (Tallon-Baudry and Bertrand 1999). These variations occurring in time window typical for P300 ERP component may suggest that the induced gamma oscillations are related to higher cognitive processes (Tallon-Baudry 2003). Deviations from typical gamma-band activity have been reported in several studies on neurological disorders, including epilepsy, Alzheimer's disease, ADHD, and autism (Herrmann and Demiralp 2005).

Our study (Baruth et al. 2010a) indicated that individuals with autism had a minimal difference in evoked gamma power between target and nontarget Kanizsa stimuli at all EEG channels of interest. In fact, evoked gamma power responses were slightly larger in response to nontarget Kanizsa stimuli relative to targets. In contrast, the control group had a significantly higher evoked gamma power to target Kanizsa stimuli compared to nontarget Kanizsa stimuli, showing clear differences in visual stimulus discrimination. Additionally, the control group showed a greater difference in evoked gamma power between frontal and parietal regions to all stimuli over the left hemisphere: controls had more frontal as compared to parietal gamma activity, while the autism spectrum disorder group showed negligible topographic differences.

These findings are similar to the findings of Grice et al. (2001) where individuals with autism did not show significant differences in frontal gamma activity during the processing of upright and inverted faces, whereas control subjects showed clear discriminative increases in frontal gamma activity when the faces were presented upright versus inverted. These findings also correspond to our previous investigation (Sokhadze et al. 2009a) where we found positive differences in gamma oscillation power (i.e., 30–80 Hz, 0–800 ms poststimulus) between target and nontarget Kanizsa stimuli were decreased, especially over the lateral frontal (F7, F8) and parietal (P7, P8) EEG sites, in adolescents and young adults with autism spectrum disorders; this was mainly due to significant increases in gamma power at all recording sites, especially evoked gamma (i.e., ~100 ms) over frontal channels, to nontarget Kanizsa stimuli compared to controls. Our results indicate that in ASD, evoked gamma activity is not discriminative of stimulus type, whereas in controls, early gamma power differences between target and nontarget stimuli are highly significant.

There are a few plausible explanations as to why the gamma response does not allow for discrimination between stimuli in ASD. It is well known that ASD is associated with amplified responses to incoming sensory information. Studies suggest that the neural systems of individuals

511

with ASD are overactivated (Belmonte and Yurgelun-Todd 2003a,b), and there is a lack of cortical inhibitory tone (Casanova et al. 2002a,b, 2006b; Rubenstein and Merzenich 2003). In a network that is overactivated and "noisy," local cortical connectivity may be enhanced at the expense of long-range cortical connections, and individuals with ASD may have difficulty directing attention. It may not be possible for them to selectively activate specific perceptual systems based on the relevance of a stimulus (i.e., target vs. nontarget).

Our previous findings investigating ERP during a visual novelty processing task further support the idea of difficulty discriminating task-relevant from irrelevant stimuli in ASD (see Sokhadze et al. 2009b). Briefly, we found that subjects with ASD showed a lack of stimulus discrimination between target and nontarget stimuli compared to controls, and this was mainly due to significantly prolonged and augmented ERP components to irrelevant distracter stimuli over frontal and parietal recording sites. Early ERP components (e.g., P100, N100) were especially increased to irrelevant distracter stimuli in the ASD group, indicating augmented responses at early stages of visual processing (i.e., ~100 ms). Early gamma components (i.e., evoked) are measured at the same time over the same cortical regions as these early ERP components. The very early burst of gamma activity between 80 and 120 ms found by Brown et al. (2005) and our findings of augmented evoked gamma (Sokhadze et al. 2009a) and early ERP responses (Sokhadze et al. 2009b) to task-irrelevant stimuli support the idea of disturbances in the activation of task-relevant neuronal assemblies and the perceptual control of attention in ASD. Although we found significant group differences in relative evoked gamma power in processing relevant and irrelevant visual stimuli in this study, it is important to mention why we did not find significantly amplified relative evoked gamma power in the ASD group compared to controls. We attribute this to the fact that relative gamma-band power is calculated in reference to the entire EEG spectrum, and in ASD, it has previously been shown that other frequency ranges are augmented as well (e.g., Dawson et al. 1995; Stroganova et al. 2007).

Studies of high-frequency oscillations in autism are accelerating at a rapid pace (Gandal et al. 2010). Gamma activity is associated with recurrent inhibition of glutamatergic pyramidal cells by GABAergic interneurons (Harada et al. 2010). Converging evidence implicates both transmitter systems in autism. Although GABA and gamma band have been related in control subjects, no studies have yet reported an association in autism.

23.5 Transcranial magnetic stimulation

Among the newly emerging neuromodulation techniques, rTMS is one of the most promising for the treatment of core symptoms in autism spectrum disorder. Transcranial magnetic stimulation (TMS) offers a noninvasive method for altering excitability of the brain. It potentially induces a short-term functional reorganization in the human cortex. The magnitude and the direction of rTMS-induced plasticity depend on the variables of stimulation (intensity, frequency, number of stimuli) and the functional state of the cortex targeted by rTMS. Since the effects of rTMS are not limited to the stimulated target cortex but give rise to functional changes in anatomically and functionally interconnected cortical areas, rTMS is a suitable tool to investigate neural plasticity within a distributed functional network (Rossi and Rossini 2004; Ziemann 2004). The lasting effects of rTMS offer new possibilities to study dynamic aspects of the pathophysiology of a variety of diseases and may have therapeutic potential in some psychiatric disorders. By convention, rTMS in the 0.3–1 Hz frequency range is referred to as "slow," whereas "fast" rTMS refers to stimulation greater than 1 Hz (Pasquale-Leone et al. 2000). This point of view is reconsidered as a certain simplification, as some studies consider the frequency of TMS as a less important factor compared to other factors related to the ability to change functional connectivity in the brain (Khedr et al. 2008; Fitzgerald et al. 2011).

Hoffman and Cavus (2002) in their review of slow rTMS studies proposed long-term depression and long-term depotentiation as models for understanding the mechanism of slow rTMS. Neocortical long-term depression and changes in the cortical excitability induced by slow rTMS appear to accumulate in an additive fashion as the number of stimulations is increased over many days. Studies of both slow rTMS and long-term depression suggest additive efficacy when higher numbers of stimulations are administered. The reversal, or depotentiation, of previously enhanced synaptic transmission due to long-term potentiation may be the most relevant model for slow rTMS when used as a therapeutic tool.

rTMS is a simple outpatient procedure lasting approximately 20–30 min. Patients are seated in a comfortable, reclining chair and are fitted with a swim cap to outline the TMS coil position and aid in its placement for each session (Figure 23.3). Before the procedure begins, the "motor threshold" (MT) is determined in each patient. "Motor threshold" is the intensity of the pulse delivered over the motor cortex that produces a noticeable motor response. Sensors are applied to the hand muscle (i.e., the first dorsal interosseous) opposite to the site of stimulation and motor responses are monitored with physiological monitoring tools on a computer. The output of the machine is gradually increased by 5% until a 50 μV deflection on the monitor (i.e., electromyograph [EMG]) or a visible twitch of the muscle is observed. Once the patient's "motor threshold" is determined, the coil is moved to the site of stimulation (e.g., the prefrontal cortex) and the pulse intensity is adjusted relative to the patient's "motor threshold."

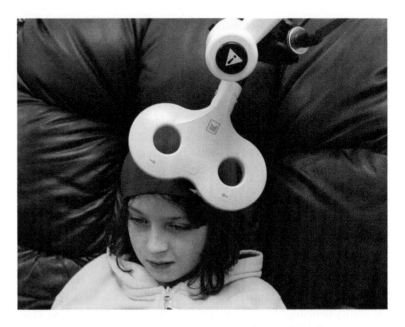

Figure 23.3 Repetitive transcranial magnetic stimulation (rTMS) procedure using an eight-shaped coil.

TMS is generally regarded as safe without lasting side effects. Reported side effects include a mild, transient tension-type headache on the day of stimulation and mild discomfort due to the sound of the pulses. There is a certain risk of inducing a seizure (Wasserman et al. 1996) and participants with epilepsy or a family history of epilepsy are generally excluded of rTMS studies, and as a safety precaution, some rTMS studies adjust the stimulation intensity below the participant's motor threshold. rTMS is generally considered safe for use in pediatric populations, as no significant adverse effects or seizures have been reported (Garvey and Gilbert 2004; Quintana 2005).

rTMS has been applied to a wide variety of psychiatric (e.g., ADHD, depression) and neurological disorders (e.g., Parkinson's disease [PD]) in adult populations and more recently rTMS has been applied in child and adolescent populations (see Croarkin et al. 2011). A number of studies report an improvement in mood after repeated frontal lobe stimulation in both depressed adults (George et al. 2010) and adolescents (Wall et al. 2011). Furthermore, it has been found that rTMS may improve certain symptoms associated with anxiety disorders, like posttraumatic stress disorder (PTSD) and obsessive-compulsive disorder (OCD) (George and Belmaker 2007). In Parkinson's disease, most studies have shown beneficial effects of rTMS on clinical symptoms (Wu et al. 2008). Currently, only rTMS-based therapy of treatment-resistant major depression has FDA approval; however, it is very likely that in the future, rTMS will be approved for the treatment of other mental and neurological disorders as well.

23.6 Inhibition defects in autism and the potential role of TMS

Recent reviews (Sokhadze et al. 2010; Oberman et al. 2013; Sokhadze et al. 2014; Casanova et al. 2015) provide a detailed account of the current status of rTMS application in autism research and treatment. Within the context of autism spectrum disorder, rTMS has unique applications as a treatment modality. A wide range of deficits in autism might be understood by an increase in the ratio of cortical excitation to cortical inhibition (Rubenstein and Merzenich 2003) and increases in local cortical connectivity accompanied by deficiencies in long-range connectivity (Rippon et al. 2007). An increased ratio of cortical excitation to inhibition and higher-than-normal cortical "noise" may explain the strong aversive reactions to auditory, tactile, and visual stimuli frequently reported in autism (Gillberg and Billstedt 2000).

Autism is associated with cortical cytoarchitectural developmental abnormalities according to "minicolumnar" hypothesis (Casanova et al. 2002a–c, 2006a,b, 2015). Reduced neuropil space (periphery of the minicolumn) reported in autism is the compartment where lateral inhibition sharpens the borders of minicolumns and increases their definition (DeFelipe et al. 1990; Favorov and Kelly 1994a,b; DeFelipe 1999). The primary source for this inhibitory effect may be derived from axon bundles of double-bouquet cells (DeFelipe et al. 1990; Favorov and Kelly 1994a). Double-bouquet cells in the peripheral neuropil space of minicolumns provide a "vertical stream of negative inhibition" (Mountcastle 1997, 2003) surrounding the minicolumnar core. Other GABAergic cells in the minicolumn, having collateral projections extending hundreds of microns tangentially, provide lateral inhibition of surrounding minicolumns on a macrocolumnar scale.

The value of each minicolumn's output is insulated to a greater or lesser degree from the activity of its neighbors by GABAergic inhibition in its peripheral neuropil space. This allows for gradations in amplitude of excitatory activity across a minicolumnar field. Rubenstein and Merzenich (2003) have posited that reductions in GABAergic inhibitory activity may explain some symptomatology of autism, including increased incidence of seizures and auditory-tactile hypersensitivity (see also Casanova et al. 2003). This hypothesis is consistent with findings of reduced minicolumnar peripheral neuropil space in the neocortex of autistics relative to controls (Casanova et al. 2002a,b). In this model, a reduction in the peripheral neuropil space would result in smaller minicolumns that would coalesce into discrete, isolated islands of coordinated excitatory activity. Significantly, by puberty, one-third of autistic patients will have exhibited at least two unprovoked seizures (Volkmar and Nelson 1995). Anecdotal case reports have shown that anticonvulsants have ameliorated autistic traits in epileptic patients (Uvebrant and Bauzienè 1994; Plioplys 1994; Childs and Blair 1997; Jambaque et al.

2000; Hollander et al. 2001). Anticonvulsants may be of some benefit on autism but at larger doses suffer from serious side effects, including stupor and coma. These side effects are due to the nonselective nature of anticonvulsants whose mechanism of action (increasing GABAergic tone) is independent of cell type (e.g., double-bouquet, small and large basket, chandelier). The effects of anticonvulsants stand in contrast to the specificity of slow rTMS. This technique induces electricity in conductors at right angles to an expanding or collapsing magnetic field (law of electromagnetic induction) (Figure 23.4). This effect may be of benefit when selectively attempting to activate the inhibitory cells and fibers surrounding the minicolumn (i.e., peripheral neuropil space) (Seldon 1981a,b). These anatomical elements have as a geometric preference for being perpendicular to the cortical surface (Casanova et al. 2003).

Ogawa et al. (2004) examined the changes in high-frequency oscillations of somatosensory-evoked potentials (SEPs) before and after slow rTMS over the right primary somatosensory cortex (0.5 Hz, 50 pulses, 80% motor threshold intensity). The HFOs, which represent a localized activity of intracortical inhibitory interneurons, were significantly increased after slow rTMS, while the SEPs were not changed. Their results suggest that slow rTMS affects cortical excitability by modulating the activity of the intracortical inhibitory interneurons beyond the time of the stimulation and that rTMS may have therapeutic effects on such disorders. This is in line with our hypothesis in which slow rTMS will increase the activity of inhibitory cells in minicolumn, which will then enhance spatial contrast needed to enhance functional discrimination.

The question remains whether rTMS is safe for application in children. Quintana (2005) evaluated studies that used TMS in persons younger than 18 years. The 48 studies reviewed involved a total of 1034 children; 35 of the studies used single-pulse TMS (980 children), 3 studies used paired TMS (20 children), and 7 studies used rTMS (34 children). The TMS studies in persons younger than 18 have been used to examine the

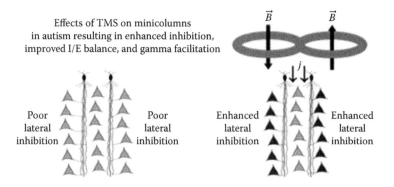

Figure 23.4 Schematic presentation of TMS effects on minicolumns in autism resulting in enhanced lateral inhibition, improved excitation/inhibition ratio, and facilitation of gamma activity.

maturation and activity of the neurons of various central nervous system tracts, plasticity of neurons in epilepsy, multiple sclerosis, myoclonus, transcallosal inhibition, and motor cortex functioning with no reported seizure risk (Lin and Pascual-Leone 2002; Garvey and Gilbert 2004). Repetitive TMS has been applied in children with psychiatric disorders such as ADHD, ADHD with Tourette's, and depression. Although there are a limited number of studies using rTMS in children, these studies did not report significant adverse effects or seizures.

Review of the state-of-the-art rTMS application in ASD treatment and research can be found in several current reviews (Oberman et al. 2013; Sokhadze et al. 2013b; Casanova and Sokhadze 2014; Casanova et al. 2015) and they all call for the need for more research clinical trials aimed to prove the efficacy of the method.

23.7 Our studies in autism using rTMS

Our studies were aimed to examine the effects of low-frequency (0.5–1 Hz) rTMS on behavioral, quantitative EEG, and ERP outcomes in children and adolescents with autism. We used rTMS over the dorsolateral prefrontal cortex (DLPFC) on a weekly basis for 6, 12, and 18 weeks in individuals with autism randomly assigned to active treatment group and waiting-list groups. We predicted that post-TMS changes in the active treatment group, as compared to the waiting-list group, can be detected during repeated tests using the same functional outcome measures (EEG, ERP, etc.) in cognitive task. Our prediction was that slow rTMS of DLPFC will result in an alteration of cortical inhibition through the activation of inhibitory GABAergic interneurons, leading to an improvement in the excitatory/inhibitory balance.

In our methodological approach, we hypothesized that contrary to other inhibitory cells (i.e., basket and chandelier), whose projections keep no constant relation to the surface of the cortex, the geometrically exact orientation of double-bouquet cells and their location at the periphery of the minicolumn (inhibitory surround) makes them the appropriate candidate for induction by a magnetic field applied parallel to the cortex. Over a course of treatment, "slow" rTMS may restore the balance between cortical excitation and cortical inhibition and lead to improved long-range cortical connectivity. Thus far, we have focused on clinical, behavioral, and neuroimaging outcome measures, in order to access the effectiveness of rTMS treatment in ASD.

In the first of our previous investigations (Sokhadze et al. 2009b), we measured the EEG gamma band in eight children with ASD and five waiting-list participants with ASD during a visual attention task, and then measured the EEG gamma band in the active treatment group after six sessions of "slow" rTMS to the prefrontal cortex. The study also used 13 age-matched typically developing children as a control group. We hypothesized that the ASD group would have excess gamma-band activity due to a lack of cortical inhibition, and treatment with "slow" rTMS would help restore inhibitory tone (i.e., reduce excess gamma-band activity). We also analyzed clinical and behavioral questionnaires assessing changes in symptoms associated with ASD after rTMS treatment. The visual attention task employed Kanizsa illusory figures, which have been shown to readily produce gamma oscillations during visual tasks.

Subjects were instructed to press a button when they see the target Kanizsa square and ignore all other stimuli: Kanizsa stimuli consist of inducer disks of a shape feature and either constitute an illusory figure (square, triangle) or not (colinearity feature); in nonimpaired individuals, gamma activity has been found to increase during the presentation of target visual stimuli compared to nontarget stimuli. We found that the power of gamma oscillations was higher in the ASD group and had an earlier onset compared to controls, especially in response to nontarget illusory figures over the prefrontal cortex. Additionally, there was less of a difference in gamma power between target and nontarget stimuli in the ASD group, particularly over lateral frontal and parietal recording sites. After six sessions of "slow" rTMS applied to the left prefrontal cortex, the power of gamma oscillations to nontarget Kanizsa figures dramatically decreased at frontal and parietal sites on the same side of stimulation, and there was more of a difference between gamma responses to target and nontarget stimuli.

According to clinical and behavioral evaluations, the ASD group showed a significant improvement on the Repetitive Behavior Scale (RBS), which assesses repetitive and restricted behavior patterns associated with ASD (e.g., stereotyped, self-injurious, compulsive, and restricted range) (Bodfish et al. 1999).

In a second study with another pool of participants (Baruth et al. 2010a; Casanova et al. 2012; Sokhadze et al. 2012), we investigated gamma-band activity in 16 subjects with ASD in rTMS group and 9 age-matched controls using Kanizsa illusory figures and assessed the effects of 12 sessions of bilateral "slow" rTMS applied to the prefrontal cortices in the TMS group of the ASD participants. In individuals with ASD, gamma activity was not discriminative of stimulus type, whereas in controls, early gamma power differences between target and nontarget stimuli were highly significant. Following rTMS individuals with ASD showed significant improvement in discriminatory gamma activity between relevant and irrelevant visual stimuli, and there was also a significant reduction in irritability and repetitive behavior as a result of rTMS.

In our most recent study (Sokhadze et al. 2014), we compared clinical, behavioral, and electrocortical outcomes in two groups of children with autism (TMS, waiting-list group, $N = 27$ per group) using 18 weekly sessions of rTMS applied bilaterally over the DLPFC. Post-TMS evaluations showed decreased irritability and hyperactivity on the aberrant behavior checklist (ABC), and decreased stereotypic behaviors on the Repetitive Behavior Scale-Revised (RBS-R). Following the rTMS course, we also found decreased ritualistic/sameness behaviors and total repetitive behaviors score. Figures 23.5 and 23.6 illustrate this outcome.

Yet one more unpublished study of our group investigated both evoked and induced gamma oscillations in a similar Kanizsa oddball task in high-functioning children with ASD ($N = 29$, mean age around 14 years). The effects of 18-session-long 0.5 Hz rTMS treatment course on both evoked and induced gamma oscillation responses in the active neurotherapy group of children with ASD were significant at the frontal (e.g., F1, F2, F3, F4) and parietal sites (e.g., P1, P2). Post-TMS changes can be described as decreased evoked gamma responses to nontarget items, along with increase of gamma power to target Kanizsa stimuli. At the parietal sites (P1, P2), we found *Stimulus × Hemisphere × Time (pre-, post-TMS)* interaction effect for evoked gamma, with effects for nontargets being more expressed at the right hemisphere. A decrease of induced gamma power to nontarget stimuli was observed at both the frontal and parietal EEG recording sites (Figures 23.7 and 23.8).

In one more pilot study on 16 children with ASD, we also reported (Hensley et al. 2014) that post-TMS gamma coherence to the target condition between F3 and T7 improved in both the evoked region (100–200 ms) and in the induced region (300–600 ms). In addition to improvement in coherence between pre- and post-TMS, differences were

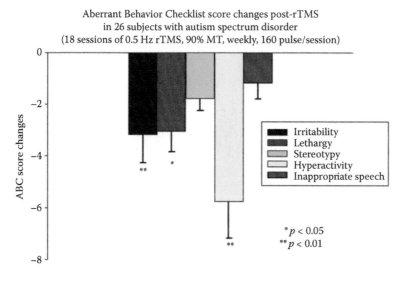

Figure 23.5 Changes of rating scores on the Aberrant Behavior Checklist (ABC) following 18-session-long rTMS course in 26 children with ASD. A statistically significant reduction was found in irritability and hyperactivity as measured by the ABC (irritability, $t = 5.44$, df = 25, $p = 0.008$; hyperactivity, $t = 3.87$, df = 25, $p = 0.001$).

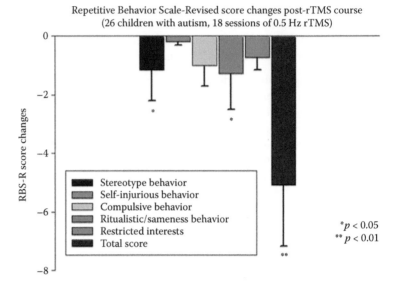

Figure 23.6 Changes of rating scores on the Repetitive Behavior Scale-Revised (RBS-R) following rTMS course in 26 children with ASD. There was a significant reduction in repetitive and restricted behavior patterns following 18 sessions of rTMS as measured by the RBS-R. (Total score decreased from 26.0 down to 20.9, $t = 3.65$, df = 26, $p = 0.001$.)

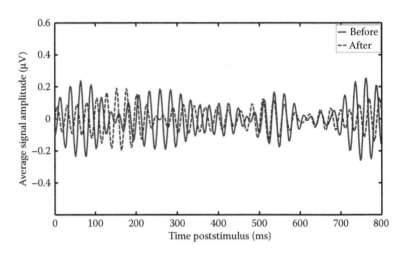

Figure 23.7 Evoked and induced gamma oscillations to nontarget Kanizsa figures in a visual oddball task with illusory figures before and after 18 sessions of 0.5 Hz rTMS course in 29 children with ASD. Gamma oscillation response averaged across two parietal sites (P1 and P2) shows lower amplitudes of both evoked and induced gamma post-TMS.

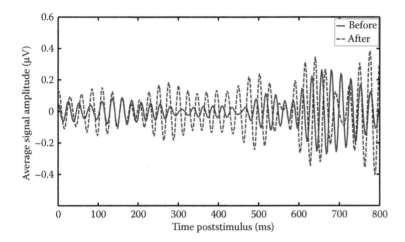

Figure 23.8 Evoked and induced gamma oscillations to target Kanizsa figures in a visual oddball task with illusory figures before and after 18 sessions of 0.5 Hz rTMS course in 29 children with ASD. Responses to targets at the parietal sites (average across P1 and P2) show higher amplitude of the late-induced gamma oscillations (within 250–400 ms window poststimulus).

also observed in the subjects' responses to target and nontarget stimuli following TMS therapy. The analysis of evoked gamma coherence between F4 and T8 to both target and nontarget stimuli indicates that before treatment, nontarget coherence was 0.43 and target coherence was 0.45, fairly similar values. However, after completion of TMS therapy, target coherence increased to 0.56 and nontarget coherence decreased to 0.42. The *p*-value of the comparison of coherence for F4–T8 between target and nontarget for both pre- and posttreatment was 0.44. These results are illustrated in Figures 23.9 and 23.10.

Another significant effect of TMS treatment was observed in evoked gamma coherence between F4 and P4. As in the case above, coherence in response to the target condition increased significantly following TMS. Coherence in response to the nontarget stimuli increased only slightly after the TMS course and it was not statistically significant. The comparison of mean coherence values for F4–P4 between target and nontarget stimuli pre- and post-TMS treatment reached significance. Children with ASD in the waiting-list group (*N* = 16) also completed two Kaniza tasks but did not receive TMS treatment between the first and second Kanizsa task. The analysis of evoked gamma coherence between F4 and T8 for those in the waiting-list group does not show significant differences in responses to target and nontarget stimuli. Similarly, no significant differences were observed in responses to target and nontarget stimuli for evoked gamma coherence between F4 and P4. The changes in evoked and induced gamma power to targets, accompanied by increased phase coherence between frontal and parietal sites,

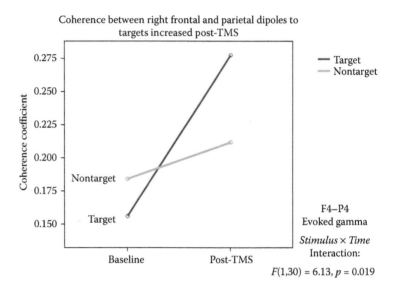

Figure 23.9 Comparison of target and nontarget evoked gamma phase coherence (between frontal F4 and parietal P4 sites as measured by BESA Coherence Module software) pre- and post-TMS therapy in 18 children with ASD. Coherence to target stimuli shows significant increase.

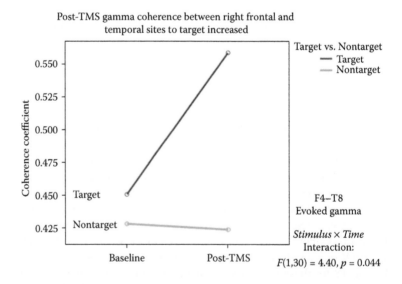

Figure 23.10 Comparison of target and nontarget evoked gamma phase coherence (between the right frontal F4 and temporal T8 sites) pre- and post-TMS therapy in 18 children with ASD. Coherence to target stimuli shows significant increase, while coherence to nontarget items did not change.

along with increased centro-parietal and parieto-occipital P100 and P300 (P3b) to targets are indicative of more efficient processing of information post-TMS treatment.

23.8 Discussion and conclusions

Recently, there were several attempts at deriving an overarching meta theory of autism that have focused on a basic abnormality of neural connectivity (Belmonte et al. 2004a,b). This model is empirically based on lack of coordinated brain activity and abnormal "binding" in the brains of autistic patients that can be detected with EEG methodology, specifically using gamma oscillations (Brock et al. 2002; Brown 2005; Rippon et al. 2007). According to Baron-Cohen and Belmonte (2005), the combination of local sensory hyperarousal and low-level overprocessing of incoming sensory stimuli concurrent with abnormalities of attention selectivity and focus may be a consequence of the overconnected low-level processing neural networks in autism spectrum disorders. In such overwired networks, signal is insufficiently differentiated from noise or task-irrelevant information, and as a result, information capacity is drastically reduced (Rubenstein and Merzenich 2003; Belmonte et al. 2004a,b; Casanova 2006). Higher-than-normal noise in cortical processes also affects the normal development of differentiated representations, because cortical response selectivity in space and time is a product of balanced inhibitory and excitatory processes. Such overrepresentation by nondifferentiated systems could plausibly account, for example, for the strong aversive reactions to auditory, tactile, and visual stimuli that are commonly recorded in autistic individuals. The abnormal long-range neural connectivity model is suggested to explain deficits in high-level complex information processing functions where rapid and integrated operation of many separate neural systems is required (Minshew et al. 1997; Welchew et al. 2005). In the autistic brain, high local connectivity may develop along with deficient long-range connectivity.

In recent years, neuropathological studies of autism have revealed abnormalities in several brain regions. Changes in brain size with widespread increases in both gray and white matter volumes suggest that the underlying pathology in autism consists of widely distributed histological abnormalities. The available neuropathological and structural imaging data suggest that autism is the result of a developmental lesion capable of affecting normal brain growth. One possible explanation for this is the recent finding of minicolumnar abnormalities in autism, in particular, demonstration of minicolumns of reduced size and increased number in the autistic brain (Casanova et al. 2002a,b, 2006a,b). The increased number of minicolumns reported in autism suggests a possible disruption during the earlier stages of neurodevelopment in the brain of an autistic patient. Furthermore, a minicolumnar abnormality may translate difficulties in the integration of information into a delay in language acquisition. In all, minicolumnar abnormalities may incapacitate a patient as a social being by distorting elements of the child's biopsychological experience.

The modular arrangement of the cortex is based on the cell minicolumn: a self-contained ecosystem of neurons and their afferent, efferent, and interneuronal connections (Mountcastle 2003). Our preliminary studies indicate that minicolumns in the brains of autistic patients are narrower, with an altered internal organization (Casanova 2006). More specifically, their minicolumns reveal less space for inhibitory local circuit projections. A defect in these GABAergic fibers may correlate with the increased prevalence of seizures among autistic patients. Based on the descriptions given thus far, it is possible to propose a disruption of the normal balance between excitation and inhibition in the columnar organization of autistic patients. In this regard, a series of noteworthy studies report that both children and adults with autism were superior to a control group in their ability to discriminate novel, highly similar stimuli (Plaisted et al. 2003). Autistic children also have a superior ability in discriminating display items in visual search tasks; such enhanced discrimination in autism results from low-level perceptual processing of incoming stimuli, and this is called the bottom-up approach.

The analysis of high-frequency EEG oscillations in patients with autism may provide additional information about potential neural deficits in autism. Abnormalities in these mechanisms have been associated with binding problems (the coactivation of neural assemblies), which may be present in both autism and schizophrenia (Grice et al. 2001; Brock et al. 2002). Oscillatory activity in the gamma band of the EEG has been related to Gestalt perception and to cognitive functions such as attention, learning, and memory (Kaiser 2003). Electrophysiological studies show strong evidence that synchronized cortical activity in the gamma frequency range could be a correlate of feature binding to form a single coherent percept. Binding of widely distributed cell assemblies by the synchronization of their gamma frequency activity is thought to underlie cohesive stimulus representation in the human brain (Kahana 2006). According to this assumption, changes in gamma EEG activity have been considered indicators of processing of Gestalt-like patterns (von Stein et al. 1999; Herrmann and Mecklinger 2000, 2001).

The "weak central coherence" (Frith and Happé 1994) in autism could result from a reduction in the integration of specialized local networks in the brain caused by a deficit in temporal binding (Brock et al. 2002). Visual and auditory perception anomalies may be attributed to a reduced coherence and synchrony of gamma activity between networks processing local features, and thus explain some of the language deficits, executive dysfunctions, and other impairments in social communication in autism. The inability to reduce gamma activity according to Brown (2005) would lead to the inability to decide which event requires attention when there are multiple choices. Excessive gamma can therefore be linked to a reduction in the ability to focus attention. The "temporal binding deficit" hypothesis of autism (Brock et al. 2002; Rippon et al. 2007) suggests that many features of autism, such as superiority in processing detail (local processing) and disadvantages in global processing, can be explained by a failure of binding between cortical areas. The analysis of evoked and induced EEG gamma oscillation can therefore significantly contribute to understanding the neurobiological nature of core autism symptoms and definitely warrant further rigorous investigations.

The chapter reviewed a series of our studies using low-frequency rTMS treatment in children with autism. It was not the aim of this chapter to be an exhaustive treatise on the state of research into rTMS application in autism spectrum disorder. A review of the current state of the art in this area was recently prepared by Oberman et al. (2013). The neuromodulation approach to autism treatment based on rTMS is a new and rapidly developing field, and substantially more information is needed about many aspects of rTMS regimen (topography, power, session frequency, etc.) and autism developmental neuropathology specifics to validate its clinical utility and efficacy.

The review of our efforts using rTMS treatment discussed our studies on the neurophysiological basis of a therapeutic intervention that targets the core symptoms of the condition with few, if any, side effects. The proposed model of clinical research using neuromodulation intervention is finely woven with the neuropathological underpinnings of autism previously described in the authors' laboratory (for review, see Casanova et al. 2012, 2013, 2015; Sokhadze et al. 2012, 2013a, 2014; Casanova and Sokhadze, 2014). Thus far, medications are being used to treat accessory problems associated to autism spectrum disorders rather than core symptoms. Many of these psychoactive drugs have serious side effects that limit their usage, primarily as applied to children. The brain's limited long-range wiring cannot directly sustain coordinated activity across arbitrary cortical locations, but it can convey patterns of synchronous activity as oscillatory neuronal fluxes, represented by local field potentials measured by EEG. Coordination of oscillations at varying interacting frequencies allows for relatively efficient and unconstrained segregation in varying forms and across hierarchical cortical levels. Disrupted patterns of coordinated oscillatory output in distributed "minicolumnar" networks might be associated with cortical "disconnection" in autism. More specifically, altered oscillatory activity in developing cortical circuits may contribute to impaired development of intra-areal and transcortical connections giving rise to a bias in short (e.g., arcuate) versus long corticocortical projections (e.g., commissural fibers).

Our approach suggests that autism reflects a global processing neurodevelopmental defect produced by an excessive local connectivity and deficient distal connectivity resulting in functional disconnectivity of networks important in behavior and social cognition. The goal of the

525

series of our studies was to test these hypotheses and further develop and test novel intervention that could become available to address behavioral, affective, and cognitive impairments in autism. The hypothesis was that rTMS will result in an improvement of multiple functions in autism, and that neuromodulation effects may help in understanding mechanisms of neuropathology underlying deficits present in autism. The cognitive tests used in our studies included recording of evoked and induced gamma oscillations and analysis of gamma coherence in children with autism and in age-matched typically developing children. The investigation of TMS effects on gamma EEG oscillations may advance neuromodulation approaches in other psychiatric and neurological disorders as well.

We would like to mention several areas we consider especially promising for future research. First of all, more comprehensive information is needed to more accurately define EEG abnormalities typical for ASD for better understanding of rTMS-induced changes in EEG outcomes. The second very important objective for the future rTMS-based treatment for autism is to conduct a randomized clinical trial using double-blind design and sham rTMS as control condition. The third principal question to be addressed is the estimation of how long rTMS-induced positive improvements last, whether they fade out after a certain period, and so on, thus emphasizing the need for follow-up studies.

In addition, it is necessary to understand whether rTMS can be used synergistically in conjunction with other conventional behavioral (ABA), biobehavioral (neurofeedback), and pharmaceutical therapies adopted in conventional ASD treatment practice. It must be admitted that current reviews call for necessity to more carefully design-controlled clinical trials to evaluate the real potential of rTMS-based treatment of autism, have it approved by FDA, and get it accepted by general practitioners and specialists in developmental disorders. With the advances made over the past several years, it is hoped that continued interest will be generated to further rTMS treatment of autism spectrum disorders.

References

Baron-Cohen, S. and M. K. Belmonte. 2005. Autism: A window onto the development of the social and the analytic brain. *Annu. Rev. Neurosci.* 28:109–26.

Baron-Cohen, S., A. M. Leslie, and U. Frith. 1985. Does the autistic child have a "theory of mind"? *Cognition* 21:37–46.

Bartos, M., I. Vida, and P. Jonas. 2007. Synaptic mechanisms of synchronized gamma oscillations in inhibitory interneuron networks. *Nat. Rev. Neurosci.* 8:45–56.

Baruth, J., M. F. Casanova, A. El-Baz, T. Horrell, G. Mathai, L. Sears, and E. Sokhadze. 2010a. Low-frequency repetitive transcranial magnetic stimulation modulates evoked-gamma frequency oscillations in autism spectrum disorders. *J. Neurother.* 14:179–94.

Baruth, J. M., M. F. Casanova, L. Sears, and E. Sokhadze. 2010b. Early-stage visual processing abnormalities in autism spectrum disorder (ASD). *Transl. Neurosci.* 1:177–87.

Baruth, J., E. Williams, E. Sokhadze, A. El-Baz, L. Sears, and M. F. Casanova. 2011. Repetitive transcranial stimulation (rTMS) improves electroencephalographic and behavioral outcome measures in autism spectrum disorders (ASD). *Autism Sci. Dig.* 1:52–7.

Başar, E., M. Schürmann, C. Başar-Eroglu, and T. Demiralp. 2001. Selectively distributed gamma band system in brain. *Int. J. Psychophysiol.* 39:129–35.

Belmonte, M. K., G. Allen, A. Beckel-Mitchener, L. M. Boulanger, R. A. Carper, and S. J. Webb. 2004a. Autism and abnormal development of brain connectivity. *J. Neurosci.* 24:9228–31.

Belmonte, M. K., E. H. Cook Jr., G. M. Anderson et al. 2004b. Autism as a disorder of neural information processing: Directions for research and targets for therapy. *Mol. Psychiatry* 9:646–63.

Belmonte, M. K. and D. A. Yurgelun-Todd. 2003a. Functional anatomy of impaired selective attention and compensatory processing in autism. *Brain Res. Cogn. Brain Res.* 17:651–64.

Belmonte, M. K. and D. A. Yurgelun-Todd. 2003b. Anatomic dissociation of selective and suppressive processes in visual attention. *NeuroImage* 19:180–9.

Bertrand, O. and C. Tallon-Baudry. 2000. Oscillatory gamma activity in humans: A possible role for object representation. *Int. J. Psychophysiol.* 38:211–23.

Bodfish, J. W., F. J. Symons, and M. H. Lewis. 1999. *The Repetitive Behavior Scale.* Morganton: Western Carolina Center.

Böttger, D., C. S. Herrmann, and D. Y. von Cramon. 2002. Amplitude differences of evoked alpha and gamma oscillations in two different age groups. *Int. J. Psychophysiol.* 45:245–51.

Brock, J., C. C. Brown, J. Boucher, and G. Rippon. 2002. The temporal binding deficit hypothesis of autism. *Dev. Psychopathol.* 14:209–24.

Brown, C. 2005. EEG in autism: Is there just too much going on in there? In *Recent Developments in Autism Research*, ed. M. F. Casanova, 109–26. New York: Nova Science Publishers.

Brown, C., T. Gruber, J. Boucher, G. Rippon, and J. Brock. 2005. Gamma abnormalities during perception of illusory figures in autism. *Cortex* 41:364–76.

Cantor, D. S., R. W. Thatcher, M. Hrybyk, and H. Kaye. 1986. Computerized EEG analysis of autistic children. *J. Autism Dev. Disord.* 16:169–87.

Carper, R. A. and E. Courchesne. 2005. Localized enlargement of the frontal cortex in early autism. *Biol. Psychiatry* 57:126–33.

Casanova, M. F. 2006. Neuropathological and genetic findings in autism: The significance of a putative minicolumnopathy. *Neuroscientist* 12:435–41.

Casanova, M. F., J. Baruth, A. S. El-Baz, G. E. Sokhadze, M. Hensley, and E. M. Sokhadze. 2013. Evoked and induced gamma-frequency oscillation in autism. In *Imaging the Brain in Autism*, eds. M. F. Casanova, A. S. El-Baz, and J. S. Suri, 87–106. New York: Springer.

Casanova, M. F., J. Baruth, A. El-Baz, A. Tasman, L. Sears, and E. Sokhadze. 2012. Repetitive transcranial magnetic stimulation (rTMS) modulates event-related potential (ERP) indices of attention in autism. *Transl. Neurosci.* 3:170–80.

Casanova, M. F., D. P. Buxhoeveden, and C. Brown. 2002c. Clinical and macroscopic correlates of minicolumnar pathology in autism. *J. Child Neurol.* 17:692–5.

Casanova, M. F., D. Buxhoeveden, and J. Gomez. 2003. Disruption in the inhibitory architecture of the cell minicolumn: Implications for autism. *Neuroscientist* 9:496–507.

Casanova, M. F., D. P. Buxhoeveden, A. E. Switala, and E. Roy. 2002a. Minicolumnar pathology in autism. *Neurology* 58:428–32.

527

Casanova, M. F., D. P. Buxhoeveden, A. E. Switala, and E. Roy. 2002b. Neuronal density and architecture (gray level index) in the brains of autistic patients. *J. Child Neurol.* 17:515–21.

Casanova, M. F., A. El-Baz, E. Vanbogaert, P. Narahari, and A. Switala. 2010. A topographic study of minicolumnar core width by lamina comparison between autistic subjects and controls: Possible minicolumnar disruption due to an anatomical element in-common to multiple laminae. *Brain Pathol.* 20:451–8.

Casanova, M. F. and E. M. Sokhadze. 2014. Transcranial magnetic stimulation: Application in autism treatment. In *Frontiers in Autism Research: New Horizons for Diagnosis and Treatment*, ed. V. W. Hu, 583–606. Hackensack: World Scientific Publishing Co.

Casanova, M. F., E. Sokhadze, I. Opris, Y. Wang, and X. Li. 2015. Autism spectrum disorders: Linking neuropathological findings to treatment with transcranial magnetic stimulation. *Acta Pediatr.* 104:346–55.

Casanova, M. F., J. Trippe 2nd, C. Tillquist, and A. Switala. 2009. Morphometric variability of minicolumns in the striate cortex of *Homo sapiens, Macaca mulatta*, and *Pan troglodytes. J. Anat.* 214:226–34.

Casanova, M. F., I. van Kooten, H. van Engeland, H. Heinsen, H. W. Steinbursch, P. R. Hof, J. Trippe, J. Stone, and C. Schmitz. 2006a. Minicolumnar abnormalities in autism. *Acta Neuropathol.* 112:287–303.

Casanova, M. F., I. van Kooten, A. E. Switala, H. van Engeland, H. Heinsen, H. W. Steinbuch, P. R. Hof, and C. Schmitz. 2006b. Abnormalities of cortical minicolumnar organization in the prefrontal lobes of autistic patients. *Clin. Neurosci. Res.* 6:127–33.

Childs, J. A. and J. L. Blair. 1997. Valproic acid treatment of epilepsy in autistic twins. *J. Neurosci. Nurs.* 29:244–8.

Chugani, D. C., O. Muzik, M. Behen, R. Rothermel, J. J. Janisse, J. Lee, and H. T. Chugani. 1999. Developmental changes in brain serotonin synthesis capacity in autistic and nonautistic children. *Ann. Neurol.* 45:287–95.

Coben, R., A. R. Clarke, W. Hudspeth, and R. J. Barry. 2008. EEG power and coherence in autism spectrum disorder. *Clin. Neurophysiol.* 119:1002–9.

Cornew L., T. P. Roberts, L. Blaskey, and J. C. Edgar. 2012. Resting-state oscillatory activity in autism spectrum disorders. *J. Autism Dev. Disord.* 42:1884–94.

Courchesne, E., R. Carper, and N. Akshoomoff. 2003. Evidence of brain overgrowth in the first year of life in autism. *JAMA* 290:337–44.

Croarkin, P. E., C. A. Wall, and J. Lee. 2011. Applications of transcranial magnetic stimulation (TMS) in child and adolescent psychiatry. *Int. Rev. Psychiatry* 23:445–53.

Daoust, A. M., E. Limoges, C. Bolduc, L. Mottron, and R. Godbout. 2004. EEG spectral analysis of wakefulness and REM sleep in high functioning autistic spectrum disorders. *Clin. Neurophysiol.* 115:1368–73.

Dawson, G., L. G. Klinger, H. Panagiotides, A. Lewy, and P. Castelloe. 1995. Subgroups of autistic children based on social behavior display distinct patterns of brain activity. *J. Abnorm. Child Psychol.* 23:569–83.

DeFelipe, J. 1999. Chandelier cells and epilepsy. *Brain* 122:1807–22.

DeFelipe, J., S. H. Hendry, T. Hashikawa, M. Molinari, and E. G. Jones. 1990. A microcolumnar structure of monkey cerebral cortex revealed by immunocytochemical studies of double bouquet cell axons. *Neuroscience* 37:655–73.

Donner, T. H. and M. Siegel. 2011. A framework for local cortical oscillation patterns. *Trends Cogn. Sci.* 15:191–9.

Engel, A. K. and W. Singer. 2001. Temporal binding and the neural correlates of sensory awareness. *Trends Cogn. Sci.* 5:16–25.

Fan, Y. T., J. Decety, C. Y. Yang, J. L. Liu, and Y. Cheng. 2010. Unbroken mirror neurons in autism spectrum disorders. *J. Child Psychol. Psychiatry* 51:981–8.

Favorov, O. V. and D. G. Kelly. 1994a. Minicolumnar organization within somatosensory cortical segregates: I. Development of afferent connections. *Cereb. Cortex* 4:408–27.

Favorov, O. V. and D. G. Kelly. 1994b. Minicolumnar organization within somatosensory cortical segregates: II. Emergent functional properties. *Cereb. Cortex* 4:428–42.

Fitzgerald, P. B., K. Hoy, R. Gunewardene, C. Slack, S. Ibrahim, M. Bailey, and Z. J. Daskalakis. 2011. A randomized trial of unilateral and bilateral prefrontal cortex transcranial magnetic stimulation in treatment-resistant major depression. *Psychol. Med.* 41:1187–96.

Fell, J., P. Klaver, K. Lehnertx, T. Grunwald, C. Schaller, C. E. Elger, and G. Fernandez. 2001. Human memory formation is accompanied by rhinal-hippocampal coupling and decoupling. *Nat. Neurosci.* 4:1259–64.

Felli, R., G. Fernandez, P. Klaver, C. E. Elger, and P. Fries. 2003. Is synchronized neuronal gamma activity relevant for selective attention? *Brain Res. Rev.* 42:265–72.

Ferri, R., M. Elia, N. Agarwal, B. Lanuzza, S. A. Musumeci, and G. Pennisi. 2003. The mismatch negativity and the P3a components of the auditory event-related potentials in autistic low-functioning subjects. *Clin. Neurophysiol.* 114:1671–80.

Fries, P. 2009. Neuronal gamma-band synchronization as a fundamental process in cortical computation. *Annu. Rev. Neurosci.* 32:209–24.

Frith, U. and F. Happé. 1994. Autism: Beyond theory of mind. *Cognition* 50:115–32.

Galambos, R. 1992. A comparison of certain gamma band 40 Hz brain rhythms in cat and man. In *Induced Rhythms in the Brain*, eds. E. Basar and T. H. Bullock, 201–16. Boston: Birkhauser.

Gandal, M. J., J. C. Edgar, R. S. Ehrlichman, M. Mehta, T. P. Roberts, and S. J. Siegel. 2010. Validating γ oscillations and delayed auditory responses as translational biomarkers of autism. *Biol. Psychiatry* 68, 1100–6.

Garvey, M. A. and D. L. Gilbert. 2004. Transcranial magnetic stimulation in children. *Eur. J. Pediatr. Neurol.* 8:7–19.

George, M. S. and R. H. Belmaker. 2007. *Transcranial Magnetic Stimulation in Clinical Psychiatry.* Arlington: American Psychiatric Publishing.

George, M. S., S. H. Lisanby, D. Avery et al. 2010. Daily left prefrontal transcranial magnetic stimulation therapy for major depressive disorder: A sham-controlled randomized trial. *Arch. Gen. Psychiatry* 67:507–16.

Gillberg, C. and E. Billstedt. 2000. Autism and Asperger syndrome: Coexistence with other clinical disorders. *Acta Psychiatr. Scand.* 102:321–30.

Gogolla, N., J. J. Leblanc, K. B. Quast, T. C. Südhof, M. Fagiolini, and T. K. Hensch. 2009. Common circuit defect of excitatory–inhibitory balance in mouse models of autism. *J. Neurodev. Disord.* 1:172–81.

Grice, S. J., M. W. Spratling, A. Karmiloff-Smith, H. Halit, G. Csibra, M. de Haan, and M. H. Johnson. 2001. Disordered visual processing and oscillatory brain activity in autism and Williams syndrome. *NeuroReport* 12:2697–700.

Grothe, B. and G. M. Klump. 2000. Temporal processing in sensory systems. *Curr. Opin. Neurobiol.* 10:467–73.

Gruber, T., A. Keil, and M. M. Muller. 2001. Modulation of induced gamma band responses and phase synchrony in a paired associate learning task in the human EEG. *Neurosci. Lett.* 316:29–32.

Hájos, N. and O. Paulsen. 2009. Network mechanisms of gamma oscillations in the CA3 region of the hippocampus. *Neural Netw.* 22:1113–9.

Happé, F. G. 1996. Studying weak central coherence at low levels: Children with autism do not succumb to visual illusions. A research note. *J. Child Psychol. Psychiatry* 37:873–7.

Happé, F. and U. Frith. 2006. The weak coherence account: Detail-focused cognitive style in autism spectrum disorders. *J. Autism Dev. Disord.* 36:5–25.

Harada, M., M. M. Taki, A. Nose, H. Kubo, K. Mori, H. Nishitani, and T. Matsuda. 2010. Non-invasive evaluation of the GABAergic/glutamatergic system in autistic patients observed by MEGA-editing proton MR spectroscopy using a clinical 3 tesla instrument. *J. Autism Dev. Disord.* 41:447–54.

Hazlett, H. C., M. Poe, G. Gerig, R. G. Smith, J. Provenzale, A. Ross, J. Gilmore, and J. Piven. 2005. Magnetic resonance imaging and head circumference study of brain size in autism: Birth through age 2 years. *Arch. Gen. Psychiatry* 62:1366–76.

Hensley, M., A. S. El-Baz, E. Sokhadze, L. Sears, and M. F. Casanova. 2014. Effects of 18 session TMS therapy on gamma coherence in autism. *Psychophysiology* 51:S16.

Herrmann, C. S. and T. Demiralp. 2005. Human EEG gamma oscillations in neuro-psychiatric disorders. *Clin. Neurophysiol.* 16:2719–33.

Herrmann, C. S. and R. T. Knight. 2001. Mechanisms of human attention: Event related potentials and oscillations. *Neurosci. Biobehav. Rev.* 25:465–76.

Herrmann, C. S. and A. Mecklinger. 2000. Magnetoencephalographic responses to illusory figures: Early evoked gamma is affected by processing of stimulus features. *Int. J. Psychophysiol.* 38:265–81.

Herrmann, C. S. and A. Mecklinger. 2001. Gamma activity in human EEG is related to highspeed memory comparisons during object selective attention. *Vis. Cogn.* 8:593–608.

Herrmann, C. S., A. Mecklinger, and E. Pfeifer. 1999. Gamma responses and ERPs in a visual classification task. *Clin. Neurophysiol.* 110:636–42.

Herrmann, C. S., M. H. Munk, and A. K. Engel. 2004. Cognitive functions of gamma-band activity: Memory match and utilization. *Trends Cogn. Sci.* 8:347–55.

Hill, E. L. 2004. Evaluating the theory of executive dysfunction in autism. *Dev. Rev.* 24:189–233.

Hoffman, R. E. and I. Cavus. 2002. Slow transcranial magnetic stimulation, long-term depotentiation, and brain hyperexcitability disorders. *Am. J. Psychiatry* 159:1093–102.

Hollander, E., R. Dolgoff-Kaspar, C. Cartwright, R. Rawitt, and S. Novotny. 2001. An open trial of divalproex sodium in autism spectrum disorders. *J. Clin. Psychiatry* 62:530–4.

Isler, J. R., K. M. Martien, P. G. Grieve, R. I. Stark, and M. R. Herbert. 2010. Reduced functional connectivity in visual evoked potentials in children with autism spectrum disorder. *Clin. Neurophysiol.* 121:2035–43.

Jambaqué, I., C. Chiron, C. Dumas, J. Mumford, and O. Dulac. 2000. Mental and behavioural outcome of infantile epilepsy treated by vigabatrin in tuberous sclerosis patients. *Epilepsy Res.* 38:151–60.

Jensen, O., J. Kaiser, and J. P. Lachaux. 2007. Human gamma frequency oscillations associated with attention and memory. *Trends Neurosci.* 30:317–24.

Just, M. A., V. L. Cherkassky, T. A. Keller, and N. J. Minshew. 2004. Cortical activation and synchronization during sentence comprehension in high-functioning autism: Evidence of underconnectivity. *Brain* 127:1811–21.

Kahana, M. J. 2006. The cognitive correlates of human brain oscillations. *J. Neurosci.* 26:1669–72.

Kahana, M. J., R. Sekuler, J. B. Caplan, M. Kirschen, and J. R. Madsen. 1999. Human theta oscillations exhibit task dependence during virtual maze navigation. *Nature* 399:781–4.

Kaiser, J. 2003. Induced gamma-band activity and human brain function. *Neuroscientist* 9:475–84.

Kanizsa, G. 1976. Subjective contours. *Sci. Am.* 235:48–52.

Keil, A., T. Gruber, and M. M. Müller. 2001. Functional correlates of macroscopic high-frequency brain activity in the human visual system. *Neurosci. Biobehav. Rev.* 25:527–34.

Keil, A., M. M. Muller, W. J. Ray, T. Gruber, and T. Elbert. 1999. Human gamma band activity and perception of a Gestalt. *J. Neurosci.* 19:7152–61.

Kemner, C., M. N. Verbaten, J. M. Cuperus, G. Camfferman, and H. Van Engeland. 1994. Visual and somatosensory event-related brain potentials in autistic children and three different control groups. *Electroencephalogr. Clin. Neurophysiol.* 92:225–37.

Khedr, E. M., J. C. Rothwell, M. A. Ahmed, and A. El-Atar. 2008. Effect of daily repetitive transcranial magnetic stimulation for treatment of tinnitus: Comparison of different stimulus frequencies. *J. Neurol. Neurosurg. Psychiatry* 79:212–5.

Koshino, H., P. A. Carpenter, N. J. Minshew, V. L. Cherkassky, T. A. Keller, and M. A. Just. 2005. Functional connectivity in an fMRI working memory task in high-functioning autism. *NeuroImage* 24:810–21.

Lazarev, V. V., A. Pontes, and L. C. deAzevedo. 2009. EEG photic driving: Right hemisphere deficit in EEG photic driving reactivity in childhood autism. *Int. J. Psychophysiol.* 71:177–88.

Lin, K. L. and A. Pascual-Leone. 2002. Transcranial magnetic stimulation and its applications in children. *Chang Gung Med. J.* 25:424–36.

Llinas, R. and U. Ribary. 1993. Coherent 40-Hz oscillation characterizes dream state in humans. *Proc. Natl. Acad. Sci. USA* 90:2078–81.

Mann, E. O. and O. Paulsen. 2007. Role of GABAergic inhibition in hippocampal network oscillations. *Trends Neurosci.* 30:343–9.

Milne, E., A. Scope, O. Pascalis, D. Buckley, and S. Makeig. 2009. Independent component analysis reveals atypical electroencephalographic activity during visual perception in individuals with autism. *Biol. Psychiatry* 65:22–30.

Minshew, N. J., G. Goldstein, and D. J. Siegel. 1997. Neuropsychologic functioning in autism: Profile of a complex information processing disorder. *J. Int. Neuropsychol. Soc.* 3:303–16.

Minshew, N. J. and T. A. Keller. 2010. The nature of brain dysfunction in autism: Functional brain imaging studies. *Curr. Opin. Neurol.* 23:124–30.

Morgan, B., M. Maybery, and K. Durkin. 2003. Weak central coherence, poor joint attention, and low verbal ability: Independent deficits in early autism. *Dev. Psychol.* 39:646–56.

Mostofsky, S. H., P. Dubey, V. K. Jerath, E. M. Jansiewicz, M. C. Goldberg, and M. B. Denckla. 2006. Developmental dyspraxia is not limited to imitation in children with autism spectrum disorders. *J. Int. Neuropsychol. Soc.* 12:314–26.

Mountcastle, V. B. 1997. The columnar organization of the neocortex. *Brain* 120:701–22.

Mountcastle, V. B. 2003. Introduction. Computation in cortical columns. *Cereb. Cortex* 13:2–4.

Mottron, L., J. A. Burack, G. Iarocci, S. Belleville, and J. T. Enns. 2003. Locally oriented perception with intact global processing among adolescents with high-functioning autism: Evidence from multiple paradigms. *J. Child Psychol. Psychiatry* 44:904–13.

Müller, M. M., J. Bosch, T. Elbert, A. Kreiter, M. V. Sosa, P. V. Sosa, and B. Rockstroh. 1996. Visually induced gamma-band responses in human electroencephalographic activity—A link to animal studies. *Exp. Brain Res.* 112:96–102.

Müller, M. M. and T. Gruber. 2001. Induced gamma-band responses in the human EEG are related to attentional information processing. *Vis. Cogn.* 8:579–92.

Müller, M. M., T. Gruber, and A. Keil. 2000. Modulation of induced gamma band activity in the human EEG by attention and visual information processing. *Int. J. Psychophysiol.* 38:283–99.

Murias, M., S. J. Webb, J. Greenson, and G. Dawson. 2007. Resting state cortical connectivity reflected in EEG coherence in individuals with autism. *Biol. Psychiatry* 62:270–3.

Nakatani, C., J. Ito, A. R. Nikolaev, P. Gong, and C. V. Leeuwen. 2005. Phase synchronization analysis of EEG during attentional blink. *J. Cogn. Neurosci.* 17:1969–79.

Oberman, L. M. and V. M. Ramachandran. 2007. The simulating social mind: The role of the mirror neuron system and simulation in the social and communicative deficits of autism spectrum disorders. *Psychol. Bull.* 133:310–27.

Oberman, L. M., V. S. Ramachandran, and J. A. Pineda. 2008. Modulation of mu suppression in children with autism spectrum disorder in response to familiar or unfamiliar stimuli: The mirror neuron hypothesis. *Neuropsychologia* 46:1558–65.

Oberman, L., A. Rotenberg, and A. Pascual-Leone. 2013. Use of transcranial magnetic stimulation in autism spectrum disorders. *J. Autism Dev. Disord.* 45:524–36. doi: 10.1007/s10803-013-960-2.

Ogawa, A., S. Ukai, K. Shinosaki, M. Yamamoto, S. Kawaguchi, R. Ishii, and M. Takeda. 2004. Slow repetitive transcranial magnetic stimulation increases somatosensory high-frequency oscillations in humans. *Neurosci. Lett.* 358:193–6.

Ogawa, T., A. Sugiyama, S. Ishiwa, M. Suzuki, T. Ishihara, and K. Sato. 1982. Ontogenic development of EEG-asymmetry in early infantile autism. *Brain Dev.* 4:439–49.

Orekhova, E. V., T. A. Stroganova, and G. Nygren. 2007. Excess of high frequency electroencephalogram oscillations in boys with autism. *Biol. Psychiatry* 62:1022–9.

Ozonoff, S. 1997. Casual mechanisms of autism: Unifying perspectives from an information-processing framework. In *Handbook of Autism and Pervasive Developmental Disorders*, eds. D. J. Cohen and F. R. Volkmar, 868–79. New York: John Wiley.

Ozonoff, S., D. L. Strayer, W. M. McMahon, and F. Filloux. 1994. Executive function abilities in autism and Tourette syndrome: An information processing approach. *J. Child Psychol. Psychiatry* 35:1015–32.

Pascual-Leone, A., V. Walsh, and J. Rothwell. 2000. Transcranial magnetic stimulation in cognitive neuroscience–virtual lesion, chronometry, and functional connectivity. *Curr. Opin. Neurobiol.* 10:232–7.

Pavlova, M., N. Birbaumer, and A. Sokolov. 2006. Attentional modulation of cortical neuromagnetic gamma response to biological movement. *Cereb. Cortex* 16:321–7.

Pfurtscheller, G. and A. Aranibar. 1977. Event-related cortical desynchronisation detected by power measurements of scalp EEG. *Electroencephalogr. Clin. Neurophysiol.* 42:817–26.

Pfurtscheller, G. and F. H. Lopes da Silva. 1999. Event-related EEG/MEG synchronisation and desynchronisation: Basic principles. *Clin. Neurophysiol.* 110:1842–57.

Plioplys, A. V. 1994. Autism: Electroencephalogram abnormalities and clinical improvement with valproic acid. *Arch. Pediatr. Adolesc. Med.* 148:220–2.

Plaisted, K., L. Saksida, J. Alcántara, and E. Weisblatt. 2003. Towards an understanding of the mechanisms of weak central coherence effects: Experiments in visual configural learning and auditory perception. *Philos. Trans. R. Soc. Lond. B* 358:375–86.

Quintana, H. 2005. Transcranial magnetic stimulation in persons younger than the age of 18. *J. ECT* 21:88–95.

Ramachandran, V. S. and L. M. Oberman. 2006. Broken mirrors: A theory of autism. *Sci. Am.* 295:62–9.

Rippon, G., J. Brock, C. Brown, and J. Boucher. 2007. Disordered connectivity in the autistic brain: Challenges for the "new psychophysiology". *Int. J. Psychophysiol.* 63:164–72.

Rizzolatti, G. and L. Craighero. 2004. The mirror-neuron system. *Annu. Rev. Neurosci.* 27:169–92.

Rodriguez, E., N. George, J. P. Lachaux, J. Martinerie, B. Renault, and F. J. Varela. 1999. Perception's shadow: Long distance synchronization of human brain activity. *Nature*, 397:430–3.

Rodriguez, R., U. Kallenbach, W. Singer, and M. H. J. Munk. 2004. Short- and long-term effects of cholinergic modulation on gamma oscillations and response synchronization in the visual cortex. *J. Neurosci.* 24:10369–78.

Rojas, D. C. and L. B. Wilson. 2014. γ-Band abnormalities as markers of autism spectrum disorders. *Biomark. Med.* 8:353–68.

Rossi, S. and P. M. Rossini. 2004. TMS in cognitive plasticity and the potential for rehabilitation. *Trends Cogn. Sci.* 8:273–9.

Rubenstein, J. L. and M. M. Merzenich. 2003. Model of autism: Increased ratio of excitation/inhibition in key neural systems. *Genes Brain Behav.* 2:255–67.

Schreg, M. 2005. *Getting Started with BESA Workshop.* Washington, DC.

Seldon, H. L. 1981a. Structure of human auditory cortex, I. Cytoarchitectonics and dendritic distributions. *Brain Res.* 229:277–94.

Seldon, H. L. 1981b. Structure of human auditory cortex. II. Axon distributions and morphological correlates of speech perception. *Brain Res.* 229:295–310.

Sheikhani, A., H. Behnam, M. R. Mohammadi, M. Noroozian, and M. Mohammadi. 2012. Detection of abnormalities for diagnosing of children with autism disorders using of quantitative electroencephalography analysis. *J. Med. Syst.* 36:957–63.

Sheikhani, A., H. Behnam, M. Noroozian, M. R. Mohammadi, and M. Mohammadi. 2009. Abnormalities of quantitative electroencephalography in children with Asperger disorder in various conditions. *Res. Autism Spectr. Disord.* 3:538–46.

Shibata, T., I. Shimoyama, T. Ito, D. Abla, H. Iwasa, K. Koseki, N. Yamanouchi, T. Sato, and Y. Nakajima. 1999. Attention changes the peak latency of the visual gamma-band oscillation of the EEG. *Neuroreport* 10:1167–70.

Shuang, M., J. Liu, M. X. Jia, J. Z. Yang, S. P. Wu, X. H. Gong, Y. S. Ling, Y. Ruan, X. L. Yang, and D. Zhang. 2004. Family-based association study between autism and glutamate receptor 6 gene in Chinese Han trios. *Am. J. Med. Genet.* 131B:48–50.

Singer, W. 1999. Neuronal synchrony: A versatile code for the definition of relations? *Neuron* 24:49–65, 111–125.

Singer, W. and C. Gray. 1995. Visual feature integration and the temporal correlation hypothesis. *Annu. Rev. Neurosci.* 18:555–86.

Sohal, V. S. 2012. Insights into cortical oscillations arising from optogenetic studies. *Biol. Psychiatry* 71:1039–45.

Sokhadze, E., J. Baruth, A. Tasman, M. Mansoor, R. Ramaswamy, L. Sears, G. Mathai, A. El-Baz, and M. F. Casanova. 2010. Low-frequency repetitive transcranial magnetic stimulation (rTMS) affects event-related potential measures of novelty processing in autism. *Appl. Psychophysiol. Biofeedback* 35:147–61.

Sokhadze, E. M., J. M. Baruth, L. Sears, G. E. Sokhadze, A. S. El-Baz, and M. F. Casanova. 2012. Prefrontal neuromodulation using rTMS improves error monitoring and correction function in autism. *Appl. Psychophysiol. Biofeedback* 37:91–102.

Sokhadze, E. M., J. Baruth, A. Tasman, and M. F. Casanova. 2013a. Event-related potential studies of cognitive processing abnormalities in autism. In *Imaging Methods in Autism*, eds. M. F. Casanova, A. El-Baz, and J. S. Suri, 61–86. New York: Springer.

Sokhadze, E., J. Baruth, A. Tasman, L. Sears, G. Mathai, A. El-Baz, and M. F. Casanova. 2009b. Event-related potential study of novelty processing abnormalities in autism. *Appl. Psychophysiol. Biofeedback* 34:37–51.

Sokhadze, E. M., M. F. Casanova, and J. Baruth. 2013b. Transcranial magnetic stimulation in autism spectrum disorders. In *Transcranial Magnetic Stimulation: Methods, Clinical Uses and Effect on the Brain*, ed. L. Alba-Ferrara, 219–31. New York: NOVA Publishers.

Sokhadze, E. M., A. El-Baz, J. Baruth, G. Mathai, L. Sears, and M. F. Casanova. 2009a. Effect of a low frequency repetitive transcranial magnetic stimulation (rTMS) on gamma frequency oscillations and event-related potentials during processing of illusory figures in autism. *J. Autism Dev. Disord.* 39:619–34.

Sokhadze, E., A. El-Baz, L. Sears, I. Opris, and M. F. Casanova. 2014. rTMS neuromodulation improves electrocortical functional measures of information processing and behavioral responses in autism. *Front. Syst. Neurosci.* 8:134.

Stieglitz Ham, H., A. Bartolo, M. Corley, G. Rajendran, A. Szabo, and S. Swanson. 2011. Exploring the relationship between gestural recognition and imitation: Evidence of dyspraxia in autism spectrum disorders. *J. Autism Dev. Disord.* 41:1–12.

Stroganova, T. A., G. Nygren, M. M. Tsetlin, I. N. Posikera, C. Gillberg, M. Elam, and E. V. Orekhova. 2007. Abnormal EEG lateralization in boys with autism. *Clin. Neurophysiol.* 118:1842–54.

Stroganova, T. A., E. V. Orekhova, A. O. Prokofyev, M. M. Tsetlin, V. V. Gratchev, A. A. Morozov, and Y. V. Obukhov. 2012. High-frequency oscillatory response to illusory contour in typically developing boys and boys with autism spectrum disorders. *Cortex* 48:701–17.

Sun, L., C. Grutzner, and S. Bolte. 2012. Impaired gamma-band activity during perceptual organization in adults with autism spectrum disorders: Evidence for dysfunctional network activity in frontal-posterior cortices. *J. Neurosci.* 32:9563–73.

Szentagothai, J. and M. A. Arbib. 1975. *Conceptual Models of Neural Organization.* Massachusetts: MIT Press.

Tallon-Baudry, C. and O. Bertrand. 1999. Oscillatory gamma activity in humans and its role in object representation. *Trends Cogn. Sci.* 3:151–62.

Tallon-Baudry, C., O. Bertrand, C. Delpuech, and J. Pernier. 1996. Stimulus specificity of phase-locked and non-phase-locked 40 Hz visual responses in human. *J. Neurosci.* 16:4240–9.

Tallon-Baudry, C., O. Bertrand, F. Peronnet, and J. Pernier. 1998. Induced gamma-band activity during the delay of a visual short-term memory task in humans. *J. Neurosci.* 18:4244–54.

Tallon-Baudry, C. 2003. Oscillatory synchrony and human visual cognition. *J. Physiol.* 97:355–63.

Tallon-Baudry, C., O. Bertrand, M. A. Henaff, J. Isnard, and C. Fischer. 2005. Attention modulates gamma-band oscillations differently in the human lateral occipital cortex and fusiform gyrus. *Cereb. Cortex* 15:654–62.

Uhlhaas, P. J. 2011. High-frequency oscillations in schizophrenia. *Clin. EEG Neurosci.* 42:77–82.

Uhlhaas, P. J. and W. Singer. 2007. What do disturbances in neural synchrony tell us about autism? *Biol. Psychiatry* 62:190–1.

Uvebrant, P. and R. Bauzienè. 1994. Intractable epilepsy in children. The efficacy of lamotrigine treatment, including non-seizure-related benefits. *Neuropediatr.* 25:284–9.

Varela, F., J. P. Lachaux, E. Rodriguez, and J. Martinerie. 2001. The brainweb: Phase synchronization and large-scale integration. *Nat. Rev. Neurosci.* 2:229–39.

Volkmar, F. R. and D. S. Nelson. 1995. Seizure disorders in autism. *J. Am. Acad. Child Adolesc. Psychiatry* 29:127–9.

Von Stein, A., P. Rappelsberger, J. Sarnthein, and H. Petsche. 1999. Synchronization between temporal and parietal cortex during multimodal object processing in man. *Cereb. Cortex* 9:137–50.

Wall, C. A., P. E. Croarkin, L. A. Sim, M. M. Husain, P. G. Janicak, F. A. Kozel, G. J. Emslie, S. M. Dowd, and S. M. Sampson. 2011. Adjunctive use of repetitive transcranial magnetic stimulation in depressed adolescents: A prospective, open pilot study. *J. Clin. Psychiatry* 72:1263–9.

Ward, L. M. 2003. Synchronous neural oscillations and cognitive processes. *Trends Cogn. Sci.* 7:563–9.

Wassermann, E. M., J. Grafman, C. Berry, C. Hollnagel, K. Wild, K. Clark, and M. Hallett. 1996. Use and safety of a new repetitive transcranial magnetic stimulator. *Electroencephalogr. Clin. Neurophysiol.* 101:412–7.

Welchew, D. E., C. Ashwin, K. Berkouk, R. Salvador, J. Suckling, S. Baron-Cohen, and E. Bullmore. 2005. Functional disconnectivity of the medial temporal lobe in Asperger's syndrome. *Biol. Psychiatry* 57:991–8.

Whittington, M. A., R. D. Traub, N. Kopell, B. Ermentrout, and E. H. Buhl. 2000. Inhibition-based rhythms: Experimental and mathematical observations on network dynamics. *Int. J. Psychophysiol.* 38:315–36.

Williams, J., A. Whiten, T. Suddendorf, and D. Perrett. 2001. Imitation, mirror neurons, and autism. *Neurosci. Biobehav. Rev.* 25:577–96.

Wilson, T. W., D. C. Rojas, M. L. Reite, P. D. Teale, and S. J. Rogers. 2007. Children and adolescents with autism exhibit reduced MEG steady-state gamma responses. *Biol. Psychiatry* 62:192–7.

Wu, A. D., F. Fregni, D. K. Simon, C. Deblieck, and A. Pascual-Leone. 2008. Noninvasive brain stimulation for Parkinson's disease and dystonia. *Neurotherapeutics* 5:345–61.

Ziemann, U. 2004. TMS induced plasticity in human cortex. *Rev. Neurosci.* 15:253–66.

Index

A

Aberrant Behavior Checklist (ABC), 518–519
Aberrant cortical connectivity in ASD, 462–463
ABIDE, *see* Autism Brain Imaging Data Exchange
Abnormal structural lateralization, 144
ACC, *see* Anterior cingulate cortex
Acquisition of "training" data, 103
AD, *see* Alzheimer's disease; Axial diffusivity
Adaptive Robot-Mediated Intervention Architecture (ARIA), 402, 403
Additive genetic variation, 17
ADHD, *see* Attention deficit hyperactivity disorder
ADI–R, *see* Autism Diagnostic Interview–Revised
Adjacency matrix, *see* Connectivity matrix A
Adolescence, 197
ADOS, *see* Autism Diagnostic Observation Schedule
ADOS-G, *see* Autism Diagnostic Observation Schedule Generic
After-the-Fact™ feature, 359
Agenesis of corpus callosum (AgCC), 163–164
Akaike information criterion (AIC), 267
Alcohol syndrome, 232–234
Alzheimer's disease (AD), 108
American Psychiatric Association (APA), 438
Amygdala abnormalities, 45–46
Anatomical atlas, 103

Anatomical connectivity of CC, 162–163
Anatomy of autism; *see also* Neurodevelopment of autism
    alteration in brain connectivity, 67–68
    alteration in neuronal volumes, 66–67
    brain size, 59–60
    brain stem, 66
    cerebellum, 65–66
    cerebral cortex, 60–64
    hippocampus, 64
    subcortical regions, 64–65
Anatomy of CC, 158–159
Animal-like robot, 399
Animal models with abnormalities of CC, 165
Animated Visual Supports for Social Skills (AViSSS), 377
ANS-dependent variables, measurement of, 384–385
ANS, *see* Autonomous nervous system
Anterior cingulate cortex (ACC), 192, 440
Anterior splenium, 158
APA, *see* American Psychiatric Association
APP, *see* Autism Phenome Project
Applied Behavior Analysis therapy, 357
AQ, *see* Autism quotient
ARIA system, *see* Adaptive Robot-Mediated Intervention Architecture
AR models, *see* Autoregressive models
ASD, *see* Autism spectrum disorder
Asperger's syndrome, 140, 223

ASR, *see* Automatic speech recognition
Attention deficit hyperactivity disorder (ADHD), 98, 109, 164, 201
Audio acquisition, 323–324
Audio signal-processing techniques, 322; *see also* Physiological signal-processing techniques; Visual signal-processing techniques
    affective speech processing, 325–326
    ASR and synthesis, 324
    audio acquisition, 323–324
    future directions and challenges, 331
    modeling interaction with speech cues, 329–331
    speech prosody, 326–329
    speech signal processing, 322–323
Auditory gamma in ASD, 479
    GBA and visual processing, 482–483
    PAC in FFA, 480
    sensory gating in high- and low-functioning ASD children, 481
    study of GBA, 479
    in visual modality, 483
Autism, 161, 172, 346; *see also* Anatomy of autism; Neurodevelopment of autism
    autism using rTMS, 517
    autonomic balance dysfunctions, 380–382
    autonomic control assessment in understanding social deficits, 382
    brain connectivity and, 249
    changes of rating scores, 519, 520
    comparison of target and nontarget evoked gamma phase coherence, 522
    cortical excitation/inhibition balance, 505–507
    effective connectivity studies, 251–255
    EST for, 425–434
    evoked and induced gamma oscillations, 507–512, 520, 521

evoked and induced gamma responses, 504–505
    functional connectivity studies, 251–255
    GABA, 505–507
    gamma activity in, 474, 502, 505–507
    inhibition defects in autism and TMS, 515–517
    minicolumnar neuropathology model, 500–501
    resting-state gamma activity, 483–485
    social engagement deficits, 383–384
    spectrum, 98
    spontaneous, resting EEG gamma, 502–503
    state of the art of VR application, 375–376
    structural connectivity studies, 249–251
    "task-free" gamma activity, 483–485
    theoretical models of, 499–500
    TMS, 512–514
    visual gamma, 475–479
    biomarkers, 101
Autism Brain Imaging Data Exchange (ABIDE), 8, 130, 199, 305
Autism data science, 2
    candidate phenotypes, 11
    data analysis, 6
    database design, 5
    data display and diagnostic limitations, 9–11
    data entry and data monitoring, 6
    data harmonization, 7–9
    data sharing, 7
    future, 7
    papers, 3
    planning next study, 7
    publication, 7
    randomization, 6
    reporting results, 12
    reproduction of central findings, 7
    sampling and screening, 5
    steps in practicing autism data science, 4
    study design, 4–5
Autism Diagnostic Interview–Revised (ADI–R), 20, 96, 253

Autism Diagnostic Observation
    Schedule (ADOS), 20, 96,
    324, 326, 363, 410
Autism Diagnostic Observation
    Schedule Generic
    (ADOS-G), 404
Autism Phenome Project (APP), 175
Autism quotient (AQ), 20, 478
Autism spectrum disorder (ASD), 17,
    38, 76, 79–80, 96, 122, 158,
    172, 190, 220, 223, 246,
    288, 320, 356, 359, 374,
    398, 425, 438, 459, 499;
    see also Twin studies
  aberrant cortical connectivity,
    462–463
  applications of MVPC, 108–111
  behavior genetics, 16–18
  body size, 177–178
  brain enlargement in subsampleof
    individuals, 175–176
  characteristics, 459–461
  clinical features, 223–224
  EEG data, 266–267
  etiology, 224
  excitation–inhibition in autism,
    461–462
  findings of GC connectivity,
    269, 272
  functional connectivity, 203–205
  GABA and, 224
  GCC analysis, 270–272
  GC in, 266
  gene expression, 226–227
  genetics, 224–226
  gold-standard diagnostic
    assessment tools, 97–99
  ICA findings, 268, 271
  imitation in, 76–77
  microcephaly, 181
  neurobiological differences with
    ASD biomarker potential,
    99–100
  neurobiology of brain
    enlargement, 178–181
  neurocognitive models, 461
  neurofunctional organization in,
    302–304
  normalization of brain size,
    178, 179
  pilot data of psychophysiological
    reactivity of children,
    384–387
  post-artifacted spectral
    analysis, 270
  research using VR, 376–378
  results, 267–269
  sex differences, 176–177
  striatal connectivity, 203
  structural connectivity, 203
  studies of macrocephaly,
    172–173
  studies of megalencephaly,
    173–174
  theory of executive dysfunction
    in, 452
  in vivo human studies, 227–229
Autistic cortex, 61
Autistic symptomatology, 288
Autistic symptoms, 96
Automatic speech recognition
    (ASR), 322
  synthesis and, 324
Autonomic balance dysfunctions in
    autism, 380
  electrodermal activity in autism,
    381–382
  HRV and phasic HR responses,
    380–381
  sympathetic overarousal in
    autism, 381–382
Autonomic control assessment in
    social deficits in autism,
    382
Autonomous level increasing of
    robotic systems, 412–413
Autonomous nervous system (ANS),
    333, 378
Autoregressive models (AR models),
    264
AViSSS, see Animated Visual
    Supports for Social Skills
Axial diffusivity (AD), 249, 298

B

"Baby-sibling" paradigm, 38
BAP, see Broader autism phenotype
Basal ganglia, 190
Bayesian information criterion
    (BIC), 267
B-cell CLL/lymphoma 2
    (BCL2), 27
BEC, see Best-estimate clinical
Behavioral intervention, 202
Behavioral phenotyping, 320

Behavioral signal processing
(BSP), 321
ASD, 320
audio signal-processing
techniques, 322–331
human-in-loop approach, 321
meta-data processing with
machine learning, 338–339
SAIL, 321–322
visual signal-processing
techniques, 331–338
Behavior Capture™, 359
Behavior Connect™, 360
Behavior-genetic analytical
approaches within ASD
research, 20
Behavior genetics, 16; see also
Twin studies
genetic influence, 17
shared and nonshared variation,
17–18
Behavior imaging (BI), 356
ASD in pharmaceutical trials, 356
Behavior Capture™, 359
Behavior Connect™, 360
data quality challenges, 361–362
educational progress of children,
356
in-field evaluation, 350–352
in natural settings, 367
NODA, 346–350
pharmaceutical R&D, 360–361
pharmaceutical trials, 363–365
proposed work flow model for
field adoption, 352
recent technology applications,
362
remote autism diagnosis, 346
for research, 357–359
retrospective evaluation of
archived video data,
365–366
technology platform, 357
Bernstein polynomials, 161
Best-estimate clinical (BEC), 338
Beta rebound, 79
BI, see Behavior imaging
BIC, see Bayesian information
criterion
Binding, 234–235
mechanism, 474
problem, 235
Biomarker, 11, 108

Biomarker and Neural Connectivity
Toolbox (BioNeCT), 260
Biostatistical models, 6
Black-box approach, 130
Blind source separation method
(BSS method), 259, 266
Blood oxygen level dependent signal
(BOLD signal), 289
Body size, ASD, 177–178
BOLD signal, see Blood oxygen level
dependent signal
Boolean values, 255
Bottom-up approach, 87–89
Brain connectivity
alteration in, 67–68
approaches, 247
in ASD, 246
autism and, 249
brain networks, 255–258
brain volume studies, 248–249
clinical applications, 273–276
connectivity explanation, 258
effective connectivity, 247–248
effective connectivity studies,
251–255
functional connectivity studies,
251–255
GC connectivity in ASD, 266–272
GC connectivity on treatment
case, 276, 277
heritable neurodevelopmental
disorders, 246
ICA findings from treatment case,
275
measuring effective connectivity
with GC, 263–266
measuring functional or effective
connectivity, 259–263
neurofeedback, 273–274
structural connectivity studies,
249–251
treatment case, 274–276
Brain-decoding methods, 101
Brain enlargement in subsample
of individuals with ASD,
175–176
Brain imaging, 79
diagnose autism by, 10–11
functional brain imaging, 101
human brain imaging studies, 196
mirror neuron activity with,
86–87
multimodal, 129

Brain network(s), 255
    anatomical connectivity, 297
    autistic symptomatology, 288
    complex fiber orientations,
        300–301
    connectivity matrix, 256
    diffusion MRI works, 297–298
    DTI struggles, 301
    findings ASD in children,
        adolescents, and adults, 298
    findings ASD in infants and
        toddlers, 299
    functional connectivity, 289–297
    motion, 301–302
    MRI techniques, 288–289
    neurofunctional organization in
        ASD, 302–304
    neuroimaging, 304–307
    organization in ASD, 288
    PCA, 258
    perspectives, 302
    small-world network, 256
    structural brain data, 255
    structural connectivity
        analysis, 257
    understanding microstructural
        underpinnings, 299–300
Brain-reading methods, 101
Brain size, 59–60
    normalization of, 178, 179
Brain stem, 66
Broader autism phenotype (BAP), 20
Broca's area, 137
Bronfenbrenner's theory, 423, 424;
        see also Ecological systems
        theory (EST)
BSP, see Behavioral signal processing
BSS method, see Blind source
        separation method
BTBR mice, 165

C

Callosal fibers, 158
Candidate phenotypes, 11
CaptureMyEmotion application, 337
Cardiac activity regulation, 382
Cardiac vagal tone, 382
Cardiovascular activity, 384–385
CAST, see Childhood Autism
        Spectrum Test
CATSS, see Child and Adolescent
        Twin Study in Sweden

Caudal-orbital prefrontal cortex,
        158
CBCL, see Child Behavior Checklist
CBS, see Computational behavioral
        science
CC, see Corpus callosum
Centers for Disease Control and
        Prevention (CDC), 438
Centralized scoring, 362
Central site (Cz site), 444
Cerebellum, 65–66, 180
    abnormalities, 44
Cerebral cortex, 60–64, 126
Cerebrospinal fluid (CSF), 43
CGI rating scale, see Clinical Global
        Impression rating scale
Child and Adolescent Twin Study
        in Sweden (CATSS),
        25–26
Child Behavior Checklist (CBCL), 26
Childhood autism, 97
Childhood Autism Spectrum Test
        (CAST), 20
CI, see Confidence interval
Clinical Global Impression rating
        scale (CGI rating scale),
        361
Cliquishness, 256
Cluster sampling design, see
        Multisite sampling design
CNTNAP2, see Contactin-associated
        protein 2
Cntnap2 deficiency, 226
CNV, see Contingent negative variation
CNVs, see Copy number variations
Cohen's classification, 448
Comorbidity, Twin studies in ASD
        and, 28–29
Computational behavioral science
        (CBS), 322
Conditional Granger causality, 265
Condition random fields (CRFs), 332
Confidence interval (CI), 444
Connectivity matrix A, 255, 256
Contactin-associated protein 2
        (*CNTNAP2*), 225
Contingent negative variation
        (CNV), 451
Continuous recording and flagging
        technology system (CRAFT
        system), 428, 429
Copy number variations (CNVs), 17,
        98, 224

Corpus callosum (CC), 6, 158, 1237
   abnormalities, 44–45
   anatomy, 158–159
   animal models with abnormalities, 165
   in idiopathic autism, 159–163
   in neurogenetic syndromes exhibiting social deficits, 163–165
Cortical excitation/inhibition balance, 505–507
Cortical inhibition, 228
Corticostriatal connectivity, 191
   functional organization of frontal cortex and striatum, 193
   specific circuits, 192–194
   tract-tracing techniques, 191–192
Cotwin control design, 19
CRAFT system, see Continuous recording and flagging technology system
CRFs, see Condition random fields
Cross-modal repetition, 83
Cross-modal adaptation, 82
Cross-sectional area and volume of CC, 159–161
CSD, see Current source density
CSF, see Cerebrospinal fluid
Current source density (CSD), 257, 259

D

Danish population-based study, 21
Data-driven approach, 103
Data analysis, 6, 441, 442–443
Database design, 5
Data display
   diagnose autism by brain imaging, 10–11
   and diagnostic limitations, 9
Data entry, 6
Data harmonization, 7
   planning multisite studies, 9
   pros and cons of meta-analysis, 8–9
Data monitoring, 6
Data quality challenges, 361–362
Data sharing, 7
DAWBA, see Development and Well-Being Assessment
DC, see Degree centrality
Deep neural networks (DNNs), 324
Default mode network (DMN), 252, 296

Degree centrality (DC), 205
De novo mutations, 18, 19, 29, 31–32
DerSimonian and Laird random-effects model, 444, 448
Development and Well-Being Assessment (DAWBA), 25
Diagnose autism by brain imaging, 10–11
Diagnostic and Statistical Manual of Mental Disorders 5th ed. (DSM-V), 223, 349, 438
Dichotic listening, 143
Diffusion tensor imaging (DTI), 46–49, 100, 110, 159, 162, 195, 247, 257, 298
Diffusion weighted MRI (dMRI), 297
DiGeorge syndrome, see Velocardiofacial syndrome (VCFS)
Directed partial coherence (DPC), 259, 266
Direct transfer function (DTF), 259, 266
Discordant MZ twin pair design, 19, 26–28
Discrimination map, 106
Dizygotic twins (DZ twins), 19
DLPFC, see Dorsolateral prefrontal cortex
DMN, see Default mode network
dMRI, see Diffusion weighted MRI
DNN-based speech processing, 324
DNNs, see Deep neural networks
Dominant genetic influence (D), 17
Dorsolateral prefrontal cortex (DLPFC), 192, 517
DPC, see Directed partial coherence
DSM-V, see Diagnostic and Statistical Manual of Mental Disorders 5th ed.
DTF, see Direct transfer function
DTI-based tractography, 250
DTI, see Diffusion tensor imaging
Dysgenesis and reduction in neuronal number, 66
Dyslexia, 137
DZ twins, see Dizygotic twins

E

Early brain overgrowth, 40–41
Early error processing (ERN), 451
Early infantile autism, 2

ECA, *see* Embodied Conversational
 Agent
ECG, *see* Electrocardiogram
Ecological systems approach
 building new bridge between
  psychology and HCI,
  422–425
 design, 420
 design in HCI and psychology
  research, 421
 EST for autism, 425–434
 reconceptualized ecological
  system, 425
Ecological systems theory (EST),
 420, 425
 for autism, 425
 chronosystem layer, 424
 family and community layers of,
  425, 428
 individual's environment, 433–434
 parents activating recording
  system, 429
 problem with social skills
  acquisitions, 431–432
 Re-Flex system, 426
 social computing, 432
 social mirror in home, 430
 solving the unlocking door
  scenario, 427
 spatial layers, 424
 therapist, 432
EDA, *see* Electrodermal activity
EEG, *see* Electroencephalography
EF, *see* Executive function
Effective connectivity; *see also*
 Functional connectivity
 method, 247–248
 neuroimaging methods, 252
 resting-state studies, 252–253
 studies, 251
 task-based studies, 253–255
E/I balance, *see* Excitation–inhibition
 balance
Electrocardiogram (ECG), 321, 333,
 334, 379
Electrodermal activity (EDA), 321,
 379, 385
 in autism, 381–382
 signal, 333, 334
Electrode/sensor-level analyses, 464
Electroencephalography (EEG), 78,
 233, 247, 374, 462, 501
 gamma, 500–501

signal, 334
 techniques, 463
 tracings, 499–500
Electromyogram (EMG), 374, 379, 513
Embodied Conversational Agent
 (ECA), 325
EMG, *see* Electromyogram
Emotion, 144
 emotional state detection and
  differentiation, 378–380
 functional lateralization for,
  145–147
 processes, 383
 reduced right hemisphere
  activation, 146
 theory of mind, 144–145
Environmental factors not shared
 (NSE), 16, 17
Environmental factors shared by
 family members (SE), 16, 17
Epigenetic mechanisms, 18
ePSPs, *see* Excitatory postsynaptic
 potentials
ERD, *see* Event-related
 desynchronization
ERN, *see* Early error processing;
 Error-related negativity
ERP, *see* Event-related potential
Error-related negativity (ERN), 440,
 444–446, 449–451
Error positivity, 444, 447–451
Error processing electrophysiology
 ASD, 438
 ERN, 444, 445–446, 449–451
 ERP study of, 440
 error positivity, 444, 447–449,
  449–451
 inclusion criteria, 441
 limitations, 452–453
 literature search, 441
 meta-analysis procedure and data
  analysis, 441, 442–443
 methods, 441
 neuroimaging technique, 440
 performance monitoring, 439–440
 results, 441
 theory of executive dysfunction in
  ASD, 452
ERS, *see* Event-related
 synchronization
ERSP, *see* Event-related spectral
 perturbation
EST, *see* Ecological systems theory

Ethnography, 420
Event-related desynchronization (ERD), 466, 502
Event-related potential (ERP), 374, 440, 508
Event-related spectral perturbation (ERSP), 502
Event-related synchronization (ERS), 466, 502
Evoked and induced gamma
    ASD, 511–512
    gamma frequencies, 510–511
    high-frequency oscillations in autism, 512
    Kanizsa illusory figures, 507–508
    oscillations using Kanizsa figures, 507
    responses in autism, 504–505
    in visual oddball task, 509–510
Excitation–inhibition balance (E/I balance), 506
    in autism, 461–462
Excitatory postsynaptic potentials (ePSPs), 230
Executive function (EF), 439
Extra-axial fluid, 43
Extrinsic functional connectivity, 195

F

FA, *see* Fractional anisotropy
Face inversion effect, 475
FACE, robotic face, 399
Faces, 147
    functional lateralization for, 149–151
    structural lateralization for, 148–149
Facial expressions, 331–332; *see also* Imitation
Facial processing, 332–333
FACS, *see* Fetal anticonvulsant syndrome
FAST-AS, *see* Fast-Fail Trials–Autism
Fast-Fail Trials (FAST), 361
Fast-Fail Trials–Autism (FAST-AS), 356
Fast Fourier transform (FFT), 385
fcMRI, *see* Functional connectivity MRI
FDA, *see* U.S. Food and Drug Administration

FEF, *see* Frontal eye fields
Fetal alcohol
    exposure, 233
    spectrum disorders, 233
    syndrome, 232–234
Fetal anticonvulsant syndrome (FACS), 220, 232–234
FFA, *see* Fusiform face area
FFT, *see* Fast Fourier transform
FMR1 knockout mice, 226, 230, 231
fMRI, *see* Functional magnetic resonance imaging
FMRP, *see* Fragile X mental retardation protein
Fractional anisotropy (FA), 162, 249, 298
Fragile X mental retardation protein (FMRP), 226, 229
Fragile X syndrome (FXS), 98, 220, 229
    clinical features and etiology, 229
    GABA and fragile X, 230–231
    human studies of GABA in, 231
Frontal eye fields (FEF), 192
Frontocentral site (FCz site), 440, 444
Fronto-insular cortex, 127–128
Fronto-temporo-parietal regions, 137, 138
Functional brain imaging, 101; *see also* Behavior imaging (BI)
Functional connectivity, 289; *see also* Structural connectivity
    approach, 247
    BOLD correlations, 293
    BOLD signal correlations, 289–290
    brain intrinsic functional connectivity, 291
    of CC, 163
    divergent findings, 290
    dynamic connectivity, 295–297
    fcMRI technique, 290–291
    GSR, 291
    methodological factors, 292–293
    neuroimaging methods, 252
    replication, 293–294
    resting state, 252–253, 294–295
    studies, 251, 253–255
Functional connectivity MRI (fcMRI), 289
Functional lateralization
    for emotion, 145–147
    for faces, 149–151
    for language, 140–144

Functional magnetic resonance
    imaging (fMRI), 10, 79,
    247, 451, 462
Fusiform face area (FFA), 254, 479
    PAC in, 480
Fusiform gyrus, 148
    hypoactivation, 149
FXS, *see* Fragile X syndrome

G

GABA, *see* Gamma-aminobutyric
    acid
GABA-T, *see* GABA transaminase
GABA transaminase (GABA-T), 221
GAD, *see* Glutamate decarboxylase
GAMMA, *see* Graphical-model-
    based multivariate analysis
Gamma abnormalities
    ASD characteristics, 459–461
    autism, gamma activity in, 474–485
    human brain, gamma activity in,
        463–474
    neurocognitive models of ASD,
        461–463
Gamma activity in autism, 474, 502,
    505–507
    auditory gamma in ASD, 479–483
    autism using rTMS, 517
    changes of rating scores on ABC,
        519, 520
    comparison of target and
        nontarget evoked gamma
        phase coherence, 522
    cortical excitation/inhibition
        balance, 505–507
    evoked and induced gamma
        oscillations, 507–512,
        520, 521
    evoked and induced gamma
        responses in autism,
        504–505
    GABA, 505–507
    gamma activity in autism,
        505–507
    inhibition defects in autism and
        TMS, 515–517
    resting-state gamma activity,
        483–485
    spontaneous, resting EEG gamma
        in autism, 502–503
    task-free gamma activity,
        483–485

TMS, 512–514
    visual gamma in ASD, 475–479
Gamma activity in human brain, 463
    functional significance of gamma
        oscillations, 474
    gamma and connectivity
        measures, 471–472
    gamma metrics, 464–471
    GBA as measure of GABA,
        473–474
    measuring gamma, 463–464
Gamma-aminobutyric acid (GABA),
    220, 458, 502, 505–507
    ASD, 223–229
    clinical implications, 235
    FACS and fetal alcohol syndrome,
        232–234
    fragile X and, 230–231
    FXS, 229–231
    gamma-band activity and feature
        binding, 234–235
    GBA as measure of, 473–474
    interneurons, 222
    metabolism, release, and
        recycling, 220–221
    minicolumns and discrimination,
        234
    in neuropsychiatric disorders, 223
    receptors, 222–223
    Rett syndrome, 231–232
    synaptic pathways responsible for
        synthesis, 221
    system dysfunction in ASD, 220
    theoretical and clinical
        implications, 234
Gamma-band activity (GBA),
    234–235, 458, 502
    as measure of GABA, 473–474
    synchronization, 474
Gamma frequencies, 464–466, 501,
    510–511
Gamma measurement, 463–464
Gamma metrics, 464
    gamma frequencies, 464–466
    task-free gamma, 471
    task-related gamma, 466–471
Gamma oscillations, functional
    significance of, 474, 501–502
Gamma rhythm, 503
Gamma waves, 235
Gaussian processes (GP), 102
GBA, *see* Gamma-band activity
GC, *see* Granger causality

GCA, *see* Granger causality analysis
Gene expression, 27
General linear model (GLM), 101
Genetic factors, 129
Genetic influence, 17
Genotype–environment
  correlation, 16
Gesture(s), 84–85, 331
  Kinect 3D face tracking, 409
  mirroring, 410
  processing, 332
  recognition module, 408–409
GLM, *see* General linear model
Global signal regression (GSR), 291
Glutamate decarboxylase (GAD), 221
GM, *see* Gray matter
Gold Standard (GS), 363
  diagnostic assessments in ASD, 96
  diagnostic assessment tools for
    ASD and limitations, 97–99
GP, *see* Gaussian processes
Granger causality (GC), 259, 264, 267
  classifier stage of BioNeCT
    analysis pipeline, 264
  conditional GC, 265
  connectivity in ASD, 266
  EEG data, 266–267
  findings of GC connectivity,
    269, 272
  GCC analysis, 270–272
  ICA findings, 268, 271
  limitations, 266
  mathematical form of, 265
  measuring connectivity, 263–264
  measuring effective connectivity
    with, 263
  method, 248
  post-artifacted spectral
    analysis, 270
  results, 267–269
  stochastic process, 264
Granger causality analysis (GCA), 264
Graphical model-based multivariate
  analysis (GAMMA), 130
Graphics over numbers, 9
Graph theory, 255, 472
  EEG data set, 261–262
  EEG recordings, 259–260
  feature selection stage of BioNeCT
    analysis pipeline, 263
  graph metric extraction, 262
  measuring functional or effective
    connectivity with, 259

statistical analyses, 262–263
thresholded connectivity
  matrix, 261
Gray matter (GM), 123, 199
GS, *see* Gold Standard
GSR, *see* Global signal regression
Gyrification of cerebral cortex, 60

H

HARDI, *see* High angular resolution
  diffusion imaging
Harmonics-to-noise ratio (HNR), 327
HCI, *see* Human–computer
  interaction
Heart rate (HR), 379, 383
  acceleration, 383
  variability, 379
Heart-rate variability (HRV), 334,
  374, 380–381
  social engagement deficits, 383–384
Hemisphere lateralization, 137
Hemispheric asymmetries in ASD
  emotion, 144–147
  faces, 147–151
  language, 137–144
Heterochronicity, 196
Heterogeneous neurodevelopmental
  conditions, 96
Heuristic challenge, 98
HF, *see* High frequency
HFA, *see* High-functioning children
  with autism
HFASD, *see* High-functioning autism
  spectrum disorder
HFOs, *see* High-frequency
  oscillations
Hidden Markov models (HMMs), 324
High frequency (HF), 380, 385
  EEG oscillations, 502
High-frequency oscillations
  (HFOs), 506
High-functioning autism spectrum
  disorder (HFASD), 425
High-functioning children with
  autism (HFA), 374
High angular resolution diffusion
  imaging (HARDI), 297
HIPAA-conforming Web portal, 346
Hippocampus, 64
HMMs, *see* Hidden Markov models
[1H]MRS, *see* Proton magnetic
  resonance spectroscopy

HNR, *see* Harmonics-to-noise ratio
HR, *see* Heart rate
HRV, *see* Heart-rate variability
5-HT, *see* 5-Hydroxytrypamine
Human-induced pluripotent stem
    cells (human-iPSCs), 229
Human brain, gamma activity in, 463
   functional significance of gamma
    oscillations, 474
   gamma and connectivity
    measures, 471–472
   gamma metrics, 464–471
   GBA as measure of GABA,
    473–474
   measuring gamma, 463–464
Human brain imaging studies, 196
Human–computer interaction
    (HCI), 420
   building new bridge with
    psychology and, 422–425
   design in, 421
Humanoid robot, 399
   NAO, 403
5-Hydroxytrypamine (5-HT), 10
Hyperparameters, 104
Hyperplane, 101
Hypotheses, 5

I

IA, *see* Inspiration wave amplitude
IADS, *see* International Affective
    Digitized Sound
IAN, *see* Interactive Autism Network
IBI, *see* Interbeat interval
ICA, *see* Independent component
    analysis
Idiopathic autism, 98
   CC in, 159
   cross-sectional area and volume of
    CC, 159–161
   functional connectivity of CC, 163
   integrity and anatomical
    connectivity of CC, 162–163
   shape and symmetry of CC, 161
iFC, *see* Intrinsic functional
    connectivity
Imitation, 79–80
   learning, 408
   system development, 408–410
   user study, 410
   user study results, 410–412
Immune process, 180

Independent component analysis
    (ICA), 259, 260, 266
Inferior premotor cortex, 158
Infrared cameras (IR cameras), 401
Inspiration wave amplitude (IA), 385
Integrity connectivity of CC, 162–163
Intelligence quotient (IQ), 199,
    444, 460
   IQ-matched controls, 123
Intent-to-treat policy (ITT policy), 5
Interactive Autism Network (IAN), 22
Interbeat interval (IBI), 334
International Affective Digitized
    Sound (IADS), 386
InterTrial Coherence (ITC), 471
InterTrial Phase Coherence
    (ITPC), 471
Intrinsic fcMRI, 289
Intrinsic functional connectivity
    (iFC), 195, 290
Inverse model approach, 259
In vivo diffusion tensor imaging
    study, 165
IQ, *see* Intelligence quotient
IR cameras, *see* Infrared cameras
ITC, *see* InterTrial Coherence
Iterative design process, 346
ITPC, *see* InterTrial Phase Coherence
ITT policy, *see* Intent-to-treat policy

K

"Keepon" robot, 401
Kinect 3D face tracking, 409

L

Language, 137–144
   functional lateralization for,
    140–144
   structural lateralization for,
    137–140
Language lateralization, 137
Lateral intraparietal area (LIP), 86
Least-to-most prompt (LTM), 404
LEDs, *see* Light-emitting diodes
Left frontal volume, 139
Left globus pallidis, 145
LF, *see* Low frequency
LFPs, *see* Local field potentials
Liability, 20
   liability-threshold model, 21, 25
   threshold parameters, 22

Light-emitting diodes (LEDs), 404
LIP, *see* Lateral intraparietal area
Local excitatory–inhibitory
    interactions, 500–501
Local field potentials (LFPs), 463
Low frequency (LF), 385
LTM, *see* Least-to-most prompt

M

Machine learning
    approaches, 96
    meta-data processing with,
      338–339
    methodsm, 122
    techniques, 106
Macrocephaly, studies of, 172–173
Magnetic resonance (MR), 8
    MR-based predictive models,
      structural, 128–129
Magnetic resonance imaging (MRI),
    96, 100, 122, 137, 159, 174,
    193, 247
Magnetic resonance spectroscopy
    (MRS), 473
Magnetoencephalography (MEG),
    78, 110, 145, 234, 247, 296,
    462, 463
MAR models, *see* Multivariant
    autoregressive models
Mass-univariate approaches, 100
Matrices, 261
Maximum margin classifier, 106
MC, *see* Mild cognitive impairment
M-CHAT, *see* Modified Checklist for
    Autism in Toddlers
MD, *see* Mean diffusivity
Mean diffusivity (MD), 249, 298
MECP2, *see* Methyl-CpG-binding
    protein 2
MEG, *see* Magnetoencephalography
Megalencephaly, studies of, 173–174
MEGAPRESS technique, 227
Mesosystems, 423
Messenger RNA (mRNA), 226
Meta-analysis
    procedure, 441, 442–443
    pros and cons of, 8–9
Meta-data processing with machine
    learning, 338–339
Methyl-CpG-binding protein 2
    (MECP2), 231
Methylation pattern, 27

Microcephaly, 181
Micromotion, 195
Microsystem level, 423
Mild cognitive impairment (MC), 108
Minicolumnar neuropathology model
    of autism, 500–501
Minicolumnopathy, 500
Mirror neurons, 77–79
Mirror neurons system (MNS),
    79–80, 499
Missouri Twin Study, 22
MNS, *see* Mirror neurons system
MoCap, *see* Motion capture
Modified Checklist for Autism in
    Toddlers (M-CHAT), 26
Modularity, 256
Monozygotic twins (MZ twins), 19, 30
Motion capture (MoCap), 333
Motor resonance phenomenon, 81
Motor threshold (MT), 513
MR, *see* Magnetic resonance
MRI, *see* Magnetic resonance
    imaging
mRNA, *see* Messenger RNA
MRS, *see* Magnetic resonance
    spectroscopy
MT, *see* Motor threshold
Multimodal brain imaging, 129; *see
    also* Behavior imaging (BI)
Multisite sampling design, 9
Multisite studies planning, 9
Multivariant autoregressive models
    (MAR models), 264
Multivariate analytical techniques,
    100–102
Multivariate autoregressive model
    (MVAR model), 259, 266
Multivariate pattern classification
    (MVPC), 101, 102
    acquisition of "training" data, 103
    applications of MVPC in ASD,
      108–111
    feature extraction, feature selection,
      and dimensionality
      reduction, 103–104
    model training and optimization,
      104
    validation using test data,
      104–105
Multivariate pattern classification
    (MVPC), 96
Multivoxel pattern analysis (MVPA),
    110, 130

"mu suppression," 79
MVAR model, *see* Multivariate
autoregressive model
MVPA, *see* Multivoxel pattern
analysis
MVPC, *see* Multivariate pattern
classification
MZ twins, *see* Monozygotic twins

N

National Center for Health Statistics
(NCHS), 173
National Database for Autism
Research (NDAR), 7
National Institute of Mental Health
(NIMH), 7
National Institutes of Health (NIH),
7, 356, 361
Naturalistic Observation Diagnostic
Assessment (NODA), 346
NODA Connect, 347–350
NODA SmartCapture, 347, 348
NCHS, *see* National Center for
Health Statistics
NDAR, *see* National Database for
Autism Research
Negative predictive value (NPV), 105
Network analysis techniques, 261
Neuroanatomy of CC, 158
Neurobiological differences with ASD
biomarker potential, 99–100
Neurobiological functions, 158
Neurobiology of brain enlargement,
178–181
Neurobiology of imitation in autism
behavioral challenge, 83–84
broken mirrors, 76
dysfunction in imitative behavior
in autism, 75
imaging challenge, 81–83
imitation in ASD, 76–77
imitation, MNS, and ASD, 79–80
mirror neurons, 77–79
noninvasive neuromodulation,
89–91
pervasive mirroring, 85–87
taking control, 84
top-down and bottom-up, 87–89
unbroken mirrors, 81
Neurochemistry, 191
Neurocognitive models of ASD,
461–463

Neurodevelopmental disorder, 160,
356, 357
Neurodevelopment of autism; *see also*
Anatomy of autism
ASD, 38
DTI, 46–49
early abnormal brain
development, 39
research on normative samples,
39–40
structural magnetic resonance
imaging, 40–46
Neurofeedback, 273
Neurofibromatosis type 1 (NF1),
163, 164
Neurofunctional organization in
ASD, 302–304
Neurogenetic disorder, 164
Neurogenetic syndromes
AgCC, 163–164
exhibiting social deficits, CC
in, 163
NF1, 164
VCFS, 164–165
WS, 165
Neuroimaging, 304–305
data, 102, 143
knowledge of subtypes, 306–307
methods, 252
rich data approach to diagnostic
prediction, 306
Neuroimaging biomarkers for
ASD; *see also* Structural
magnetic resonance
imaging
advances in multivariate analytical
techniques and predictive
modeling, 100–102
applications of MVPC in ASD,
108–111
gold-standard diagnostic
assessment tools for ASD,
97–99
limitations to classification
approaches, 111–115
MVPC, 102–105
neurobiological differences with
ASD biomarker potential,
99–100
SVM, 106–108
Neuronal circuit dysfunction in
ASD, 462
Neuronal volumes, alteration in, 66–67

549

Neuropsychiatric disorders, GABA
     in, 223
Neurotypically developing (NTD),
     327
NF1, *see* Neurofibromatosis type 1
NIH, *see* National Institutes of Health
NIH Research Domain Criteria
     (RDoC), 11
NIMH, *see* National Institute of
     Mental Health
NODA, *see* Naturalistic Observation
     Diagnostic Assessment
Nonadditive genetic variance, 17
Noninvasive neuromodulation, 89–91
Nonshared variation, 17–18
Nonspecific SCR (NS.SCR), 379, 382
Nonsyndromic autism, 98
Normalization, 174
     of brain size, 178, 179
NOT-OD-16-011, 7
NPV, *see* Negative predictive value
NSE, *see* Environmental factors not
     shared
NS.SCR, *see* Nonspecific SCR
NTD, *see* Neurotypically developing
Nucleus accumbens septi, 191

O

Obsessive-compulsive disorder
     (OCD), 514
Oculus rift, 373
Orbitofrontal cortex (OFC), 192

P

PAC, *see* Phase–amplitude coupling
Parasympathetic inputs, 383
Parietocentral site (Pz site), 444
Parkinson's disease (PD), 514
Partial directed coherence
     (PDC), 259
Parvalbumin
     parvalbumin-expressing
          interneurons, 62
     parvalbumin-immunoreactive
          interneurons, 64
     parvalbumin+ GABA
          interneurons, 222, 231
     PV+ cells, 234
Path length, 256
PCA, *see* Principal component
     analysis

PCAST, *see* President's Council of
     Advisors on Science and
     Technology
PCC, *see* Posterior cingulate cortex
PD, *see* Parkinson's disease
PDC, *see* Partial directed coherence
PDD-NOS, *see* Pervasive
     developmental disorder not
     otherwise specified
Peak respiration frequency
     (PFRQ), 385
Pe amplitude, 438, 441, 444, 448,
     449, 451
Pearson correlation coefficient, 257
Pervasive developmental disorder not
     otherwise specified (PDD-
     NOS), 438
Pervasive mirroring, 85–87
PET, *see* Positron emission
     tomography
PFRQ, *see* Peak respiration frequency
Pharmaceutical
     R&D, 360–361
     trials, 356, 357, 363–365
Phase-locking factor (PLF), 471
Phase-locking value (PLV), 471
Phase–amplitude coupling (PAC),
     459, 480
Phase-locking statistic (PLS), 257
Phasic heart-rate responses, 383
Phasic HR responses, 380–381
Photoplethysmogram (PPG), 379
Physiological signal-processing
     techniques, 333, 335–336;
     see also Audio signal-
     processing techniques;
     Visual signal-processing
     techniques
     collecting physiological signals,
          334–335
     EDA, 333–334, 336
     signal fundamentals, 334
Pilot data of psychophysiological
     reactivity of children, 384
     measurement of ANS-dependent
          variables, 384–385
     results, 385–387
     standard emotional responses, 384
PLF, *see* Phase-locking factor
PLS, *see* Phase-locking statistic
PLV, *see* Phase-locking value
Pneumogram (PNG), 384
PNG, *see* Pneumogram

Point-of-view (POV), 332
Polymorphisms, 10
Positive predictive value (PPV), 105
Positron emission tomography (PET),
        11, 96, 110, 227, 289
Posterior cingulate cortex (PCC), 252
Posterior protuberance, 172
Posterior superior temporal gyrus, 138
Postmortem studies, 500
Posttraumatic stress disorder
        (PTSD), 514
POV, *see* Point-of-view
PPG, *see* Photoplethysmogram
PPV, *see* Positive predictive value
Predictive modeling to neuroimaging
        data, 100–102
President's Council of Advisors on
        Science and Technology
        (PCAST), 360
Primary outcome measure, 4–5
Principal component analysis (PCA),
        258, 262
Proton magnetic resonance
        spectroscopy ([¹H]MRS),
        227, 231, 235
Psychology, 420
    building new bridge with HCI
        and, 422–425
    research, 421
Psychophysiological measures,
        emotional state detection
        and differentiation, 378–380
PTSD, *see* Posttraumatic stress
        disorder
Publication, 7
Pulse volume (PV), 379, 385
PV, *see* Pulse volume
Pz site, *see* Parietocentral site

Q

Quantitative dimensional
        approach, 108

R

Radial diffusivity (RD), 47, 249, 298
Randomization method, 6
Rapid serial visual presentation
        (RSVP), 254
RATSS, *see* Roots of Autism and
        ADHD Twin Study in
        Sweden
RBB, *see* Restricted and repetitive
        behaviors
RBS, *see* Repetitive Behavior Scale
RD, *see* Radial diffusivity
RDoC, *see* NIH Research Domain
        Criteria
Re-Flex system, 426, 429
Refl-Ex Authoring and Critiquing
        Tool system (REACT
        system), 432, 433
Regional cortical differences in
        overgrowth, 41–43
Regions of interest (ROIs), 462
    ROI-based methods, 122
    ROI-based morphometry, 122–124
    techniques, 247, 250
Reinforcement learning (RL), 439
Relative recurrence risk (RRR), 21
Repetitive Behavior Scale (RBS), 518
    RBS-R, 519
Repetitive restricted behaviors
        (RRB), 197, 200
Repetitive transcranial magnetic
        stimulation (rTMS), 273, 498
    EEG gamma, 500–501
    functional significance of gamma
        oscillations, 501–502
    gamma activity findings in
        autism, 502–523
    minicolumnar neuropathology
        model of autism, 500–501
    theoretical models of autism,
        499–500
Reproduction of central findings, 7
Respiration rate (RESP), 385
Respiratory activity, 385
Respiratory sinus arrhythmia (RSA),
        see Heart-rate variability
        (HRV)
Respiratory volume (RV), 379
Resting-state functional MRI
        (rsfMRI), 165
Resting-state gamma, *see*
        Task-free—gamma
Resting-state studies, 252–253
Restricted and repetitive behaviors
        (RBB), 253
Retinoic acid-related orphan receptor
        alpha (RORA), 27
Retrospective evaluation of archived
        video data, 365–366
Rett syndrome, 98, 220, 231–232
Right fusiform gyrus, 147

RL, *see* Reinforcement learning
Robot-mediated intervention
    generalization, 413–414
Robot-mediated joint attention
    training, 402
    habituation study, 406–408
    system development, 402–405
    user study results, 405–406
Robot-mediated skill training
    for children with ASD, 402
    imitation learning, 408–412
    robot-mediated joint attention
      training, 402–408
Robotic platform development,
    399–400
Robots impact on children with ASD
    increasing autonomous level of
      robotic systems, 412–413
    large group study, 413
    patterns of robot–children
      interactions, 401–402
    potential cost effectiveness, 398
    robot-mediated intervention
      generalization, 413–414
    robotic platform development,
      399–400
    unrestricted interaction
      environment, 413
ROIs, *see* Regions of interest
Roots of Autism and ADHD
    Twin Study in Sweden
    (RATSS), 28
RORA, *see* Retinoic acid-related
    orphan receptor alpha
Rostral-caudal axis, 161
RRB, *see* Repetitive restricted
    behaviors
RRR, *see* Relative recurrence risk
rsfMRI, *see* Resting-state functional
    MRI
RSVP, *see* Rapid serial visual
    presentation
rTMS, *see* Repetitive transcranial
    magnetic stimulation
RV, *see* Respiratory volume

S

SAIL, *see* Signal Analysis and
    Interpretation Lab
Sampling, 5
SATSA, *see* Swedish Adoption/Twin
    Study of Aging

SCIT, *see* Social Communication
    Interaction Test
SCL, *see* Skin conductance level
SCQ, *see* Social Communication
    Questionnaire
SCR, *see* Skin conductance responses
Screening, 5
SD, *see* Standard deviation
SDHR, *see* Standard deviation of HR
SE, *see* Environmental factors shared
    by family members
SEF, *see* Supplementary eye fields
Select archiving device, 359
Selection bias type, 6
SEPs, *see* Somatosensory-evoked
    potentials
Serotonin, 10
Sex differences, ASD, 176–177
Shape absent stimuli, 475
Shape present stimuli, 475
Shared variation, 17–18
Shprintzen syndrome, *see*
    Velocardiofacial syndrome
    (VCFS)
Signal-processing
    practice, 321
    technologies, 337
Signal-to-noise ratio (SNR), 323
Signal Analysis and Interpretation
    Lab (SAIL), 321–322
Single-photon emission computed
    tomography (SPECT), 227
Single nucleotide polymorphisms
    (SNP), 103, 224
Single nucleotide variants (SNVs), 17
16 p11.2 deletion syndrome, 163
Skin conductance level (SCL), 334, 374
Skin conductance responses (SCR),
    295, 334, 377
Skin temperature (SKT), 379
sLORETA, *see* Standardized
    low-resolution brain
    electromagnetic
    tomography
SMA, *see* Supplementary motor area
Small-world network, 256
Small wireless remote control
    device, 359
SNP, *see* Single nucleotide
    polymorphisms
SNR, *see* Signal-to-noise ratio
SNVs, *see* Single nucleotide variants
Social brain network, 100

Social Communication Interaction Test (SCIT), 363
Social Communication Questionnaire (SCQ), 404
Social engagement deficits in autism and HRV, 383–384
Social Responsiveness Scale (SRS), 20, 404
Somatic markers, 384
Somatosensory-evoked potentials (SEPs), 516
Source density signals, 266
Spatial filters, 259
Spatial Laplacians, 266
SPECT, see Single-photon emission computed tomography
Speech, 331
    cues, BSP modeling interaction with, 329–331
    prosody, 326–329
    signal-processing applications, 322
Speech processing
    affective, 325–326
    DNN-based, 324
Spindle neurons, see von Economo neurons (VEN)
Spontaneous gamma oscillations, 503
Spontaneous, resting EEG gamma in autism, 502–503
SRS, see Social Responsiveness Scale
SSR, see Steady-state response
Standard deviation (SD), 123, 441
Standard deviation of HR (SDHR), 385
Standardized low-resolution brain electromagnetic tomography (sLORETA), 259
Statistical methods, 247
Steady-state response (SSR), 468
STG, see Superior temporal gyrus
Stratified psychiatry, 11
Striatal abnormalities, 197
Striatal imaging in ASD, 197
    functional imaging, 200–201
    inhibitory control, 202
    regional striatal studies, 198
    reward, 201–202
    task-based fMRI studies, 197–198
    volumetric studies, 198–199
    voxel-based morphometry, 199–200
Striatum, 190
    studies in humans, 194–195

Striatum imaging in ASD
    ASD striatal connectivity, 203–205
    corticostriatal connectivity, 191–194
    nonhuman primates, 191
    striatal anatomy and neurochemistry, 191
    striatal development, 196
    striatal imaging in ASD, 197–202
    striatum, 190
    studying striatum in humans, 194–195
Structural brain network, 127–128
Structural connectivity; see also Functional connectivity
    approaches, 247
    studies, 249–251
Structural covariance analysis, 127
Structural lateralization for language, 137–140
Structural magnetic resonance imaging; see also Neuroimaging biomarkers for ASD
    amygdala abnormalities, 45–46
    of ASD, 122
    cerebellum abnormalities, 44
    corpus callosum abnormalities, 44–45
    developments, 129–130
    early brain overgrowth, 40–41
    extra-axial fluid, 43
    neurodevelopment of autism, 40
    regional cortical differences in overgrowth, 41–43
    ROI-based morphometry, 122–124
    structural brain network, 127–128
    structural MR-based predictive models, 128–129
    surface-based morphometry, 126
    surface area and cortical thickness, 41
    tensor-based morphometry, 126–127
    VBM, 124–125
STS, see Superior temporal sulcus
Subcortical regions, 64–65
Superior temporal gyrus (STG), 43, 200, 202
Superior temporal sulcus (STS), 43, 145
Supplementary eye fields (SEF), 192
Supplementary motor area (SMA), 192

Support vector machine (SVM), 102, 106–108, 130
Surface-based morphometry, 122, 126
Surface area and cortical thickness, 41
SVM, *see* Support vector machine
Swedish Adoption/Twin Study of Aging (SATSA), 19
Sympathetic overarousal in autism, 381–382
Syndromic autism, 98

T

Task-based
    fMRI, 195, 197–198
    studies, 253–255
Task-free
    functional imaging, 195
    gamma, 471
    gamma activity, 483–485
Task-related gamma, 466–471
TBS, *see* Theta burst stimulation
TBSS, *see* Tract-based spatial statistics
TBV, *see* Total brain volume
TD, *see* Typically developing
TDC, *see* Typically developing controls
TEDS, *see* Twin early development study
Tensor-based morphometry, 122, 126–127
Testing phase, 101
TFR, *see* Time–frequency response
Theory of executive dysfunction, 439
    in ASD, 452
Theory of mind (ToM), 439
    deficit in autism, 499
Theta burst stimulation (TBS), 89
Thresholding, 261
Time–frequency response (TFR), 466
TMS, *see* Transcranial magnetic stimulation
ToM, *see* Theory of mind
Tonic heart-rate responses, 383
Top-down approach, 87–89
Total brain volume (TBV), 198
Tourette's disorders, 197
Tract-based spatial statistics (TBSS), 162, 298
Tract-tracing techniques, 191–192
Traditional statistical analysis methods, 128

Training phase, 101
Transcranial magnetic stimulation (TMS), 78, 228, 231, 512–514
    inhibition defects in autism and, 515–517
Triggers, 359
Tuberous sclerosis, 98
Turner syndrome, 163
T1-weighted structural MRI, 122
22 q11.2 deletion syndrome, *see* Velocardiofacial syndrome (VCFS)
Twin-based designs, 18
Twin early development study (TEDS), 22, 25
Twin studies
    ASD, 18
    and ASD heritability estimates, 23–25
    BAP, 20
    behavior-genetic analytical approaches within ASD research, 20
    CATSS, 25–26
    and comorbidity, 28–29
    as continuous trait, 22
    Danish population-based study, 21
    discordant MZ twin pair design in ASD research, 26–28
    etiological overlap between different domains of symptoms, 29–30
    ICD-10 criteria, 21
    liability threshold parameters, 22
    limitations, 30–31
    Missouri Twin Study, 22
    symptoms in toddlers, 26
    TEDS, 22, 25
    twin designs, 18–19
Typically developing (TD), 292
    individuals, 172
    persons, 246
Typically developing controls (TDC), 198

U

Underconnectivity theory, 289
Unweighted graph, 255
U.S. Food and Drug Administration (FDA), 361

V

Validation using test data, 104–105
Valproic acid (VPA), 473
VBM, *see* Voxel-based morphometry
VCFS, *see* Velocardiofacial
syndrome
Velocardiofacial syndrome (VCFS),
158, 163, 164–165
VEN, *see* von Economo neurons
Ventral intraparietal area (VIP), 86
Ventromedial prefrontal cortex
(vmPFC), 193
Very-low-frequency (VLF), 385
Vesicular inhibitory amino acid
transporter (VIAAT), 221
VIAAT, *see* Vesicular inhibitory
amino acid transporter
Video capture system, 357
Video recording, 362–363
VIP, *see* Ventral intraparietal area
Virtual environments, 377
Virtual reality (VR), 373
in ASD, 376–378
autonomic balance dysfunctions
in autism, 380–382
autonomic control assessment, 382
emotional state detection and
differentiation, 378–380
environment, 398
phasic and tonic heart-rate
responses, 383
pilot data of psychophysiological
reactivity, 384–387
social engagement deficits in
autism and HRV, 383–384
state of the art of VR application
in autism, 375–376
Virtual simulators, 376
Visual gamma in ASD, 475–479
gamma TFR, 476
GBA and visual processing, 479
source power in high gamma
band, 478

Visual search (VS), 254
Visual signal-processing techniques,
331; *see also* Audio signal-
processing techniques;
Physiological signal-
processing techniques
BSP for physiological data,
336–338
facial expressions, 331–332
facial marker positions, 333
facial processing techniques,
332–333
gesture processing, 332
physiological signal-processing
techniques, 333–338
VLF, *see* Very-low-frequency
vmPFC, *see* Ventromedial prefrontal
cortex
Volumetric brain enlargement, 99
von Economo neurons (VEN), 62
Voxel, 101
Voxel-based morphology, *see* Voxel-
based morphometry
Voxel-based morphometry (VBM),
122, 124–125, 194,
199–200, 298
Voxel-wise analysis, 122
VPA, *see* Valproic acid
VR, *see* Virtual reality
VS, *see* Visual search

W

Weak central coherence (WCC), 439
Weighted graph, 255
Weight vector, 106
Wernicke's area, 137
White matter (WM), 123
Williams syndrome (WS), 158,
163, 165
Within-twin pair differences
design, 19
World Health Organization
(WHO), 173

Printed and bound by CPI Group (UK) Ltd, Croydon, CR0 4YY

01/11/2024

01782601-0011